Roxburgh's Common Skin Diseases

19th Edition

D1330515

Ayşe Serap Karadağ, MD

Department of Dermatology and Venereology
Istanbul Arel University, School of Medicine
Memorial Health Group Atasehir and Sisli Hospital
Istanbul, Turkey

Lawrence Charles Parish, MD, MD (Hon)

Department of Dermatology and Cutaneous Biology
Sidney Kimmel Medical College at Thomas Jefferson University
and Jefferson Center for International Dermatology
Philadelphia, PA, USA

Jordan V. Wang, MD, MBE, MBA

Department of Dermatology and Cutaneous Biology
Sidney Kimmel Medical College at Thomas Jefferson University
Philadelphia, PA
and Laser & Skin Surgery Center of New York
New York, NY, USA

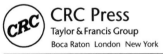

CRC Press
Taylor & Francis Group
Boca Raton London New York

CRC Press is an imprint of the
Taylor & Francis Group, an **informa** business

Nineteenth edition published 2022
by CRC Press
6000 Broken Sound Parkway NW, Suite 300, Boca Raton, FL 33487–2742

and by CRC Press
2 Park Square, Milton Park, Abingdon, Oxon, OX14 4RN

© 2022 Taylor & Francis Group, LLC

Eighteenth edition published 2011

CRC Press is an imprint of Taylor & Francis Group, LLC

This book contains information obtained from authentic and highly regarded sources. While all reasonable efforts have been made to publish reliable data and information, neither the author[s] nor the publisher can accept any legal responsibility or liability for any errors or omissions that may be made. The publishers wish to make clear that any views or opinions expressed in this book by individual editors, authors or contributors are personal to them and do not necessarily reflect the views/opinions of the publishers. The information or guidance contained in this book is intended for use by medical, scientific or health-care professionals and is provided strictly as a supplement to the medical or other professional's own judgement, their knowledge of the patient's medical history, relevant manufacturer's instructions and the appropriate best practice guidelines. Because of the rapid advances in medical science, any information or advice on dosages, procedures or diagnoses should be independently verified. The reader is strongly urged to consult the relevant national drug formulary and the drug companies' and device or material manufacturers' printed instructions, and their websites, before administering or utilizing any of the drugs, devices or materials mentioned in this book. This book does not indicate whether a particular treatment is appropriate or suitable for a particular individual. Ultimately it is the sole responsibility of the medical professional to make his or her own professional judgements, so as to advise and treat patients appropriately. The authors and publishers have also attempted to trace the copyright holders of all material reproduced in this publication and apologize to copyright holders if permission to publish in this form has not been obtained. If any copyright material has not been acknowledged please write and let us know so we may rectify in any future reprint.

Library of Congress Cataloging-in-Publication Data
Names: Karadağ, Ayşe Serap, editor. | Parish, Lawrence Charles, editor. | Wang, Jordan V., editor. | Marks, Ronald. Common skin diseases.
Title: Roxburgh's common skin diseases / [edited] by Ayşe Serap Karadağ, Lawrence Charles Parish, Jordan V Wang.
Other titles: Common skin diseases
Description: Nineteenth edition. | Boca Raton : CRC Press, 2021. | Preceded by Common skin diseases 18th ed. / Ronald Marks, Richard Motley. 2011. | Includes bibliographical references and index.
Identifiers: LCCN 2021037604 (print) | LCCN 2021037605 (ebook) | ISBN 9780367614997 (hardback) | ISBN 9780367614980 (paperback) | ISBN 9781003105268 (ebook)
Subjects: MESH: Skin Diseases
Classification: LCC RL71 (print) | LCC RL71 (ebook) | NLM WR 140 | DDC 616.5—dc23
LC record available at https://lccn.loc.gov/2021037604
LC ebook record available at https://lccn.loc.gov/2021037605

ISBN: 978-0-367-61499-7 (hbk)
ISBN: 978-0-367-61498-0 (pbk)
ISBN: 978-1-003-10526-8 (ebk)

DOI: 10.1201/9781003105268

Typeset in Palatino
by Apex CoVantage, LLC

Contents

Preface

When Archibald Cathcart Roxburgh (1886–1954) created *Common Skin Diseases* in 1932,[1] we doubt that he had any idea that the book would now be in its 19th edition. Some later editions were edited by Peter Forbes Borrie (1918–1984),[2] John D. Kirby, and Ronnie Marks (1935–2020).[3] This may well be a record for a dermatology textbook and rivals such textbooks of medicine as those by Cecil[4] and Harrison.[5] There have been several dermatology books that have had multiple editions but none approaching two score.

What makes *Common Skin Diseases* such a perennial favorite among students and practitioners may be that it is not encyclopedic and that it is straightforward. It does not intend to be as all-encompassing as the works by Rook[6] or Bologna;[7] rather, it follows in the role of the *Manual of Dermatology*,[8] written during World War II for the medical corps, or the *Handbook of Diseases of the Skin* created by the Suttons.[9] Although it was once possible for a single physician to create an inclusive textbook, this is no longer feasible nor realistic. This was recognized by Donald M. Pillsbury (1902–1980) at the University of Pennsylvania in Philadelphia, who created the first modern multi-authored dermatology book in 1956. [10]

Roxburgh was an exacting author and sometime editor of the *British Journal of Dermatology*, where he seems to have been an equally exacting editor. According to one obituary, he wrote his textbook in the hours before breakfast, and he took all the pictures for his book himself, processing them as well.[11] *The Lancet* referred to his text as "a practical vade-mecum for the dermatologist."[12]

In creating this edition, we have built on the excellence of the previous versions. The contributors, whom we invited from several international centers, were asked to follow a suggested outline for the chapters. The mere complexities of modern medicine—and dermatology is no exception—often does not permit a uniform format nor did we wish to discuss every affliction of the skin. We have included color pictures where appropriate and have limited the additional reading to but ten items.

REFERENCES

1. Roxburgh AC. Common skin diseases, London: H. K. Lewis.1932.
2. Obituary: Peter Forbes Borrie, MD, MC Cantab, FRCP. Lancet. 1984; ii:415.
3. Finlay AY. Obituary: Professor Ronald Marks, 1935–2020. Br J Dermatol. 2020; 183:598–599.
4. Goldman L, Schafer AI, Cecil RL. Goldman-Cecil medicine. 26th edition/ed, Philadelphia, PA: Elsevier.2020: 2 volumes.
5. Harrison TR. Principles of internal medicine, Philadelphia, PA: Blakiston.1950.
6. Rook A, Wilkinson DS, Ebling FJG. Textbook of dermatology, Oxford; Edinburgh: Blackwell Scientific.1968.
7. Bolognia J, Jorizzo JL, Rapini RP. Dermatology, Edinburgh: Mosby.2003.
8. Pillsbury DM, Sulzberger MB, Livingood CS, et al. Manual of dermatology, Philadelphia, London: W.B. Saunders Company.1942.
9. Sutton RL. Handbook of diseases of the skin, St. Louis: C. V. Mosby Co.1949.
10. Pillsbury DM, Shelley WB, Kligman AM. Dermatology, Philadelphia, PA: Saunders.1956.
11. Obituary: Dr. A. C. Roxburgh. Br J Dermatol. 1955; 67:33–34.
12. Archibald Cathcart Roxburgh, MA, MD (Camb.), F.rRC.P. Lancet. 1954; ii:1237–1238.

Contributors

José Wilson Accioly Filho, MD, PhD
Sector of Dermatology
School of Medicine and University Hospital
Federal University of Ceará
Fortaleza, Brazil

Saira N. Agarwala, MD
Department of Dermatology
Lewis Katz School of Medicine at
Temple University
Philadelphia, PA, USA

Necmettin Akdeniz, MD
Department of Dermatology and
Venereology, Memorial Health Group
Şişli and Ataşehir Hospitals
Department of Dermatology
Istanbul, Turkey

Hasan Aksoy, MD
Department of Dermatology and
Venereology
Istanbul Medeniyet University
School of Medicine
Prof. Dr. Suleyman Yalcin City Hospital
Istanbul, Turkey

Christian Albornoz, MD
Department of Dermatology and Cutaneous
Biology
Sidney Kimmel Medical College at Thomas
Jefferson University
Philadelphia, PA, USA

Albert Alhatem, MD
Department of Pathology, Immunology, and
Laboratory Medicine
Rutgers-New Jersey Medical School
Newark, NJ
Department of Dermatology, St Louis
University School of Medicine
St Louis, MO

Sam Allen, FRCP, FFTM-RCPS(Glasg)
Infectious Diseases
NHS Ayrshire & Arran
Scotland, UK

Ozge Askin, MD
Department of Dermatology
Istanbul University
Cerrahpasa Medical Faculty, Fatih
Istanbul, Turkey

Laura Atzori, MD
Unit of Dermatology
Department of Medical Sciences and
Public Health
University of Cagliari, Italy

Robert Baran, MD
Nail Disease Centre
Cannes, France

Cynthia Bartus, MD
Department of Dermatology
Lehigh Valley Health Network
Allentown PA, USA

Mark Biro, MD
Department of Dermatology
Georgetown University School of Medicine
Washington, DC, USA

**Christopher B Bunker, MA(Hons)(Cantab),
MD(Cantab), FRCP**
Department of Dermatology
University College London and Chelsea and
Westminster Hospital
London, UK

Sueli Carneiro, MD, PhD
Department of Dermatology
School of Medical Sciences and University
Hospital
State of Rio de Janeiro University and Sector
of Dermatology
School of Medicine and University Hospital
Federal University of Rio de Janeiro
Rio de Janeiro, Brazil

Charles Cathcart, MBChB, PG, Med Ed Cert
Department of Dermatology
Liverpool University Hospitals NHS
Foundation Trust
Liverpool, UK

Emily Chea, DO
Department of Dermatology
Lehigh Valley Health Network
Allentown, PA, USA

Kayla A. Clark, BS
Department of Dermatology
University of Illinois at Chicago
College of Medicine
Chicago, IL, USA

Emily Correia, BS
Department of Dermatology and Cutaneous
Biology
Sidney Kimmel Medical College at Thomas
Jefferson University
Philadelphia, PA, USA

Annie Dai, BA
Department of Dermatology
Baylor College of Medicine
Houston, TX, USA

Razvigor Darlenski, MD, PhD
Clinic of Dermatology and Venereology
Acibadem-City Clinic, Tokuda Hospital
Sofia, Bulgaria

Abdullah Demirbaş, MD
Department of Dermatology and
Venereology
Kütahya Health Sciences University
School of Medicine
Kütahya, Turkey

Kossara Drenovska, MD, PhD
Department of Dermatology and
Venereology
Medical Faculty
Medical University
Sofia, Bulgaria

Robert Duffy, MD
Division of Dermatology
Cooper Medical School of Rowan University
Camden, NJ, USA

Ömer Faruk Elmas, MD
Department of Dermatology and
Venereology
Kırıkkale University
School of Medicine
Kırıkkale, Turkey

Nurimar Conceição Fernandes, MD, PhD
Sector of Dermatology
School of Medicine and University Hospital
Federal University of Rio de Janeiro
Rio de Janeiro, Brazil

Caterina Ferreli, MD
Unit of Dermatology
Department of Medical Sciences and Public
Health
University of Cagliari, Italy

Warren Heymann, MD
Division of Dermatology
Cooper Medical School of Rowan University
Camden, NJ
Department of Dermatology
Perelman School of Medicine
University of Pennsylvania
Philadelphia, PA, USA

Uta-Christina Hipler, PhD
Department of Dermatology
University Hospital
Jena, Germany

Madeline Hooper, BA
Department of Dermatology
Lehigh Valley Health Network
Allentown, PA, USA

Sylvia Hsu, MD
Department of Dermatology
Lewis Katz School of Medicine at Temple
University
Philadelphia, PA, USA

Tara Jennings, MD
Division of Dermatology
Cooper Medical School of Rowan University
Camden, NJ, USA

Virginia A. Jones, MD, MS
Department of Dermatology
University of Illinois at Chicago College of
Medicine
Chicago, IL, USA

Melek Aslan Kayıran, MD
Department of Dermatology and
Venereology
Istanbul Medeniyet University
School of Medicine
Prof. Dr. Suleyman Yalcin City Hospital
Istanbul, Turkey

Jana Kazandjieva, MD, PhD
Department of Dermatology and Venerology
Medical University
Sofia, Bulgaria

Matthew Keller, MD
Department of Dermatology and Cutaneous
Biology
Sidney Kimmel Medical College at Thomas
Jefferson University
Philadelphia, PA, USA

Chelsea Kesty, MD
Department of Dermatology
Lehigh Valley Health Network
Allentown, PA, USA

Soo Jung Kim, MD, PhD
Department of Dermatology
Baylor College of Medicine
Houston, TX, USA

Wei-Liang Koh, MBBS, MRCP, FAMS
Department of Dermatology
Changi General Hospital
Singapore

Shalini Krishnasamy, MD
Department of Dermatology and Cutaneous
Biology
Sidney Kimmel Medical College at Thomas
Jefferson University
Philadelphia, PA, USA

Muriel W. Lambert, PhD
Department of Pathology
Immunology and Laboratory Medicine and
Department of Dermatology
Rutgers-New Jersey Medical School
Newark, NJ, USA

W. Clark Lambert, MD, PhD, FRCP(Edin)
Department of Pathology
Immunology and Laboratory Medicine and
Department of Dermatology
Rutgers-New Jersey Medical School
Newark, NJ, USA

**Michael Joseph Lavery, MBBCh, BAO,
MRCP(UK)**
Division of Dermatology
Phoenix Children's Hospital
Phoenix, AZ, USA

Jason B Lee, MD
Department of Dermatology and Cutaneous
Biology
Sidney Kimmel Medical College at Thomas
Jefferson University
Philadelphia PA, USA

Shari Lipner, MD, PhD
Department of Dermatology
Weill Cornell Medical College
New York, NY, USA

Erin McClure, BS
Department of Dermatology
Lehigh Valley Health Network
Allentown, PA, USA

Liam Mercieca, MD, MRCP(UK)
University Department of Dermatology
Mater Dei Hospital
Msida, Malta

Pietro Nenoff, MD
Laboratory for Medical Microbiology
Mölbis, Germany

Alexander V. Nguyen, BA
Department of Dermatology
Baylor College of Medicine
Houston, TX, USA

Neda Nikbakht, MD, PhD
Department of Dermatology and Cutaneous
Biology
Sidney Kimmel Medical College at Thomas
Jefferson University
Philadelphia, PA, USA

Ivy M. Obonyo, BS
Department of Dermatology
University of Illinois at Chicago College of
Medicine
Chicago, IL, USA

**Joseph Pace, MD, FRCP(Edin), FRCP(Lond),
KM**
University Department of Dermatology
Mater Dei Hospital
Msida, Malta

Allison Perz, BS
Division of Dermatology
Cooper Medical School of Rowan University
Camden, NJ, USA

Vesna Petronic-Rosic, MD, MSc, MBA
Department of Dermatology
Cook County Hospital
Chicago, IL, USA

Marcia Ramos-e-Silva, MD, PhD
Oral Dermatology Clinic and Sector of
Dermatology
School of Medicine and University Hospital
Federal University of Rio de Janeiro
Rio de Janeiro, Brazil

Franco Rongioletti, MD
Unit of Dermatology
Department of Medical Sciences and Public
Health
University of Cagliari, Italy

Kristen Russomanno, MD
Department of Dermatology
MedStar Washington Hospital Center and
Georgetown University Hospital
Washington, DC, USA

Robert A Schwartz, MD, MPH, DSc(Hon), FRCP(Edin)
Department of Pathology
Immunology and Laboratory Medicine and
Department of Dermatology
Rutgers-New Jersey Medical School
Newark, NJ, USA

Saloni Shah, BS
Department of Dermatology and Cutaneous
Biology
Sidney Kimmel Medical College at Thomas
Jefferson University
Philadelphia, PA, USA

Alexander Sherban, BM
Department of Dermatology and Cutaneous
Biology
Sidney Kimmel Medical College at Thomas
Jefferson University
Philadelphia, PA, USA

Nanette Silverberg, MD
Department of Dermatology
Icahn School of Medicine at Mount Sinai
New York, NY, USA

Rodney Sinclair, MBBS, MD
Sinclair Dermatology
Melbourne, Australia

Roselyn Stanger, MD
Department of Dermatology
Icahn School of Medicine at Mount Sinai
New York, NY, USA

Aspen R. Trautz, MD
Department of Dermatology
Lewis Katz School of Medicine at Temple
University
Philadelphia, PA, USA

Nikolai Tsankov, MD, PhD
Clinic of Dermatology and Venerology
Acibadem-City Clinic
Tokuda Hospital, Sofia, Bulgaria

Maria M. Tsoukas, MD
Department of Dermatology
University of Illinois at Chicago College of
Medicine
Chicago, IL, USA

Yalçın Tüzün, MD
Department of Dermatology
Istanbul University
Cerrahpasa Medical Faculty, Fatih
Istanbul, Turkey

Serap Utaş, MD
Department of Dermatology
Fulya Acıbadem Hospital
Istanbul, Turkey

Aarthy K Uthayakumar, BA(Hons)(Cantab), MBBS, MRCP
Department of Dermatology
University College London Hospitals NHS
Foundation Trust
London, UK

Tugba Kevser Uzuncakmak, MD
Department of Dermatology
Istanbul University
Cerrahpasa Medical Faculty
Fatih, Istanbul, Turkey

Snejina Vassileva, MD, PhD
Department of Dermatology and
Venereology, Medical Faculty
Medical University
Sofia, Bulgaria

Shyam Verma, MBBS, DVD, FRCP(London)
Department of Dermatology
Nirvana Skin Clinic
Vadodara, Gujarat, India

Shayan Waseh, BS, MPH
Department of Dermatology and Cutaneous
Biology
Sidney Kimmel Medical College at Thomas
Jefferson University
Philadelphia, PA, USA

Uwe Wollina, MD
Department of Dermatology and
Allergology
Städtisches Klinikum Dresden
Germany

Sherry Yang, MD
Department of Dermatology and Cutaneous
Biology
Sidney Kimmel Medical College at Thomas
Jefferson University
Philadelphia, PA, USA

1 Glossary of Dermatologic Words and Terms

Lawrence Charles Parish

Each medical specialty has its own vocabulary, and dermatology is no different. Sometimes, the use of words or terms relating to the skin may seem different from those used in other fields. Other times, the Latinate form of the word may appear questionable.

Our purpose in creating this glossary is to make the chapters uniform and to be understandable to the reader being introduced to the field of dermatology. Where appropriate, we have used the American spelling and nomenclature. Synonyms are included, but an exhaustive listing is not provided.

Abscess: a tender, red 2–3 cm lesion that is inflamed with walled-off purulent material
Acantholysis: separation of epidermal cells due to loss of their connections
Acanthosis: diffuse thickening of the epidermis
Acneiform: resembling acne with somewhat pointed lesions that might include comedones, papules, and pustules
Allergic: an altered reaction to which the patient has been previously exposed
Alopecia: hair loss
Annular: ring-shaped, often with central clearing
Atopic: condition that includes asthma, hay fever, and atopic dermatitis
Atopy: strange-like
Auspitz sign: pinpoint bleeding when the scale is removed
Autoimmune: an altered reaction to one's own body
Barbae: relating to the beard
Biopsy: to take a living specimen for microscopic examination, as opposed to an autopsy (dead specimen)
Blaschko's line: the invisible lines of normal embryonic development that are whorls on the chest and flanks, "V" shaped on the back, and wavy appearance on the scalp
Bleb: a flaccid blister, as in a bulla
Blister: small (>0.5-cm) vesicle; larger (<0.5-cm) bulla
Bohn's nodule: a small nodule found in the ear canal or mouth of a newborn.
Bulla: a blister generally over 1.0 cm, as opposed to a small blister or vesicle and a pustule; bullae (plur)
Burow's solution: an astringent comprised of aluminum triacetate. It is usually diluted with water to make a 1:40 solution
Burrow: a superficial epidermal tunnel due to scabies
Café au lait: the color of coffee with milk or cream added
Carbuncle: an abscess with one opening
Casal's necklace: reddish pigmentation on the neck, resembling a collar, and due to pellagra
Cellulitis: redness, edema, and tenderness without a purulent opening
Chadwick's sign: bluish discoloration of the labia, vagina, or cervix that occurs during pregnancy
Chromonychia: abnormal discoloration of a nail except for white
Circinate: a round lesion-like circle
Clubbing: enlargement of the terminal digit of the fingers that creates a rounding down of the nail and may be associated with underlying disease, sometimes pulmonary malignancy
Comedo: occlusion of the pilosebaceous duct; comedones (plural)
Condyloma: a warty lesion found in the genital region
Confluent: lesions that have merged
Congenital: appearing at birth, not necessarily inherited
Crowe's sign: axillary freckling
Cutis marmarota: a red or blue mottled appearance of the skin due to cold exposure
Cyst: an elevated lesion with an epithelial lining
Dactylitis: sausage finger, swelling of an entire finger or toe, as found in psoriasis
Dandruff: scurf, white scale on the scalp
Darier sign: swelling of the skin after scratching the skin
Decubitus: lying down leading to loss of skin and subcutaneous material, that is, decubitus ulcer
Defluvium: flowing or falling off
Dermatitis: inflammation of the skin; dermatitides (plural)

DOI: 10.1201/9781003105268-1

Dermatographism: a red elevation of the skin due to scratching the skin

Desquamation: peeling of the skin, often in sheets, as occurs following a sunburn

Diascopy: a test that shows the vascular or non-vascular characteristics of a lesion when pressure is applied

Discoid: a round or nummular lesion

Eczema: inflammation of the skin; dermatitis is the preferred American term

Eczematoid: resembling eczema, that is, dermatitic-like

Ecchymosis: black and blue, due to bleeding under the epidermis

Eclabium: a deformity of the lips with the outward turning

Ectropion: an abnormal outward turning of either the upper or lower eyelid

Edema: swelling of tissue due to abnormal amounts of fluid

Emperipolesis: inclusion of a cell within the cytoplasm of another cell

Ephelids: freckles

Epithelioma: an older term used for describing basal cell carcinoma or squamous cell carcinoma

Eponym: use of a proper name to describe a disease

Epstein's sign: small elevated lesions in a newborn 's mouth

Eruption: a rapidly appearing lesion

Erosion: wearing away of the surface

Erythroderma: redness and subsequent shedding of scales, affecting most of the body's surface area

Erythronychia: reddish discoloration of the nail

Excoriation: picking or scratching to eliminate a lesion or an imaginary lesion

Exudate: fluid that has leaked from blood vessels into the surrounding tissue; when due to an infectious process, it is considered a purulent process or pus

Exfoliation: peeling off the skin

Factitial: artificial, self-created lesion

Familial: occurring within family members; not necessarily due to heredity

Flaccid: soft, no longer firm

Folliculitis: inflammation of the hair follicle

Freckle: a small brown lesion, that is, ephelids

Furuncle: an abscess with several openings

Fusiform: spindle-shaped

Futcher's line: also known as Voight's line; a normal demarcation between a darker and lighter area

Genodermatosis: disease with abnormal skin findings due to heredity

Goodell's sign: softening of the cervix, occurring after four weeks of gestation

Goosebump: horripilation, piloerection of the hair follicles due to emotions, temperature change, or fright, frequently observed on the forearms

Granuloma: packed collection of inflammatory cells

Granulomatous: resembling a granuloma

Gulliver's sign: an indication in a patient with pyoderma gangrenosum that the inflammation is being con trolled.

Gyrate: round or circular

Hematoxylin and eosin stain: abbreviated as H&E, where hematoxylin stains the nuclei purplish-blue and eosin stains the cytoplasm pinkish

Hereditary: inherited, as opposed to acquired

Herpetic: a group of lesions with central pustules, resembling the lesions of *Herpes simplex* or *Herpes zoster* infection

Hive: a reddish elevated lesion, that is, urticaria

Horripilation: see *goosebump*

Hutchinson's sign: vesicular eruption on the nose preceding eye involvement due to viral infection of the trigeminal nerve

Ichthyosiform: resembling ichthyosis or fish scale–like

Impetiginized: resembling impetigo with oozing, crusting, and scaling

Id reaction: development or stimulation of acute dermatitis or lesions in a distant location from the initial site, usually on the hands induced by most often due to a superficial fungal infection on the feet

Immunofluorescence: using fluorescence to stain the antibody. Direct immunofluorescence stains the antibody. Indirect immunofluorescence permits the antigen to react with the antibody, after which the non-antibody globulin is washed away, and the tissue is bathed with fluorescein-labeled anti-rabbit globulin

Impetiginization: superficial bacterial infection superimposed upon an underlying dermatitis

Isomorphic response: creation of additional lesions of the same characteristics as the original lesion, that is, Koebner phenomenon

Itch: an irritable feeling that can be associated with hives or many other skin conditions causing one to scratch

Jacuemier's sign: purplish discoloration of the vagina occurring early in the pregnancy

Kamino bodies: dull pinkish bodies found at the tip of the dermal papillae

Keratinization: creating additional skin or scale

Keratolysis: separation of sheets of epidermal cells

Keratosis: excessive horny material

Koebner phenomenon: see *isomorphic response*

Koilonychia: spoon-shaped nails

Lamellar: sheets of cells

Lentigo: a small brown lesion

Lesion: a characteristic change in the structure of the skin

Leukonychia: white streaks or dots in the nail

Lichenified: thickening of the skin, as in lichens

Linea: formation of a line

Lisch nodule: an elevated tannish nodule on the iris

Livedo: bluish color due to venous congestion

Lunula: the whitish half-moon area often seen at the base of the nail

Lupus: wolflike appearance

Maceration: softening of the skin leading erythema, oozing, and scaling

Macrophage: a cell that surround bacteria or other organisms. It can provide antigens to T cells that release cytokines that can start an inflammatory process

Macular: resembling a macule

Macule: a lesion that is flat with color change

Melanotic: a dark, blackened appearance

Melanonychia: brown or black streaks or dots in the nail

Microbiome: the bacteria, viruses, or fungi found in areas of the body

Morbilliform: red lesions resembling measles

Mottled: irregular discoloration

Multiforme: many different shapes

Nikolsky's sign: slight rubbing of the skin leading to peeling of the superficial layers

Nodule: a larger elevated lesion

Nummular: coin-shaped

Onychodystrophy: defective nail formation

Onychomadesis: shedding of the nail

Onychorrhexis: longitudinal ridging of then ail

Ophiasis: hair loss at the edges of the scalp

Palmar: pertaining to the ventral surface of the hand

Papular: resembling a papule

Papule: a smaller elevated firm lesion, varying in area up to 1 cm

Paraneoplastic: signs and symptoms occurring elsewhere in the body due to chemical signaling from a malignancy

Paronychia: inflammation of the nail fold that leads to a painful, sometimes, pruritic area

Patch: a large macule

Pathergy: an exaggerated response to an injury that exacerbates the underlying condition and may create new lesions

Pautrier microabcess: an accumulation in the epidermis of at least four atypical lymphocytes as found in mycosis fungoides

Peau d'orange: resembling the peel of an orange

Pityriasis: a scaly condition

Plantar: pertaining to the sole

Plaque: a small thickened area

Polymorphic: many different shaped lesions

Prurigo: an older term for an itching condition

Pruritic: an itchy condition

Pruritus: itching

Purpuric: extravasated red blood cells giving a purplish color

Pustule: a lesion containing white to yellow, somewhat viscous fluid
Rash: a term that should be avoided when possible, eruption
Reticulated: resembling a net
Retiform: netlike
Russell's sign: callouses on the dorsal aspect of the hand, associated with self-induced vomiting
Scale: exfoliated skin
Scaling: a lesion containing scale
Seborrheic: a term whose original meaning had to with the sebaceous gland
Serous: a watery yellowish fluid
Serpiginous: having a wavy appearance, like a snake moving
Sisaipho: ophiasis spelled backward to reflect a reversed hair pattern loss with the hair remaining at the edges of the scalp
Sign: a clinical manifestation that can be seen or elicited on examination
Syndrome: a group of signs and/or symptoms to describe a condition
Symptom: an abnormal feeling experienced by the patient that cannot be seen
Stria: a superficial atrophic line
Targetoid: resembling a target shape
Test results: a positive test result, such as pathogenic growth on a bacterial culture, confirms the diagnosis, whereas a reactive serologic test result only suggests the diagnosis
Tinea: a scaling fungal eruption
Trachyonychia: longitudinal ridging with brittle grayish nails, split ends, and a rough surface
Transudate: an edematous process due to increased pressure on blood vessels causing fluid to accumulate in the surrounding tissue leading to swelling of the tissue
Trichodystrophy: defective hair growth often leading to alopecia
Trichomalacia: distorted hair shafts due to repeated twisting, occurring in trichodystrophy
Tumor: abnormal skin growth, often connoting a skin cancer
Tzanck smear: a smear taken from moist tissue that is stained with Giemsa or toluidine blue that will show nucleic bodies; that is, in *Herpes simplex* or *Herpes zoster* infection with multi-nucleated giant cells that have ballooned
Ulcer: a defect that descends from the skin surface
Ulcerated: the result of an ulcer, a depression from the surface
Ungual: related to the nail
Verrucous: wartlike
Vesicle: a small blister
Voight's line: see *Futcher's line*
Xeropthalmia: decrease in tears
Xerotic: resembling dry skin
Xerostomia: decrease in saliva
Wart: a verruca
Wheal: a red elevated lesion, that is, hive
Welt: a red elevated lesion, that is, hive
Wood light: a diagnostic tool that uses long-wave ultraviolet light appearing as a black light to diagnose skin infections and disorders
Woronoff ring: a round, blanched area surrounding a psoriatic lesion in the shape of a girdle, resembling the lesions of *Herpes zoster* infection

ADDITIONAL READINGS

Burgdorf WH, Hoenig LJ. Favorite Animal Names in Dermatology. JAMA Dermatol. 2013;149:997.
Buxton PK. ABC of Dermatology. Introduction. Br Med J (Clin Res Ed). 1987;295:830–834.
Griffith RD, Falto-Aizpurua LA, Nouri K. Dermatologic Etymology: Primary morphology of skin lesions. JAMA Dermatol. 2015;151:69.
Grzybowski A, Parish LC. The Dermatologist and Color. Skinmed. 2018;16:376–378.
Leider M, Rosenblum M: A Dictionary of Dermatological Words, Terms and Phrases. New York, McGraw-Hill, 1968, 440 pp.
Milam EC, Mu EW, Orlow SJ. Culinary Metaphors in Dermatology: Eating Our Words. JAMA Dermatol. 2015;151:912.
Parish LC, Wallach D. Cutaneous Morphology: The basic tool of dermatology. Skinmed. 2003;2:76–77
Parish LC, Witkowski JA. Updating the Dermatologic Nomenclature: Names that are good or bad. Skinmed. 2010;8:199–200.
Parish LC, Lambert WC. Speaking Good (and Safe) Dermatologic English. Skinmed. 2019 29;17:90–91.
Sprecher E. What's in a Disease Name? Br J Dermatol. 2014;170:1005–1007

2 Diagnosing Skin Disease

Shayan Waseh and Jason B. Lee

CONTENTS

DIAGNOSING SKIN DISEASE

Skin diseases represent a vast and heterogeneous body of disorders that can vary greatly in their clinical presentations, manifesting signs, and associated symptoms. Adopting a systematic and methodic approach is essential to the effective and accurate diagnosis of skin disease. This systematic approach, when combined with the responsible utilization of appropriate diagnostic aids, can serve to secure the diagnosis in a wide variety of dermatologic conditions.

SIGNS AND SYMPTOMS

Signs

Many of the characteristics that define skin diseases are fundamentally visual in nature given the externality of the skin. The distribution, color, and morphology of skin lesions are all integral components of the description of dermatologic conditions and serve as a foundational component of the diagnostic process.

Color

The color of the skin is determined by the interaction of a variety of internal and exogenous factors, including the production of melanin pigment by resident melanocytes, the functional activity of skin vasculature, and many external forces, such as ultraviolet radiation and manipulation of the skin. Color changes related to these factors often manifest as hyperpigmentation, hypopigmentation, or erythema. Discoloration can be a source of significant distress for patients, especially when widespread or highly visible areas, such as the face, are involved. This is particularly true in dark-skinned patients, in whom the contrast between normal and affected skin may be dramatic, such as the depigmentation of vitiligo and hyperpigmentation of resolved lichen planus.

The pigmentation of the skin is primarily determined by the function of skin melanocytes in the production and distribution of melanin pigment. This process is responsible for the determination of skin type in normal skin, but it is also implicated in the pigmentary changes associated with many dermatologic conditions. Inflammation, ultraviolet radiation, and cryotherapy all can cause significant changes to skin color (Figure 2.1). Melanocytes are highly sensitive to cold temperatures, and cryotherapy may lead to post-treatment hypopigmentation, particularly in patients with darker skin. Inversely, exposure to ultraviolet radiation activates melanocytes to produce and

DOI: 10.1201/9781003105268-2

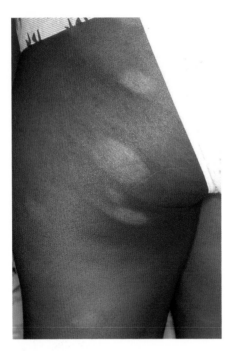

Figure 2.1 Hypopigmented and subtle erythematous plaques of sarcoidosis in a dark skin patient.

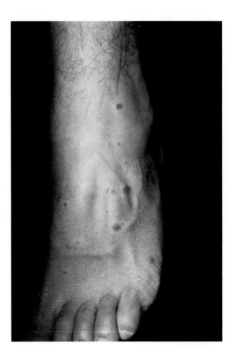

Figure 2.2 Non-scaly erythematous papules of early lesions of psoriasis.

distribute melanin granules more effectively, which can lead to skin tanning as part of an evolutionarily honed response.

A variety of other pigments can less commonly contribute to changes in skin color at a localized or generalized level. Systemic disorders in metabolic or endocrine function can cause generalized changes in skin pigmentation. For example, the buildup of homogentisic acid in connective tissue and cartilage in alkaptonuria leads to skin darkening, especially on the ears where cartilage is closely opposed to the skin. Prolonged systemic therapy, such as hydroxychloroquine, may result in widespread slate-gray discoloration.

Erythema is a visual manifestation of most inflammatory skin diseases, which is determined by the number, caliber, flow rate, oxygenation status, and body site of the skin's blood vessels. Other factors that determine the specific hue and shade include the density of the inflammatory infiltrate and epidermal changes. In turn, the specific characteristics of erythema, such as shade of color and border definition, can provide significant clinical insight into the disease process unfolding within the skin (Figure 2.2). A plaque of psoriasis, for example, has a characteristic, bright red hue that is well circumscribed (Figure 2.3), while a plaque of pityriasis rubra pilaris has a characteristic erythema with an orange hue that is less well-circumscribed. Additionally, the extravasation of red blood cells from the vasculature can lead to striking changes in skin color, referred to as purpura. This presence of palpable purpura is associated with a variety of vasculitides and vasculopathies. In darker skin individuals, erythema may be subtle, harder to detect than in fair skin individuals, and often have a duskier hue (Figures 2.4 and 2.5).

Texture

The texture of healthy skin should mostly be smooth and soft. When the normal function and life cycle of skin cells are disturbed, their texture can become profoundly altered. Coarseness, excessive scale, and dryness can each indicate a disruption of normal functioning and serve to indicate the presence of an underlying pathologic process.

The replacement rate of the cornified cells in the stratum corneum, the outermost layer of the epidermis, is approximately 2 weeks with some variation by body site and age. This turnover normally occurs incrementally through the shedding of individual cornified cells throughout the

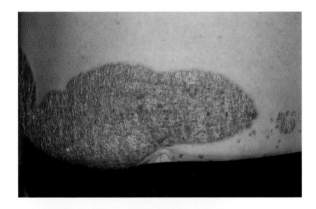

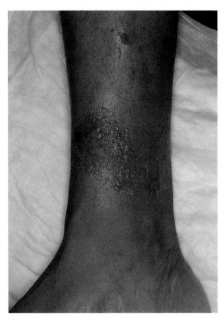

Figure 2.3 Scaly large erythematous plaque of psoriasis.

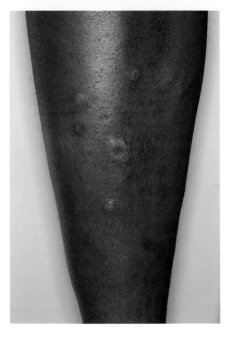

Figure 2.4 Flat-topped hyperpigmented papules with the violaceous border of lichen planus.

Figure 2.5 Hyperpigmented plaque surrounded by a cluster of vesicles due to allergic contact dermatitis from using an antibiotic ointment.

course of daily life. This process is largely imperceptible in healthy skin, but it can become apparent when the process of normal keratinization is disrupted. Should this occur, a significant scale can form on the surface of the skin, which results in visual and textural changes. This disruption of skin function can be the result of a variety of underlying conditions that can range from genetic abnormalities, such as ichthyosis, to inflammatory changes, such as psoriasis, to the exogenous influence of factors, such as medication application and repetitive friction.

Morphology: Primary and Secondary Skin Lesions

An appreciation of the essential attributes of color, size, shape, and thickness is vital to the process of describing and understanding skin lesions and, in turn, underlies the accurate diagnosis of dermatologic conditions. Traditionally, skin lesions have been divided into primary and secondary lesions, where a primary skin lesion represents the initial or primary appearance before any treatment, manipulation, or changes due to the natural history of the disease process. A secondary lesion represents the appearance after the evolution of the skin disease process, treatment, or manipulation of the primary lesion.

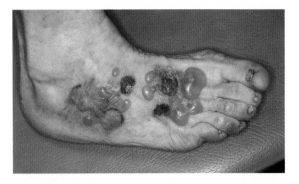

Figure 2.6 Tense vesicles and bullae of bullous pemphigoid.

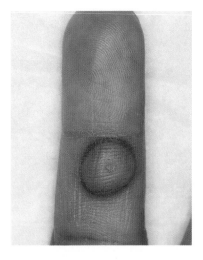

Figure 2.7 Tense hemorrhagic vesicle from cryotherapy of a wart.

Primary lesions have been categorized predominantly based on size and palpability. Although different size references have been applied, a 10-mm size threshold rather than 5 mm has been consistently applied. For example, macules, papules, and vesicles are 10 mm or less in diameter.

- *Macule/patch:* Flat, usually nonpalpable skin lesion

- *Papule/plaque:* Mesa or table-like elevated skin lesion

- *Vesicle/bulla:* Blisters that can be intraepidermal, subepidermal, or both

Some contour descriptors of a papule and plaque—flat-topped, dome-shaped, acuminate, papillated, digitated, and umbilicated—are strongly associated with specific skin conditions, such as the flat-topped papules of lichen planus (Figure 2.4), acuminate vesicles of dyshidrotic dermatitis, and the umbilicated papules of molluscum contagiosum. In addition, nodule (1–2 cm) and tumor (>2 cm) have been referred to as primary lesions that are larger and more elevated than plaques.

A variety of causes are associated with blistering dermatosis, including autoimmune, infectious, and inflammatory etiologies. Autoantibodies against desmogleins 1 and 3, which are components of desmosomes that keep keratinocytes attached to one another, resulting in acantholysis, or a loss in intercellular connections, and can lead to intraepidermal blisters. In contrast, autoantibodies against components of hemidesmosomes of the dermo-epidermal junction in bullous pemphigoid result in subepidermal blisters (Figure 2.6). Herpesvirus infection of the epidermis may result in acantholysis and varying degrees of epidermal necrosis, which can lead to intraepidermal or subepidermal blisters. Significant intercellular edema in allergic contact or nummular dermatitis results in intraepidermal blisters. Any process that weakens the dermo-epidermal junction may result in a subepidermal blister (Figure 2.7). Severe dermal edema from a variety of sources may also result in a subepidermal blister (e.g., lymphedema blister, bullous insect bite, and bullous Sweet syndrome). Depending on the severity and acuity, most interface dermatitides, which are associated with a variable degree of necrosis of keratinocytes at the dermo-epidermal junction, have a subepidermal bullous expression. Examples include bullous erythema multiforme, bullous lichen planus, and bullous fixed-drug eruption.

The location of these blisters within the epidermis determines their behavior and longevity. Intraepidermal blisters tend to be flaccid and evolve into erosions in a short amount of time, while subepidermal blisters tend to be tense and generally last longer before rupturing (Figure 2.6). Whether a blister is tense or flaccid, however, will ultimately depend on the size and speed at which it forms.

Secondary skin lesions include impetiginization, pigmentary changes, scale-crust that can be purulent and/or hemorrhagic, lichenification, fissures, erosion, ulceration, and scar formation. A patient with atopic dermatitis may manifest a variety of secondary skin lesions, all of which are due to manipulation of the skin, including rubbing, scratching, and picking by the patient due to persistent pruritus. The presence of secondary changes offers insight into the symptomatology

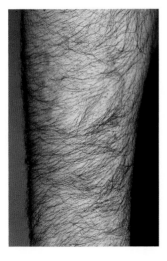

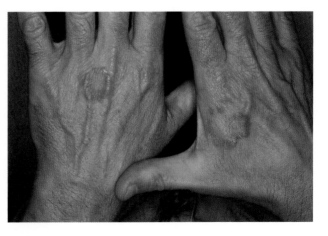

Figure 2.9   Annular non-scaly plaques of granuloma annulare.

Figure 2.8   Scaly annular patch of tinea corporis.

of the patient's disease and provides useful information on the clinical course and characteristics of the condition. Inversely, they may also obscure the primary findings that would help identify the underlying skin disease; therefore, an awareness of the presence of secondary skin changes is important to adjusting clinical expectations during the assessment of primary lesions.

Dermatologic disorders can manifest in any variety of shapes, from the linear configuration associated with allergic contact dermatitis to polygonal papules with lichen planus (Figure 2.4) to scaly and non-scaly annular plaques associated with tinea corporis (Figure 2.8) and granuloma annulare (Figure 2.9). The demarcation of shape can be well-defined, such as psoriasis (Figure 2.3) and vitiligo, or it can be ill defined and blend into the surrounding normal skin, such as nummular dermatitis. Additionally, it is important to be aware that shape is not only limited to external skin changes but also includes depth of involvement, particularly in malignant skin conditions. This includes melanoma, where the depth of extension has profound prognostic implications, and basal cell carcinoma, where the insidious process of infiltration can cause significant distortion of surrounding tissue over time.

Distribution

The distribution of skin findings in dermatologic disorders is an important diagnostic tool. Diseases of the skin can present in a generalized manner or be localized to one or several specific body sites. Although the varicella-zoster virus causes the appearance of vesicles in both chickenpox disease and shingles, these two clinical entities vary considerably, as the former is characterized by a generalized eruption, and the latter is typically limited to the localized dermatome. Skin cancer is most commonly found on chronically sun-exposed sites, while necrobiosis lipoidica is almost always localized to the shin. Additional examples include erythema multiforme characteristically involving the palms and bilateral extremities (Figure 2.10), dermatitis herpetiformis involving bilateral elbows, knees, buttocks, and scalp, and warfarin-induced skin necrosis usually involving fatty areas, such as the abdomen and thigh. When encountering a hospitalized patient with a suspicion of drug reaction, the presence of mucosal involvement can be a clinically significant indicator of life-threatening diseases, such as Stevens-Johnson syndrome or toxic epidermal necrolysis requiring a higher acuity of care. In sum, careful assessment of the overall distribution of skin lesions should be performed routinely since it can provide important diagnostic information.

SYMPTOMS

Dermatologic conditions are often associated with a variety of subjective symptoms, including pruritus, pain, and discomfort. Awareness of the presence of these symptoms is an important component of clinical care, because these symptoms play a significant role in influencing the patient's quality of life and well-being.

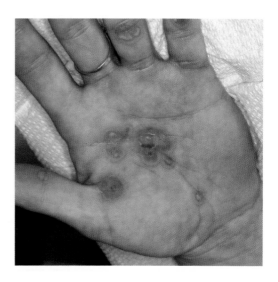

Figure 2.10 Targetoid macules and patches of erythema multiforme.

Pruritus

Pruritus, or itch, is a common symptom found in a wide variety of dermatologic disorders, including atopic dermatitis, urticaria, allergic contact dermatitis, nummular dermatitis, scabies, and dermatitis herpetiformis.

Pruritus is fundamentally characterized as an uncomfortable sensation linked to a desire to scratch. The degree of pruritus associated with these dermatologic conditions and other systemic disorders can vary from mild to debilitating. The presence of pruritus can be associated with significant skin changes, or it can be found in seemingly normal skin. Pruritus can be exacerbated by many different factors, including low humidity, frequent bathing, aging skin, and irritating substances. These factors can aggravate underlying skin disease, since they can incite pruritus, particularly in the diseases listed earlier.

Pruritus can also lead to the development of new skin lesions through the traumatic effect of scratching. For example, atopic dermatitis has been colloquially referred to as the "itch that rashes." Sites of repetitive scratching can also become infected, which can further exacerbate the disease. In some cases, new lesions of the underlying dermatologic disease can occur focally at the site of scratching, which is known as the Koebner phenomenon.

In addition to recognizing the impact that pruritus has on the quality of life and well-being of patients, a focused evaluation of the chronicity and behavior of pruritus symptoms can be a helpful diagnostic clue in the workup of dermatologic conditions. As an example, the pruritus in urticaria is typically transient and migratory, while it can be more chronic and exacerbated by drier seasons in atopic dermatitis.

Pain

The presence or absence of pain can be an important differentiating factor in the diagnosis of dermatologic disorders. Pyoderma gangrenosum and calciphylaxis are both classically characterized as being extremely painful. Additionally, the subjective symptom of pain is often associated with the presence of acute inflammation as seen in cellulitis, panniculitis, infected cysts, and even seborrheic keratoses when they become irritated. In the case of skin malignancies, the presence of pain may indicate perineural invasion.

Importantly, pain can be a significant detractor in the quality of life of patients with chronic dermatologic conditions. In severe atopic dermatitis and other diseases, fissuring of the skin can lead to significant pain and discomfort. In patients with irritant contact dermatitis from workplace exposure, pain can sometimes necessitate alterations in their workplace or work habits; therefore, pain represents a significant source of morbidity for patients with painful dermatologic diseases.

Disability

Dermatologic disorders can carry a profound degree of disability and morbidity into the lives of patients in a variety of ways. Many skin disorders are associated with significant cosmetic concerns that can interfere with physical and mental well-being. There is a nearly universal human aversion to diseased skin, and it is challenging to prevent and overcome these feelings. One theory proposes that this aversion is rooted in the infectious nature of some dermatologic conditions and, therefore, serves as an evolutionarily protective mechanism. In the modern era, these prejudices are maladaptive and can interfere with interpersonal relationships and even employment. As examples, acne can be a significant stressor in the lives of adolescents and adults, and the nail and scalp changes seen in psoriasis can be embarrassing for patients who work in occupations requiring social contact. An appreciation of the impact that dermatologic disorders can have on the physical and mental well-being of patients is an integral component of providing patient-centered care.

The location of dermatologic disease can also be an important determinant of the degree of disability that it causes. Although the severity of most dermatologic conditions is correlated with the body surface area of involvement, even small and localized lesions on the palms and soles can be debilitating given their functional importance. For example, patients with dactylitis in psoriasis and psoriatic arthritis may be unable to work with their hands as effectively, if at all. Plantar warts and clavus can likewise cause discomfort during ambulation, which can limit mobility. Diseases, such as atopic dermatitis, can also cause fissuring around joints, which can result in discomfort with movement and subsequent immobilization.

Additionally, lesions affecting the face and other exposed areas of the skin can significantly impact self-esteem and self-confidence in patients who interact with others daily. The treatment of choice for various skin conditions may also vary based on the site of involvement. High-potency steroids are often prescribed for plaques on the body but seldom for the face and other areas of thin skin. Therefore, an appreciation of the distribution of lesions on a patient's skin is an important factor in understanding the patient's experience with their disease and in providing effective and appropriate clinical care.

Importantly, the impact of dermatologic conditions on health and well-being on a global and societal scale cannot be understated. Dermatologic conditions represent the fourth-leading cause of disability worldwide among nonfatal conditions. In the United States, one in four people are impacted by skin disease, and the estimated annual cost for medical care alone approaches $100 billion each year. The global health burden of some dermatologic disorders, such as psoriasis, has continued to rise over recent decades, which indicates a greater need for public and global health efforts to address dermatologic disease.

Common aids: The foundation of diagnosis in dermatologic disease is the clinical history and physical examination. An appreciation of the patient's demographic factors, history of present illness, and general medical status are all important components in understanding the patient's disease process. The presence or absence of associated systemic symptoms is an important data point that may indicate an urgent need for more acute and comprehensive care. Additionally, an informed and focused physical examination that accurately defines and describes the lesions of concern is a uniquely powerful diagnostic tool in the practice of dermatology; however, dermatologic diseases can manifest in a variety of ways, and even a single condition can have multiple different presentations that may overlap with other clinical entities. An armamentarium of diagnostic aids and tools has been developed to assist in the often-challenging endeavor of identifying skin lesions when history and physical examination alone are unable to definitively do so.

Lighting

The availability of bright and consistent environmental lighting is essential in evaluating skin disorders. Sunlight from examination room windows as a source of lighting should be avoided because it provides a highly variable lighting that depends on the time of day, weather conditions, and room orientation. Bright overhead ambient lighting provides more consistent and standardized illumination for skin examinations, while the additional implementation of sidelights can assist with minimizing light distortion and shadow.

More complicated light-based tools are also readily available in many clinical settings. The Wood's lamp is one such valuable tool that has found use in a variety of dermatologic conditions, such as vitiligo and bacterial and fungal infections. A Wood's lamp, which emits wavelengths in the 320–450-nm range, can assist in differentiating pigmentary changes, highlighting fungal and bacterial infections, such as tinea versicolor and erythrasma, and identifying systemic diseases, such as porphyria.

BEDSIDE DIAGNOSTIC TESTS

Diascopy

Diascopy is a useful technique that assesses the blanchability of a skin lesion through the application and pressing of a glass slide over the lesion. This simple test allows for the differentiation of erythema into vascular etiologies related to blood vessel dilation, which are blanchable, and hemorrhagic etiologies, which do not exhibit blanching. Diascopy can also be used in other clinical contexts, such as the identification of lupus vulgaris involving the skin, which exhibits an apple jelly color on testing.

Magnification

Although the naked eye can collect a significant amount of information regarding the morphology of a skin lesion, magnification tools can yield meaningful additional information. A simple magnifying glass can highlight features not readily seen on gross examination, such as small telangiectasias in a lesion suspicious for basal cell carcinoma.

Evaluation of skin scrapings prepped with potassium hydroxide under simple light microscopy is the classic diagnostic test utilized in the diagnosis of dermatophytosis. Using a blue stain, such as toluidine blue, microscopic evaluation of vesicle scrapings—referred to as the Tzanck smear—can be performed to diagnose herpesvirus infection. A mineral oil prep involves the examination of skin scrapings of burrow under light microscopy to identify the presence of scabies mites.

Skin Testing

The unique accessibility of the skin allows for the utilization of a variety of tests that can be readily carried out in the clinical setting. Manipulation of the skin by a clinician is one such test that can yield useful diagnostic information. In the case of Darier's sign, vigorous rubbing of the patient's skin can support the diagnosis of mastocytosis when it results in significant swelling, itch, and erythema. The presence of Auspitz's sign, which is the appearance of punctate bleeding after the scraping of scaly lesions, can be indicative of psoriasis. Additionally, the shearing of skin with rubbing, known as the Nikolsky sign, can be a clinically useful diagnostic finding in the evaluation of blistering skin disorders, such as pemphigus and toxic epidermal necrolysis.

More complex forms of skin testing are also available and can serve to either support or refute a variety of diagnoses. In the case of allergic contact dermatitis, the application of potential causative agents to the surface of the skin through a patch test can yield a hypersensitivity reaction that supports the suspicion of hypersensitivity to a certain substance. The clinical application of this test allows for it to be carried out in a more supervised and controlled setting with lower concentrations of the suspected allergen than otherwise possible.

A similar principle is applied in prick testing for anaphylactic reactions, which involves piercing the skin with a needle laden with a low concentration of the suspected allergen in a controlled and closely monitored setting with anaphylaxis treatment readily available. Additionally, the application of various biochemically active substances to the skin can help in identifying a variety of skin lesions; for example, acetic acid is commonly applied to suspected warts on genital areas and can result in significant whitening that serves to highlight the lesion of concern.

Dermatoscopy

With the advent of portable handheld dermatoscopes, the practice of dermatoscopy has become ubiquitous in dermatology. The technique involves rendering the cornified layer translucent either by using polarized light or immersion contact with the skin, thereby exposing subsurface structures that can be better visualized (Figure 2.11). The most widely utilized dermatoscope consists of polarized light capable of 10× magnification. Special attachments and adaptors for cameras and smartphones allow easy capture and sharing of dermatoscopic images.

Dermatoscopic diagnostic criteria have been developed for a variety of skin diseases, which include inflammatory, neoplastic, and infectious diseases. Its utility has been promoted for evaluating pigmented lesions, especially in the early detection of melanomas and their simulators, such as melanocytic nevi, seborrheic keratoses, dermatofibromas, and solar lentigines. In melanocytic lesions, assessment of subsurface structures, such as typical and atypical pigment networks, dots, and globules, allows for differentiating a nevus from a melanoma. Additionally, a variety of nonmalignant pigmented skin lesions exhibit characteristic appearances under dermatoscopy. A seborrheic keratosis, which can occasionally be difficult to distinguish from melanoma, often exhibits characteristic comedo-like openings on dermatoscopic evaluation. In vascular lesions, dermatoscopy allows for a greater definition of the specific vascular structures (e.g., lagoons) and

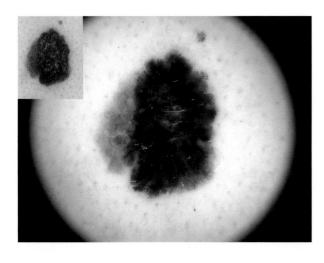

Figure 2.11 Dermatoscopy of melanoma showing multicomponent pattern: blue-gray veil, dark blotch, and asymmetric peripheral distribution of globules.

morphology present within the lesion. Since significant time and effort are needed to become proficient in dermatoscopy, early and strategic immersion in mastering this technique is recommended. Sources of learning material include books, internet sites, and courses.

Medicine is entering the era of artificial intelligence-augmented practice, and dermatology is expected to fully embrace this transformative technology. This is particularly true within the domain of skin cancer detection, where the application of artificial intelligence and machine learning has been increasingly developed. As dermatoscopes and other forms of visualization assist dermatologists in diagnosing skin conditions, advanced machine learning algorithms can process digital macroscopic or dermatoscopic images to identify patterns that differentiate lesions. The deployment of these technologies as diagnostic aids and supplementary tools has been shown to increase the diagnostic accuracy of dermatologists in the differentiation of skin cancers. The era of artificial intelligence–augmented practice is expected to provide more efficient and accessible care of skin diseases.

Laboratory studies: Although the externality of skin allows for the unique ability of clinicians to evaluate conditions through visual inspection and physical manipulation, there are a variety of contexts in which laboratory studies are indicated in the evaluation, diagnosis, and management of skin diseases. Laboratory studies can assist in the initial workup of dermatologic conditions, especially in cases where there is systemic involvement or potential involvement of internal organs. They may be helpful in the initial evaluation of symptoms, such as generalized pruritus when there are no readily apparent dermatologic causes. Laboratory studies are often indicated to monitor adverse reactions of high-risk systemic medications, such as isotretinoin and methotrexate, requiring baseline and serial laboratory studies to monitor the functional status of the liver, kidneys, and other organs.

A variety of laboratory tests are available for dermatologists to establish or confirm a specific diagnosis. In women with hirsutism, hormone levels can be obtained to confirm hyperandrogenism. Venereal disease research laboratory or rapid plasma reagin tests may be obtained in patients suspected of syphilis. Antinuclear antibody testing and tissue antibodies are often reported through titers and can support the diagnosis of diseases, such as systemic lupus erythematosus and a variety of vasculitides. The clinical interpretation of these tests can often be challenging when patients present in an atypical manner or results are borderline. Enzyme-linked immunosorbent assay tests are available to aid in the diagnosis of several autoimmune blistering diseases, such as pemphigus, pemphigoid, and dermatitis herpetiformis. In the case of pemphigus, the detection and level of anti-desmoglein antibodies can contribute to confirming a diagnosis and monitoring the disease course.

There are many examples of dermatologic diseases in which comorbid or associated diseases may need to be excluded via laboratory studies. A patient with alopecia areata may require a check of thyroid disease status, while a patient with oral lichen planus may require checking of viral hepatitis status. A diagnosis of Sweet syndrome requires the exclusion of some time-associated leukemias.

Dermatopathology: The function of dermatopathology—that is, the microscopic examination, description, and interpretation of skin biopsies—is essential to the practice of dermatology.

Through the use of microscopy in conjunction with a variety of histochemical and immunochemical stains, dermatopathology can offer significant insight into the underlying pathology for a wide variety of dermatologic conditions.

Biopsy of the skin is a necessary initial step in the process of dermatopathology evaluation. The selection of the biopsy site is an important decision that can have a profound impact on the utility and sensitivity of histologic evaluation. Depending on the suspected disease process, factors influencing the selection of an ideal biopsy site include lesion age, stage of development, and morphology.

Skin biopsy techniques include shave, punch, incision, and excision. In shave biopsies, a thin superficial portion of the skin is shaved off with a blade, whereas punch biopsies involve the use of a cylindrical cutting device that is rotated down to the level of the subcutaneous tissue before the base of the tissue is cut with scissors to release the specimen. Although a shave biopsy or removal is better suited for superficial epidermal skin lesions, such as superficial basal cell carcinomas, a punch biopsy allows for a more complete microscopic evaluation of the various layers of the skin, which is better suited for inflammatory dermatoses. Finally, an excisional biopsy typically involves the creation of an elliptical excision around the lesion of concern and can result in the greatest quantity of tissue removed for evaluation, which is particularly suited for suspected melanomas. A less optimal incisional biopsy may be warranted when lesions are too large for an excisional biopsy. The most appropriate method of biopsy is directly related to the clinical entity under investigation.

Since errors in the procurement of a skin biopsy specimen are not uncommon, steps to minimize the common errors should be implemented. This should include verification of patient name and site, especially when multiple sites are involved. An appropriate volume of fixative is matched for the size of the sample, for which the ratio of fixative to the specimen should be 15–20:1. The most common stain used in pathology and dermatopathology is the hematoxylin and eosin stain, also known as the H&E stain. This stain highlights the nuclei, cytoplasm, and extracellular matrix, which allows for visualization of individual cells forming the various components of the skin, including their nuclei.

Ancillary stains are often utilized when H&E-stained slides do not provide sufficient diagnostic information. In modern dermatopathology, the development of immunohistochemical stains has allowed for precise evaluation of specific epitopes within the skin. Immunohistochemical stains that target specific protein epitopes are available, which include those used to detect syphilis spirochetes and human herpesvirus 8 associated with Kaposi sarcoma.

For neoplasms that may be benign or malignant, a skin biopsy can often help provide a specific diagnosis, such as seborrheic keratosis, basal cell carcinoma, and melanoma. For inflammatory dermatoses, a biopsy can often demonstrate a histopathologic pattern that is associated with more than one disease, thus requiring clinical pathologic correlation. A spongiotic dermatitis, for example, is associated with nummular or allergic contact dermatitis, so the clinician should correlate this with the clinical findings to arrive at a specific diagnosis. A histologic description of the subepidermal blister with numerous neutrophils, which pattern observed in dermatitis herpetiformis, linear IgA dermatosis, and bullous lupus erythematosus, narrows the differential diagnosis and guides the clinician to pursue specific additional testing (Figure 2.12). In other instances,

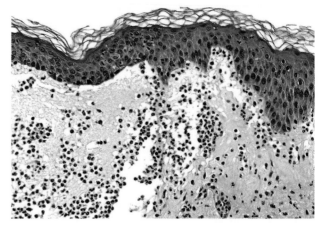

Figure 2.12 A subepidermal blister with neutrophils that may be seen in bullous lupus erythematosus, linear IgA dermatosis, and dermatitis herpetiformis.

a skin biopsy may show nonspecific changes. In these cases, depending on the clinical context, either additional biopsy or watchful waiting for more specific lesions to develop can be a reasonable course of action.

FINAL THOUGHT

As a visual specialty, physical examination in dermatology continues to play a critical role in diagnostic assessment. Accurate assessment of color, texture, morphology, and distribution is essential in the evaluation of dermatologic diseases. Becoming proficient in diagnosing skin diseases requires exposure to the wide spectrum of presentations of dermatologic disorders, especially those that are common, with follow-up and feedback—the necessary required steps toward expertise. An experienced dermatologist will rarely require additional diagnostic aids other than a physical examination. If further diagnostic confirmation is needed, a variety of diagnostic tests are available that include dermatoscopy, skin biopsy, and, shortly, artificial intelligence–augmented assessment of skin diseases.

ADDITIONAL READINGS

Elston DM, Stratman EJ, Miller SJ. Skin biopsy: biopsy issues in specific diseases. J Am Acad Dermatol. 2016;74:1–16.

Grzybowski A, Parish LC, Wollina U. The color of skin. Clin Dermatol. 2019;37:389–606.

Happle R, Kluger N. Koebner's sheep in Wolf's clothing: does the isotopic response exist as a distinct phenomenon? J Eur Acad Dermatol Venereol. 2018;32:542–543.

Jackson R. Morphological Diagnosis of Skin Disease: A Study of the Living Gross Pathology of the Skin. Grimsby, ON, Canada: Manticore; 1998.

Lee JB. Diagnostic and therapeutic instrumentation in dermatology. Clin Dermatol. 2021;39.

Micali G, Lacarrubba F. Alternative use of dermatoscopy. Dermatol Clin. 2018;36:345–502.

Tintle SJ, Cruse AR, Brodell RT, et al. Classic findings, mimickers, and distinguishing features in primary blistering skin disease. Arch Pathol Lab Med. 2020;144:136–147.

Trayes KP, Savage K, Studdiford JS. Annular lesions: diagnosis and treatment. Am Fam Physician. 2018;98:283–291.

Tüzün Y, Wolf R. Fold dermatoses. Clin Dermatol. 2015;33:411–508.

Wolf R, Parish LC, Parish JL. The rash: part I. Clin Dermatol. 2019;37:85–172. The rash: part II. Clin Dermatol. 2020;38:1–121.

Yang TB, Kim BS. Pruritus in allergy and immunology. J Allergy Clin Immunol. 2019;144:353–360.

3 Adnexal Diseases

Hasan Aksoy, Jordan V. Wang, and Ayşe Serap Karadağ

CONTENTS

ACNE

Definition: Acne vulgaris (acne) is a chronic, inflammatory disorder of the pilosebaceous unit, which affects about 85% of adolescents and young adults. The disease may result in permanent scars and often causes immense psychologic burdens, such as poor self-image, anxiety, and depression.

Overview: Four cardinal pathogenic factors of acne are follicular hyperkeratinization, sebum overproduction, bacterial colonization by *Cutibacterium acnes*, and inflammation.

Clinical presentation: Acne lesions arise on the sebaceous gland–rich areas of the face, chest, shoulders, and back. The primary lesions include open and closed comedones, papules, pustules, and abscesses or cysts. Plugging of the follicles with sebum and keratin can form skin-colored lesions that can oxidize to create blackheads.

Inflammation associated with the rupture of follicles can cause papules and pustules to form (Figure 3.1). Nodules (abscesses) are larger, deep-seated, and tender lesions that can be seen as the inflammation progresses. In severe cases, there may be deep, fluctuant, cystic lesions, which contain liquefied material (e.g., pus, blood), called pseudocysts. Lesions may subsequently evolve into transient erythema, post-inflammatory hyperpigmentation, and persistent scarring. Acne scars can be atrophic (e.g., icepick, rolling, boxcar), hypertrophic, and keloidal.

ACNE CONGLOBATA AND ACNE FULMINANS

Acne conglobata is a severe form of acne presenting with numerous inflamed papules, grouped comedones, painful nodules, cysts, sinus tracts, and severe scars, which predominantly involve the face and trunk. Acne conglobata is a component of the follicular occlusion tetrad, which is also composed of hidradenitis suppurativa, dissecting cellulitis of the scalp, and pilonidal sinus.

DOI: 10.1201/9781003105268-3

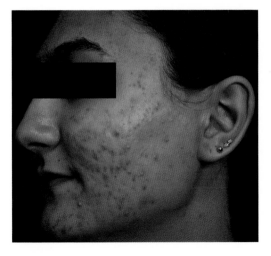

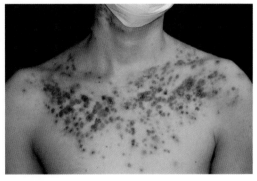

Figure 3.2 Acne fulminans; ulcerating, hemorrhagic, and crusted papules and nodules with scars on the chest and neck.

Source: Courtesy of Istanbul Medeniyet University Dermatology Clinic.

Figure 3.1 Multiple closed comedones, papules, and pustules on the cheek, chin, and forehead.

Source: Courtesy of Istanbul Medeniyet University Dermatology Clinic.

Acne fulminans is a rare and severe variant of acne, which presents with painful, ulcerating, hemorrhagic, crusted, necrotizing, and destructive papules, pustules, and nodules that eventually heal with scarring (Figure 3.2). This variant primarily affects male adolescents. Unlike acne conglobata, it is typically accompanied by systemic symptoms, such as fever, arthralgia, myalgia, and weakness, and systemic findings, including leukocytosis, anemia, and osteolytic bone lesions of the sternum and clavicles.

DRUG-INDUCED ACNE

Drug-induced acne is an acneiform eruption caused by medications, dietary supplements, herbal products, and systemic steroids (Table 3.1). It often has a good prognosis, which may not require cessation of the culprit drug. Development of lesions due to epidermal growth factor inhibitors (e.g., cetuximab, erlotinib, lapatinib) is often an indicator for successful treatment response.

Laboratory studies: Patients with post-adolescent acne or accompanying clinical signs of hyperandrogenism can be screened for potential alteration in serum levels of dehydroepiandesterone

Table 3.1 Common Culprits of Drug-Induced Acne

Topical, oral, systemic steroids
Hormones containing progesterone
Antiepileptic drugs (e.g., carbamazepine, phenytoin, phenobarbital)
Isoniazid
Lithium
Cyclosporine
Azathioprine
Halogens (iodides and bromides)
Disulfiram
Propylthiouracil
Quinidine
B vitamins (B6 and B12)
Tumor necrosis factor (TNF)-inhibitors
Epidermal growth factor receptor (EGFR) inhibitors

Table 3.2 Common Treatment Regimens for Acne Vulgaris

	Comedonal acne	Mild Papulopustular Acne	Moderate Papulopustular Acne	Severe Papulopustular Acne	Severe Nodulocystic Acne
First step	• Topical retinoid • Benzoyl peroxide	• Topical antibiotic and topical retinoid and/or benzoyl peroxide	• Topical antibiotic and topical retinoid and/or benzoyl peroxide • Oral antibiotic and topical retinoid and/or benzoyl peroxide	• Oral antibiotic and benzoyl peroxide and/or topical retinoid	• Oral isotretinoin • Oral antibiotic and topical retinoid and/or benzoyl peroxide
Second step	• Alternative topical retinoid • Azelaic acid • Salicylic acid	• Alternative topical combination therapy • Azelaic acid • Salicylic acid • Topical dapsone	• Alternative topical combination therapy • Consider a change in oral antibiotic	• Oral isotretinoin	

sulfate (DHEA-S) total and free testosterone, luteinizing hormone/follicle-stimulating hormone (LH/FSH) ratio, prolactin, and 17-OH progesterone. Acne fulminans may requires testing for inflammatory markers and blood counts. Histopathologic examination is rarely required.

Differential diagnosis: Acne is typically diagnosed clinically with relative ease; however, acne-iform eruptions may sometimes be confused with acne.

Management: This is based on the severity of the disease and type of lesions (Table 3.2).

TOPICAL TREATMENT

Topical Retinoids

Topical retinoids regulate follicular keratinization, which can reduce microcomedo formation and offer comedolytic activity. They are also anti-inflammatory and can reduce pigmentation and scar formation. Topical retinoids include tretinoin, isotretinoin, tazarotene, adapalene, and trifarotene.

Benzoyl Peroxide

Benzoyl peroxide is not an antimicrobial, but it has bactericidal effects and can reduce the bacteria within follicles. It can help prevent antibiotic resistance from topical and systemic antibiotic therapy.

Other Topical Agents

Topical antibiotics include clindamycin and erythromycin, which can reduce the bacterial load; however, the resistance of up to 80% of *C. acnes* strains to erythromycin has been reported. These should be used in combination with other topical agents to prevent resistance. Azelaic acid can also inhibit bacterial overgrowth, regulate hyperkeratinization, and lighten post-inflammatory hyperpigmentation. Dapsone is another topical that works through anti-inflammatory and anti-bacterial effects, which can help with inflammatory lesions.

SYSTEMIC TREATMENT

Oral Antimicrobials

Systemic antibiotics are indicated in severe scarring acne or when topical treatment is difficult to apply. Tetracyclines (e.g., doxycycline, minocycline) are preferred due to their antibacterial and anti-inflammatory effects and lower antibiotic resistance. Doxycycline is often the first choice, with traditional dosing ranging from 100–200 mg/day. Recent evidence suggests that sub-antimicrobial dose may also be sufficient. The most important side effects are photosensitivity and gastrointestinal upset.

Oral Isotretinoin

Isotretinoin is mainly used for the treatment of recalcitrant, severe papulopustular, and nodular acne. Isotretinoin is regarded as the most effective acne treatment; however, recurrence may develop in one-fourth of cases. Recent evidence has suggested higher cumulative doses than the traditional 120–150 mg/kg in more severe cases. Isotretinoin has many mucocutaneous side effects, including cheilitis and xerosis. Serum levels of cholesterol, triglycerides, and transaminases can elevate. The most important side is teratogenicity; therefore, effective contraception and frequent pregnancy testing are important in women of childbearing potential.

Hormonal Therapies

Hormonal therapies (i.e., antiandrogens) can be helpful in women with acne, regardless of whether hyperandrogenism is present. The most commonly used agents are combined oral contraceptive pills and spironolactone. Spironolactone can cause irregular menses, breast tenderness, headaches, nausea, and hypotension. Hyperkalemia is rare, and monitoring serum potassium is not indicated in low-risk individuals.

MAINTENANCE TREATMENT

In some patients, cure can be achieved with isotretinoin. Despite appropriate treatment, acne is a chronic and recurrent disease, and therefore, maintenance treatment is often required. The most suitable agents are topical retinoids and benzoyl peroxide.

Course: Acne vulgaris is a chronic disease that commonly manifests in adolescence. The disease has a relapsing-remitting course and may persist into adulthood. Although it has a good prognosis and usually is not associated with systemic involvement, severe acne variants should be considered in the presence of accompanying systemic symptoms or signs.

Final comment: This is a chronic disease that can manifest with visible lesions, dyspigmentation, or scarring; therefore, it has a psychosocial impact and should be treated appropriately. Although its use is limited by teratogenicity, oral isotretinoin is the most effective therapeutic agent.

FOLLICULITIS

Definition: This is inflammation of the hair follicle, which presents with erythematous papules or pustules in hair-bearing areas. It has superficial and deep forms, and it is typically caused by infectious agents, irritants, or medications.

Overview: Based on etiology, common forms of folliculitis include superficial bacterial folliculitis, gram-negative folliculitis, fungal folliculitis, viral folliculitis, and *Demodex* folliculitis.

Clinical Presentation

Bacterial Folliculitis

Overview: Clusters of pustules surrounded by an erythematous rim can manifest on the head (scalp and beard area), neck, trunk, groin, and extremities (Figure 3.3). Lesions usually heal in

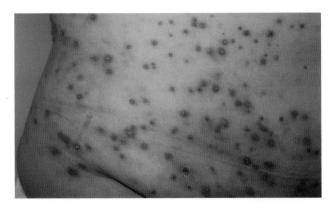

Figure 3.3 Bacterial folliculitis with numerous pustules with an erythematous rim on the trunk.

Source: Courtesy of Istanbul Medeniyet University Dermatology Clinic.

7–10 days but may also transform into furuncles. Nasal carriage of the most common pathogen, *Staphylococcus aureus*, is an important predisposing factor.

Management: Treatment with tetracyclines, especially for acne, may cause gram-negative folliculitis, which can be due to *Klebsiella, Enterobacter, Escherichia,* and *Proteus* species. It usually involves the face and is confused with acne. Hot-tub folliculitis is caused by *Pseudomonas aeruginosa* and primarily involves the trunk. This develops due to exposure to contaminated water.

Fungal Folliculitis

Overview: Dermatophytic folliculitis typically presents with follicular pustules on the surface of a red, firm, exudative, and extending plaque. It can develop in association with tinea barbae, tinea capitis, or tinea corporis. Lesions of folliculitis in tinea barbae involve the beard or mustache area. Trichophytic (Majocchi) granuloma classically occurs in women shaving their legs or when tinea corporis is first treated with topical corticosteroids. *Malassezia* (Pityrosporum) folliculitis commonly affects young males and presents with follicular papules and pustules involving the trunk, shoulders, neck, or extensor aspects of the arms. Candidal folliculitis appears as satellite pustules around the flexural lesions of candidiasis, especially in diabetics.

Demodex *Folliculitis*

Overview: *Demodex* normally lives in the pilosebaceous unit, but overgrowth can be associated with folliculitis. *D. folliculorum* and *D. brevis* can cause rosacea-like eruption, perioral dermatitis, or pityriasis folliculorum, especially on the zygomatic, periorbital, and nasal regions.

Laboratory studies: Histologically, superficial bacterial folliculitis demonstrates neutrophilic infiltration enclosing the follicular infundibulum and subcorneal/infundibular abscess formation. In KOH examination, hyphae and spores can be seen. *Demodex* mites can be demonstrated by direct microscopy of both superficial skin biopsy and KOH preparation.

Differential diagnosis: The differential diagnosis of folliculitis is listed in Table 3.3. The conditions mentioned in this chapter can easily mimic each other.

Management

Bacterial Folliculitis

Topical antibiotics, such as mupirocin, are used as first-line treatment. Oral antibiotics, such as dicloxacillin or cephalexin, are often required for furuncles or carbuncles. Nasal/skin decontamination can be achieved with a 5-day course of intranasal mupirocin application (twice daily) and chlorhexidine gluconate bathing. In gram-negative folliculitis, culprit antibiotics should be stopped, and oral isotretinoin has been shown to offer help.

Table 3.3 Differential Diagnosis of Folliculitis

• Bacterial folliculitis	• Acne vulgaris
• Gram-negative folliculitis	• Papulopustular rosacea
• Dermatophytic folliculitis	• Perioral dermatitis
• *Malassezia* folliculitis	• Drug-induced folliculitis
• Candidal folliculitis	• Hidradenitis suppurativa
• Herpetic folliculitis	• Scabies
• *Demodex* folliculitis	• Disseminate and recurrent infundibulofolliculitis
• Irritant folliculitis	• Pseudofolliculitis barbae
• Ofuji disease	• Acne keloidalis
• Immunosuppression-associated eosinophilic folliculitis	• Folliculitis decalvans
	• Keratosis pilaris
• Eosinophilic pustular folliculitis of infancy	• Fox-Fordyce disease
	• Idiopathic follicular mucinosis
	• Perforating folliculitis

Fungal Folliculitis

Dermatophytic folliculitis is treated with oral antifungals such as terbinafine, griseofulvin, or itraconazole. Antifungal shampoo (e.g., ketoconazole) can be used to prevent the spread of spores. *Malassezia* folliculitis usually responds well to topical azoles or shampoos with selenium sulfide. In patients with candidal folliculitis, the use of steroids or antibiotics should be discontinued. Topical azoles and/or oral fluconazole can be used.

Demodex *Folliculitis*

Therapeutic options for *Demodex* folliculitis include topical permethrin 5% cream, topical ivermectin 1% cream, and oral ivermectin. Permethrin cream can be considered as initial treatment, and in recalcitrant cases, oral agents can be added.

Course: Most forms of folliculitis are curable conditions with a good prognosis. Recurrence of infective folliculitis can be prevented by proper hygienic measures and skin decontamination.

Final comment: Folliculitis refers to a heterogeneous group of conditions that may occur due to infection or irritation or as a manifestation of inflammatory skin disease. Different types of folliculitis should be properly diagnosed to clarify preventive and therapeutic recommendations.

ROSACEA

Definition: This is a chronic, inflammatory skin disease that typically affects the central face. It is characterized by persistent erythema, papules, pustules, telangiectasias, and recurrent flushing.

Overview: Rosacea commonly affects middle-aged women who are Fitzpatrick skin types I–III. Proposed pathophysiologic mechanisms include activation of the cutaneous innate immune system, neurovascular dysregulation, and increase in density of *Demodex* mites. Ultraviolet radiation is a contributing factor.

Clinical presentation: Rosacea has four clinical subtypes: erythematotelangiectatic, papulopustular, phymatous, and ocular (Table 3.4). Rosacea often presents earlier on as the erythematotelangiectatic subtype, which is characterized by persistent erythema, recurrent flushing, and telangiectasias on mid-face (Figure 3.4). Flushing can be triggered by physical, nutritional, or psychologic factors.

In the papulopustular subtype, patients have several small, dome-shaped erythematous papules and pustules on the mid-face. Unlike acne, rosacea is not typified by comedones (Figure 3.5).

Overview: In the phymatous form, sebaceous gland hypertrophy and fibrosis are present (Figure 3.6). Phyma primarily occurs in men and commonly affects the nose (rhinophyma) but may also be seen on the chin, ears, forehead, and eyelids.

Ocular involvement is present in 50–60% of patients who have rosacea, which can manifest with nonspecific symptoms, such as dryness, tearing, gritty sensation, styes, blepharitis, and itching.

Table 3.4 **Summary of Clinical Subtypes of Rosacea**

Clinical Subtype	Characteristics
Erythematotelangiectatic rosacea	• Recurrent flushing and fixed centrofacial erythema • Midfacial edema and/or telangiectasia • Skin sensitivity
Papulopustular rosacea	• Fixed centrofacial erythema, intermittent red papules, and pustules • No comedones • Persistent midfacial edema caused by intermittent inflammation
Phymatous rosacea	• Sebaceous gland hypertrophy and fibrosis • Flesh-colored, soft, irregular nodules • Nose: Rhinophyma; Chin: Gnathophyma; Ear: Otophyma; Forehead: Metophyma; Eyelid: Blepharophyma
Ocular rosacea	• Strongly suggestive: Lid margin telangiectasia, interpalpebral conjunctival injection, spade-shaped infiltrates in the cornea, scleritis, and sclerokeratitis • Nonspecific: Burning, stinging, light sensitivity, and foreign object sensation

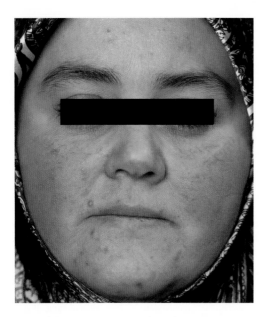

Figure 3.4 Erythematotelangiectatic rosacea. Erythema and telangiectasias are seen on the cheeks with a few papules in the perioral region.

Source: Courtesy of Istanbul Medeniyet University Dermatology Clinic.

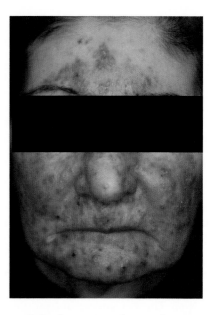

Figure 3.5 Severe papulopustular rosacea. Numerous papules and pustules with crust on an erythematous base can be seen on the forehead, nose, cheeks, and chin.

Source: Courtesy of Istanbul Medeniyet University Dermatology Clinic.

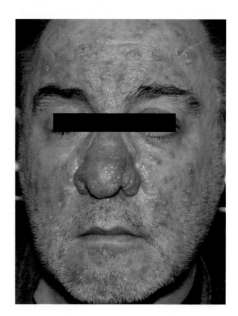

Figure 3.6 Papulopustular and rhinophymatous rosacea.

Source: Courtesy of Istanbul Medeniyet University Dermatology Clinic.

There is no correlation between the presence of ocular involvement and the severity of skin disease. Ocular rosacea is historically underdiagnosed.

Rosacea fulminans (i.e., pyoderma faciale, rosacea conglobata) is a severe form that is more common in young women. In addition to diffuse facial erythema, there is sudden onset, and coalescing papules, pustules, purulent nodules, and sinuses are often seen. Short-term use of systemic corticosteroids can be helpful.

Granulomatous rosacea is a clinical variant that presents with monomorphous, 1–3-mm-sized yellow-brown or red papules or nodules on the cheeks or periorificial areas. There is an

Table 3.5 Differential Diagnosis of Rosacea

Erythematotelangiectatic rosacea	Actinic damage
	Photoaging with telangiectasias
	Seborrheic dermatitis
	Contact dermatitis
	Keratosis pilaris rubra
	Malar rash
	Flushing
Papulopustular rosacea	Acne
	Demodex folliculitis
	Acneiform eruption
Phymatous rosacea	Lupus pernio
	Discoid lupus erythematosus
	Lupus vulgaris
Ocular rosacea	Seborrheic dermatitis
	Drug-induced ocular rosacea

Table 3.6 General Skin Care Measures in the Management of Rosacea

Avoidance of triggers, such as environmental factors (e.g., cold, heat, humidity), exercise, stress, diet, spices, histamine-rich food, alcohol, hot food

Use of broad-spectrum sunscreen with ultraviolet-A, ultraviolet-B, and visible-light protection

Cleansing using lukewarm water and soap-free cleansers

Moisturizing using non-oily moisturizers

Avoidance of topical corticosteroids

Avoidance of cosmetic products, such as waterproof make-up, skin toners, astringents, and abrasive exfoliators

Avoidance of cosmetic ingredients, such as sodium lauryl sulfate, strong fragrances, fruit acids, glycolic acids, alcohol, menthols, camphor, witch hazel, peppermint, and eucalyptus oil

"apple-jelly" appearance on diascopy as in sarcoidosis or lupus vulgaris, and dermal noncaseating granulomas are present histologically. This variant may cause permanent scarring.

Laboratory studies: Skin biopsy is rarely required for diagnosis and can be nonspecific.

Differential diagnosis: This can be organized according to subtype (Table 3.5). Papulopustular rosacea may resemble acne, but there are typically no comedones or scarring in rosacea. Some clinical features of acne, such as truncal distribution, hyperseborrhea, and adolescent-onset are not observed in rosacea. Actinic damage can be confused with erythematotelangiectatic rosacea; however, actinic damage commonly affects the periphery of the face and neck, upper chest, and postauricular region.

Management: Management of rosacea involves general skincare practices listed in Table 3.6 and pharmacologic intervention.

In patients with erythematotelangiectatic rosacea, topical α-adrenergic agonists, such as brimonidine (α_2) or oxymetazoline ($\alpha_{1A}+\alpha_2$), can help improve erythema by causing peripheral vasoconstriction. Carvedilol is a nonselective beta-blocker and is effective in the treatment of flushing and persistent erythema. Vascular lasers (e.g., pulsed dye laser) and intense pulsed light (IPL) can also be used to treat telangiectasias and erythema.

Papulopustular rosacea should be treated with topical agents, systemic antibiotics, or oral isotretinoin. First-line topicals include metronidazole, ivermectin, and azelaic acid. Topical metronidazole is often initially preferred. Ivermectin cream demonstrates slightly higher efficacy than metronidazole in terms of reduction in inflammatory lesions. Other topical options are listed in Table 3.7.

In patients with moderate to severe inflammatory lesions, systemic antibiotics, such as doxycycline, tetracycline, or azithromycin can be used. Low-dose (0.3 mg/kg/day) oral isotretinoin is recommended for patients with moderate to severe recalcitrant papulopustular rosacea. Systemic treatments are outlined in Table 3.8.

Table 3.7 Topical Agents Used in the Treatment of Rosacea

Drug	Mechanism	Subtype
Metronidazole	Anti-inflammatory Antioxidant Antibacterial Antiparasitic	Papulopustular Erythematotelangiectatic
Azelaic acid	Anti-inflammatory Antioxidant Antibacterial Anti-keratinizing	Papulopustular Erythematotelangiectatic
Ivermectin	Anti-inflammatory Antioxidant Antiparasitic	Papulopustular Erythematotelangiectatic *Demodex* mite
Brimonidine	α-2 adrenergic receptor agonist Vasoconstriction	Persistent erythema
Oxymetazoline	α-1 adrenergic receptor agonist Vasoconstriction	Persistent erythema
Sodium sulfacetamide + sulfur	Antibacterial Anti-inflammatory	Papulopustular
Permethrin	Antiparasitic	*Demodex* mite
Pimecrolimus	Inhibits T-cell activation	Granulomatous rosacea
Tacrolimus	and proinflammatory cytokines	Steroid-induced rosacea
Tretinoin	Anti-inflammatory Anti-keratinizing Inhibits TLR2	Erythematotelangiectatic Papulopustular

Table 3.8 Systemic Medications Used in the Treatment of Rosacea

Drug	Mechanism	Subtype
Doxycycline Tetracycline	Reduction of MMPs Preventing kallikrein-5 Reduction of ROS and NO Vasoconstriction Anti-inflammatory	Papulopustular Granulomatous Ocular Phymatous
Ivermectin	Reduction of MMPs Preventing kallikrein-5 Reduction of ROS and NO Anti-inflammatory Antiparasitic	Papulopustular Granulomatous Ocular Phymatous
Isotretinoin	Anti-inflammatory Antioxidant Anti-keratinizing Reduction of sebaceous gland volume	Papulopustular Granulomatous Ocular Phymatous
Carvedilol	α1, β1, β2 antagonist Vasoconstriction Antioxidant Anti-inflammatory	Erythematotelangiectatic
Metronidazole	Anti-inflammatory Antioxidant Antibacterial Antiparasitic	Papulopustular Granulomatous Ocular

Abbreviations: MMPs, matrix metalloproteinases; ROS, reactive oxygen species, NO: nitric oxide.

Phyma may respond to low-dose isotretinoin if it is inflamed. In rhinophyma, isotretinoin may reduce the nasal volume and prevent progression. Severe and fibrotic forms can only be treated with physical modalities, such as surgical excision, electrosurgery, ablative lasers, and dermabrasion.

For ocular rosacea, lavage of eyelids twice daily with warm water and baby shampoo, use of eye drops, and referral to an ophthalmologist are recommended. Oral antibiotics, such as doxycycline, are helpful in most cases.

Course: It is a benign skin disease with a good prognosis that has no systemic complications. Since its chronic and recurrent nature, treatment is often required for both exacerbations and maintenance.

Final comment: This is an inflammatory syndrome affecting the midface with or without eye involvement. Management of rosacea aims to prevent symptoms, improve cosmesis, and maintain remission and involves patient education, appropriate skincare, avoidance of sunlight, and topical/oral anti-inflammatory medications, as well as interventions.

PERIORIFICIAL DERMATITIS

Overview: It is characterized by multiple papules and pustules localized around the mouth, nose, or eyes. It is commonly seen in young women and children. It is often associated with topical, nasal, or inhaled steroids, fluorinated toothpaste, mouthwashes, soaps, and cosmetics. It can be more common in atopic individuals. The exact cause is not understood.

Clinical presentation: There are many tiny pustules and pink papules, or thin plaques with desquamation in perioral, perinasal, and/or periocular areas (Figure 3.7). Lesions can spread around the lip, but there is typically an unaffected zone of 5 mm from the vermilion line.

Management: Periorificial dermatitis is usually treated with topical medications, which can include metronidazole, erythromycin, clindamycin, tacrolimus, and pimecrolimus. Systemic tetracyclines (e.g., doxycycline, minocycline) can be used for initial improvement. Any topical steroid use should be stopped.

HIDRADENITIS SUPPURATIVA

Synonym: Acne inversa

Definition: Hidradenitis suppurativa (HS) is a chronic, inflammatory disorder characterized by deep-seated and tender nodules, cysts, sinus tracts, and scarring in intertriginous areas. It is often misdiagnosed as folliculitis, furuncles, or carbuncles in the early stages. The disease shows female predominance and commonly arises in the second or third decade.

Overview: Aggravation of the disease is strongly associated with two major risk factors: smoking and obesity. Hyperkeratosis, occlusion, and destruction of the follicle and inflammation of the apocrine glands are implicated in the pathogenesis.

Clinical presentation: HS lesions are primarily located in the apocrine gland–bearing areas, such as axillae and inguinal folds. Further localizations include anogenital, gluteal, sternal, mammary, submammary, and retroauricular regions. Inflamed and noninflamed nodules can progress into the characteristic multiheaded comedones or coalesce to form sinus tracts with scarring

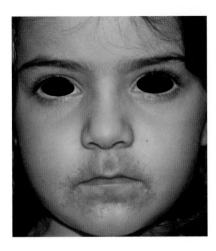

Figure 3.7 Multiple tiny papules and pustules in perioral and periocular regions.

Source: Courtesy of Istanbul Medeniyet University Dermatology Clinic.

(Figure 3.8). Deep-seated nodules can extend to develop abscesses in which suppuration drains to the skin surface (Figure 3.9). The discharged fluid consists of serous exudate, blood, and pus. As the disease progresses, bridged scars, fibrosis, contracture, and hardening of the skin may develop. Secondary infections can cause malodor.

Patients often report stinging, burning, itching, and warmth a few days before active lesions appear. Inflamed nodules, cysts, and sinuses are usually painful. Disease severity can be assessed with grading systems, such as the Hurley staging system.

HS is a component of the follicular occlusion tetrad in addition to acne conglobata, dissecting cellulitis, and pilonidal cyst. The disease is associated with several systemic conditions, such as Crohn's disease, pyoderma gangrenosum, diabetes mellitus, metabolic syndrome, polycystic ovary syndrome, and arthritis.

Laboratory studies: Diagnosis of HS is made clinically. Histopathology demonstrates a mixed inflammatory cell infiltrate in the deeper dermis, poral occlusion, inflammation, and fibrosis of the follicles and sweat glands. Later stages can show abscesses draining to the skin surface through a channel, tract formation containing inflammatory cells and keratin, and granulation tissue. As the disease progresses, fibrosis becomes more prominent.

Differential diagnosis: In the early stages, HS may be confused with furunculosis; however, nodules of furuncles have a central punctum and are not interconnected to form tracts. Acne, pilonidal disease, and dermoid/epidermoid cysts are also included in the differential of early lesions. Cutaneous Crohn's disease can present with perianal/genital fistulae, abscesses, and scars similar to HS, but there are no comedones, and the fistulae are linked to the gastrointestinal tract.

In advanced stages, the nodular, draining, ulcerating, indurated, and scarring lesions of HS may resemble infectious/granulomatous skin diseases, such as cutaneous tuberculosis, syphilis, granuloma inguinale, lymphogranuloma venerium, tularemia, actinomycosis, nocardiosis, and cat-scratch disease.

Management: This includes lifestyle modifications, treatment with topical or systemic pharmacologic agents, and surgical or laser interventions. The severity of the disease determines the therapeutic approach.

General measures include weight reduction, smoking cessation, reducing friction by wearing loose clothing, and skin decontamination using antiseptic scrubs or antibacterial soaps. Warm compresses can be beneficial. Patients should be screened for accompanying metabolic conditions.

Topical clindamycin is preferred as a first-line treatment in cases with mild to moderate inflammatory lesions. Topical dapsone or resorcinol can be used for their anti-inflammatory effects. Oral antibiotics (e.g., doxycycline, tetracycline, clindamycin, rifampin) are another first-line treatment option, and combination therapy is commonly required.

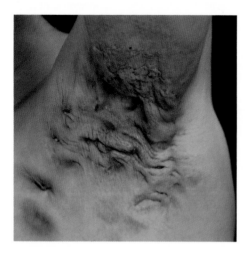

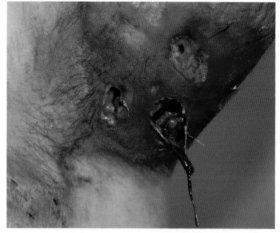

Figure 3.8 Multiheaded comedones, sinus tracts, draining sinuses, and scarring in the axilla.

Source: Courtesy of Istanbul Medeniyet University Dermatology Clinic.

Figure 3.9 Abscess with sinus tracts that drain to the skin surface.

Source: Courtesy of Istanbul Medeniyet University Dermatology Clinic.

Antiandrogenic therapy is considered second-line treatment, especially for women with mild or moderate HS. Spironolactone can be used in women who experience hormonal flares. Metformin can inhibit the production of pro-inflammatory cytokines, reduce insulin resistance, and exert anti-androgenic effects.

Intralesional triamcinolone acetonide injection is an effective adjunctive therapy for individual lesions when inflamed. Oral retinoids do not appear to be effective enough. The results of the case series regarding the use of isotretinoin in HS have been disappointing.

Biologic agents can be considered in moderate to severe cases that are recalcitrant to conventional therapies. TNF-α inhibitors used for the treatment of HS include adalimumab and infliximab. Other biologic therapies have been utilized with varying degrees of success.

Surgery involves either limited or extensive excision and aims to improve the quality of life. It is non-curative and does not replace medical treatment, but it can offer benefit in severe, recalcitrant disease that includes scarring and sinus tracts. Deroofing of the sinus tracts, cysts, or abscesses is associated with fewer overall complications; however, wide excision has been shown to have lower rates of recurrence. Nd: YAG and carbon dioxide laser treatment have offered significant improvement in several studies.

Course: HS is a chronic, recurring, and debilitating disorder that is associated with poor quality of life and significant psychosocial morbidity. HS has many complications, including secondary amyloidosis, anemia, fistulae to the urinary or gastrointestinal tract, and lymphedema. Squamous cell carcinoma can rarely arise in sites of chronic lesions.

FINAL THOUGHT

HS is an unpleasant disease for both the patient and the physician. Lesions are often tender, draining, suppurating, and malodourous. Because HS is incurable, treatment is often difficult; however, proper disease management can offer improvement, especially in the quality of life.

ADDITIONAL READINGS

Alikhan A, Lynch PJ, Eisen DB. Hidradenitis suppurativa: a comprehensive review. J Am Acad Dermatol. 2009;60:539–563.

Dessinioti C, Antoniou C, Katsambas A. Acneiform eruptions. Clin Dermatol. 2014;32:24–34.

Gallo RL, Granstein RD, Kang S, et al. Standard classification and pathophysiology of rosacea: the 2017 update by the National Rosacea Society Expert Committee. J Am Acad Dermatol. 2018;78:148–155.

Goldburg SR, Strober BE, Payette MJ. Hidradenitis suppurativa: current and emerging treatments. J Am Acad Dermatol. 2020;82:1061–1082.

Laureano AC, Schwartz RA, Cohen PJ. Facial bacterial infections: folliculitis. Clin Dermatol. 2014;32:711–714.

Lee GL, Zirwas MJ. Granulomatous rosacea and periorificial dermatitis: controversies and review of management and treatment. Dermatol Clin. 2015;33:447–455.

Luelmo-Aguilar J, Santandreu MS. Folliculitis: recognition and management. Am J Clin Dermatol. 2004;5:301–310.

Saunte DML, Jemec GBE. Hidradenitis suppurativa: advances in diagnosis and treatment. JAMA. 2017;318:2019–2032.

van Zuuren EJ. Rosacea. N Engl J Med. 2017;377:1754–1764.

Williams HC, Dellavalle RP, Garner S. Acne vulgaris. Lancet. 2012;379:361–372.

4 Papulosquamous Diseases

Melek Aslan Kayıran, Jordan V. Wang, and Ayşe Serap Karadağ

CONTENTS

PSORIASIS

Definition: This is a chronic, systemic inflammatory disease that affects the skin and is the most common papulosquamous disease. Numerous systemic effects, such as hyperlipidemia, cardiovascular disease, diabetes mellitus, depression, inflammatory bowel disease, nonalcoholic fatty liver disease, and metabolic syndrome may accompany it.

Overview: Psoriasis can be seen in every age, gender, and race; however, it peaks between 16–22 and 57–60 years of age. Although its frequency varies by country, it is estimated to be between 0.09–11.8% of the general population.

Psoriasis is a multifactorial genetic disease that has been associated with many genes and pathways, especially HLA-CW*06, interleukin (IL)4, IL23/17 axis, and NF-κB signaling. Stress, humid and cold weather, trauma, smoking, obesity, HIV infection, beta-blockers, lithium, antimalarials, antidepressants, antivirals, and nonsteroidal anti-inflammatory medications are among the potential triggers. Streptococcal pharyngitis is known to initiate guttate psoriasis, especially in pediatric patients.

Clinical presentation: Psoriasis has different forms, such as psoriasis vulgaris (PV), pustular psoriasis, guttate psoriasis, inverse psoriasis, erythrodermic psoriasis, and palmoplantar psoriasis, which can be associated with psoriatic arthritis.

The most common form is PV and accounts for 80–90% of all cases. Lesions are often symmetric, well-demarcated, pink, scaly plaques (Figure 4.1). Lesions may differ in size and shape. Knees, elbows, scalp, and sacral region are frequently involved; however, lesions can be observed in all areas of the body (Figure 4.2).

There are a number of phenomena that can help to diagnose PV. For the "wax spot phenomenon," when the lesion is scraped with the blunt tip of a scalpel, the scale sheds in thin white layers, which indicates parakeratotic hyperkeratosis. If the lesion continues to be scraped, a sticky and wet layer is reached; this is the lowest layer of the dermal papillae, and this finding is called as the "last membrane phenomenon." When the lesion is scraped even further, bleeding foci are seen

Table 4.1 Pathogenesis of Psoriasis

Keratinocyte Hyperproliferation	Vasodilation in Dermal Capillaries	Proinflammatory Mediator Release
• Acceleration in cell turnover	• Angiogenesis	• Increased release of interleukin, endothelin, IFN-ϒ, TNF-α, and vascular endothelial growth factor
• Rapid desquamation of keratinocytes	• Lymphocyte and neutrophil penetration into the skin	
• Abnormal maturation and thickening of the stratum corneum		• T-cell activation
		• Immune response onset

DOI: 10.1201/9781003105268-4

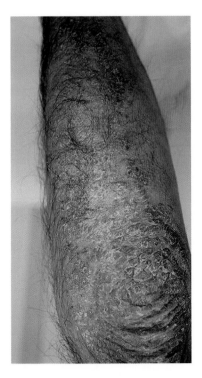

Figure 4.1 Psoriasis vulgaris with erythematous scaly plaques on the elbow and arm.

Source: Courtesy of Istanbul Medeniyet University Dermatology Clinic.

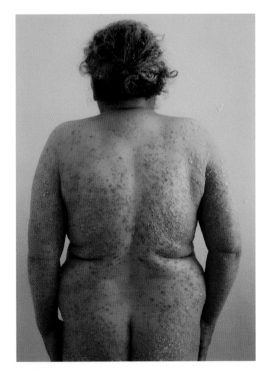

Figure 4.2 Psoriasis vulgaris with erythematous scaly papules and plaques on the back and arms.

Source: Courtesy of Istanbul Medeniyet University Dermatology Clinic.

as tiny pinheads. This finding is the "Auspitz sign" and indicates papillomatosis in the dermal papilla. While the lesions are healing, they can be surrounded by a hypopigmented ring, called the "Woronoff ring."

Guttate psoriasis is more common in children and young adults. Lesions are in the form of multiple, small, erythematous, scaly plaques that are 0.5–1.5 cm in diameter. Streptococcal throat infection is believed to precede many cases. A relationship has been found with HLA-CW*0602.

Inverse psoriasis is a variant that involves the retroauricular region, axillae, inframammary, inguinal, and intergluteal areas. It can be seen alone or together with other forms of psoriasis. It appears as well-defined, wet, erythematous plaques, and scale is not expected.

Pustular psoriasis is a clinical variant in which pustules are located on erythematous areas, which can be generalized or localized. It is seen at the rate of 1.2–1.8% among all forms of psoriasis. Its acute generalized form is also called von Zumbusch disease (Figure 4.3). Patients typically have fever, and pustules appear suddenly. It is more common between 30–50 years and in women. Its etiology includes drugs, such as terbinafine, amoxicillin, sulfonamides, and lithium, as well as infection, pregnancy, hypoparathyroidism, hypocalcemia, and ultraviolet radiation. Occasionally, it can emerge as a result of the sudden discontinuation of treatments in patients with psoriasis. Eye and nail involvement, along with a geographic tongue, can be observed. Fever, arthralgia, myalgia, malaise, and abdominal pain are common.

In localized pustular forms, fingers are typically involved (Figure 4.4), which has been called acrodermatitis continua of Hallopeau, acropustulosis, pustular acrodermatitis, acrodermatitis perstans, and dermatitis repens. It is common in middle-aged women. It starts in the form of sterile pustules in the nail folds and beds. The pustules combine to form pustule ponds that may open and form painful erosions. Onychodystrophy and anonychia may develop due to nail bed and matrix involvement. It usually starts on a few fingers and then extends onto the hands, forearm, and feet over time. Hand involvement is more common.

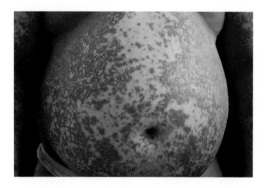

Figure 4.3 Pustular psoriasis with multiple pustules located on erythematous plaques on the chest, abdomen, flanks, and arms.

Source: Courtesy of Istanbul Medeniyet University Dermatology Clinic.

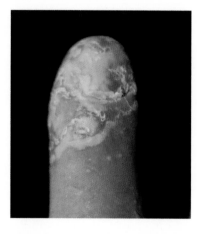

Figure 4.4 Localized pustular psoriasis, acropustulosis.

Source: Courtesy of Istanbul Medeniyet University Dermatology Clinic.

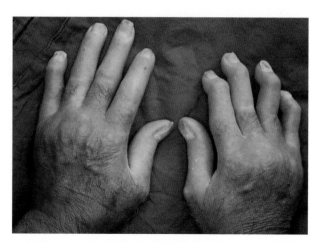

Figure 4.5 Psoriatic arthritis with asymmetric oligoarthritis of the hands.

Source: Courtesy of Istanbul Medeniyet University Dermatology Clinic.

Palmoplantar psoriasis can be encountered alone or in combination with other forms. Lesions are well-defined, hard, and thick scaly plaques, especially in the plantar region, which are sometimes accompanied by thick fissures. Erythema can be seen but is not always expected. It may be painful.

The most common comorbidity is psoriatic arthritis. which is a seronegative arthritis (Figure 4.5). It accompanies 5–7% of patients and can reach nearly 30% in those with severe psoriasis. It is seen equally in both genders. Although it can be positive, HLA-B27 is typically negative. Asymmetric oligoarthritis is the most common clinical presentation, and dactylitis and enthesitis can be seen. Joint pain and swelling, heel pain, and morning stiffness are common symptoms, and nail involvement is common.

Laboratory studies: Clinical findings are generally sufficient for diagnosis. In ambiguous cases, histopathologic examination can be helpful, which shows an elongation of the rete ridges and dermal papillae, edema of the dermal papillae, enlargement of blood vessels, thinning of the suprapapillary plates, parakeratosis, compact orthokeratosis, spongiform pustules, microabscesses caused by neutrophil accumulation in the upper portion of the epidermis, and regular acanthosis. Dilated capillaries and keratinocyte proliferation are expected in all stages.

Dermatoscopy can reveal red dot and globules; diffuse, patched, polygonal, and twisted vessels; and diffuse, patched, central, or peripheral scale.

Table 4.2 Nail Changes Seen in Psoriasis

Inflammation of the nail matrix	Inflammation in the nail bed	Hyponychium and proximal nail fold
Pitting	Onycholysis	Irregularly dispersed and tortuous veins
Onychomadesis	Splinter hemorrhages	
Leukonychia	Subungual hyperkeratosis	
Beau's lines	Oil-drop (salmon) patches	
Red spots on lunula		
Separation in nail plate		

Blood tests may be abnormal due to comorbidities, but laboratory findings are generally normal. Hyperuricemia can be seen in patients with extensive lesions. In psoriatic arthritis, C-positive protein (CRP) and erythrocyte sedimentation rate (ESR) can be elevated. In the generalized form of pustular psoriasis, leukocytosis, hypoalbuminemia, hypocalcemia, and elevated CRP and ESR can be observed.

Patients should be screened at regular intervals for comorbidities, such as metabolic syndrome, diabetes mellitus, hypertension, cardiovascular disease, inflammatory bowel disease, and liver dysfunction.

Differential diagnosis: This includes nummular dermatitis, seborrheic dermatitis, pityriasis rosacea, pityriasis rubra pilaris, syphilis, atopic dermatitis, pityriasis lichenoides chronica, parapsoriasis, and mycosis fungoides. In pustular forms, acute generalized exanthematous pustulosis, IgA pemphigus, and pustular drug eruption should be considered. In localized pustular forms, bacterial paronychia, herpetic whitlow, chronic candidiasis, and acrodermatitis enteropathica can be considered.

Management: Treatment decision depends on the clinical type, severity, extent, duration, response to previous treatments, and psychosocial status of the patient.

Topical Treatment

Topical treatments are typically sufficient in mild to moderate cases. Corticosteroids are anti-inflammatory, antiproliferative, and immunosuppressive. Treatment with high-potency corticosteroids is often started initially followed by lower potency formulations for maintenance as needed. Stronger corticosteroids should generally not be used for more than a few weeks at a time. For thick scaly plaques, it is useful to combine them with a keratolytic agent, such as salicylic acid, urea, or a retinoid (e.g., tazarotene), in order to increase penetration. Low- or medium-potency steroids should be used in inverse areas and on the face.

Anthralin and coal tar have been used with some benefit, but they have largely been replaced with topical steroids and steroid-sparing agents, such as calcipotriol and calcineurin inhibitors. Anthralin is mostly preferred in plaque psoriasis and used in short-term contact or combined preparations. Coal tar can be effective in reducing the thickness of scale in scalp psoriasis. Calcipotriol is a vitamin D analogue that suppresses inflammation and reduces the proliferation of epidermal keratinocytes in psoriasis. It is available alone or in combination with corticosteroids. Topical calcineurin inhibitors include tacrolimus and pimecrolimus. They can be particularly effective as maintenance treatment and in children.

Systemic Treatment

Systemic treatments are preferred in moderate to severe cases and those resistant to topical therapy or phototherapy. Agents include acitretin, methotrexate, cyclosporine, biologic agents, and steroids.

Acitretin can be used in all types of psoriasis and can be especially helpful in pustular psoriasis. Response can be observed after 4–6 weeks, but maximal effect is typically seen after 3–4 months. Once the disease stabilizes, the dose can be reduced for maintenance. Side effects are generally dose dependent and include skin dryness, cheilitis, palmoplantar desquamation, irritation, myalgia, hair loss, increased triglycerides, and increased liver function markers. Acitretin should not be used in women of childbearing age due to its teratogenicity.

Methotrexate works by inhibiting DNA synthesis through affecting dihydrofolate reductase. It reduces keratinocyte proliferation and has anti-inflammatory and immunomodulatory effects. Generally, 7.5–25 mg/week is sufficient for psoriasis treatment. It is helpful in PV, pustular, erythrodermic, and arthropathic psoriasis and affects nail findings. Patients should be given 1 mg/day of folate supplementation 48–72 hours after taking the medication to reduce gastrointestinal side effects. Before treatment, hepatitis markers, blood count, liver and kidney function tests, chest radiography, and complete urinalysis can be examined. Testing can be performed regularly for monitoring.

Cyclosporine suppresses IL-2 production and has immunosuppressive effects. It can be preferred in cases, where rapid remission is desired or in cases recalcitrant to other therapies. It is started by dividing 2.5 mg/kg/day into two doses and can be increased up to 4–5 mg/kg/day. In erythrodermic forms, treatment can be initiated with higher doses. Recurrence is common with discontinuation, especially abrupt cessation. Maintenance treatment is recommended, and patient can be slowly transitioned. Cyclosporine is nephrotoxic; if serum creatinine increases by 30% and glomerular filtration rate decreases below 30%, the treatment is discontinued. Side effects include hypertension, hyperlipidemia, electrolyte disturbance, myalgia, paresthesia, headache, flu-like syndrome, nausea, and vomiting. Blood pressure should be checked regularly.

Various biologic agents can target specific molecules and pathways in the psoriasis pathway. They generally have more systemic side effects and risks than other systemic immunosuppressant regimens. Common biologic agents include tumor necrosis factor-alpha inhibitors (e.g., adalimumab, etanercept, certolizumab), IL-17 inhibitors (e.g., secukinimab, ixekizumab, brodalumab), IL-12/23 inhibitors (e.g., ustelkinumab) and IL-23 inhibitors (e.g., guselkumab, risankizumab). Biologic treatments are mainly approved for psoriasis vulgaris and psoriatic arthritis and are generally not as effective for pustular psoriasis.

Systemic corticosteroids are not routinely used in the treatment of psoriasis. Despite rapid response from treatment, flaring can be rapid and severe when the steroid is discontinued; however, in severe erythrodermic psoriasis and generalized pustular psoriasis, prednisone 30–60 mg/day can be considered for a short time to allow for improved control, especially as a biologic agent is administered and begins to take effect. Systemic steroids should be slowly decreased and discontinued as soon as possible.

Phototherapy

Overview: Phototherapy can be helpful in moderate to severe cases of plaque psoriasis and guttate psoriasis, where topical treatments may be impractical. It can reduce epidermal hyperproliferation and suppress T-cell apoptosis and cytokines. Phototherapy is typically administered three days a week and continued for an average of 6–8 weeks with titration. The most common regiments use narrowband ultraviolet (UV) B (311–313 nm), which is believed to be the most effective spectrum in the treatment of psoriasis. UVA (320–400 nm) can be effective, especially in extremity-localized thick plaques; however, it comes with greater risk of carcinogenesis and cannot be used in pregnancy and childhood.

Course: Psoriasis is a chronic and recurring disease without cure. With appropriate use of topical and systemic agents and thorough patient education regarding treatment strategies, psoriasis can be managed. Severe forms, such as pustular psoriasis and erythrodermic psoriasis, may be life-threatening if not treated appropriately. In these patients, appropriate treatment should be initiated as soon as possible.

Final comment: Psoriasis is a lifelong disease that is associated with various comorbidities. When treating patients, it is important to not only treat skin findings but also to screen for other related systemic conditions. When indicated, a multidisciplinary approach should be adopted.

LICHEN PLANUS

Definition: Lichen planus (LP) is a chronic and often recurring inflammatory skin disease that can involve skin and mucosa. The most common presentation is characterized by small, itchy papules. The cause is not yet fully understood.

Overview: While the prevalence of skin involvement varies between 0.2–1%, oral involvement is more common (1–4%); however, both are commonly seen together. The mean age at diagnosis is 50–60 years for oral lesions and 40–45 years for skin lesions. LP is 1.5 times more common in women compared to men. There is a strong association between hepatitis C infection and LP. HCV seropositivity is detected five times more in LP than the normal population.

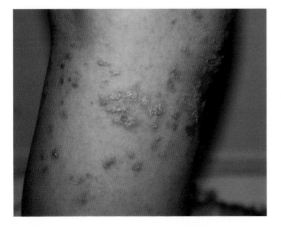

Figure 4.6 Lichen planus with lattice-like white lines, termed Wickham striae, on the papules.

Source: Courtesy of Istanbul Medeniyet University Dermatology Clinic.

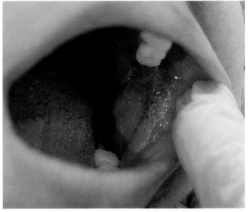

Figure 4.7 Mucosal involvement of lichen planus with reticular lesions on the buccal mucosa.

Source: Courtesy of Istanbul Medeniyet University Dermatology Clinic.

Clinical presentation: Generally, the flexural part of the wrists, the dorsum of hands, ankles, and waist are involved, but lesions can also be seen on the hips, trunk, and neck. When the axillae, inguinal, and inframammary areas are involved, it is called inverse LP. Lesions are typically violaceous, flat-topped, polygonal papules, which can have lattice-like white lines, termed Wickham striae (Figure 4.6). Although the disease can be significantly pruritic, itching is not observed in 20% of patients. As lesions resolve, they usually leave behind a gray to brown hyperpigmentation, especially in dark-skinned individuals.

Mucosal involvement is often in the form of reticular lesions on the buccal cheeks, which have a white lattice-like appearance (Figure 4.7). Other lesion types include erosive, papular, plaque-like, atrophic, ulcerative, and bullous. Erosive and ulcerative lesions are considered to be premalignant, and squamous cell carcinoma (SCC) development has been reported in 1% of patients.

Nail involvement alone is rare, but nails are affected in 25% of lichen planus patients (Table 4.3).

LP has clinically different types. These include the actinic form in sun-exposed areas, annular form in which papules combine to form plaques, linear form in which papules are aligned linearly due to the Koebner phenomenon, hyperpigmented form in which the lesions are darker and brownish purple, and inverse form that involves the intertriginous areas.

Laboratory studies: LP can often be diagnosed clinically; however, a biopsy may be necessary. Histopathologically, LP is characterized by hyperkeratosis without parakeratosis, apoptotic bodies

Table 4.3 Nail Changes Seen in Lichen Planus

Nail Plate	Matrix	Nail Bed	Bad Prognosis
Longitudinal streaking	Trachyonychia	Onycholysis	Nail bed anomalies
Fragmentation on nail plate	Pitting	Chromonychia	Longitudinal streaking
Onychatrophy	Pterygium	Splinter hemorrhages	Nail loss
Nail loss	Erythema of the lunula	Subungual hyperkeratosis	
	Irregularly dispersed and tortuous veins		

(Civatte bodies), and wedge-shaped hypergranulosis with a sawtooth appearance in rete ridges. There can also be vacuolar degeneration of keratinocytes, a characteristic band-like lymphocytic accumulation at the dermo epidermal junction, and pigment incontinence. In cases that do not improve despite treatment, a biopsy should be performed to exclude dysplasia and SCC. Patients can be screened for hepatitis C, especially if they have oral lesions or are at risk.

Differential diagnosis: LP can often be difficult to differentiate from lichenoid drug eruption, in which lesions are more frequently symmetrically distributed in sun-exposed areas with less oral involvement and without Wickham striae. Medication history in the last 2 years should be questioned. Common drugs include gold salts, antimalarials, beta-blockers, angiotensin-converting-enzyme inhibitors, penicillamine, nonsteroidal anti-inflammatory drugs, thiazide diuretics, spironolactone, and furosemide.

The differential also includes lupus erythematosus, guttate psoriasis, erythema dyschromicum perstans, secondary syphilis, pityriasis rosea, lichen amyloidosis, graft versus host disease, and pityriasis lichenoides chronica. For oral lesions, the differential includes leukoplakia, candidiasis, and morsicatio buccarum.

Management: This varies according to the number and localization of lesions. Because lesions tend to heal spontaneously, topical corticosteroids can be administered to hasten resolution and relieve itching. In oral involvement, potent topical corticosteroids are recommended as first-line treatment. When topical corticosteroids are insufficient, systemic corticosteroids can be used for several weeks. After improvement, slow tapering is often necessary in order to prevent abrupt recurrence of lesions. In resistant cases, other options include phototherapy and systemic retinoids.

Course: In the majority of patients, skin lesions resolve spontaneously within 1–3 years. Systemic steroids can lead to resolution with several weeks in many cases; however, recurrence is common. As lesions resolve, they typically leave behind transient hyperpigmentation. Spontaneous recovery is rare in oral involvement. Patients with chronic or ulcerative oral cases should be closely followed to monitor for potential malignancy, such as squamous cell cancer.

Final comment: LP is an inflammatory skin disease that can involve both skin and mucosa. Although skin lesions can improve spontaneously, treatment can hasten improvement. Mucosal involvements should be monitored for squamous cell cancer development.

PITYRIASIS RUBRA PILARIS

Definition: Pityriasis rubra pilaris (PRP) is an inflammatory and papulosquamous skin disease characterized by follicular and palmoplantar hyperkeratosis and orange-pink scaly plaques.

Overview: This appears in men and women at nearly equal rates. Although it peaks in childhood (1–10 years old) and adulthood (50–60 years old), it can be seen at any age.

Its etiology is not yet fully understood. Viral or bacterial infections and autoimmune diseases may be potential triggers.

Clinical presentation: PRP is divided into 6 groups according to age of onset, clinical manifestations, morphologic characteristics, and prognosis.

Type I (classic adult type): The majority of patients (55%) are type I. This type typically starts in the upper half of the body with a cephalocaudal spread (Figure 4.8). It begins as perifollicular papules with keratotic plugs, and diffuse salmon-colored plaques appear over time (Figure 4.9). Between these plaques, there are unaffected skin islets. After a few weeks to months, palmoplantar keratoderma in the form of thick orange scale emerges (Figure 4.10). Nail involvement may accompany. The condition can acutely turn into erythroderma. Within 3 years, about 80% of patients with this type regress spontaneously.

Type II (atypical adult type): In this type, there is no cephalocaudal progression. Palmoplantar involvement is accompanied by ichthyosiform dermatitis and lamellar scaling is seen. Alopecia can be seen on the scalp. Only 20% of patients regress within 3 years, and most conditions continue for many years.

Type III (classic juvenile type): This type is seen in children, who are 5–10 years old. It constitutes 10% of all cases. It has a clinical presentation similar to Type 1. Type III typically regresses spontaneously within 1 year.

Type IV (circumscribed juvenile type): This is the most common type in the 3–10-year age range. Sharply circumscribed, follicular, hyperkeratotic areas and erythema, especially on the knees and elbows, are observed. Of all cases, 25% are from this group. Remission can be seen within 3 years; however, relapse is frequent.

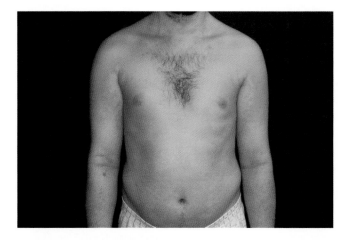

Figure 4.8 Pityriasis rubra pilaris with diffuse salmon-colored plaques and islands of sparing.

Source: Courtesy of Istanbul Medeniyet University Dermatology Clinic.

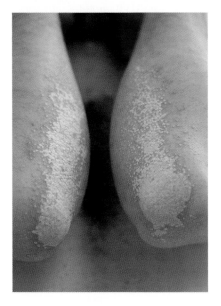

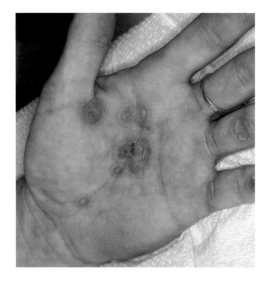

Figure 4.9 Pityriasis rubra pilaris with perifollicular papules with keratotic plugs, so-called nutmeg grater papules.

Source: Courtesy of Istanbul Medeniyet University Dermatology Clinic.

Figure 4.10 Pityriasis rubra pilaris with orange-colored palmoplantar keratoderma appearing as if it was dipped in wax.

Source: Courtesy of Istanbul Medeniyet University Dermatology Clinic.

Type V (atypical juvenile type): This type is seen between the ages of 0–4 years. It constitutes 5% of all cases. Hereditary forms are generally of this type. Follicular hyperkeratosis and ichthyosiform dermatitis are seen. Type V has an early onset and a chronic course.

Type VI (HIV-associated type): Similar to type 1, follicular plugs with spicules are seen. Erythroderma frequently develops. Lesions can be seen together in the setting with acne conglobata, hidradenitis suppurativa, and lichen spinulosus. It is often chronic.

PRP can sometimes be observed together with seronegative arthritis, alopecia, ectropion, and loss of sweating. Of all patients with PRP, more than 80% of cases have palmoplantar keratoderma, and 45% can progress to erythroderma.

Laboratory studies: Histopathologic examination demonstrates irregular psoriasiform acanthosis of the epidermis, parakeratosis and orthokeratosis in "checkerboard" pattern, follicular plugs accompanied by shoulder parakeratosis, thickening and neutrophil loss in the stratum corneum, and mild superficial perivascular lymphohistiocytic infiltration. Epidermal spongiosis and focal acantholytic dyskeratosis are rare but can be seen.

HIV infection must be investigated in generalized and rapid erythrodermic types.

Differential diagnosis: Classic psoriasis and pityriasis lichenoides should be considered. When erythroderma develops, psoriasis, atopic dermatitis, drug reactions, cutaneous T-cell lymphoma, congenital ichthyosis, paraneoplastic phenomenon, and graft versus host disease should be excluded.

Because ichthyosiform changes are observed in types II and V, which are atypical forms, PRP is differentially diagnosed with acquired and congenital ichthyosis and lichen spinulosus. Keratosis pilaris should also be considered when spiny follicular papules are seen.

Management: Because most cases are self-limiting and asymptomatic, treatment may not be required.

Topical moisturizers, keratolytic agents (e.g., urea 5–10%, salicylic acid 1–3%, alpha hydroxy acid), corticosteroids, retinoids, calcineurin inhibitors, and calcipotriol can be used to help with inflammation and scaling.

For systemic treatment, high-dose vitamin A (200,000–1,000,000 U/g) and acitretin (0.5 mg/kg/day) can be used in children, while isotretinoin (0.5–1 mg/kg/day) and UVB phototherapy can be used those older than age 12. Methotrexate, cyclosporine, azathioprine, and TNF-alpha inhibitors can be administered in resistant cases. Acitretin (0.5 mg/kg/day), isotretinoin (1–1.5 mg/kg/day), and methotrexate (5–30 mg/week) are first line treatments in adults. UVB and UVA1 or photo-chemotherapy (PUVA) can be tried. In resistant cases, cyclosporine (<5 mg/kg/day), TNF-alpha inhibitors, azathioprine (50–200 mg/day), secukinumab, ustekinumab, infliximab, fumaric acid, and intravenous immunoglobulin treatment can be trialed.

Antiretroviral treatment should be given in association with HIV.

Course: In most cases, PRP is a self-limiting and asymptomatic disease that does not require treatment. Of all type I PRP cases, 80% recover spontaneously within 3 years. Although types II and V have a chronic course, type III often enters remission after 1 year. The course of types IV and VI is uncertain.

Final comment: PRP, which has distinctive findings, such as follicular involvement, orange color, waxlike keratoderma, and islands of sparing, is generally a self-limiting disease. Due to its atypical forms, erythroderma, and thick scaling, it can often cause significant disruption to a patient's life and difficulties in diagnosis and treatment.

PITYRIASIS LICHENOIDES

Definition: According to the clinical features, course, and response to treatment, pityriasis lichenoides includes a group of inflammatory skin diseases classified as pityriasis lichenoides et varioliformis acuta (PLEVA) and pityriasis lichenoides chronica (PLC).

Overview: The etiology, prevalence, and incidence of pityriasis lichenoides (PL) are not fully clarified. Disease has been shown to peak in the third decade, and the majority of cases are diagnosed before the age of 50 years. PL typically appears in late childhood and young adulthood; however, it can be seen in all ages, races, and geographic regions. It is thought to be slightly more common in men. Cases of PLEVA can also be seen during pregnancy.

Clinical presentation: PLEVA has an acute-subacute onset. Multiple 2–3-mm erythematous macules rapidly evolve into papules and then into polymorphic lesions (Figure 4.11). Papules have a thin mica-like scale that thicken over time, moves away from the periphery, and clings to the center. In time, the middle of the papules collapses and vesiculopustules (papules covered with hemorrhagic crusts and superficial necrotic ulcers) can be seen. They heal within weeks and months and can leave hypo/hyperpigmentation or varioliform scars. Lesions tend to involve the trunk's anterior aspect, flexural surfaces, and proximal extremities, but they can also be generalized. Skin lesions may rarely burn or itch and be accompanied by systemic symptoms, such as fever and fatigue.

PLC is the most common disease in the PL group. The lesions begin as erythematous, maculo-papular lesions, which gradually evolve into small, dull erythematous-brown papules with shiny mica-like scale in the center (Figure 4.12). Necrotic lesions are not expected. The lesions regress within weeks and heal with hyperpigmentation. As in PLEVA, lesions can be polymorphic. The proximal trunk and extremities are involved, but acral or segmental involvement may also occur. It is generally asymptomatic.

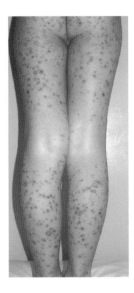

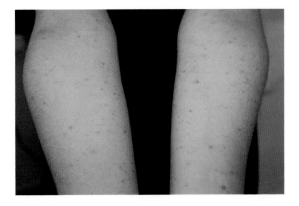

Figure 4.12 Pityriasis lichenoides chronica with maculopapular lesions on the arms.

Source: Courtesy of Istanbul Medeniyet University Dermatology Clinic.

Figure 4.11 Pityriasis lichenoides et varioliformis acuta with polymorphic lesions consisting of macules, papules, and plaques with some covered with hemorrhagic crust.

Source: Courtesy of Istanbul Medeniyet University Dermatology Clinic.

Febrile ulceronecrotic Mucha-Habermann disease (FUMHD) is a rarely seen type. It may have sudden onset or develop gradually from PLEVA or PLC. It is more common in males between the ages of 10–30 years. In the aggressive and generalized form, purpuric-black, ulceronecrotic and crusted plaques can suddenly appear and tend to merge. Hemorrhagic bullae and pustules may accompany them. Painful, extensive skin necrosis and secondary infection of ulcers can be observed. As a result, fulminant sepsis and hypertrophic and atrophic scars can develop. It may involve oral and genital mucosa. Pain, itching, high fever, weakness, fatigue, sore throat, diarrhea, abdominal pain, pneumonia, splenomegaly, arthritis, and conjunctival ulcers can be observed.

Laboratory studies: For PLEVA, histopathologic features include parakeratosis, spongiosis, dyskeratosis, acanthosis, lymphocytic exocytosis in the basal layer, erythrocytes in the epidermis, apoptotic and necrotic keratinocytes, neutrophilic inclusions, vacuolization in the basal layer, and focal necrosis in the form of diffuse peripheral necrosis in the dermis. Subepidermal vesicles and dermal sclerosis may accompany previous lesions.

In PLC, histopathology can reveal focal parakeratosis, acanthosis, focal spongiosis, minimal keratinocyte necrosis, hemorrhage and minimal vacuolar degeneration of the basal layer, lymphocyte and erythrocyte focal invasion, and superficial, band-like perivascular lymphocytic infiltration covering the dermo epidermal junction locally.

With FUMHD, biopsy can demonstrate a deep and intense inflammatory infiltration, epidermal and dermal ulceration, leukocytoclastic vasculitis, and apoptotic and necrotic keratinocytes. Leukocytosis, anemia, hyperalbuminemia, and hypoalbuminemia can be seen, as well as elevated erythrocyte sedimentation, C reactive protein, lactate dehydrogenase, liver enzymes, and IL-2 receptor levels.

Differential diagnosis: This can include lymphomatoid papulosis, guttate psoriasis, LP, tinea versicolor, Gianotti-Crosti syndrome, pityriasis rosea, drug eruptions, varicella and other viral eruptions, generalized arthropod bite, erythema multiforme, small vessel vasculitis, secondary syphilis, papulonecrotic tuberculid, polymorphous light eruption, generalized folliculitis, dermatitis herpetiformis, toxic epidermal necrolysis, and graft-versus-host disease.

Management: There is no current standard treatment protocol for PL; however, treatments are generally selected based on type of lesions, distribution, scarring, and systemic symptoms. Phototherapy (UVB, narrow-band UVB, PUVA, UVA1) can be considered as first-line treatment, especially in PLC and generalizes presentation. UVB is effective in the pediatric age group. If an underlying etiology is detected, treatment of this is recommended. Tetracyclines, erythromycin, dapsone, and acyclovir may be considered especially in infections. Tetracyclines and erythromycin can also provide benefit with their anti-inflammatory effect, but it is recommended to be discontinued gradually due to recurrence following cessation. Antiretroviral treatment should be given in HIV-positive cases.

Topical corticosteroids can reduce inflammation and itching in mild to moderate cases. Antihistamines and moisturizers can also be added. Although these treatments provide symptomatic relief, they do not change the course of the disease.

In severe cases, including those with fever, arthritis, and myalgia, systemic corticosteroids (prednisone 40–60 mg/day started and slowly reduced), methotrexate, oral calciferol, pentoxifylline, thiobendazole, dapsone, 4-diaminodiphenyl-sulfone, intravenous γ-globulin, cyclosporine, and retinoids can be used. Systemic corticosteroids and methotrexate have proven to offer benefit in FUMDH, especially in children. Tumor necrosis alpha inhibitors may be useful.

Course: PLEVA is generally self-limiting within weeks to occasionally years, but remissions can be seen. In PLC, generalized lesions typically heal within months, but they can continue for years. FUMHD can be serious. Mortality can occur in up to 25% of cases, especially in immunosuppressed and elderly individuals; therefore, the disease should be treated as soon as it is diagnosed.

Final comment: PL is a disease group with an undefined etiology, and its treatment has not yet been clarified. Although PLC is a chronic but milder form, FUMHD can be serious; therefore, patients should be followed closely with particular clinical presentations.

PITYRIASIS ROSEA

Definition: Pityriasis rosea (PR) is a skin disease with sudden onset, which is characterized by papulosquamous lesions. Although its etiology has not been clearly elucidated, it has been associated with human herpesvirus (HHV-6 and HHV-7) infections.

Overview: The incidence of PR is estimated to be between 0.5–2%. Of all cases, 75% are diagnosed between the ages of 10–35 years. PR is less common under 10 years of age and peaks between the ages of 20–29 years. It is relatively more common in women. Although PR is generally more frequent in winter months, there are also a few studies reporting no seasonal variation. In some patients, there may be a recent history of upper respiratory tract infection before lesions appear.

Clinical presentation: Although PR generally has a typical presentation, an atypical presentation can be seen in 20% of cases. Atypical morphology is seen in papular, urticarial, erythema multiforme-like, vesicular, purpuric, hemorrhagic, follicular, hypopigmented, circinata and marginata, and irritated types, while atypical distribution is seen in inverse, unilateral, extremity dense, mucosal, and acral forms.

In typical PR cases, annular lesions are prominent. The first emerging lesion is called the "herald patch," which is frequently seen on the trunk. The herald patch is an ovoid, erythematous, scaly annular plaque with slightly raised edges and a diameter of 2–10 cm (Figure 4.13). After this lesion present, erythematous, ovoid plaques with a diameter of 5–10 mm emerge after 3–4 days in children and 1–2 weeks in adults. These lesions have a slightly gray peripheral collarette of scale (Figure 4.14). These typically form along the Langer's lines of the trunk and proximal extremities, which can resemble a pine tree of a *Christmas tree* pattern. Pruritus can be seen in 25% of patients. Before skin lesions appear, some patients may experience weakness, anorexia, mild fever, and enanthema.

In pregnant women, some complications may develop with PR. It has been reported that intrauterine fetal infection, and, consequently, congenital defects, fetal hydrops, and fetal death, can be seen with PR in pregnancy. Pregnant women with high HHV-6, especially those with PR lesions starting before the 15th gestational week and those with enanthema, are considered in the major risk group for fetal complications, while those with constitutional symptoms and involvement of more than 50% of the body surface area are considered in the minor risk group.

Laboratory studies: Histopathologic examination may be helpful in cases that cannot be clinically diagnosed. Perivascular superficial dermatitis with lymphocytes, histiocytes, and eosinophils, hyperplasia, focal spongiosis, focal parakeratosis, irregular acanthosis, elongated rete ridges, endothelial and papillary dermal edema, and extravascular erythrocytes can be seen.

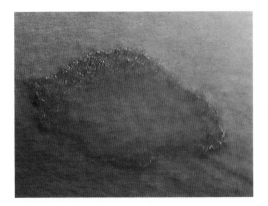

Figure 4.13 Pityriasis rosea with herald patch.

Source: Courtesy of Istanbul Medeniyet University Dermatology Clinic.

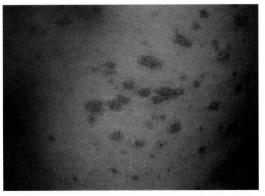

Figure 4.14 Pityriasis rosea with erythematous ovoid plaques with grayish peripheral collarette.

Source: Courtesy of Istanbul Medeniyet University Dermatology Clinic.

Differential diagnosis: This includes tinea corporis, nummular dermatitis, and erythema annulare centrifugum for single lesions, while secondary syphilis, guttate psoriasis, annular lichen planus, tinea versicolor, tinea corporis, parapsoriasis, erythema dyschromicum perstans, and erythema multiforme are considered for generalized lesions.

Management: Even if the disease is not treated, PR is self-limiting. Oral antihistamines and topical corticosteroids may help with pruritus. Systemic corticosteroids, phototherapy, acyclovir, or cidofovir may be useful in severe and resistant cases. Low-dose acyclovir (800 mg/day, three times daily for 1 week) treatment can be used in high-risk pregnant women with early onset of disease and systemic symptoms. Bed rest should be recommended for these pregnant women.

Course: The lesions typically resolve in 6–8 weeks without any scarring. In some patients, it can take 5–6 months. Temporary hypopigmentation or hyperpigmentation can be seen as lesions heal. Although recurrence is not often expected, this can be seen by 1.8–3.7% of cases.

Final comment: PR is a papulosquamous disease that is often seen in adolescents and young adults. It is generally self-limiting. In treatment-resistant cases, it is useful to confirm the diagnosis. PR is believed to be associated with HHV-6 and HHV-7 infections.

ERYTHRODERMA

Synonym: exfoliative erythroderma

Definition: Thesis defined by diffuse erythema or edema covering more than 90% of body surface area. In erythroderma, anatomic, physiologic, barrier, and metabolic functions of the skin are impaired. There are various causes, including inflammatory diseases, infections, drug eruptions, and underlying malignancy. Because there are high rates of morbidity and mortalities, it should be promptly diagnosed and with rapid initiation of treatment.

Overview: The incidence is not clearly known and varies according to geography. It has been reported as very different rates of approximately between 1–44/100,000. It is rare in the neonatal period and is more common between the ages of 40–60 years. It is two to four times more common in men.

Clinical presentation: Erythroderma may emerge due to primary skin diseases, infections, drug use, and malignancies. In approximately half of cases, it is idiopathic.

The most common cause of erythroderma is psoriasis. Other cutaneous diseases, such as atopic dermatitis, seborrheic dermatitis, contact dermatitis, PRP, LP, acquired ichthyosis, subacute lupus erythematosus, bullous pemphigoid, pemphigus foliaceus, actinic dermatoses, sarcoidosis, dermatomyositis, and graft versus host, are among other causes. Infections include staphylococcal scalded skin syndrome, toxic shock syndrome, crusted scabies, dermatophytosis, and congenital cutaneous candidiasis. In 1% of patients, there is an underlying malignancy. This can include mycosis fungoides, cutaneous T-cell lymphoma, diffuse cutaneous mastocytosis, B-cell chronic

Table 4.4 Common Causes of Erythroderma

Neonatal-Infant	Childhood	Adult
Congenital	Infections	Inflammatory skin diseases
• Ichthyoses	• Staphylococcal scalded skin syndrome	• Psoriasis vulgaris/pustular psoriasis
• Omen syndrome	• Crusted scabies	• Contact dermatitis
• Congenital cutaneous candidiasis	• Dermatophytoses	• Atopic dermatitis
• Diffuse cutaneous mastocytosis		• Pityriasis rubra pilaris
• Staphylococcal scalded skin syndrome		• Lichen planus
		• Chronic actinic dermatitis
	Drugs*	• Acquired ichthyosis
	Existing dermatologic diseases	
	• Atopic dermatitis	
Non-congenital	• Psoriasis vulgaris/pustular psoriasis	
• Seborrheic dermatitis	• Pityriasis rubra pilaris	
• Psoriasis vulgaris		Drugs*
• Atopic dermatitis		Malignancies
• Staphylococcal scalded skin syndrome		• Cutaneous T cell lymphomas (Sezary syndrome, Mycosis fungoides)
		• Internal malignancies (often gastric, esophageal, colon, liver, prostate, renal, lung cancer)
		• Leukemias
Drugs*		Infections
Metabolic diseases		• Staphylococcal scalded skin syndrome
		• Crusted scabies
		• Dermatophytoses
		• Toxic shock syndrome
		Bullous diseases
		• Pemphigus foliaceus
		• Bullous pemphigoid
		• Paraneoplastic pemphigus
		Connective tissue diseases
		• Dermatomyositis
		• Subacute lupus erythematosus)
		Blood disorders
		• Hypereosinophilic syndrome
		• Mastocytosis
		• Graft versus host disease

Note: *Most common drugs: Vancomycin and ceftriaxone in neonatal; antiepileptics, amoxicillin, sulfonamide, and antituberculosis drugs in childhood; antiepileptics, antibiotics, and nonsteroidal anti-inflammatory drugs in adults

lymphocytic leukemia, and solid organ cancers. In newborns, ichthyosiform diseases may result from primary immune deficiencies and metabolic diseases. It is accepted to be idiopathic when the cause cannot be determined.

In erythroderma, the skin is generally covered with bright red erythematous patches and/or plaques, and a yellowish-white scale can emerge over time (Figure 4.15). The patient may feel hardening of the skin due to edema and lichenification. Itching often accompanies it. Patients may experience fever, weakness, fatigue, muscle and joint pain, nausea, and vomiting. There may be lymphadenopathy, splenomegaly, and hepatomegaly. Hair loss and nail findings, such as subungual hyperkeratosis, onycholysis, and dry and brittle nails can be observed.

Clues related to the underlying disease may be seen in patients. The presence of psoriatic plaques due to psoriasis and the presence of intact islets of skin are in favor of PRP and mycosis

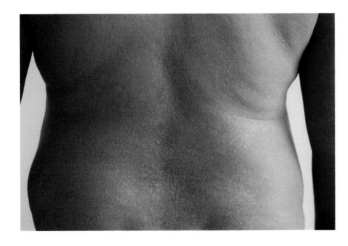

Figure 4.15 Erythroderma with bright red erythematous plaques covering the body.

Source: Courtesy of Istanbul Medeniyet University Dermatology Clinic.

Table 4.5 Clinical Clues to Possible Causes of Erythroderma

Disease	Scale of Skin Lesions	Early Involved Sites	Primary Lesion	Tips
Psoriasis	Diffuse Erythematous Thin or thick Pustular ponds	Groin and periumbilical regions in newborns Knee/elbow in adults	Papule Plaque Pustule	Typical nail findings History of psoriasis Existing psoriatic plaques
Pityriasis rubra pilaris	Bran-like Small husk-like Dry	Scalp, face, palmoplantar area	Follicular hyperkeratotic papules	Islands of sparing Thick, waxy keratoderma Nutmeg-grater-like lesions
Staphylococcal scalded skin syndrome	Exfoliation Perioral radial crust-fissures	Face and flexural folds	Erythema	Skin sensitivity Positive Nikolsky sign
Pemphigus foliaceus	Raised edges Cornflake-like	Seborrheic regions	Vesicle Bulla	Malodorous intertriginous areas Positive Nikolsky sign
Drug reactions	Exfoliation	Any location	All lesion types	Facial edema Purpuric rash Sudden onset
Seborrheic dermatitis	Yellow-colored Oily	Seborrheic regions	Papule Plaque	Frequent in Neonatal, HIV+ patients
Mycosis fungoides	Gray-colored	Hips Legs Bathing-suit distribution	Infiltrated plaque Nodule	Slow development Lymphadenopathy
Atopic dermatitis	Thin	Flexural regions in adults Face, extensor regions in children	Plaque	Flexural areas in children Pruritic intertriginous and groin areas in newborn
Crusted scabies	Hyperkeratotic Fine	Interdigital Finger and toe webs Wrists Periumbilical Periareolar Penis	Excoriated papule	Pruritus Excoriations Burrows

fungoides (MF). Drug etiology should be investigated in erythroderma with sudden onset; it typically improves rapidly after discontinuation of the offending agent. Cutaneous T-cell lymphomas and visceral malignancies should be considered in erythroderma that develops slowly over an extended duration of time.

Laboratory studies: Histopathologic examination frequently does not reveal the underlying cause. Commonly observed findings include perivascular dermal infiltration, acanthosis, hyperkeratosis, and parakeratosis. Direct immunofluorescence can be useful in determining whether there is an underlying bullous disease or connective tissue disorder. KOH, mineral oil, and gram-staining can be considered to look for possible infectious etiologies.

In the majority of patients, the levels of ESR and CRP are elevated. Anemia, leukocytosis, eosinophilia, and disturbances in serum protein levels and fluid electrolyte balance can be seen.

Necessary testing for malignancy should be checked if clinically indicated, including peripheral smear, chest radiography, and abdominal ultrasonography (USG).

Differential diagnosis: It is easy to diagnose erythroderma, but finding the underlying cause is not always easy. Help can be obtained from the patient's history, clinical presentation, histopathologic and immunofluorescent examination, and laboratory findings.

Management: Finding the responsible disease process is important for prompt treatment and follow-up. If the underlying cause can be detected, then the appropriate treatment should be initiated based on the diagnosis. If it is thought to result from drugs, then all potential culprits should be stopped, if possible. Because it is a severe condition, there should be a low threshold to hospitalize patients. The hemodynamics of patients should be checked, and fluid and electrolyte balance should be maintained. Wet dressings, topical corticosteroids, and moisturizers may be recommended. Oral antihistamines can have benefit for pruritus, and systemic antibiotics can be administered for secondary infections. Systemic corticosteroids, methotrexate, azathioprine, and phototherapy can be administered in idiopathic cases when there are no contraindications.

Course: Erythroderma often has high morbidity and mortality. Mortality often results from related causes, such as heart failure due to fluid–electrolyte imbalance, sepsis, and pneumonia from secondary infection. Response to treatment varies according to the underlying cause and time of initiation for treatment. In drug-related cases, discontinuation of the culprit can help to quicken recovery. In erythroderma that is secondary to malignancy, is necessary to identify and treat the underlying cause, but the erythroderma is generally more severe and progressive. Oftentimes, skin disease may progress parallel to the course of the underlying malignancy. Idiopathic erythroderma may recur. In recurrent cases, malignancy screening should be repeated.

FINAL THOUGHT

This is one of the frequent emergencies in dermatology. As soon as the cause of the disease is established, it is important to intervene and start treatment as soon as possible. Clues regarding the underlying primary disease must be reviewed in order to offer better treatment and prevent recurrence with necessary precautions.

ADDITIONAL READINGS

Bellinato F, Maurelli M, Gisondi P, et al. A systematic review of treatments for pityriasis lichenoides. J Eur Acad Dermatol Venereol. 2019;33:2039–2049.

Halper K, Wright B, Maloney NJ, et al. Characterizing disease features and other medical diagnoses in patients with pityriasis rubra pilaris. JAMA Dermatol. 2020:e203426.

Husein-ElAhmed H, Gieler U, Steinhoff M. Lichen planus: a comprehensive evidence-based analysis of medical treatment. J Eur Acad Dermatol Venereol. 2019;33:1847–1862.

Inamadar AC, Ragunatha S. The rash that becomes an erythroderma. Clin Dermatol. 2019;37:88–98.

Mahajan K, Relhan V, Relhan AK, et al. Pityriasis rosea: an update on etiopathogenesis and management of difficult aspects. Indian J Dermatol. 2016;61:375–384.

Rapalli VK, Waghule T, Gorantla S, et al. Psoriasis: pathological mechanisms, current pharmacological therapies, and emerging drug delivery systems. Drug Discov Today. 2020;25:2212–2226.

Roenneberg S, Biedermann T. Pityriasis rubra pilaris: algorithms for diagnosis and treatment. J Eur Acad Dermatol Venereol. 2018;32:889–898.

Rothe MJ, Bialy TL, Grant-Kels JM. Erythroderma. Dermatol Clin. 2000;18:405–415.

Svoboda SA, Ghamrawi RI, Owusu DA, et al. Treatment goals in psoriasis: which outcomes matter most? Am J Clin Dermatol. 2020;21:505–511.

Wolf R, Parish LC, Parish JL. Emergency Dermatology. 2nd ed. London: CRC Press; 2017.

5 Dermatitides

Allison Perz, Tara Jennings, Robert Duffy, and Warren Heymann

CONTENTS

Definition: The dermatitides are a group of eczematous disorders characterized by inflammation of the epidermis. They present clinically as a spectrum of acute, subacute, and chronic lesions, including pruritic vesicles, erythematous papules, and/or lichenified plaques (Table 5.1). While *eczema* is the preferred term in the United Kingdom, *dermatitis* is used in the United States.

ATOPIC DERMATITIS

Synonyms: Eczema

Definition: Atopic dermatitis (AD) is a complex immune-mediated skin disorder that presents with intense pruritus and, most commonly, erythematous, often-lichenified papules and plaques on the face and flexural surfaces of infants and children. The word *atopy* means strange.

Overview: The etiology of AD is complex and not yet fully elucidated. There is a strong genetic component with contributing environmental factors. AD is characterized by elevated IgE levels, impaired epidermal barrier function, immune dysregulation with an imbalance of suppressive and inflammatory T-cell subtypes, and alterations in the skin microbiome. Impaired skin barrier function, oftentimes due to mutations in the filaggrin protein, results in penetration of the stratum corneum by environmental irritants and allergens. This leads to an abnormal immune response and both acute and chronic inflammation. Transepidermal water loss aggravates the xerosis, and changes of the acid mantle result in abnormal cutaneous bacterial colonization. Intense pruritus leads to scratching and further impairment of the skin barrier, which puts patients at greater risk for skin infection, specifically with *Staphylococcus aureus*.

AD is part of the "atopic triad" of asthma, AD, and allergic rhinitis, which are thought to share similar hypersensitive immunologic etiology. AD typically presents first, followed by asthma in childhood and allergic rhinitis in adolescence. This is referred to as the *atopic march*. AD is also often comorbid with food allergies; however, the association between the two is unclear. Food allergies are generally not considered a cause or trigger of AD even when allergen-specific IgE tests are positive.

Clinical presentation: Patients typically present in infancy and childhood with pruritus and erythematous papules and plaques on the face and flexural surfaces, including the wrists, forearms, antecubital fossae, neck, and popliteal fossae. Infants are more likely to present with lesions on the face and extensor surfaces. Patients experience intense pruritus and typical rub and scratch their skin, which causes lesions to become excoriated. Chronic lesions of AD are often lichenified and may demonstrate post-inflammatory hyper- or hypopigmentation. In patients with darker skin tones, follicular papules may be the dominant morphology (Figures 5.1–5.4).

DOI: 10.1201/9781003105268-5

Table 5.1 Types of Dermatitis

Type	Synonyms	Age Group	Classic Clinical Findings	Distribution
Anogenital pruritus	Pruritus ani, pruritus vulvae	Adults	Erythema and lichenification with excoriation	Perineal, perianal, and genital skin
Ashy Dermatitis	Erythema dyschromicum perstans	Adults and children	Blue-grey macules and patches	Trunk, neck, and extremities
Atopic dermatitis	Atopic eczema	Children > Adults	Acute: Erythema, vesicles, weeping and crusting. Subacute: Erythematous plaques or patches with overlying scale. Chronic: Lichenified plaques with hyper/hypopigmentation	Infants: Face, scalp, extensor surfaces of extremities. Children/adults: Flexural aspects of extremities. All ages: Generalized disease possible
Id reaction	Autoeczematization	Children and adults	Pruritic, erythematous papules, and/or vesicles	Extensor surfaces of the arms, face, trunk, and legs
Contact dermatitis	Occupational dermatitis	Children and adults	Well-demarcate, geometric erythema with weeping vesicles in the early stages and lichenification in chronic disease	Anywhere on the body
Dyshidrotic dermatitis	Pompholyx, palmoplantar eczema	Adults and children	Pruritic pustules	Hands and feet, particularly the lateral surfaces
Keratosis pilaris	Gooseflesh	Children, young adults > Adults	Small monomorphic skin-colored papules	Proximal arms and legs, buttocks
Lichen simplex chronicus	Circumscribed neurodermatitis	Adults	Well-demarcated leathery plaques of thickened skin with accentuated skin markings	Shins, scalp, nape, wrists, vulva, scrotum
Nummular dermatitis	Discoid eczema	Children and adults	Coin-shaped scaly plaques possibly with erosions or crusting	Trunk and extremities
Prurigo nodularis		Adults > children	Hyperpigmented to violaceous papules and nodules with scaling or crusted centers; the center of lesions is often excoriated and can appear dark gray or hypopigmented	Extremities > trunk
Seborrheic dermatitis		Children and adults	Erythematous, fine, greasy scaling patches and plaques	Scalp, eyebrows, nasolabial folds, chest, ears
Stasis dermatitis	Venous eczema, gravitational eczema	Adults	Erythematous, scaly, fissured patches and plaques that may demonstrate a "woody" edema and brown pigmentation secondary to hemosiderin deposition	Legs
Xerosis	Eczema craquelé, winter itch	Adults	Erythematous, polygonally cracked skin with horizonal and vertical fissuring	Trunk and extremities

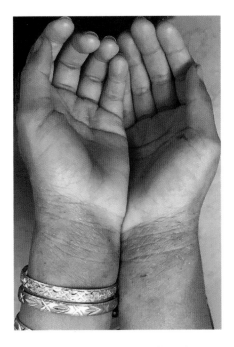

Figure 5.1 Erythematous and patchy, hyperpigmented, lichenified plaques on both wrists of a woman with severe AD.

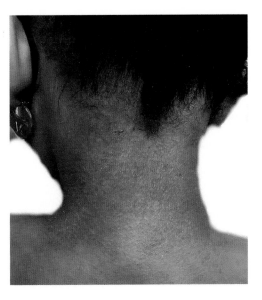

Figure 5.2 A hyperpigmented, slightly lichenified plaque with overlying fine scale on the nape of a girl with AD.

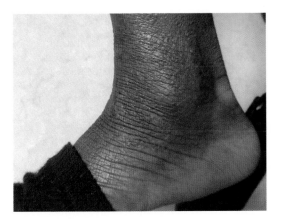

Figure 5.3 Hyperpigmented, lichenified plaque in AD.

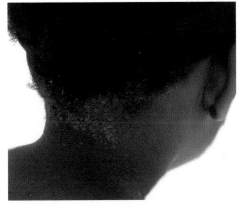

Figure 5.4 Hyperpigmented lichenified plaque with prominent scaling along the hairline on the nape of a girl with AD.

The lesions of AD have a propensity to become impetiginized, presenting with a crusted, scaly appearance. Patients often have widespread xerosis and may have comorbid asthma or allergic rhinitis. AD may present in adulthood; however, when it does, it tends to have more localized lesions with a predilection for the hands.

A thorough history should be taken, because a family history of atopy is a risk factor for AD. The single line that occurs under the eyes is known as Dennie's line.

Laboratory studies: A biopsy is not necessary for diagnosis, but dermatopathologic study will reveal varying degrees of spongiosis, parakeratosis, epidermal thickening, and an inflammatory infiltrate, depending on whether the disease is acute, subacute, or chronic. Patch testing can be considered to rule out an irritant or contact dermatitis, particularly if a patient is not responding to treatment.

Differential diagnosis: AD may be confused with allergic or irritant contact dermatitis, psoriasis, tinea corporis, or even scabies.

Management: AD is a chronic disorder that is prone to flares, particularly with environmental triggers. Management includes both medication and lifestyle changes. Topical corticosteroids applied twice daily as needed are the mainstay of treatment, such as topical hydrocortisone 2.5%, topical fluticasone 0.05%, or more potent steroids, such as topical clobetasol 0.05%. Tacrolimus ointment, pimecrolimus cream, or topical crisaborole can be used on the face and intertriginous areas.

In addition to treatment, prevention has been shown to be an effective therapeutic strategy with recent research supporting the use of calcineurin inhibitors, such as tacrolimus ointment, to prevent flares in atopic dermatitis. Because many atopic patients are allergic to lanolin, Cetaphil® lotion or cream is the recommended lubricating agent. Occasionally, bleach or tar baths may be helpful. For more severe disease, a biologic (dupilumab, a monoclonal antibody targeting the IL-4α receptor) may be indicated. Other modalities include cyclosporine, mycophenolate mofetil, methotrexate, or phototherapy.

Course: AD follows a chronic course with intermittent flares. It typically improves by late childhood, but it may persist into adulthood and even appear for the first time later in life.

CONTACT DERMATITIS

Synonyms: Occupational dermatitis

Definition: Contact dermatitis is an inflammatory reaction that can either be an irritant type, resulting from contact with a directly irritating substance, or an allergic type, resulting from a delayed hypersensitivity reaction to an environmental substance. A third idiopathic type may also be considered.

Clinical presentation: Primary irritant contact dermatitis results from the direct toxic effect of an irritant substance coming in contact with the skin. Trichloracetic acid would be an example of an agent that causes an irritant contact dermatitis. Patients with primary irritant contact dermatitis typically present with cracked, fissured skin accompanied by erythema and pain.

In contrast, allergic contact dermatitis is a delayed hypersensitivity reaction to an environmental substance, such as nickel or lanolin. When a substance breaches the barrier of the stratum corneum, it is consumed by Langerhans cells in the epidermis. The Langerhans cells present the antigenic substance to T-cells in what is known as the "sensitization" phase of allergic contact dermatitis. On a sensitized patient's next contact with the substance, T-cells elicit a cytokine-mediated response that is responsible for the clinical picture. Allergic contact dermatitis typically presents as pruritic, well-demarcated, erythematous papules or plaques with characteristically sharp, geometric margins. Acute lesions may be red and vesicular. Chronic lesions may be crusted and lichenified (Figures 5.5–5.7).

Both primary irritant contact and allergic contact dermatitides have photosensitive counterparts. Phototoxic reactions occur when a substance becomes directly toxic to the skin upon exposure to light, and photoallergic reactions occur when an antigen stimulates an immune response upon exposure to light. Both of these will appear similar to their non-photosensitive counterparts but are limited to areas exposed to light, oftentimes the face, décolletage, and forearms.

Laboratory studies: With comprehensive investigation, the history and lesion distribution may disclose the culprit. If allergic contact dermatitis is suspected, patch testing may reveal the offending agent. During patch testing, antigens from substances that most commonly cause allergic reactions are applied to a patient's skin in an attempt to identify the potential offending agent (Figure 5.8). Additional history may be needed to determine if the results of the patch test correspond with the disease presentation. A biopsy is generally not needed, but, if performed, will reveal characteristic dermatitic findings.

Differential diagnosis: On occasion, bacterial or fungal infection may be confused with contact dermatitis. AD can closely resemble contact dermatitis, especially the allergic type. Rarely, the initial presentation may mimic psoriasis.

Management: Identification and avoidance of the offending agent is the most important step in managing contact dermatitis. This can be quite difficult, as patients may be sensitized to common household chemicals, so counseling is of the utmost importance. Patients with occupational

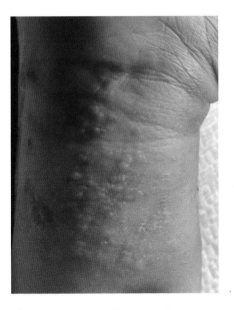

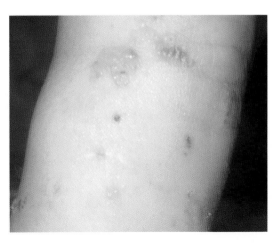

Figure 5.6 Streaks of erythematous, weeping vesicles on the forearm of a patient with allergic contact dermatitis to poison ivy.

Figure 5.5 Well-demarcated erythematous patch with vesicles on the ventral aspect of the wrist of a patient with allergic contact dermatitis to poison ivy.

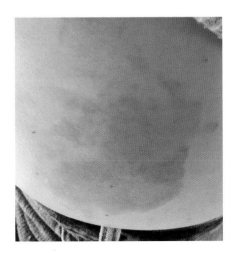

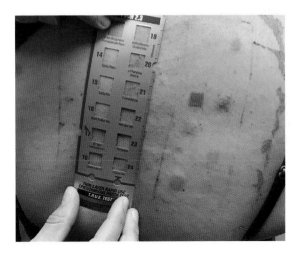

Figure 5.7 Erythematous, urticarial plaque on a patient with allergic contact dermatitis.

Figure 5.8 Positive patch testing for a woman with allergic contact dermatitis. A positive finding usually reveals erythema, induration, and vesiculation.

exposure can try to use protective clothing; however, a change in role or occupation may be required. Topical corticosteroids are appropriate treatment. Occasionally, oral antihistamines are needed. There are barrier creams, such as silicone, that may act as preventatives. Avoiding contact with the culprit, such as nickel in silver or low-karat gold or latex in gloves or underwear, is important. A latex allergy, when severe, can be life-ruining.

Prognosis: Contact dermatitis will usually clear when the culprit is eliminated; however, reexposure with contact to the culprit will induce a flare.

NEURODERMATITIS

Synonyms: Lichen simplex chronicus, prurigo nodularis

Definition: Neurodermatitis (ND) is an umbrella term for an eruption caused by repeated rubbing and scratching. This can be further differentiated into different clinical entities, with the two most common being lichen simplex chronicus (LSC) and prurigo nodularis (PN).

Overview: By definition, ND has no known cause. If an etiology is found, the diagnosis is changed to correspond to the inciting agent, such as contact dermatitis (CD). ND starts as an eczematous eruption that then leads to pruritus causing a patient to scratch. The scratching results in further pruritus, which starts an itch–scratch cycle that is difficult to overcome.

Clinical picture: History and patient observation are key in making this diagnosis. Patients may report intense pruritus and the urge to scratch, but others may not be cognizant of their behavior or scratch mainly while sleeping. While interviewing a patient, watching them for unconscious scratching may provide clues to the diagnosis.

Patients with LSC typically present with well-demarcated, lichenified erythematous plaques. If the lesions become chronic, the plaques may become significantly thickened and hyperpigmented (Figures 5.9–5.11).

Patients with PN present with erythematous, hyperkeratotic papules and nodules. All lesions in the ND family are typically located on easily accessible areas of the body, such as the scalp, extensor surfaces of arms, and genitalia. They may demonstrate overlying excoriation or scale. The itching is often intense, and the urge to scratch may be uncontrollable.

Laboratory studies: ND is diagnosed by history and observing the characteristic lesions. Dermatopathologic examination will show hyperkeratosis with focal parakeratosis, hypergranulosis, and vertical thickened collagen bundles in the superficial dermis. If fungal infection is considered, a KOH scraping is indicated.

Differential diagnosis: Other red and scaly conditions may be considered, such as psoriasis, AD, contact dermatitis, mycosis fungoides, tinea cruris, candidosis (especially in the genital region), or lichen planus.

Management: Treatment of ND typically involves high-potency topical corticosteroids, such as clobetasol. Immunomodulators, such as tacrolimus or pimecrolimus, have also been shown to be effective for some patients who do not respond to topical steroids. Oral antihistamines, such as hydroxyzine 25 mg every 6–8 hours, may be added for the antipruritic effect.

Prognosis: LSC may improve with treatment, but many patients have a chronic dermatitis that is unresponsive to treatment.

NUMMULAR DERMATITIS

Synonyms: Nummular eczema, discoid dermatitis

Definition: Nummular dermatitis is an eczematous eruption characterized by pruritic, scaly disc-shaped plaques that are located mainly on the extremities.

Overview: The cause is unclear, and it is probably multifactorial. It is associated with dry skin, low humidity, and exposure to external or environmental irritants. There is some suggestion that nummular dermatitis may be associated with allergic contact dermatitis.

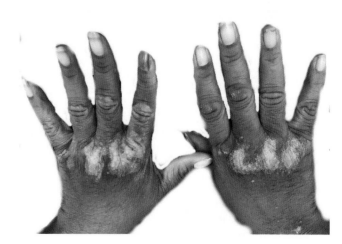

Figure 5.9 Lichenified plaques on the dorsal surfaces.

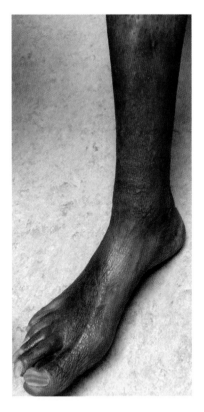

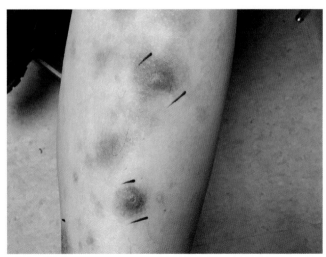

Figure 5.11 Hyperpigmented nodules with overlying scale and central erosion on the right leg, representing prurigo nodularis.

Figure 5.10 Hyperpigmented lichenified plaques on the right leg and foot.

Clinical picture: Patients present with multiple scaly, erythematous, discrete disc-shaped plaques of the extremities and/or trunk (Figure 5.12). These lesions are often pruritic. Papulovesicular lesions may precede the formation of plaques, and round erosions and crusting can often be seen within lesions. It is most common in middle-aged and older patients. A particular type of nummular dermatitis is Sulzberger-Garbe disease (chronic exudative and discoid dermatitis).

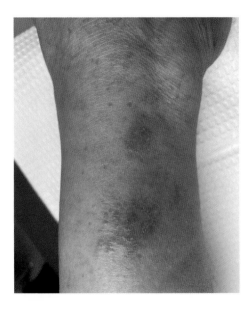

Figure 5.12 Coin-shaped erythematous lesions with overlying scale on the leg.

Laboratory studies: This is a clinical diagnosis. Patch testing can be performed to rule out an associated contact dermatitis. Histologically, acute lesions will demonstrate spongiosis, and chronic lesions will reveal hyperkeratosis and acanthosis.

Differential diagnosis: Other diseases that may be similar include psoriasis, contact dermatitis, tinea corporis, or xerosis.

Management: Therapy includes mid- or high-potency topical corticosteroids applied to lesions twice daily. This may be complemented with lubricating lotions or creams.

Prognosis: This condition is usually chronic and may follow an intermittent course with flares often occurring during the winter months.

STASIS DERMATITIS

Synonyms: Venous eczema, gravitational dermatitis

Definition: Stasis dermatitis is an eczematous eruption occurring on the legs due to venous hypertension.

Overview: Stasis dermatitis occurs when venous hypertension causes extravasation of fluid, red blood cells, and plasma from the underlying vessels, which leads to inflammation of the skin and subsequent eczematization.

Clinical picture: The condition is pruritic with chronic changes, erythema, hyperpigmentation, scaling, and lichenification. There is often accompanying edema. Sometimes, there is skin breakdown (stasis ulcer).

Laboratory studies: This is a clinical diagnosis. Although generally unnecessary, a biopsy will demonstrate nonspecific epidermal changes, such as spongiosis, hyperkeratosis, and acanthosis with extravasated red blood cells, hemosiderin-laded macrophages, and fibrosis in the dermis.

Differential diagnosis: Although the diagnosis is usually obvious, contact dermatitis may be a co-diagnosis. Cellulitis is unlikely to occur on both legs, and induration is infrequent with stasis dermatitis.

Management: Contributing factors must be addressed, including management of lower extremity edema with compression stockings and leg elevation. Topical corticosteroids are effective in many cases. Local wound care with occlusive dressings may be needed if the patient presents with an ulcer. When there is secondary infection, oral antimicrobials, such as doxycycline 150 mg twice a day or sulfamethoxazole/trimethoprim twice a day for 10–14 days may be needed.

Prognosis: Stasis dermatitis is a chronic condition that may flare, even when venous hypertension is controlled.

XEROSIS

Synonyms: Asteatotic eczema, eczema craquelé, winter itch, xeroderma,

Definition: Xerosis is a chronic skin disorder characterized by inflamed, dry skin and pruritus.

Overview: Xerosis is most common in older patients and typically occurs during the winter months due to cold dry air. Decreased activity of sebaceous and sweat glands may contribute to the dry skin, which contributes to increased transepidermal water loss and fissuring. Pruritus incited by the dry skin then causes the patient to scratch, leading to further disturbance of the skin barrier.

Clinical picture: Patients present with dry, rough skin and may demonstrate superficial fissuring, cracking, and bleeding (Figure 5.13). The chronic itching may lead to oozing and crusted fissures that are often painful rather than itchy.

Laboratory studies: The diagnosis is usually obvious; otherwise, careful medical history should be taken to rule out other causes of pruritic dry skin, such as hypothyroidism or malignancy, which is referred to as acquired ichthyosis. A biopsy will demonstrate nonspecific spongiosis and acanthosis, sometimes with a superficial lymphocytic infiltrate and a diminished granular layer.

Differential diagnosis: Stasis dermatitis, contact dermatitis, and AD may be considered.

Management: The most important recommendation is to limit soap to the critical areas (face, hands, feet, axillae, buttocks, groin). Use of a washcloth or loofah should be avoided. Lubricating lotions are the foundation of treatment, with the purpose of maintaining cutaneous moisture. For persistent pruritus, topical corticosteroids, such as hydrocortisone 2.5% or fluticasone cream, can be used.

Prognosis: Xerosis typically responds to treatment but may flare in winter months due to dry heat or harsh environments.

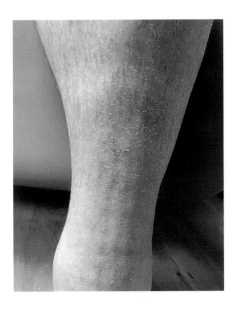

Figure 5.13 Characteristic appearance of xerosis on the leg. When severe, there may be a "crazed appearance" due to scaling and polygonally cracked skin.

OTITIS EXTERNA

Synonyms: Swimmer's ear

Definition: This is an inflammatory process affecting the outer ear that is caused by infection or a chronic eczematous process.

Overview: Otitis externa can either be an infectious process, typically secondary to *Pseudomonas aeruginosa* or *S. aureus* infection, or a noninfectious inflammatory process, secondary to dermatologic conditions, such as atopic dermatitis, seborrheic dermatitis, or psoriasis. The pathophysiology typically involves disruption of the protective barrier of the skin and decreased cerumen, which protects the ear from external factors. Otitis externa is sometimes referred to as *swimmer's ear*, because moisture from exposure to water can create a favorable environment for bacterial growth and infection.

Clinical picture: Otitis externa typically presents with exquisite pain, edema, and erythema of the outer ear. If the etiology is infectious, then warmth, exudate, and discharge may be present. A variation of otitis externa is infectious eczematoid dermatitis, where the external ear oozes with crusting and becomes tender.

Laboratory studies: This is a clinical diagnosis.

Differential diagnosis: Other diagnoses to be considered include tympanic membrane rupture, otitis media, seborrheic dermatitis, and even psoriasis.

Management: Topical antibiotics, such as neomycin or mupirocin, may be applied twice daily. Sometimes, otic drops with an antimicrobial, such as ciprofloxacin, may be needed. If an inflammatory process is suspected, otic formulations of steroids are available for patient use.

Prognosis: Otitis externa usually responds to treatment, unless there is an underlying cause that should be addressed.

SEBORRHEIC DERMATITIS

Definition: Seborrheic dermatitis (SD) is a common disorder characterized by redness and scaling on the scalp.

Overview: SD may be an inflammatory response to the overgrowth of the normal skin yeast *Malassezia*; however, this has not been proved. Possible overactivity of the sebaceous glands may also play a contributory role. Severe cases of SD may be observed in patients with Parkinson disease or HIV infection.

Clinical picture: Patients present with a spectrum of often pruritic lesions, ranging from mild white scale and flaking to more severely inflamed, greasy pink or yellow crusted plaques (Figure 5.14). The locations for this often-recalcitrant dermatitis include the scalp, postauricular area, glabella, paranasal area, axillae, sternum, umbilicus, and, less commonly, the groin. Seborrhea, being the oiliness found on the scalp, may also be present. It also has an unclear etiology.

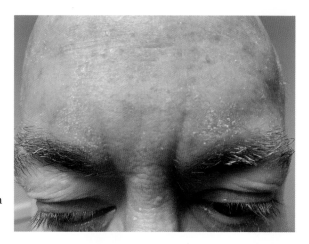

Figure 5.14 Erythematous patches with fine, greasy scale on the eyebrows and glabella.

Laboratory studies: This is a clinical diagnosis. In patients who present with severe and sudden onset, consider obtaining an HIV test.

Differential diagnosis: SD, in general, may be confused with a dermatophyte infection. The scaling on the scalp may suggest psoriasis, but the absence of plaque formation on the elbows and knees, for example, would point against it; however, sometimes the distinction is difficult. In these situations, the diagnosis of sebo-psoriasis can be made. When presenting on the face, rosacea can appear similar, but it also has papules and pustules. Intertrigo in the groin can also appear clinically similar, but it is characterized by its location within intertriginous areas.

Management: For SD of the scalp, shampooing with a tar, selenium sulfate, ketoconazole, salicylic acid, or zinc pyronate shampoo can help to control the condition. A topical corticosteroid solution may be needed for occasional use to control breakthrough redness and itching. Elsewhere on the body, a topical corticosteroid, such as hydrocortisone 2.5% or fluticasone cream, applied two times per day for the redness and itching can offer control.

Prognosis: SD is a chronic condition that can be controlled but not cured. Fortunately, it eventually burns itself out in most cases.

ANOGENITAL PRURITUS

Synonyms: Pruritus vulvae, pruritus ani, scrotal pruritus

Definition: Anogenital pruritus refers to acute or chronic itch of the genital region, including the vulvar, scrotal, and perianal skin.

Overview: Acute presentations are most commonly caused by infection or contact dermatitis; however, it can also be caused by locoregional factors, including fissures or hemorrhoids. Chronic presentations are often idiopathic with an unclear etiology. There is also the possibility of lumbo-sacral radiculopathy.

Clinical picture: There may be erythema and eczematous changes, including excoriations and lichenification in chronic cases. Many times, there is only intractable pruritus.

Laboratory studies: This condition is often without signs. In acute cases, infection with fungal (tinea cruris) or parasitic species, particularly pinworms, in children should be considered. In chronic cases, underlying malignancy or systemic illness should be excluded.

Differential diagnosis: The differential diagnosis includes dermatophytosis, pinworm infection, contact dermatitis, and intertrigo. Extramammary Paget's disease and lichen sclerosus are considerations if the condition is long-standing and recalcitrant to treatment.

Management: Topical corticosteroids can be used. For a fungal cause, topical antifungal cream should be used. Often, the most potent, such as clobetasol cream, is required to control the itching. Pruritis vulvae may require a gynecologic consultation, while external and/or internal hemorrhoids may indicate the need for a gastrointestinal consultation.

Prognosis: Unfortunately, this condition may be chronic and have intermittent flares.

KERATOSIS PILARIS

Definition: Keratosis pilaris (KP) is a common, benign disorder characterized by the presence of multiple small, skin-colored rough papules on the proximal arms and legs.

Overview: The papules of KP are caused by keratotic plugging of follicles. Its etiology is multi-factorial, and there is likely a heritable component. It can be associated with atopic dermatitis.

Clinical picture: Patients present with multiple small, monomorphic, skin-colored papules distributed symmetrically on the upper arms and occasionally the legs and/or buttocks. Underlying xerosis or atopic dermatitis is common. It often presents in childhood and persists through young adulthood.

Diagnosis: The diagnosis of KP is based on its clinical presentation.

Differential diagnosis: The differential diagnosis includes atopic dermatitis, folliculitis, and lichen nitidus.

Management: The appearance of KP can be improved through the regular use of exfoliation and keratolytics, such as lactic acid or salicylic acid. Patients should be encouraged to moisturize their skin regularly, since xerosis is often a contributing component.

Prognosis: KP is a chronic condition that can improve with regular treatment but does not completely resolve. It may improve with age.

DYSHIDROTIC DERMATITIS

Synonyms: Pompholyx, palmoplantar eczema

Definition: This affliction of the palms and soles is characterized by the presence of small, pruritic vesicles.

Overview: The cause of this eccrine gland disorder is unknown.

Clinical picture: There are recurrent crops of vesicles on the palms and soles, accompanied by intense itching.

Laboratory studies: The diagnosis is made clinically. Histopathologic confirmation is not generally required.

Differential diagnosis: This condition may mimic palmoplantar pustolosis, contact dermatitis, or pustular psoriasis.

Management: A high-potency topical corticosteroid, such as clobetasol 0.05%, should be used. Sometimes, the intense itching can be quelled by icy-water soaks. Dupilumab and botulinum toxin injections can be considered for recalcitrant cases.

Prognosis: Dyshidrotic dermatitis typically follows a chronic, relapsing course.

ASHY DERMATOSIS

Synonyms: Erythema dyschromicum perstans

Definition: This is a disorder of hypermelanosis characterized by the development of blue-grey macules and patches distributed widely across the body.

Overview: While the cause is unclear, genetic and environmental factors are suspected.

Clinical presentation: It presents as asymptomatic, progressively enlarging, blue-gray macules and patches distributed symmetrically on the trunk, neck, arms, and legs. The lesions may have a raised, erythematous border, and they typically appear in photo-protected areas. Ashy dermatosis is most common in patients of Hispanic and Asian descent and often develops in the second or third decade of life.

Laboratory studies: The diagnosis often requires clinicopathologic correlation. Histopathologic study will show basal vacuolar degeneration and edema of the papillary dermis. Older lesions can have pigmentary incontinence.

Differential diagnosis: Lichen planus pigmentosus and post-inflammatory hyperpigmentation may resemble the condition.

Management: There is no consistently efficacious treatment. Occasionally, tacrolimus ointment or hydroquinone 4% cream can offer some clinical improvement, as may oral dapsone, clofazimine, or isotretinoin.

Prognosis: This is a chronic, progressive disorder with few effective treatment options. When it occurs in children, it typically resolves spontaneously within 2–3 years.

ID REACTION

Synonym: Autoeczematization

Definition: An id reaction is characterized by the occurrence of inflammatory reaction in an area that is not affected by the primary lesions or process.

Overview: Id reactions occur as a secondary reaction to a number of primary dermatoses, including fungal or bacterial infections, stasis dermatitis, or contact dermatitis. Id reactions associated with primary fungal reactions, such as tinea capitis and tinea pedis, are called dermatophytid reactions. Pustular bacterid refers to id reactions secondary to primary bacterial infection, commonly streptococcus. The exact mechanism by which id reactions occur has not yet been elucidated, but it is thought to be a delayed-type hypersensitivity reaction precipitated by a primary inflammatory dermatitis.

Clinical presentation: In adults, id reactions typically present as eruptions of small, erythematous, monomorphic papules and/or vesicles. They occur in a location unaffected by the primary dermatosis and are most commonly distributed on the extensor surfaces of the forearms, trunk, face, or legs. In children, id reactions are often secondary to tinea capitis and/or kerion, and eruptions on the face are therefore common. Pustular bacterid presents as pustules located on the lateral aspects of the hands and feet, which can resemble dyshidrotic dermatitis. Because id reactions occur subsequent to a primary dermatosis, skin changes related to the primary dermatosis may be visualized. Pruritus is common.

Laboratory studies: Diagnosis can be made clinically. A thorough physical examination or history may reveal the primary dermatosis, such as tinea pedis or contact dermatitis.

Differential diagnosis: Other dermatitides to consider include atopic dermatitis, contact dermatitis, and dyshidrotic dermatitis.

Management: Treatment of the primary dermatosis will often eliminate the id reaction; however, lesions may persist. Topical corticosteroids can be used.

Prognosis: The id reaction will typically resolve when the primary dermatitis is eliminated.

FINAL THOUGHT

Dermatitides affect all age groups. Causes may be exogenous, such as an allergic contact dermatitis, or endogenous, such as stasis dermatitis. An accurate diagnosis is needed for the patient to avoid aggravating factors and/or to use appropriate treatment.

ADDITIONAL READINGS

Billings SD. Common and critical inflammatory dermatoses every pathologist should know. Mod Pathol. 2020;33(Suppl 1):107–117.

Chu C, Marks JG Jr, Flamm A. Occupational contact dermatitis: common occupational allergens. Dermatol Clin. 2020;38:339–349.

Fenner J, Silverberg NB. Skin diseases associated with atopic dermatitis. Clin Dermatol. 2018;36:631–640.

Fernandez K, Long KA, Zhang A, et al. Clinical features of idiopathic anogenital pruritus in adult males: a case-control study. J Am Acad Dermatol. 2020;20:S0190-9622(20)32837-1. https://doi.org/10.1016/j.jaad.2020.10.025.

Lipman ZM, Yosipovitch G. Substance use disorders and chronic itch. J Am Acad Dermatol. 2021;84:148–155.

Sidbury R, Kodama S. Atopic dermatitis guidelines: diagnosis, systemic therapy, and adjunctive care. Clin Dermatol. 2018;36:648–652.

Sundaresan S, Migden MR, Silapunt S. Stasis dermatitis: pathophysiology, evaluation, and management. Am J Clin Dermatol. 2017;18:383–390.

Williams KA, Huang AH, Belzberg M, et al. Prurigo nodularis: pathogenesis and management. J Am Acad Dermatol. 2020;83:1567–1575.

Wollina U. Pompholyx: a review of clinical features, differential diagnosis, and management. Am J Clin Dermatol. 2010;11:305–314.

Wu A, Vaidya S. Literature review of treatment outcomes for lichen planus pigmentosus, erythema dyschromicum perstans, and ashy dermatosis. J Cutan Med Surg. 2018;22:643–645.

6 Bacterial, Mycobacterial, and Spirochetal (Nonvenereal) Infections

Liam Mercieca and Joseph Pace

CONTENTS

Some commensal bacteria live on skin as part of the normal skin flora without causing any harm. They can, however, also become pathogenic and cause a wide variety of skin presentations. Some are easily treatable, while others can cause serious life-threatening infections.

STREPTOCOCCAL AND STAPHYLOCOCCAL SKIN INFECTIONS

Definition: The vast majority of bacterial skin infections are caused by gram-positive cocci that can lead to a number of different skin manifestations.

Folliculitis, Furuncles (Boils), and Carbuncles

Overview: Folliculitis refers to inflamed hair follicles, which can be secondary to bacterial infection, most commonly staphylococci.

Clinical presentation: It results in tender erythematous papules and pustules occurring on any site where hairs are present, such as the chest, back, and buttocks. Furuncles, also known as boils, are a deep form of bacterial folliculitis with one pustular opening, while carbuncles refer to a cluster of boils (Figure 6.1). Furuncles generally have one pustular surface, whereas carbuncles contain several pustules.

Laboratory studies: Diagnosis is usually based on the clinical presentation, and bacterial cultures are useful to identify the organism and antibiotic sensitivities; however, cultures are not always necessary. In recurrent or severe skin infections, such as carbuncles, investigations to rule out an underlying contributory factor, such as diabetes mellitus, is necessary.

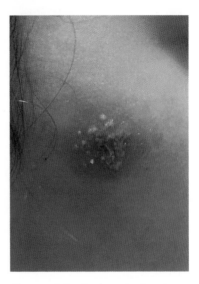

Figure 6.1 Carbuncle showing a cluster of boils.

DOI: 10.1201/9781003105268-6

Management: Treatment includes antiseptic washes (e.g., chlorhexidine 2–4%) as well as topical or oral antibiotics, such as flucloxacillin at a dose of 250–500 mg taken four times a day for 7–14 days. Cephalosporins (e.g., cefazolin, cephalothin, and cephalexin) provide a reasonable alternative to penicillin, but clindamycin, lincomycin, and erythromycin have an important therapeutic role in less serious infections or those with penicillin-hypersensitivity in whom cephalosporins are best avoided. Inpatient treatment with intravenous vancomycin at a dose of 2 g divided either as 500 mg every 6 hours or 1 g every 12 hours remains the gold standard for more serious infections. Assessing nasal carriage of staphylococci and eradicating the organism with topical antimicrobials (e.g., mupirocin ointment applied twice daily for 5 days) is important in preventing recurrent outbreaks; however, recurrence is frequent.

Impetigo

Overview: Impetigo is a highly contagious superficial bacterial skin infection commonly found in children (Figure 6.2). It is typically caused by staphylococcal organisms and less commonly by streptococcal bacteria. **Ecthyma** is a deeper form of impetigo that can lead to crusted sores and ulcers (Figure 6.3). This is usually caused by *Streptococcus pyogenes* and *Staphylococcus aureus*.

Clinical presentation: Impetigo presents acutely with red sores or blisters, which can burst and leave behind crusty yellowish patches. They usually affect exposed areas, such as the hands and face, and can rapidly enlarge and spread to other body parts. Impetiginization refers to a superficial secondary skin infection of an underlying skin condition, such as dermatitis.

Management: Treatment with topical antiseptics and oral antibiotics usually leads to resolution within 7–10 days. Topical antiseptics, such as povidone-iodine, hydrogen peroxide 1% cream, and chlorhexidine, can be used. Beta-lactam drugs are a good initial choice (e.g., flucloxacillin 500 mg four times a day for 7–10 days) although resistance is increasing. Other options include trimethoprim/sulfamethoxazole, clindamycin, or doxycycline. Topical antibiotics should be avoided in generalized cases and used with caution due to the emergence of resistant bacterial strains.

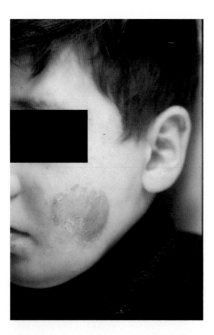

Figure 6.2 Impetigo on the face of a child.

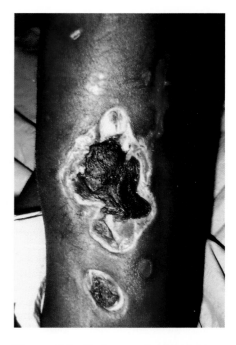

Figure 6.3 Ecthyma affecting the leg.

Cellulitis

Overview: Cellulitis is a skin infection that affects the upper portion of the dermis and subcutaneous layers of the skin.

Clinical presentation: It starts with a small area of redness and increased warmth, before spreading to involve larger areas within a few days. The skin becomes swollen, tender, and painful and can be associated with systemic symptoms, such as fever, chills, and rigors (Figure 6.4). **Erysipelas** (more often streptococcal) is considered a superficial form of cellulitis.

Laboratory studies: Bacterial cultures from open areas can help to identify the organism involved and guide the administration of an appropriate antibiotic. Blood tests can reveal an elevated white cell count and inflammatory markers.

Management: Prompt treatment with oral or intravenous antibiotics, usually penicillin-based (e.g., flucloxacillin 500 mg every 6 hours for 7–14 days) or cephalosporins, is essential to prevent complications, such as sepsis. There is no place for topical antibiotics in this case. *Methicillin-resistant staphylococcal aureus* (MRSA) leading to cellulitis is on the increase, and alternative antibiotics should be chosen based on local guidelines. Other treatment considerations include bed rest, elevation where possible, wet dressings, anti-inflammatory drugs, and analgesia when needed. It is important to check for entry sites and underlying risk factors, such as tinea pedis, insect bites, and trauma, in cellulitis of the legs.

Necrotizing Fasciitis

Overview: Necrotizing fasciitis is a serious bacterial infection of the fascia and soft tissue and represents a medical/surgical emergency.

Clinical presentation: Toxins and enzymes released by a variety of bacterial organisms lead to thrombosis and necrosis of the fascial layers, which may not be immediately apparent on the skin surface. This can rapidly progress to involve large areas. Initially, the area can be exquisitely painful and accompanied by systemic symptoms, such as nausea, fever, and lethargy. After a few days, the affected area becomes swollen and violaceous, which leads to necrosis. This can ultimately lead to sepsis and death. Worsening of the patient's general condition, increasing pain, and fever will all point to an increasing possibility of necrotizing fasciitis being present, with all the consequent implications on treatment and outcome.

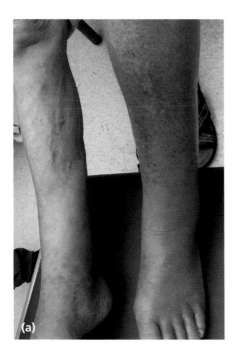
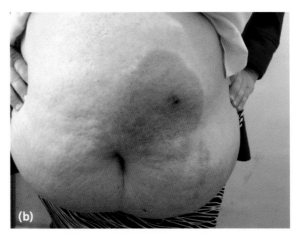

Figure 6.4 (a) Cellulitis of the left leg and onychomycosis; (b) cellulitis on the abdomen.

Laboratory studies: Blood tests will show high white cell counts and raised inflammatory markers, muscle enzymes, and urea. Imaging studies can help identify the extent of involvement.

Management: Treatment includes supportive care in an intensive therapy unit; high-dosage broad-spectrum intravenous antimicrobials should be started immediately and changed according to bacterial cultures and sensitivities. Prompt surgical debridement of all necrotic tissue is essential. Other considerations include hyperbaric oxygen therapy and intravenous immunoglobulins.

Staphylococcal Scalded Skin Syndrome

Overview: Staphylococcal scalded skin syndrome (SSSS) is a disorder caused by two exotoxins (epidermolytic toxins A and B), which cause a reaction with the desmosomes (a cell structure important in cell-to-cell adhesion) that leads to cellular separation.

Clinical presentation: It presents as a red, painful, and blistering eruption and resembles—and has been mistaken for—a burn. This is followed by desquamation of skin in large sheets (Figure 6.5). SSSS occurs mostly in children younger than 5 years old, particularly newborn babies. It is uncommon in older children and adults, since exposure leads to development of protective antibodies against staphylococcal exotoxins. Immunocompromised individuals and individuals with kidney disease, regardless of age, may also be at risk of SSSS. The differential diagnosis includes bullous impetigo, pemphigus or other blistering disorders, Steven Johnson syndrome, toxic erythema of the newborn, and thermal burns.

Laboratory studies: Investigations include bacterial culture from skin, blood, urine, or umbilical cord sample (in a newborn baby). A Tzanck smear (scraping of an ulcer base to look for acantholytic cells, dyskeratosis, no or little inflammation, cocci, and absence of abundant neutrophils) can be a useful, simple, low-cost rapid test to aid diagnosis.

Management: Early treatment with systemic antimicrobials, such as nafcillin 100 mg/kg/day intravenously in 4 divided doses or 50 mg/kg/day in 4 divided doses orally × 7–10 days, and general care usually leads to resolution; however, if left untreated or in the presence of debilitating factors, it can lead to pneumonia, sepsis, and death. The outcome is more serious in adults.

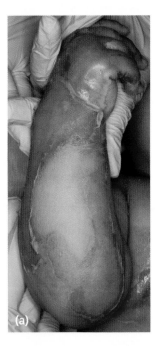 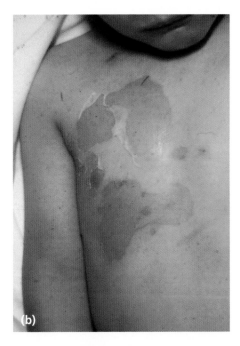

Figure 6.5 (a) Staphylococcal scalded skin syndrome right arm; (b) staphylococcal scalded skin syndrome on the chest.

Source: (a) is from Tsujimoto M, Makiguchi T, Nakamura H, et al., Staphylococcal scalded skin syndrome caused by burn wound infection in an infant: A case report, Burns Open 2018; 2(3): 139–43, with permission); (b) is from the personal collection of Prof. Joseph Pace.

Toxic Shock Syndrome and Scarlet Fever

Overview: Toxic shock syndrome (TSS) is a rare medical emergency. It presents with fever, a widespread erythematous eruption, and possible organ failure.

Clinical presentation: Exotoxins released from staphylococcal and streptococcal bacteria act as superantigens. Toxic shock syndrome, particularly but not exclusively, have affected menstruating women 3–5 days after a surgical procedure, especially those using superabsorbent tampons. It has also been described, albeit rarely, postoperatively in men and children.

The Centers for Disease Control and Prevention (CDC) case definition for toxic shock syndrome requires presence of the following 5 clinical criteria:

1. Temperature ≥ 38.9°C

2. Low blood pressure (including fainting or dizziness on standing)

3. Widespread, red, flat eruption

4. Shedding of skin, especially on palms and soles, 1–2 weeks after onset of illness

5. Abnormalities in 3 of the following:

   - Gastrointestinal: vomiting or diarrhea

   - Muscular: severe muscle pain

   - Hepatic: decreased liver function

   - Renal: raised urea or creatinine levels

   - Hematologic: bruising due to low blood platelet count

   - Central nervous system: disorientation or confusion

   - Mucous membranes: red eyes, mouth, and vagina due to increased blood flow to these areas

Laboratory studies: Investigations include bacterial swabs from infected site of origin and blisters, blood cultures, and various blood tests, including a complete blood count, renal and liver function, creatine kinase, and coagulation screen.

Differential diagnosis: The CDC case definition for the clinically similar, but streptococcus-related TSS requires isolation of group A streptococci and hypotension with 2 or more of the following clinical criteria: (1) renal impairment: decreased urine output; (2) coagulopathy: bleeding problems; (3) liver problems; (4) dermatitis that may shed, especially on palms and soles, 1–2 weeks after onset of illness; (5) difficulty breathing; and (6) soft tissue necrosis including necrotizing fasciitis, myositis, and gangrene.

Management: Treatment includes removing the source of infection, such as infected tampons, and when indicated, surgical debridement of infected wounds and inpatient general systemic support. Intravenous antimicrobials with penicillins or cephalosporins are appropriate first-line options or vancomycin in penicillin-allergic patients.

Scarlet fever is caused by toxins produced by streptococcal organisms. It is characterized by an exudative pharyngitis, fever, and bright erythematous eruption. The characteristic eruption usually appears 12 to 48 hours after the onset of fever. Patients present with tiny pink-red spots usually starting cranially and descending to the chest, axillae, and groin and then spreading to the rest of the body. As the eruption progresses, it becomes more widespread and resembles a sunburn with a bright red eruption. The tongue can be red and bumpy and is described as a *strawberry tongue*. Antimicrobials, usually penicillin for 10 days, is the mainstay of treatment.

Final comment: Staphylococcal and streptococcal infections cause a wide variety of skin manifestations as outlined. This can lead to significant morbidity and rarely, mortality, which underscores the importance of early recognition and appropriate management.

MYCOBACTERIAL SKIN INFECTIONS

Definition: There are over 190 different mycobacterial species, and most are innocuous; however, some of these species are pathogenic. Mycobacterial species, other than *Mycobacterium tuberculosis* and *Mycobacterium leprae* causing tuberculosis and leprosy respectively, are classified as atypical mycobacteria. There are a number of pathogenic atypical mycobacteria, such as *Mycobacterium marinum* and *Mycobacterium ulcerans*, which can lead to uncommon skin manifestations

Tuberculosis

Overview: Cutaneous tuberculosis is uncommon, even in countries where pulmonary tuberculosis is rife; hence, a high index of suspicion is needed, especially in immunocompromised patients (e.g., HIV, intravenous drug users, malignancy, long-term immunosuppressive medication, including monoclonal antibodies, alcoholism), where drug-resistant tuberculosis is prevalent, and in ethnic communities in deprived situations.

Clinical presentation: *M. tuberculosis* generally affects the lungs but can also attack any part of the body and cause a variety of skin presentations (Figure 6.6). Some of these are rare nowadays due to better treatments and eradication programs. These presentations should always be considered in an increasingly global world with migration routes from endemic countries. Clinical presentations are summarized in Table 6.1.

Laboratory studies: A skin biopsy will reveal granulomas, consisting of giant cells with central caseating necrosis. These contain acid-fast bacilli that can be detected by tissue staining, culture, and polymerase chain reaction. Chest x-rays and sputum cultures are indicated to detect pulmonary tuberculosis. Interferon gamma release assays (Quantiferon) are serum blood tests that can measure a person's immune reactivity to tuberculosis. A positive result need not necessarily indicate active infection but could also be due to latent tuberculosis.

Differential diagnosis: Cutaneous tuberculosis should be included in the differential diagnosis of any unexplained lesions, especially if in high-risk groups. Atypical mycobacterial infections can be similar to a tuberculous chancre or scrofuloderma. Crohn's disease and syphilis can resemble orificial tuberculosis, while leprosy and sarcoidosis can look similar to lupus vulgaris.

Management: Patients with pulmonary tuberculosis should be isolated in order to prevent spread. Antibiotic regimens include isoniazid, rifampin, pyrazinamide, and either ethambutol or streptomycin and are usually given for 6 months dosed according to weight. Treatment of cutaneous

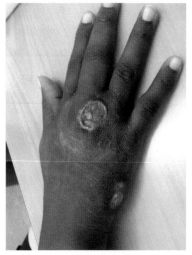

Figure 6.6 Ulcers caused by *Mycobacterium tuberculosis* infection.

Table 6.1 Types and Features of Cutaneous Tuberculosis

Types of Cutaneous Tuberculosis	Features
Miliary tuberculosis	• Occurs due to an acute hematogenous spread of tuberculosis • Results in diffuse, tiny, erythematous papules, ulcers, and abscesses • Usually arises in immunosuppressed patients and has poor prognosis
Tuberculid	• Is a cutaneous immunologic reaction to *Mycobacterium tuberculosis* in patients with a high degree of immunity • Presents as a generalized exanthem with papular-necrotic lesions
Tuberculosis verrucosa cutis	• Presents as small, erythematous papules • Appear a few weeks after direct inoculation of *M. tuberculosis* in an immunocompetent individual who was previously infected
Lupus vulgaris	• Is the most common form of cutaneous tuberculosis • Starts as a soft brownish-red papule or nodule that gradually expands into irregularly shaped plaques and progresses over time to form a well-defined skin-colored to erythematous plaque with an "apple jelly nodule" appearance • Historically, its appearance was compared to damage caused by wolf bites (lupus)
Scrofuloderma	• Results from the direct extension of tuberculosis infection from underlying lymph nodes, joints, or bones • Presents as firm, painless nodules that can become ulcerated

tuberculosis as recommended in the guidelines by the World Health Organization, consist of an intensive phase for 2 months (isoniazid, 5 mg/kg/day; rifampin, 10 mg/kg/day; ethambutol, 15 mg/kg/day; and pyrazinamide, 25 mg/kg/day) followed by a maintenance phase for 4 months (isoniazid and rifampicin).

Leprosy

Synonym: Hansen's disease

Overview: Leprosy is a chronic bacterial infection due to *M. leprae*, which manifests in different forms depending on the immune response of the host. It primarily affects the skin, mucous membranes, eyes, peripheral nervous system, and testes. It can affect all ages and is curable with early treatment avoiding morbidity. Historically, patients with leprosy were isolated, and the disease carried a strong negative social stigma. Transmission is thought to occur via droplet spread, and prolonged contact over many months is needed to contact the disease.

Clinical presentation: The cutaneous manifestations of leprosy vary depending on patient immunity and can include single or multiple lesions with various morphology (e.g., macules, papules, nodules) that can be hyper- or hypopigmented. Typically, the skin lesion shows a decreased sensation to pain and touch. Peripheral nerves can be thickened and become easily palpable, which can lead to muscle weakness and atrophy. Leprosy has traditionally been classified into two major types: tuberculoid and lepromatous leprosy. Patients with tuberculoid leprosy (TT; high resistance) have limited disease and few bacteria in the skin and nerves, while patients with lepromatous leprosy (LL; low resistance) have widespread disease and large numbers of bacteria (Figure 6.7).

Indeterminate leprosy refers to a very early form of leprosy that consists of a single skin lesion with slightly diminished sensation to touch. It will usually progress to one of the major types of leprosy.

In addition, recognized variants of the major types include the following:

Borderline tuberculoid leprosy which presents with similar lesions to TT but larger in size, more numerous (5–20), and can be less well defined. Anesthesia over the lesions is less pronounced compared to TT. Peripheral nerves are affected in an asymmetrical pattern and can cause deformity and disability.

Borderline lepromatous leprosy is characterized by widespread bilaterally symmetrical lesions of variable size and shape. There is no loss of sensation, but peripheral nerves can be extensively involved with resulting glove and stocking numbness.

Laboratory studies: Investigations include a

- Skin smear test for acid-fast bacilli; a small slit is made using a blade over the skin on the forehead, earlobe, or lesional skin. The exposed dermis is smeared onto a glass slide looking for acid fast bacilli under microscopy. Patients showing negative smears at all sites are grouped as paucibacillary leprosy (PB), while those showing positive smears at any site are grouped as having multibacillary leprosy (MB).

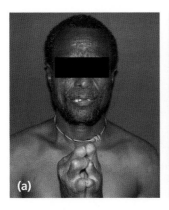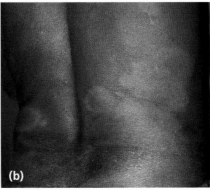

Figure 6.7 (a) Lepromatous leprosy with characteristic leonine facies and finger deformities and (b) tuberculoid leprosy showing hypopigmented patches.

Source: Courtesy of Valeska Padovese, MD

- Skin biopsy; from lesional skin that can show the bacilli with a modified Ziehl-Neelson stain (Wade-Fite) and histologic features depending on the type of leprosy.

- Serologic assays and DNA polymerase chain reaction (PCR) for *M. leprae*.

Differential diagnosis: There are a number of possible differentials due to the various presentations of leprosy. The hypopigmented macules can resemble pityriasis versicolor or pityriasis alba, while raised pigmented lesions can be similar to leishmaniasis, yaws, or lupus vulgaris.

Management: A combination of rifampin, clofazimine, and dapsone is the mainstay of treatment. Dosing depends on the age group, and duration depends on whether it is MB leprosy (1 year) or PB leprosy (6 months). The aim of treatment is to stop active infection and avoid deformities. Surgical correction of any permanent deformities might be needed.

Mycobacterium marinum (Fish Tank/Swimming Pool Granuloma)

Definition: *M. marinum* is an atypical mycobacterium that can cause skin and soft tissue infection (Figure 6.8). It is also known as fish tank granuloma.

Overview: *M. marinum* is a slow-growing organism commonly found in bodies of fresh or saltwater in many parts of the world. Skin infections with this organism are uncommon, and they are usually acquired through contact and inoculation of contents of aquariums or fish, especially when cleaning the former.

Clinical presentation: This infection presents as nodules, plaques, or ulcers typically found on the extremities. These can spread in a sporotrichoid pattern (subcutaneous nodules that progress along lymphatic vessels) and are usually painless.

Laboratory studies: A biopsy of the skin lesion can be sent for culture of the atypical mycobacteria. Histologic analysis typically demonstrates tuberculoid granulomas with varying degrees of abscess formation. PCR of tissue biopsies is another diagnostic option.

Differential diagnosis: This includes infections with other atypical mycobacteria, sporotrichosis, leishmaniasis, and foreign body granuloma.

Management: Combination antimicrobial therapy for prolonged periods is needed to eliminate the organism. For treatment of superficial papules, monotherapy with the following antibiotics is appropriate: clarithromycin 500 mg twice daily, minocycline 100 mg twice daily, and doxycycline 100 mg twice daily. In deeper infections, combination therapy is needed, such as clarithromycin 500 mg twice daily and rifampicin 600 mg once a day. Treatment duration is generally 3 to 4 months.

Buruli Ulcer

Synonym: *Mycobacterium ulcerans* ulcer

Overview: This atypical mycobacterium can be found in fish and amphibians. Infection with this organism is commonly found in Central and West Africa, but it can occur in travelers, as well.

Clinical presentation: Lesions start as solitary, painless nodules that can ulcerate and spread rapidly to cause large ulcers. If not treated promptly, it can cause permanent deformities and functional impairment. Osteomyelitis can also occur.

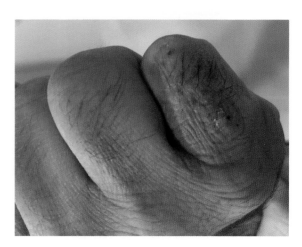

Figure 6.8 Fish tank granuloma.

Laboratory studies: A direct smear stained with Ziehl-Neelson stain shows the acid-fast bacilli under microscopy. PCR of swabs or soft tissue can confirm the infection. Culture of the organism from a tissue culture is also possible, although this takes weeks to be reported. A skin biopsy shows diffuse coagulative necrosis of subcutaneous tissues.

Differential diagnosis: Other skin conditions that can look similar include actinomycosis infection, leprosy, leishmaniasis, pyoderma gangrenosum, tuberculosis, and yaws.

Management: The mainstay of treatment is an 8-week course of combination antibiotics, such as rifampin and streptomycin or ciprofloxacin. It is important to start this early on. There may be an immune response and flare-up when commencing antibiotics, at which time oral prednisone can be added. Surgical intervention of necrotic areas and correction of deformities might be needed.

CORYNEBACTERIAL SKIN INFECTIONS

Definition: These are gram-positive infections caused by bacteria that are more often commensal microorganisms.

Erythrasma

Definition: This skin infection is caused by *Corynebacterium minutissimum*, which is a normal skin commensal but can lead to a chronic superficial infection.

Clinical presentation: It usually involves the intertriginous areas, creating reddish brown, well-demarcated macular patches that may be asymptomatic or mildly pruritic. The lesions usually have a fine scale, and the skin has a wrinkled appearance. It commonly coexists with other bacteria, yeasts, and dermatophytes and can persist for many years if left untreated.

Laboratory studies: Although this is a clinical diagnosis, Wood lamp examination will reveal atypical fluorescent coral-pink color. This is attributed to coproporphyrin III secreted by the bacteria. Bacterial culture will yield gram-positive filamentous rods.

Differential diagnosis: This includes fungal infections with candida or dermatophytes, acanthosis nigricans, irritant contact dermatitis, and intertrigo.

Management: Topical treatment includes antimicrobials, such as erythromycin or clindamycin cream, applied twice daily for about 10 days. Oral antimicrobials are rarely required.

Pitted Keratolysis

Definition: This is a bacterial skin infection of the feet characterized by pitting in weightbearing areas and malodor.

Clinical presentation: Several bacteria, including *Corynebacteria* and *Kytococcus sedentarius*, *Dermatophilus congolensis*, and *Actinomyces*, are able to proliferate on the palms and soles, which is aggravated by excessive sweating. This can be exacerbated by prolonged use of occlusive footwear. These organisms secrete protease enzymes that destroy the stratum corneum, which can create multiple small craters and pits (Figure 6.9). Sulfur compounds produced by these organisms cause

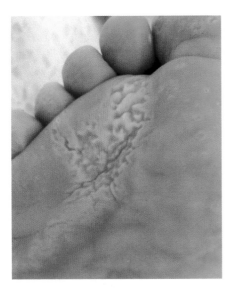

Figure 6.9 Pitted keratolysis.

the characteristic malodor that can persist on footwear. The affected areas can have a whitish appearance, which is more noticeable after bathing. The pits can coalesce to form larger craters. At times, walking precipitates itching and tenderness.

Laboratory studies: Cultures show gram-positive coccobacilli or bacilli. KOH scrapings may exclude tinea pedis of the lesions.

Differential diagnosis: This includes tinea pedis, contact dermatitis, keratolysis exfoliativa, porokeratosis, and palmoplantar keratoderma.

Management: The condition responds fairly rapidly to a variety of topical agents applied twice daily for about two weeks. Topical preparations include benzoyl peroxide, clindamycin, erythromycin, fusidic acid, or mupirocin. Oral erythromycin or clindamycin are rarely required. Preventive measures include keeping shoes well aerated and using applications of topical antiperspirants.

Trichomycosis Axillaris

Definition: This is due to a superficial bacterial colonization of the axillary hair by the overgrowth of *Corynebacterium* species or *Serratia marcescens*. This often occurs in patients who are obese with hyperhidrosis and poor hygiene. The term *trichomycosis* is misleading, because this is a bacterial infection and not a fungal infection

Clinical presentation: It is characterized by yellowish, and less commonly red or black, concretions along the hair shaft. It occurs with warmth in the intertriginous areas found in humid and hot climates, where it can more commonly affect other areas, including the pubis hair.

Laboratory studies: A Wood lamp examination shows a pale yellow fluorescence, although the diagnosis is usually clinical.

Differential diagnosis: This includes piedra, hair casts, pediculosis pubis, and artifacts from soaps, creams, or deodorants.

Management: Treatment includes shaving the affected areas and application of topical clindamycin, erythromycin, or fusidic acid. Antiperspirants may be used as a preventative measure.

Gram-Negative Bacterial Infections

Gram staining is a common technique used to differentiate two major groups of bacteria based on their cell wall properties. Gram-positive bacteria stain violet, while gram-negative bacteria stain pink or red. Gram-negative bacteria include *Pseudomonas aeruginosa, Escherichia coli, Serratia marcescens, Klebsiella*, and *Proteus* species.

These gram-negative bacteria can all cause soft tissue infections and should always be considered in cellulitis, nonhealing infected ulcers, and abscesses. Multidrug resistant strains are emerging due to inappropriate and prolonged antibiotic use, leading to significant morbidity and mortality. Bacterial culture and sensitivities are therefore important in such cases, and empiric treatment should be guided by local protocols.

Pseudomonas aeruginosa Infection

Overview: This gram-negative organism may lead to a variety of different skin presentations, ranging from infected wounds to skin ulcers, which can cause a characteristic pungent smell.

Clinical presentation: There are a number of cutaneous manifestations, such as nail infection leading to green nail syndrome (Figure 6.10), interdigital infection, folliculitis, ear infections, subcutaneous nodules, ecthyma gangrenosum, and severe skin and soft tissue infection. Spa-pool or hot-tub folliculitis represents follicular inflammation due to bathing in heated and infected water. This can create a red, itchy, tender, and pustular dermatitis within a few hours or days. Immunocompromised individuals have occasionally developed bacterial emboli that create hemorrhagic erythematous lesions. They can create gangrenous ulcerations with a black scab and surrounding erythema (Figure 6.11).

Laboratory studies: For hot-tub folliculitis and *Pseudomonas* nail infection, a bacterial culture may be helpful, but the diagnosis is typically clinical.

Differential diagnosis: The folliculitis may resemble acne or folliculitis due to other types of bacteria, while the green nail may also be associated with monilial paronychia.

Management: For the folliculitis, topical antibiotics, such as bacitracin or polymyxin B, can be applied two to four times per day; however, treatment may not be necessary. Use of a benzoyl peroxide wash in the shower may be a useful adjunct. For the nail infection, applications of topical thymol 4% in absolute alcohol four times per day can be effective, as can be antimicrobial solutions.

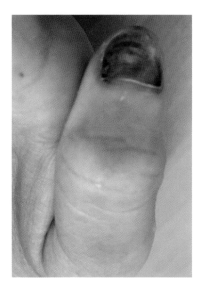

Figure 6.10   Green nail secondary to *Pseudomonas* infection.

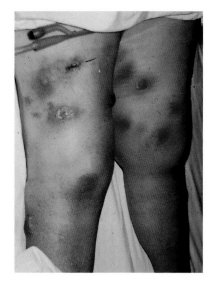

Figure 6.11   Ecthyma gangrenosum and *Pseudomonas* septicemia.

SPIROCHETAL NONVENEREAL SKIN INFECTIONS

Definition: Spirochetes refers to a group of spiral-shaped bacteria that can be pathogenic in humans.

Bejel

Overview: Nonvenereal syphilis (bejel- *T. pallidum endemicum*) was first reported by Ellis H. Hudson (1890–1992) in 1928 in Deir az Zawr, Syria, when he found that syphilis was rampant among the poorest groups, especially nomads, while uncommon among townspeople. A nonspecific flocculation test for syphilis was widely positive, but the Bedouins, with their strict code of life, refuted the possibility of a venereal disease, instead calling it bejel and not the French disease (*marad fransi*). Nonvenereal syphilis (bejel) historically antedated the emergence of sexually transmitted syphilis and is also caused by *Treponema pallidum subsp. endemicum*. It is associated with poor living conditions and consequently was expected to gradually disappear with the change from nomadic to a settled lifestyle with better basic services, including water supply, drainage, and health, leaving sexual transmission as the remaining important mode of transmission.

   Clinical presentation: The majority of cases present during childhood. Initially, the infection causes a mucous patch on the buccal mucosa followed by papulosquamous and erosive papular lesions of the trunk and extremities. Periostitis of the bones of the lower limbs and deforming gummatous lesions of the nose and soft palate are seen in later stages. Nowadays, this is rare with early treatment.

   Differential diagnosis: The diagnosis should be considered in patients with unexplained reactive treponemal tests. Patients fit the following diagnostic profile, although serologic testing does not differentiate between venereal and nonvenereal syphilis. The diagnostic clinical profile includes low or absent serologic titer, no suggestion of sexual transmission, absence of cases of congenital syphilis, transmission in childhood by contact/drinking vessels, no central nervous system/cardiovascular involvement, bone pain, long bone involvement with sabre tibia appearance, collapsed nasal septum, and perforation of the palate.

   Management: Treatment with intramuscular penicillin may help reduce the progression of the disease. One dose of penicillin benzathine 1.2 million units (or 600,000 units in children <45kg) is the preferred treatment. Other options include doxycycline 100 mg twice a day for 2 weeks in penicillin-allergic patients. It is important not to mistakenly suggest sexually transmitted disease in these patients.

Yaws

Definition: Yaws is caused by *Treponema pallidum pertenue*, which belongs to the same family of bacteria as *T. pallidum*.

Overview: It is a tropical infection characterized by a rapidly growing ulcer with surrounding lymphadenopathy. It was nearly eradicated in the past; however, there has been a resurgence in poor areas of West and Central Africa, Indonesia, Papua New Guinea, and the Solomon Islands.

Clinical presentation: Yaws usually affects children and is spread via direct contact from infected persons. It initially presents with a papule at the site of inoculation a few weeks later. It then grows and ulcerates and can cause localized lymphadenopathy. The painless ulcer, known as parangi and paru, usually heals on its own. If left untreated, yaws can affect the joints and bones and lead to disabling deformities.

Laboratory studies: Dark field microscopy from the skin lesion can show the spirochaetes. Nontreponemal tests (rapid plasma reagin, venereal disease research laboratory) are usually non-specific but can be helpful for monitoring the progress of the infection and clearance. Treponemal tests (Treponema pallidum hemagglutination [TPHA], enzyme immunoassay [EIA]) detect antibodies to past or present infections even after treatment and are reactive in both yaws and syphilis. PCR testing can distinguish between yaws and syphilis, although these are usually not readily available.

Differential diagnosis: This includes other treponemal infections, arthropod bites, tuberculosis, leprosy, leishmaniasis, and blastomycosis.

Management: Yaws is easily treatable with a single intramuscular injection of benzathine penicillin 0.6 million units (children younger than 10 years of age) or 1.2 million units (older 10 years of age). Another option is a single oral dose of azithromycin (30 mg/kg up to a maximum of 2g)

Lyme Disease (Lyme Borreliosis)

Definition: Lyme disease is caused by the spirochaete known as *Borrelia burgdorferi*. It was originally described in Lyme, Connecticut.

Overview: It is transferred via an *Ixodes* tick bite, which is usually present on animals, such as deer. It is estimated to affect 300,000 people per year in the United States and is also common in Europe and Asia. The incubation period from infection to onset of clinical manifestations is typically 1–2 weeks.

Clinical presentation: Signs and symptoms of the disease vary depending on the stage. In the early stage, the site of the tick bite develops a distinct circular, targetoid, erythematous eruption, known as erythema migrans in approximately 80% of patients. Fever, lethargy, muscle pains, and chills can develop. It can disseminate and present with lymphadenopathy, conjunctivitis, myocarditis, nerve palsies, and meningitis. If left untreated, it may also cause arthritis.

Laboratory studies: The diagnosis is confirmed by testing enzyme-linked immunosorbent assay antibody titers to *B. burgdorferi*. If this is positive, a Western blot test is usually done to confirm the diagnosis.

Management: Treatment includes a 3-week course of antibiotics, such as doxycycline 100 mg twice a day, amoxicillin, or cefuroxime. Intravenous antibiotics are usually reserved in central nervous system involvement.

FINAL THOUGHT

In all skin infections, especially if recurrent or persistent, the possibility of an underlying bacterial cause should be considered, especially in patients with underlying conditions, such as poorly controlled diabetes mellitus. Antimicrobials are the mainstay of treatment in bacterial skin infections; however, their misuse has led to the emergence of resistant strains. It has been suggested that by 2050, more people will die from infections with antibiotic-resistant bacteria than due to a malignancy. Great importance is correctly being attributed to appropriate use of antimicrobials with emphasis on patient compliance and adherence to local antibiotic guidelines to reduce the potential for developing resistance. Topical antimicrobials and their long-term use should be avoided. In an increasingly global world with extensive travel and varying migratory routes between different countries, one should always keep in mind any exotic infections.

ADDITIONAL READINGS

Bolognia J, Schaffer J, Cerroni L, et al. Chapter 74—Bacterial diseases. In: Dermatology. 4th ed. Philadelphia: Elsevier; 2017. p. 1187–1221.

Chiller K, Selkin B, Murakawa G. Skin microflora and bacterial infections of the skin. J Investig Dermatol Symp Proc. 2001;6:170–174.

Dorff G. Pseudomonas septicemia. Illustrated evolution of its skin lesion. Arch Intern Med. 1971;128:591–595.

Franco-Paredes C, Marcos L, Henao-Martínez A, et al. Cutaneous mycobacterial infections. Clin Microbiol Rev. 2018;32:1–25.

Griffiths C, Barker J, Bleiker T, et al. Chapter 26—Bacterial infections. In: Rook's Textbook of Dermatology. 9th ed. Chichester, West Sussex: John Wiley & Sons Inc.; 2016. p. 667–751.

Hudson EH. Treponematosis among the Bedouin Arabs of the Syrian desert. Naval Med Bull. 1928;26:817–824.

Hundi G, Pinto M, Bhat R, et al. Clinical and epidemiological features of coryneform skin infections at a tertiary hospital. Indian Dermatol Online J. 2016;7:168–173.

Lastória J, Abreu M. Leprosy: review of the epidemiological, clinical, and etiopathogenic aspects—part 1. An Bras Dermatol. 2014;89:205–218.

Pace J, Csonka G. Endemic non-venereal syphilis (bejel) in Saudi Arabia. Sex Transm Infect. 1984;60:293–297.

Sukumaran V, Senanayake S. Bacterial skin and soft tissue infections. Aust Prescr. 2016;39:159–163.

7 Viral Infections

Soo Jung Kim and Annie Dai

CONTENTS

Definition: Viral infections encompass a wide variety of conditions. Such dermatologic manifestations can be caused by either the direct infection of the skin or the body's reaction to a viral infection. It is important to recognize the clinical characteristics and appropriate treatments.

HERPES SIMPLEX

Synonyms: Herpes, cold sore, fever blister, sun sore

Overview: Herpes simplex is a DNA viral infection by the *Herpes simplex* virus (HSV) resulting in mucocutaneous lesions. Infections can be caused by type 1 (HSV-1) and type 2 (HSV-2). HSV-1 is the main cause of orolabial herpes and is more prevalent than HSV-2, the main cause of genital herpes.

Clinical presentation: The initial primary infection of HSV-1 is spread through direct contact with contaminated body fluids. This may be asymptomatic or with prodromal symptoms and signs, such as malaise, lymphadenopathy, and fever, followed by mucocutaneous lesions, which resolves without sequelae in 1–2 weeks. The recurrent infections can occur due to latent virus in sensory ganglia neurons (Figure 7.1). These are often triggered by stress and sunlight, being preceded by localized pain, burning, and tenderness. The common locations are near or on the lip and present as characteristic painful, uniform grouped vesicles on an erythematous base (Figure 7.2). These will progress into grouped pustules and crusted ulcers that will heal spontaneously.

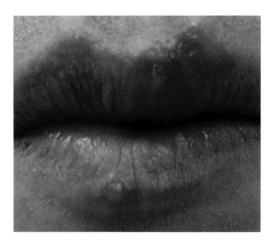

Figure 7.1 Herpes labialis.

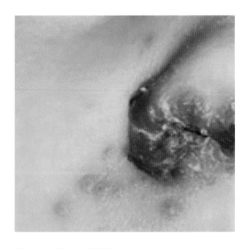

Figure 7.2 HSV lesions of grouped vesicles on an erythematous base.

Source: Courtesy of Raegan D. Hunt, MD, PhD.

DOI: 10.1201/9781003105268-7

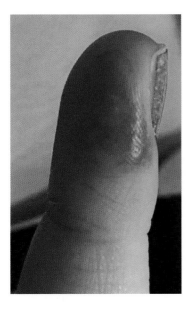

Figure 7.3 Herpetic whitlow involving the finger.

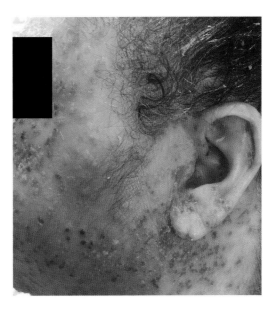

Figure 7.4 Eczema herpeticum involving the face.

The first episode of genital herpes usually occurs through sexual contact and can present on the penis in men (on the glans or shaft of penis and buttocks), and the vulva, vagina, or cervix, as well as on the perineum, in women; it often co-occurs with inguinal lymphadenopathy. *Herpes simplex* infection may occur on the fingers (herpetic whitlow; Figure 7.3), on hair follicles (herpetic sycosis), and the lateral side of the neck in wrestlers (herpes gladiatorum). Eczema herpeticum can occur most commonly in atopic patients and those with other skin diseases, such as pemphigus vulgaris, Darier disease, and Hailey-Hailey disease. It may present with monomorphic blisters along with fever. This can be widely disseminated throughout the body (Figure 7.4).

Laboratory studies: The diagnosis is made clinically. This can be confirmed with a variety of studies, including polymerase chain reaction (PCR) testing, direct fluorescent antibody test (DFA), viral culture, serologies, and a Tzanck smear. Histopathologic evaluation shows intraepidermal vesicles with ballooning degeneration of multinucleate keratinocytes, acantholysis, and ground-glass inclusions.

Differential diagnosis: These tests can assist in the differential diagnosis of HSV, including aphthous stomatitis and herpangina in orolabial herpes, and syphilis and chancroids in genital herpes.

Management: This can be divided into treatment and prevention (suppressive therapy), depending on the severity of the disease. Most patients with the mild disease do not require treatment. Oral antivirals acyclovir, valacyclovir, and famciclovir are commonly used and can shorten the duration and lessen the symptoms if started early. Suppressive therapy can be used for frequent herpetic recurrences and has the added benefit of decreasing viral shedding. Suggested dosing regimens of the three antivirals are listed in Table 7.1.

Table 7.1 Genital Herpes Medication Dosing in Healthy Patients

	Acyclovir	Valacyclovir	Famciclovir
HSV First Infection	400 mg TID × 10 days	1000 mg BID × 10 days	250 mg TID × 10 days
HSV Recurrent Infection	400 mg TID × 5 days	500 mg BID × 3 days or 1000 mg daily × 5 days	125 mg BID × 5 days
HSV Suppressive Therapy	400 mg BID	500 mg daily for <10 outbreaks/year or 1000 mg daily for ≥10 outbreaks/year	250 mg BID

Abbreviations: HSV: *Herpes simplex* virus; TID: three times a day; BID: two times a day.

If untreated, the lesions generally heal without scarring within weeks for immunocompetent individuals. For immunosuppressed patients, it is important to begin therapy, as patients can have extracutaneous symptoms and severe complications without treatment.

Final comment: Overall, HSV is one of the most prevalent infections worldwide. Recognition and proper patient counseling about reducing transmission are important in treating and preventing this infection. Research is currently devoted to creating a vaccine for HSV.

HERPES ZOSTER

Synonym: Shingles

Overview: Herpes zoster and chickenpox (varicella) are caused by the varicella-zoster virus (VZV). The primary infection is chickenpox (varicella) during infancy or childhood. Once the patient is infected, this DNA virus stays latent in the sensory dorsal root ganglion cells. Herpes zoster is caused by reactivation of VZV. The incidence of herpes zoster increases with age and immunosuppression, especially hematologic malignancy, and HIV infection, is another risk factor.

Clinical presentation: Before cutaneous signs of herpes zoster appear, patients can experience prodromal symptoms of pain, pruritis, burning, and/or hyperesthesia in the affected skin for a few days before the appearance of the skin eruption. Rarely, patients will only have pain without any later dermatologic manifestations (Zoster sine herpete). The eruptive phase is characterized by edematous, erythematous plaques in which vesicles develop. Vesicles become pustules or bullae and heal with crusts. Lesions are in a dermatomal distribution (Figure 7.5), confined to the skin innervated by the dorsal primary roots, and the thoracic dermatomes are the most commonly affected. Involvement of one of the branches of the trigeminal nerve is the most common single nerve involved with lesions in the distribution of the maxillary, mandibular, or ophthalmic sensory nerves.

Disseminated herpes zoster (>20 vesicles in the primary/adjacent dermatomes) can occur in the elderly or immunocompromised individuals. The lesions may be hemorrhagic (Figure 7.6) or gangrenous. The infection can also spread to visceral organs, including the liver, lungs, and the central nervous system.

Herpes zoster ophthalmicus occurs when the fifth cranial nerve (ophthalmic branch) is affected, and vesicles can develop on the tip of the nose (Hutchinson sign). These patients with ocular involvement (most commonly uveitis and keratitis) should also be seen immediately by the ophthalmologist. Ramsay Hunt syndrome, also known as herpes zoster oticus, occurs when the facial and auditory nerves are affected. Patients can present with auditory symptoms and facial paralysis, when herpes zoster involves the external ear or tympanic membrane.

Laboratory studies: The diagnosis of herpes zoster is usually clinical, and a history of previous varicella and vaccine status should be obtained. To confirm the diagnosis, PCR, DFA, and Tzanck smear can be completed. Viral culture and serology of rising titers are not useful, because both

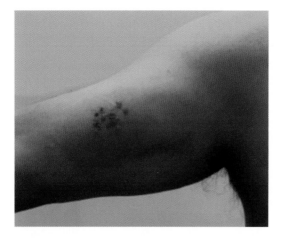

Figure 7.5 Herpes zoster erythematous vesicles in a dermatomal distribution.

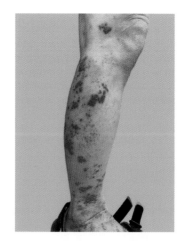

Figure 7.6 Hemorrhagic herpes zoster in an immunocompromised individual.

Table 7.2 Herpes Zoster Medication Dosing

	Acyclovir	Valacyclovir	Famciclovir
Herpes Zoster Immunocompetent	800 mg 5 times daily × 7–10 days	1000 mg TID × 7 days	500 mg TID × 7 days
Herpes Zoster Immunocompromised	800 mg 5 times daily × 7–10 days or 10 mg/kg IV q8h × 7 days	1000 mg TID × 7–10 days	500 mg TID × 7–10 days

Abbreviations: TID: three times a day; q8h: every 8 hours.

take a while to obtain the results. Histologically, skin lesions are indistinguishable from *Herpes simplex* lesions, as both are characteristic for intraepidermal blisters with multinucleate epithelial cells (balloon cells) and inclusion bodies.

Differential diagnosis: Physical examination and history can assist in the differential diagnosis of herpes zoster, including HSV, bacterial skin infections, and contact dermatitis.

Management: Treatment for herpes zoster infection includes restricting physical activities in elderly patients and local heat application. Antiviral therapy (e.g., acyclovir, valacyclovir, famciclovir) should ideally be initiated within 72 hours of the eruption or onset of pain to accelerate healing time and decrease the severity of zoster-associated pain. Immunocompromised individuals should be treated due to increased risk of dissemination and potential complications. Recommended dosages are listed in Table 7.2. Two vaccines have been developed for a Herpes zoster infection: Zostavax® (the first-generation vaccine, live attenuated vaccine) and Shingrix® (newer recombinant zoster vaccine). Shingrix® is the preferred vaccine due to its increased and sustained efficacy and is recommended for adults 50 years and older, whether or not the patient has had zoster. The vaccines will decrease the incidence of zoster, and if zoster still develops, they can decrease the rate of postherpetic neuralgia and shorten the duration of disease.

It is important to counsel patients with herpes zoster that infection is transmissible through contact for local disease and contact and airborne route for disseminated disease. Covering lesions and maintaining distance from nonimmunized, immunocompromised patients are important to reduce transmission.

In younger immunocompetent patients, the total duration of the disease is generally 2–3 weeks, while in elderly patients, it can take greater than 6 weeks for lesions to heal. Pain can last after skin lesions resolve and is called postherpetic neuralgia (PHN); the duration and severity of PHN are variable and often age-dependent. Treatments for postherpetic neuralgia are topical therapy (e.g., lidocaine, capsaicin), tricyclic antidepressants, gabapentin and pregabalin, venlafaxine, and oral analgesics, including opiates.

Final comment: With such a large prevalence worldwide of VZV, it is important to recognize the signs and symptoms of reactivation leading to herpes zoster. To help reduce the incidence, there is the need for vaccination for both VZV and herpes zoster.

VERRUCAE

Synonyms: Warts

Overview: Verrucae are benign skin growths caused by human papillomaviruses (HPV) infecting the skin. HPV is a DNA virus with over 150 genotypes. Some antigenic types are associated with specific clinical types of warts and the relationships are listed in Table 7.3.

Clinical presentation: Common warts (verrucae vulgaris) are most commonly found on the hands but can be anywhere on the skin. Meat handlers (butchers) and fish handlers have a high

Table 7.3 Verrucae and Commonly Associated Human Papillomavirus (HPV) Genotypes

Verrucae Subtype	Common HPV Genotypes
Common warts (verrucae vulgaris), palmar and plantar warts	1, 2, 4, 27, 57
Flat warts (verrucae plana)	3, 10
Anogenital warts (condylomata acuminata)	6, 11

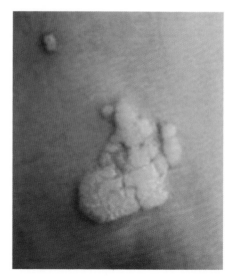

Figure 7.7 Hyperkeratotic common warts on the ankle.

Source: Courtesy of Grace L. Lee, MD.

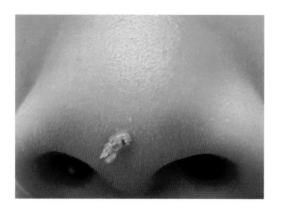

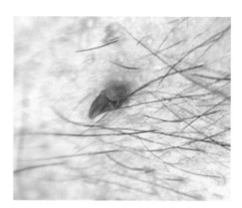

Figure 7.8 (a) Filiform wart with spiky projections from the base; (b) close-up of the filiform wart.

Source: Courtesy of Audrey J. Chan, MD.

incidence of verrucae on their hands. Warts begin as skin-colored smooth papules and progress into gray-brown hyperkeratotic, exophytic growths (Figure 7.7). Growths characteristically have black dots (thrombosed dilated capillaries) on the surface, which hemorrhage into the stratum corneum. Such viral infections can also be transmitted through close contact. Different presentations include filiform and digitate warts, which are skin-colored projections with small spikes coming from a narrow or broad base (Figure 7.8). They are most commonly found on the scalp and around the mouth, eyes, and nose.

Flat warts can vary in color from pink to brown and are flat-topped papules (Figure 7.9). They occur mainly as grouped or linear lesions around the mouth, forehead, hands, and shaved areas. Flat warts are seen most commonly in young adults and children. Autoinoculation is often seen through shaving.

Plantar and palmar verrucae are thick warts of the soles and palms and usually occur at pressure points (Figure 7.10). On the feet, they commonly present on the heels or the head of the metatarsal bones and are painful due to pressure from walking. They are often covered by a callus. These warts can be grouped or fused to appear as one "mosaic" wart.

Anogenital warts (condylomata acuminata) are the most frequently encountered sexually transmitted disease and are most commonly caused by low-risk genital HPV 6 and 11. These are associated with genital cancers, including cervical and anal cancer, which are induced by oncogenic HPV 16 and 18. They characteristically appear as multifocal, sessile, lobulated papules

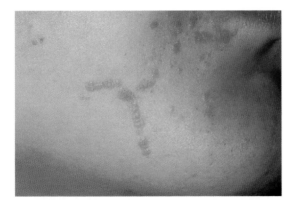

Figure 7.9 Flat warts located on the face.

Source: From Gawkrodger DJ, Ardern-Jones MR, Viral infections—Warts and other viral infections, in Dermatology: An Illustrated Colour Text, 6th edition, 54–55, Elsevier Ltd (2017), used with permission.

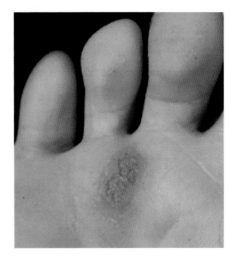

Figure 7.10 Plantar wart.

Source: Courtesy of Raegan D. Hunt, MD, PhD.

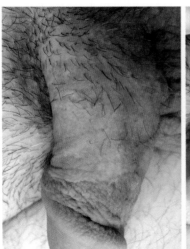
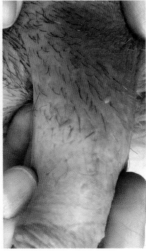

Figure 7.11 Anogenital warts on the penis.

Source: Courtesy of Soo Jung Kim, MD, PhD.

(Figure 7.11). Warts can appear on the penis, anus, vulva, or cervix and can be skin-colored, brown, or white. The verrucae can also be flat and are known as condylomata plana (flat cervical warts).

Laboratory studies: The diagnosis is easy to make. The black dots in warts help differentiate it from other diagnoses such as corns or calluses. Besides, skin lines (dermatoglyphics) will stop at the base of the wart, whereas they are more prominent in calluses. Wiping the area with vinegar will reveal warts as white lesions (acetowhitening). Dermatoscopy often shows grouped papillae with dotted vessels/hemorrhagic points surrounded by a white halo. Genital verrucae can have a mosaic pattern of grouped vessels in the center of dermatoscopy. A biopsy can be used to confirm the diagnosis and rule out various dysplasias and other growths including malignancies. Histopathologic observation of verrucae generally shows hyperkeratosis, granular cell layers with irregular enlarged basophilic granules, and koilocytes.

Differential diagnosis: Verrucae can present similarly to other skin lesions. Differential diagnoses of common warts can be broad and include seborrheic keratoses, actinic keratoses, cutaneous horns, keratoacanthomas, squamous cell carcinomas, and even other neoplasms and inflammatory conditions. For plantar warts, the differential diagnosis includes corns and black heels (talon noir). Corns have a well-demarcated hard central core, whereas plantar warts have black dots with a soft central core. Black heels, from ruptured capillaries or petechiae, would have skin lines, and the condition will self-resolve in weeks. Anogenital warts can look similar to condyloma lata associated with syphilis and molluscum contagiosum.

Management: Many nongenital warts in healthy individuals can spontaneously regress. Almost all common warts (~90%) resolve within 5 years. Treatment is initiated based on patient preference. Multiple treatment rounds or methods may be needed for a satisfactory resolution. Genital warts have high recurrence rates likely secondary to surrounding subclinical infection. Treatment modalities include two approaches: destruction and induction of local immune reactions. Destruction methods include topical treatments, cryotherapy, curettage, and light electrocautery, intralesional bleomycin, laser, and surgical removal. Topical treatments, such as salicylic acid preparations, podophyllin, cantharidin, and 5-fluorouracil (5-FU) cream, have shown success for common warts. For genital warts, topical treatments such as podophyllotoxin, imiquimod, sinecatechins, and trichloroacetic (TCA) acid are used. Immunotherapy to induce a local immune reaction in common warts includes topical dinitrochlorobenzene (DNCB), squaric acid, diphencyprone, imiquimod, and intralesional candida, mumps antigen, or bacillus Calmette Guérin (BCG). Imiquimod is Food and Drug Administration (FDA)–approved to treat genital warts.

Prevention of genital warts is also crucial. The HPV quadrivalent vaccine (brand name Gardasil 9®) can be given from ages 9–45 to protect against HPV types 6, 11, 16, 18, 31, 33, 45, 52, and 58 and has led to a significant reduction in anogenital warts and carcinomas. Due to high-risk strains of HPV (16, 18, 31, 33) associated with cervical cancer, women with anogenital warts should have routine gynecologic screening.

Final comment: Ultimately, HPV is an extremely common viral infection causing verrucae in different anatomic locations of the body. Treatment methods should be individualized for each patient.

MOLLUSCUM CONTAGIOSUM

Overview: Molluscum contagiosum (MC) is a common viral infection caused by the poxvirus. The infection spreads via direct skin-to-skin or sexual contact. It holds the distinction of the first disease to have a proven infectious origin.

Clinical presentation: MC is characterized by skin or pink-colored dome-shaped papules with the characteristic central umbilication (Figure 7.12). The lesions can appear anywhere on the skin but are most commonly found being grouped in skin folds or on the trunk, thighs, buttocks, and genital region. Young children, sexually active adults, and immunocompromised individuals (e.g., HIV patients) are the groups primarily affected by MC.

In young children, the lesions are generalized on the face, trunk, and extremities. Molluscum dermatitis (mild, eczematous eruption) surrounding the MC lesions can be seen more commonly in atopic children. Other forms of inflammatory reaction characterized by erythema, swelling, sometimes with pustular formation can occur as well, indicating the resolution of MC. If MC is limited on genital areas in children, this can be a sign of sexual abuse. In adults, MC is sexually

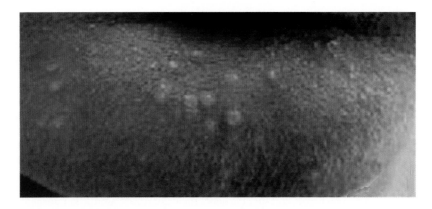

Figure 7.12 Umbilicated skin-colored molluscum lesions.

Source: Courtesy of Audrey J. Chan, MD.

transmitted disease (STD), and other STDs may coexist. If there are numerous, widespread, and/or giant-sized lesions present on the face and trunk in an adult, an underlying HIV infection should be ruled out.

Laboratory studies: The diagnosis can be made clinically. To confirm the clinical diagnosis of MC or rule out other diagnoses, the histopathologic examination can be used. The microscopic examination would show the characteristic large intracytoplasmic inclusion bodies (i.e., molluscum bodies, Henderson-Patterson bodies) within the keratinocytes that compress the nucleus.

Management: MC infection and lesions self-resolve in immunocompetent children, with individual lesions lasting months, and the duration of infection is about 2 years. Treatment can be determined individually, but deciding not to treat may be practical. Methods include curettage to remove small papules, forceps to remove the central core of lesions, surgical tape, cryosurgery, topical cantharidin, and trichloroacetic acid (TCA) peels. Molluscum dermatitis can be treated with a topical corticosteroid. In immunocompromised individuals, especially in HIV patients, management is more difficult. Treating HIV with antiretroviral therapy (ART) has been shown to resolve lesions. Treatment should be initiated for genital lesions to decrease the risk of transmission through sexual contact. Cryotherapy or curettage is very effective.

Final comment: Overall, MC is a self-limited condition in young children and certain subpopulations of adults. Treatment should be individualized based on patient preference.

VARICELLA (CHICKEN POX)

Synonym: Chicken pox

Overview: Varicella is a very common infection in children caused by VZV.

Clinical presentation: This common childhood ailment is transmitted by the respiratory route (droplets) and less likely by direct contact. The incubation period is 14–21 days, and patients are infectious 1–5 days before cutaneous lesions appear until all vesicles have crusted over.

Most patients experience prodromal signs (e.g., fever, malaise, headache). The vesicular eruption initially occurs on the trunk and then spreads centrifugally to the face, scalp, and extremities in successive crops. The characteristic feature of this viral exanthem is the "teardrop" vesicles on an erythematous base (rose petal), which progress to pustules and vesicles followed by crusting, often leaving scars. Different stages of lesions are present at the same time, which is another characteristic finding (Figure 7.13). Vesicles in the oral cavity easily rupture to form aphthae-like ulcers.

Lesions generally heal without scarring within 7–10 days in immunocompetent individuals. The severity of the disease is age-dependent, with adults having more severe disease and a greater risk of visceral disease. For immunocompromised adults, varicella infection is more diffuse and can involve the lungs, liver, and central nervous system. These patients may have hemorrhagic and purpuric lesions. Pregnant women also have an increased risk of adverse outcomes with varicella infection, including pneumonia, spontaneous abortion, and fetal death.

Laboratory studies: Like herpes zoster, the diagnosis of chickenpox is typically made clinically. A Tzanck smear, PCR, and DFA can aid in making the diagnosis. Tzanck smear would show multinucleated cells, as in HSV; therefore, it cannot differentiate between VZV and HSV. A viral

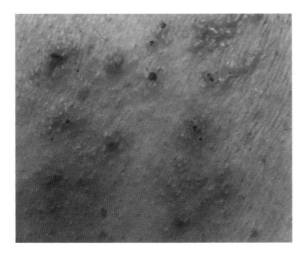

Figure 7.13 Varicella vesicles surrounded by erythematous halos. Lesions are in different stages of development.

Source: Courtesy of Annie Dai.

culture is rarely used since VZV grows poorly and slowly. The use of PCR has increased with the advantage of high sensitivity and specificity.

Differential diagnosis: This can include vesicular viral exanthems (e.g., coxsackieviruses, smallpox), drug eruptions, pityriasis lichenoides et varioliformis acuta (PLEVA), bullous insect bites, scabies, and disseminated HSV infections. In smallpox, patients would have had more severe systemic findings and would have had lesions on the palms and soles, which are rarely involved in varicella. The viral exanthems of smallpox are in the same stages.

Management: In immunocompetent children, routine antiviral therapy is not recommended, and varicella can be treated symptomatically with antipyretics, antihistamines, and topical anti-pruritic lotions. Aspirin should be avoided in children because it increases the risk of Reye syndrome. Antiviral agents are FDA-approved treatments for children >2 years and adults. Antivirals initiated within 24–72 hours of lesion onset would have maximum benefit with the decrease in the severity of symptoms and time to healing. Acyclovir at 20 mg/kg (800 mg maximum) four times a day for 5–7 days or valacyclovir 20 mg/kg TID (1000 mg maximum) for 5 days are the recommended dosages. The varicella vaccine, which is a live attenuated vaccine given at 12–15 months and 4–6 years, has been crucial in decreasing rates of varicella and preventing severe disease.

The most common complication of varicella is secondary bacterial infection leading to round, depressed scarring. For healthy children, varicella is a benign disease and self-limited with lesions healing within 10 days. In adolescents and adults, more severe complications are often seen, including increased incidence of pneumonia. Immunocompromised individuals can develop pneumonia, hepatitis, and encephalitis resulting in a fatal infection. Varicella infection during the first 20 weeks of pregnancy can result in congenital varicella syndrome, which is associated with cutaneous scarring, hypoplastic arms and legs, and ocular anomalies. After the primary infection, the virus stays latent in the dorsal root sensory ganglia and can reactivate anytime, as herpes zoster

Final comment: Overall, varicella is a common and contagious infection with characteristic pruritic dermatologic manifestations. Therapy is indicated for certain populations and is ideally started promptly. Counseling about viral transmission and emphasizing prevention through vaccination is key in reducing incidence and complications. The incidence of varicella has decreased with the varicella vaccine.

HAND-FOOT-MOUTH DISEASE

Overview: Hand-foot-mouth disease (HFMD) is a viral exanthem characterized by eruptions on the palms and soles with mouth ulcers. It is caused by multiple serotypes of the coxsackievirus, which is an RNA enterovirus, and most commonly Coxsackievirus A16. Enteroviruses are spread person-to-person, the fecal-oral route, respiratory route, or through direct inoculation. Outbreaks frequently occur during the summer and the fall.

Clinical presentation: Infection primarily occurs in young children. After the incubation period (3–7 days), patients develop fever and oral ulcerating vesicles with an erythematous halo on the buccal mucosa, tongue, palate, uvula, and the anterior tonsillar pillars. Lesions on the hands and feet (more commonly on the palms and soles) are asymptomatic red papules that evolve into grayish vesicles with a red halo (Figure 7.14). They often run parallel to the skin lines on the

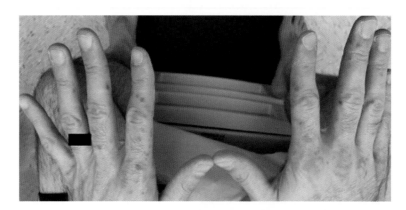

Figure 7.14 Hand-foot-mouth disease vesicles with surrounding erythematous halo.

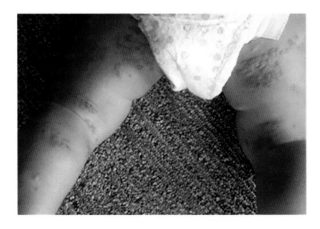

Figure 7.15 Coxsackie dermatitis on a child with atopic dermatitis.

fingers and toes. In children wearing diapers, these vesicles can also be present on the perineum and buttocks.

The atypical variant, commonly caused by Coxsackievirus A6, is a more widespread eruption of HMFD with lesions located periorally and on the trunk as well as the more typical locations. Children with atopic dermatitis may develop vesicular eruptions in the areas of dermatitis, called eczema coxsackie (Figure 7.15). More severe variants of HMFD have been identified. Enterovirus 71 infection is associated with the central nervous system and cardiopulmonary complications.

Laboratory studies: The diagnosis is made clinically. PCR or viral cultures can be used from vesicle samples if the diagnosis needs to be confirmed for atypical cases. Serologic testing is not of much utility due to multiple serotypes of coxsackievirus. A skin biopsy is usually not needed, but the histopathology would show epidermal necrosis and intraepidermal blisters with no inclusion bodies or multinucleated giant cells.

Differential diagnosis: This may include herpangina and varicella. In herpangina, another disease caused by a coxsackievirus, there is no viral exanthem, and oral lesions are primarily located in the posterior oropharynx. For varicella, the spread of the lesions is distinct from HMFD and is concentrated on the trunk and extremities with various stages of exanthem and vesicles that quickly crust over.

Management: For mild illness, the condition is generally self-limiting, and infections usually resolve within 1 week. Treatment is typically not needed except for supportive measures.

Approximately 1–2 months after HFMD, some patients will develop onychomadesis, which is the shedding of the proximal nails due to a temporary arrest of the matrix.

Final comment: HMFD is an extremely prevalent viral infection in children with characteristic features of stomatitis and cutaneous lesions. It is mostly a benign condition with only supportive treatment needed, but some serotypes cause atypical presentations, and some are associated with more systemic complications.

ERYTHEMA INFECTIOSUM

Synonym: Fifth disease, slapped cheek

Overview: This is a viral exanthem caused by the DNA virus, human parvovirus B19. The virus is spread through the respiratory route and can also be transmitted through blood products and vertically from mother to fetus. Infections rates are highest in late winter and early spring and occur most commonly in young children.

Clinical presentation: Erythema infectiosum appears in three stages. The incubation period lasts around 4–14 days and prodromal findings of headache, runny nose, myalgias, and low-grade fever can precede the dermatologic manifestations. The first stage presents as diffuse and macular erythema of the cheeks, hence the name "slapped cheek" disease. The eruption is asymptomatic and generally spares the perioral area, nasal bridge, eyelids, and chin (Figure 7.16). Within 1–4 days, patients will progress to the second stage, where erythematous macules and papules form on the extremities and the trunk, forming a lacy or reticulated pattern (Figure 7.17). The third stage is considered the recurring stage in which the exanthem is reduced or not visible but only recurs due to heat/sunlight or due to crying and exercise. The viral exanthem will typically resolve in 1–3 weeks. A minority (7%) of children will also experience arthralgias, whereas a majority (80%)

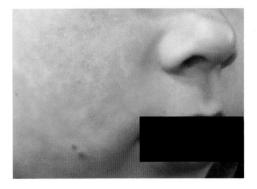

Figure 7.16 "Slapped cheek" rash of erythema infectiosum.

Source: Courtesy of Oleg E. Akilov, MD, PhD.

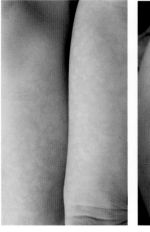
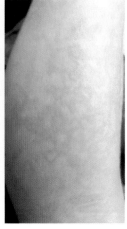

Figure 7.17 Lacy, reticulated erythema infectiosum pattern on arms (left) and leg (right).

Source: Courtesy of Oleg E. Akilov, MD, PhD.

of adults will experience arthralgias but have no skin findings. One of the systemic complications is a transient aplastic crisis in patients with hemoglobinopathies. Infection of pregnant women, especially before 20 weeks of gestation, is associated with fetal infection complications, including self-limited anemia, hydrops, spontaneous miscarriage, or still-birth.

Less commonly, parvovirus B19 can cause papular-purpuric gloves and socks syndrome (PPGSS). It occurs mainly in young adults and teenagers and presents as edema and erythema of the hands and feet associated with fever, petechiae, purpura, pruritis, and mucosal involvement (Figure 7.18). The condition is self-limiting, and spontaneous resolution occurs within 2 weeks.

Laboratory studies: The diagnosis is typically easy to make clinically because the exanthem is characteristic of erythema infectiosum. If needed, PCR for the virus or serology to detect anti-B19 IgM antibodies can be used to confirm the diagnosis. A skin biopsy is generally not needed.

Differential diagnosis: This may include scarlet fever, enteroviral infection, and rubella.

Management: Erythema infectiosum is generally self-resolving, and there is no specific antiviral therapy for Parvovirus B19. Therapy is supportive. If patients are experiencing arthralgias, then nonsteroidal anti-inflammatory drugs can be used. Patients with aplastic crises may need red blood cell transfusions depending on anemia severity. For pregnant women, fetal ultrasonography and monitoring are recommended.

Final comment: Parvovirus B19 is a common seasonal viral infection, and the "slapped cheek" exanthem is characteristic of the disease. It is generally self-limiting, but diagnosis is important, especially in those who are at high risk for developing complications from the infection.

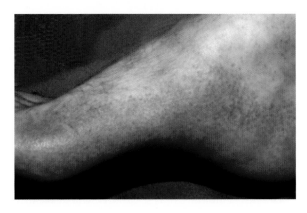

Figure 7.18 Papular-purpuric gloves and socks syndrome with erythema and petechiae on the foot.

Source: From Andrew's Diseases of the Skin, 13th edition, James WD, Elston DM, Treat JR, et al, Viral diseases, 362–420, Elsevier Inc (2020), used with permission.

COVID-19

Overview: Coronavirus disease 2019 (COVID-19) is a viral respiratory infection first reported in late 2019. It is caused by the novel coronavirus, severe acute respiratory syndrome coronavirus 2 (SARS-CoV-2). In 2020, COVID-19 was declared a pandemic by the World Health Organization. Systemic symptoms of COVID-19 range from asymptomatic to multi-organ failure or septic shock leading to death.

Clinical presentation: The most common presenting symptoms include fever, fatigue, shortness of breath, and dry cough. A wide range of skin manifestations of COVID-19 have been reported, including acral pernio-like lesions (i.e., "COVID toes"; Figure 7.19), erythema multiforme-like eruption, a maculopapular eruption (morbilliform and papulosquamous eruption), petechiae, urticaria, vesicles, livedo reticularis exanthem, vascular lesions (retiform [angulated] purpura and acro-ischemia; Figure 7.20), and hair loss (androgenetic alopecia and telogen effluvium).

Pernio-like red-purple macules/papules (i.e., "COVID toes") have been seen in young, healthy asymptomatic individuals and can present with pain/burning and/or pruritis (Figure 7.21). An erythema multiforme-like eruption can be seen in children with a milder course. In contrast, some children have presented with the serious multisystem inflammatory syndrome in children (MIS-C). MIS-C can resemble Kawasaki disease clinically with the main features of a viral exanthem and/or mucocutaneous involvement, myocardial dysfunction, hypotension, coagulopathy, and gastrointestinal upset. Other cutaneous COVID-19 presentations include a morbilliform, urticarial, petechial, vesicular eruption on the trunk and extremities and livedo reticularis. These often occur

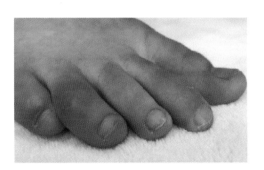

Figure 7.19 Acral edematous, erythematous, red-purple macules of a COVID-19 patient.

Source: From Freeman EE, McMahon DE, Lipoff JB, et al, The spectrum of COVID-19-associated dermatologic manifestations: an international registry of 716 patients from 31 countries, Journal of the American Academy of Dermatology, 83(4), 1118–1129 (2020), Elsevier Inc, used with permission.

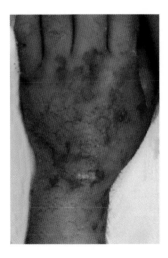

Figure 7.20 Netlike pattern of retiform purpura on the hand of a COVID-19 patient.

Source: From Freeman EE, McMahon DE, Lipoff JB, et al, The spectrum of COVID-19-associated dermatologic manifestations: an international registry of 716 patients from 31 countries, Journal of the American Academy of Dermatology, 83(4), 1118–1129 (2020), used with permission.

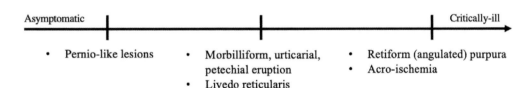

Figure 7.21 Severity of COVID-19 based on dermatologic manifestations.

after the onset of COVID-19 findings and are generally seen in moderately sick patients. Retiform (angulated) purpura on the extremities and buttocks at pressure sites and acro-ischemia have been seen in critically ill hospitalized patients. The retiform purpura and acro-ischemia mostly occur after other COVID-19 findings and are likely due to thrombotic disease/vasculopathy via activation of the complement pathway.

Laboratory studies: The diagnosis is confirmed by using reverse transcription PCR (RT-PCR) to detect SAR-CoV-2 RNA from nasopharyngeal/oropharyngeal swabs, tracheal aspirate, or bronchoalveolar lavage. Serologic studies can be utilized to detect SARS-CoV-2 antibodies in the blood, documenting a previous infection. Other abnormal serology findings include increased C-reactive protein, D-dimer, and ferritin. Characteristic computed tomography findings include ground-glass opacities in the lungs.

Differential diagnosis. The specificity of the current dermatologic manifestations of COVID-19 is not well understood, and many cutaneous findings are also present in many viral infections. However, skin findings may be one of the first signs of the infection, it is important to monitor other signs and symptoms that point to a COVID-19 diagnosis.

Management: Treatment of COVID-19 has been the target of many studies. Various treatments, including baricitinib and remdesivir, tocilizumab, antibody cocktails, and convalescent plasma therapy, are being investigated as potential therapeutic options. Corticosteroids have shown benefit in severely ill patients and Pfizer-BioNTech and Moderna messenger RNA vaccines have been authorized by the FDA to prevent COVID-19 by encoding the virus's spike protein. Anticoagulation is often initiated for hospitalized patients for venous thromboembolism prophylaxis and to treat patients with thrombotic cutaneous manifestations. For MIS-C, intravenous immunoglobulin and steroids are used as treatment.

The prognosis of the disease is worse in older adults or those with obesity or underlying medical conditions, such as chronic lung disease and diabetes. Major complications that can develop include acute respiratory distress syndrome, thromboembolic complications, and acute cardiac injury.

FINAL THOUGHT

The severe impact of COVID-19 has been observed worldwide, and further investigation will help to reveal more information about systemic and dermatologic manifestations of the disease as well as better treatments.

ADDITIONAL READINGS

Bolognia JL, Schaffer JV, Cerroni L, eds. Dermatology. 4th ed. Philadelphia: Elsevier; 2018. p. 1383–1446.

Calonje E, Brenn T, Lazar AJ, et al., eds. McKee's Pathology of the Skin. 5th ed. Philadelphia: Elsevier; 2020. p. 826–975.

Dinulos JGH. Habif's Clinical Dermatology. 7th ed. Philadelphia: Elsevier; 2021. p. 413–482.

Freeman EE, McMahon DE, Lipoff JB, et al. The spectrum of COVID-19-associated dermatologic manifestations: an international registry of 716 patients from 31 countries. J Am Acad Dermatol. 2020;83:1118–1129.

Gawkrodger DJ, Ardern-Jones MR. Dermatology: An Illustrated Colour Text. 6th ed. China: Elsevier Limited; 2017. p. 54–57.

James WD, Elston DM, Treat JR, et al. Andrew's Diseases of the Skin. 13th ed. Philadelphia: Elsevier; 2020. p. 362–420.

Jiang L, Tang K, Levin M, et al. COVID-19 and multisystem inflammatory syndrome in children and adolescents. Lancet. 2020;20:e276–88.

Pascarella G, Strumia A, Piliego C, et al. COVID-19 diagnosis and management: a comprehensive review. J Intern Med. 2020;288:192–206.

Piccolo V. Update on dermoscopy and infectious skin diseases. Dermatol Pract Concept. 2020;10:e2020003.

Wollina U, Karadag AS, Rowland-Payne C, et al. Cutaneous signs in COVID-19 patients: a review. Dermatol Ther. 2020;33:e13549.

Wolverton S, Wu J, eds. Comprehensive Dermatologic Drug Therapy. 4th ed. Philadelphia: Elsevier; 2021. p. 114–125.

8 Fungal Infections

Uwe Wollina, Pietro Nenoff, Shyam Verma, and Uta-Christina Hipler

CONTENTS

SUPERFICIAL FUNGAL INFECTIONS

Candidosis

Definition: Cutaneous candidosis is a common skin disease caused by the yeast genus *Candida*, often associated with diabetes mellitus, wet occupational work, and neutropenia.

Overview: *Candida spp.* are common commensal organisms of the mouth mucous membranes and gut microbiota. The most common isolated species is *Candida albicans*, but the prevalence of *Candida spp.* varies considerably depending on geographic location. *C. albicans* is a ubiquitous, diploid, dimorphic yeast. In disseminated candidosis with maculopapular cutaneous lesions, *C. tropicalis* was dominant, while nodular and papular lesions were caused mainly by *C. krusei*. Preferred infected body areas are oral and genital mucosae and intertriginous skin (groins, axillae, submammary folds). In *Candida* paronychia and onychomycosis, *C. parapsilosis* represents the most frequently isolated causative agent.

Cutaneous candidosis appears as cutaneous granulomatous candidosis, maculopapular disseminated candidosis, erythema mycoticum infantile, erosio interdigitalis blastomycetica (EIB) affecting the third webspace of digits, *Candida* intertrigo, "diaper dermatitis," *Candida* cheilitis, candidal paronychia and onychia, and candida onychomycosis (see the following discussion and Figure 8.1).

Oral candidosis is characterized by whitish removable plaques, sometimes erosions, and erythema. *Candida* cheilitis (Perlèche) can be painful due to fissures and rhagades of the mouth angels.

Erosions, well-defined erythematous macules, and satellite lesions are typical for *Candida* intertrigo; sometimes, papules and pustules develop.

Clinical presentation: EIB most commonly consists of a central erythematous erosion surrounded by a rim of white macerated skin involving at least one interdigital webspace.

Candida paronychia is painful, with purulent discharge resembling bacterial infections.

In contrast to other forms of candidosis, vulvovaginal candidosis is a disease of immunocompetent and otherwise healthy women. It is very common during reproductive years and is characterized by vaginal itching, burning, pain, and redness, being accompanied by a vaginal discharge and cheesy odor (Figure 8.2).

DOI: 10.1201/9781003105268-8

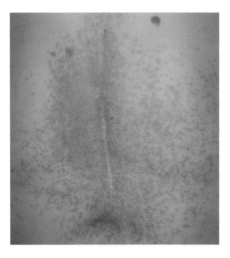

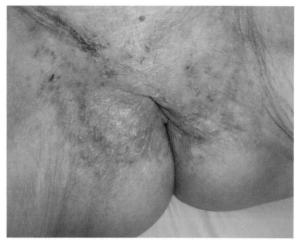

Figure 8.1 Candidosis in a patient with diabetes mellitus.

Figure 8.2 Candida vulvitis and peri-vulvitis in an elderly woman.

Chronic mucocutaneous candidosis (CMC) is characterized by recurrent or persistent symptomatic mucocutaneous infections caused by *Candida spp.*, affecting the (finger) nails, skin, oral cavity, and genital mucosa. Most cases of CMC are sporadic and secondary to medical conditions, including HIV infection, diabetes, immunosuppressive, or antimicrobial treatment. There are rare presentations due to a primary immunodeficiency associated with genetic disorders. In addition to cutaneous candidosis, mucosal-cutaneous, visceral, and disseminated infections can occur.

Differential diagnosis: This may include (irritant) contact dermatitis, erythrasma, inverse psoriasis, bacterial infection (i.e., impetigo), and leukoplakia (mucosal lesions).

The diagnosis is made by clinical examination in addition to scrapings and fungal culture. For confirmation, skin scrapings, hair, or nail clippings obtained with sterile instruments dissolved with 20% KOH for 20 minutes, may show characteristic round and elongated yeast cells and filamentous cells due to dimorphism. The area used for diagnosis should be cleansed with 70% alcohol to avoid bacterial overgrowth in culture.

Management: Topical treatment by azole drugs (econazole, clotrimazole, ketoconazole, miconazole, sertaconazole), ciclopirox amine, or polyene antifungal drugs (nystatin, amphotericin B, natamycin) are effective. In case of mucosal infections or chronic mucocutaneous candidosis, oral treatment with itraconazole 100–200 mg/day and fluconazole 100–400 mg/day is recommended. Primary drug resistance to fluconazole has been recorded with some *C. albicans spp.*, *C. krusei*, *C. dubliniensis*, *C. glabrata*, and *C. auris*. Second-line treatment consists of voriconazole and posaconazole.

Dermatophytosis

Synonyms: Tinea, ringworm

Definition: Tinea is a superficial infection of skin, hair, and nail due to dermatophytes. Both anthropophilic species and zoophilic species can be responsible. Infection due to geophilic fungi is rare.

Clinical presentation: This is often made clinically. For confirmation, skin scrapings, hair, or nail clippings dissolved with 20% KOH for 20 minutes may show characteristic spores and/or hyphae (Table 8.1). Fluorescence microscopy with calcofluor white allows quick identification of dermatophytes in skin or nail scrapings.

Cultures on Sabouraud's medium can take up to 3 weeks to grow out and may be positive in only about 75% of cultures. Macromorphology, color, and microscopy of colonies are used for species identification (Figure 8.3). Recently, real-time polymerase chain reaction (PCR) or PCR-microarray for dermatophyte DNA detection have become available for a quick diagnosis based on genomic Sanger sequencing of the internal transcribed spacer (ITS) region and the translation elongation factor (TEF)-1α gene.

Table 8.1 Common Species in Dermatophytosis

Species	Clinical Presentations
Antropophilic fungi	
• *Trichophyton rubrum*	Tinea capitis, corporis and pubogenitalis, palmo-plantar skin, scaling ringworm lesions, Majocchi's granuloma, onychomycosis, "two feet–one hand" syndrome
• *T. soudanense*	Tinea capitis—black dot pattern, scaling ringworm lesions on the body, endothrix hair infection, onychomycosis,
• *T. interdigitale*	Tinea capitis, corporis, cruris, and pedis, plus onychomycosis
• *T. tonsurans*	Tinea capitis and barbae with endothrix hair infection, rarely bullous lesions, tinea pedis, highly infectious
• *Epidermophyton floccosum*	Tinea corporis, cruris and capitis have become rare
• *Microsporum audouinii*	Tinea capitis in children, moth-eaten pattern, ectothrix hair infection
Zoophilic species	
• *T. mentagrophytes*	Highly variable ringworm lesions, tinea barbae, tinea genitalis profunda, "Indian" type with terbinafine- and/or fluconazole-resistance
• *T. benhamiae*	Tinea capitis and corporis in children, pubogenital tinea, deep abscessing mycosis
• *T. verrucosum*	Highly inflammatory lesions, pustules, plaques often also lymphadenopathy, tinea capitis, barbae, faciei and corporis, endothrix hair infection, sometimes life-threating
• *T. violaecum*	Tinea capitis in children of either seborrhoeic pattern, "black dot" and "gray patch" type, or highly inflammatory Kerion Celsi, endothrix hair infection
• *T. equinum*	Tinea capitis and corporis with scaling ringworm lesions, onychomycosis
• *T. erinacei*	Tinea faciei and corporis, scaly erythematous partly erosive lesions, seropapules, bullae, crusts
• *M. canis*	Tinea capitis, facei, corporis, cruris, and pedis, scaling ringworm lesions, ectothrix hair infection
• *M. ferrugineum*	Tinea capitis, gray patch pattern, seldom Majocchi's granuloma
Geophilic fungi	
• *Nannizzia gypsea*	Tinea manus and pedis, scaling ringworm lesions
• *N. praecox*	Mainly seen in equestrians, tinea corporis with ringworm lesions
• *N. incurvata*	Favus and tinea corporis

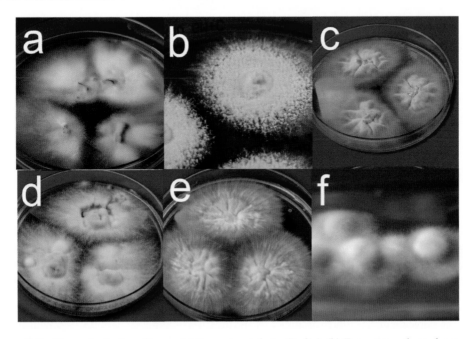

Figure 8.3 Dermatophyte cultures: (a) *T. mentagrophytes* (India), (b) *T. mentagrophytes* from tinea corporis, (c) *T. benhamiae* from tinea genitalis, (d) *T. tonsurans*, (e) *M. canis*, and (f) *T. rubrum* (Sabauroud agar).

Tinea Corporis

Clinical presentation: Patients commonly present with itchy, erythematous circular or ovoid patches and plaques on the exposed skin. These annular lesions demonstrate sharp margins with a raised erythematous scaly edge which may contain vesicles. The lesions advance centrifugally from a core, leaving a central clearing and mild residual scaling, giving rise to the term "ringworm" (Figure 8.4). When a deep purulent folliculitis forms, often on the legs, this granulomatous infection, usually due to *T. rubrum*, is called Majocchi's granuloma.

T. rubrum is the most common species worldwide. Differential diagnoses include atopic dermatitis, irritant, and allergic contact dermatitis, seborrheic dermatitis, and psoriasis.

In circumscribed cases, topical treatment with either clotrimazole 1%, miconazole 2%, ciclopirox olamine 1%, or terbinafine 1% applied topically twice daily or with ketoconazole 2%, naftifine 1% is possible. Larger areas, multiple lesions, and more severe inflamed tinea should be treated orally. A *T. mentagrophytes* "Indian ITS genotype VIII" has been identified as responsible for a chronic-relapsing and therapy-refractory superficial dermatophytosis on the Indian subcontinent with terbinafine-resistance and partial resistance to itraconazole and voriconazole. Currently, this new *T. mentagrophytes* Type VIII is spreading worldwide.

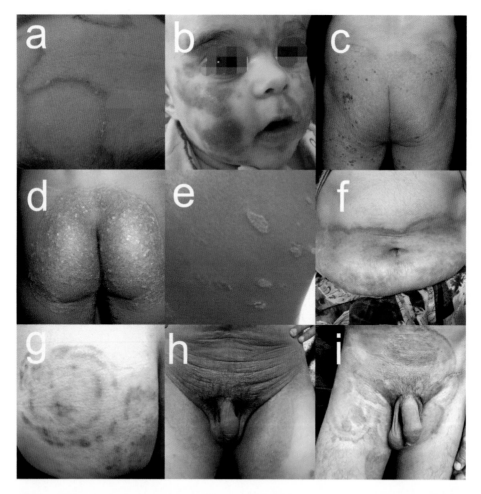

Figure 8.4 (a) Tinea faciei on the forehead. (b) Highly inflammatory tinea faciei in a toddler treated initially as atopic dermatitis (tinea incognito). (c) and (d) Tinea corporis of the buttocks demonstrating the tendency to hyperpigmentation in darker skin types. (e) Tinea corporis in skin type V. (f) Tinea corporis with elevated hyperpigmented margin. (g)–(i) Tinea pseudoimbricata with concentric rings. (h) Heavy hyperpigmentation and infiltration due to misuse of topical corticosteroids.

Tinea Manuum

Clinical presentation: Ringworm of the hands is less common than tinea pedis. It presents with erythema and mild scaling on the dorsal aspect of the hands or as chronic, dry, scaly hyperkeratosis of the palms. When the palms are infected, the feet are also commonly involved. The most common fungus is *T. rubrum*. A typical pattern of involvement is either one hand (mostly the left) and both feet are also known as two-feet-one-hand-syndrome.

Tinea Pedis

Synonym: Athlete's foot

Clinical presentation: This represents the most common dermatophyte infection. It is usually related to hyperhidrosis and the use of occlusive footwear. Middle-aged men are most frequently affected. The infection often presents as white, macerated areas in the third or fourth toe webs (Figure 8.5). The "moccasin type" occurs on the dorsal surface of the foot or as chronic dry, scaly hyperkeratosis of the soles and heels due to *T. rubrum* infection. It may be associated with vesicles. Vesicles often found on the palms, known as an id reaction, are infrequent today.

Tinea Cruris

Synonym: Jock itch

Clinical presentation: This is a superficial fungal infection of the genital, pubic, perineal, and perianal skin that affects about 20% of the world population. It is caused by dermatophytes of the three genera *Trichophyton*, *Epidermophyton*, and *Microsporum*, with *Trichophyton spp.* being the most common. Risk factors include excessive perspiration, occlusive clothing, improper hygiene, diabetes mellitus, immunocompromised status, and lower socioeconomic status. Clinical presentation is symmetrical with the development of well-defined erythematous, slightly itching lesions with elevated scaling borders.

Differential diagnosis: This includes intertrigo, seborrheic dermatitis, flexural psoriasis, and erythrasma. In recent years, tinea profouna of the genital area has been seen more often due to genital shaving, so bacterial infections and hidradenitis suppurativa should be considered.

Tinea Capitis

Clinical presentation: This is highly variable depending on the fungal species and immune status of the host. Zoophilic *Microsporum canis* and anthropophilic *T. tonsurans* are the most common species. The infection of the hair shaft can be either ectothrix (*M. canis* and *M. audouinii*), which

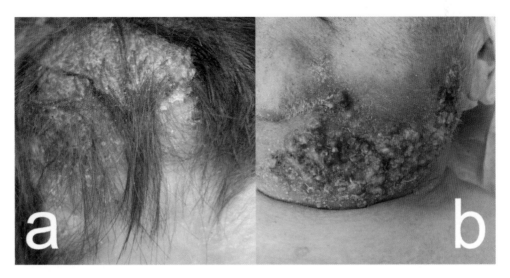

Figure 8.5 (a) Kerion celsi due to *T. mentagrophytes var. asteroids*; (b) purulent tinea barbae due to *T. verrucosum*.

Source: From Wollina et al. (2018), used with permission.

fluoresce with the Wood's light, or endothrix (*T. tonsurans, T. violaceum, T. soudanense*). In the latter case, the hair cuticle remains intact, but the inner part is filled with spores leading to the black-dot ringworm appearance on dermatoscopy. A moth-eaten pattern can be caused by *M. audouinii* or *T. violaceum*. Endothrix infections are less immunogenic and sometimes asymptomatic. Scaling may be psoriasiform.

Microsporum-caused tinea capitis is a non-purulent hair follicle infection causing a greenish fluorescence under Wood light. The hair shafts break, leaving round-shaped lesions of very short hair covered by a wheat-dust-like scaling (gray patch tinea). In dermatoscopy, comma hairs (Caucasians, Asians) or corkscrew hairs (Africans) are observed.

Ringworm infections of the deep follicles cause follicular pustules and massive purulent secretions, fever, and lymph node swellings (Kerion Celsi; Figure 8.5a). Bacterial infections should be ruled out.

Treatment: Delayed treatment of deep follicular ringworm of the scalp can lead to scarring alopecia. Treatment has to be systemic, and topical antifungal preparations should not be used. Terbinafine is effective against *Trichophyton spp.*, itraconacole and griseofulvin are more effective against *Microsporum spp./Nannizzia spp.* The initial treatment should be prescribed for at least 4 weeks.

Tinea Barbae

Clinical presentation: This type of dermatophyte infection of the beard area is generally seen in men (Figure 8.5b). Transmission of the zoophilic fungi leads to deep follicular infections with pronounced inflammation. This is usually due to contact with infected dogs or cats. Oral antifungals are warranted.

Tinea Unguis

Synonym: Onychomycosis

Clinical presentation: This is the most common nail disorder. Risk factors include age, peripheral vascular disease, diabetes, and systemic immunosuppression, but tinea ungium may occur in many patients, in whom the toes nails have thickening, disintegration, color changes, and hardening (Figure 8.6). Onychomycosis can be due to infection with dermatophytes (tinea unguis, in about 80% of cases), molds, or yeasts. Onychomycosis occasionally may be a risk factor for bacterial soft tissue infections.

Differential diagnosis: This includes traumatic nail dystrophy and nail psoriasis.

Management: This should be with oral antifungal agents for approximately 2 months for fingernails and 3 months for toenails. Fingernails take 6 months to grow out, and toenails, 9 months.

Tinea Incognito

Overview: Tinea incognito is a misnomer for steroid modified atypical ringworm caused by inappropriate use of topical and sometimes systemic corticosteroids. This can lead to chronic widespread and occasionally deep cutaneous tinea with delayed diagnosis and treatment.

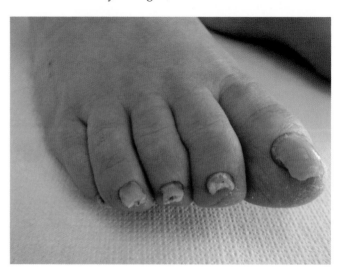

Figure 8.6 Toenail onychomycosis due to *T. rubrum* infection.

Tinea Versicolor

Synonym: TV, pityriasis versicolor

Clinical presentation: This occurs worldwide with the highest prevalence of about 50% in tropical regions. It represents a superficial cutaneous infection more frequently seen in adolescents and young adults. Clinical features include either hyperpigmented or hypopigmented finely scaly macules on the trunk, neck, and arms (Figure 8.7). The causative agent is *Malassezia spp.*, which is the most abundant fungus on many human skin sites.

Laboratory studies: Fourteen species have been identified including *M. globosa*, *M. restricta*, and *M. sympodialis*. Because they are part of the normal skin microbiome, the condition may recur.

The diagnosis is made clinically. In doubtful cases, examination by Wood light (coppery-orange fluorescence) and microscopic examination of scales with 20% potassium hydroxide may be helpful. The latter can be stained by ink blue to provide a better contrast to identify grape-like clusters of yeast cells and middle long hyphae. Curiously, patients with juicy ear wax are more prone to this condition.

Differential diagnosis: This includes vitiligo, tinea corporis, nummular and seborrheic dermatitis, and psoriasis.

Management: Treatment is most effective with fluconazole 150 mg or itraconazole 200 mg given once weekly for 5 weeks. The scaling disappears in about a month and the pigmentation in about 5 months. Pigmentary changes are caused by the fungus, which is generating Trp-derived indole pigments by transaminase 1 (TAM 1). Cycloserine is a TAM inhibitor capable to inhibit pigment production in vitro. The condition can recur annually for upward of 20 years.

Deep Skin and Soft Tissue Fungal Infections

Overview: These are uncommon. Systemic immunosuppression including HIV-infection is the major risk factor. These, sometimes life-threatening, infections are seen more in tropical and subtropical regions of the world. Systemic endemic mycoses occur after the inhalation of fungal spores, while the cutaneous endemic mycoses enter the host via traumatic inoculation into the skin. For treatment, see Table 8.2.

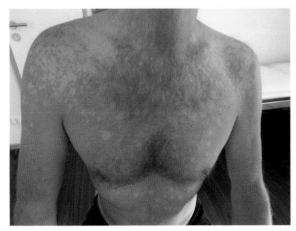

Figure 8.7   Tinea versicolor.

Table 8.2 **Treatment of Deep and Soft Tissue Mycosis**

Disease	First-Line Treatment	Second-Line Treatment
Cryptococcosis	up to 400 mg fluconazole/ once a day	0.7 mg amphotericin B/kg/d
Histoplasmosis	3 × 200 mg itraconazole/d	amphotericin B, in HIV patients liposomal amphotericine B (higher response rate)
Blastomycosis	itraconazole, fluconazole, and posaconazole	amphotericin B
Paracoccidioido-mycosis	itraconazole	trimethoprim- sulfamethoxazole, voriconazole, amphotericin B

Cryptococcosis

Overview: Cryptococcosis is caused by two yeasts: *Cryptococcus neoformans* and *Cryptococcus gattii*.

Clinical presentation: The mucocutaneous form is the result of the spread of infection from other foci in patients with disseminated disease. It presents as subcutaneous papules and nodules on the face and neck, with a preference for patients with advanced AIDS.

Histoplasmosis

Overview: Histoplasmosis is an endemic mycosis caused by *Histoplasma capsulatum*.

Clinical presentation: Demolition, construction, working with bird or bat droppings, and farming have been associated with an increased risk of infection. Endemic areas include Central and South America, the western United States, and southern Mexico. There may be disseminated papules, ulcers, and crusts, especially in immunocompromised patients.

Laboratory studies: Direct examination of Giemsa-stained tissue specimens will show characteristic intracellular yeast forms surrounded by a halo simulating a capsule. The fungi can be isolated in body fluids and tissue specimens for culture. Identification is also possible by molecular techniques, including PCR analysis of fungal DNA.

North American Blastomycosis

Synonym: Gilchrist's disease

Clinical presentation: Blastomycosis is caused by a dimorphic fungus endemic in soil with a high prevalence in the Midwest of the United States. The asexual form is known as *Blastomyces dermatitidis*, while the sexual phase is called *Ajellomyces dermatitidis*. Primary cutaneous blastomycosis is rare, while secondary spread to the skin by pulmonary blastomycosis is seen in up to 30% of patients. North American cutaneous blastomycosis typically evolves from papules that develop into crusted, vegetative plaques often with central clearing or ulceration. Lymphangitis and lymphadenopathy may be present. It occurs also in immunocompetent patients and can be diagnosed by culture, direct visualization of the yeast in affected tissue by silver or periodic acid Schiff (PAS) stains and/or antigen testing.

South American Blastomycosis

Synonym: Paracoccidioidomycosis

Clinical presentation: This is a chronic or subacute granulomatous endemic systemic mycosis, caused by *Paracoccidioides brasiliensis* and *Paracoccidioides lutzii* in South America. Risk factors include lymphoma, organ transplantation, and HIV infection. *P. brasiliensis* affects mucous membranes of the mouth and nose, causing ulceration with subsequent spreading through the lymphatic system. Nodular cutaneous lesions occur that can become necrotic or result in subcutaneous cold abscesses (Figure 8.8).

Laboratory studies: The diagnosis is established by the growth of *P. brasiliensis* in culture. Early identification can be established from infected tissue specimen stained with silver methenamine or PAS stains, showing budding yeasts that resemble a "mariner's wheel" or from secretions treated with calcofluor white.

Differential diagnosis: This includes leishmaniasis, sporotrichosis, histoplasmosis, tuberculosis, non-Hodgkin's lymphoma, and vasculitis.

OTHERS

Other deep skin and soft tissue fungal infections are shown on Table 8.3, and relatively common ones are described in the section.

Sporotrichosis

Clinical presentation: This is a subacute or chronic infection caused by dimorphic fungi. Lymphocutaneous sporotrichosis starts as a painless purple or blackish nodule on exposed skin that erodes into a small ulcer (sporotrichotic chancre) with swollen edges, a painful granulomatous center, and minimal discharge. This is followed by lymphangitis with secondary nodules along the line of lymphatic drainage that can progress to ulcers (sporotrichoid spread). Fixed sporotrichosis characterized by the presence of a solitary lesion. The disease is limited and presents as a slow growing verrucous plaque.

Chromoblastomycosis or chromomycosis is a chronic polymorphic fungal infection of the skin and subcutaneous tissue. It is caused by several species of melanized or dematiaceous fungi,

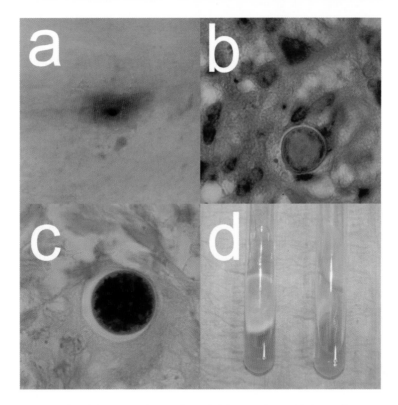

Figure 8.8   Paracoccidioidomycosis due to *Coccidioides posadassii*: (a) Secondary cutaneous manifestation on the abdominal skin; (b) histology overview; (c) spherules of *Coccidioides posadasii*—detail (hematoxylin-eosin × 130); (d) culture of *Coccidioides posadasii* on Sabouraud agar after 10 days incubation.

Source: From Wollina U, Hansel G, Vennewald I, et al. Successful treatment of relapsing disseminated coccidioidomycosis with cutaneous involvement with posaconazole. J Dtsch Dermatol Ges. 2009;7(1):46–9. doi: 10.1111/j.1610–0387.2008.06863.x. PMID: 18759738. Used with permission.

Table 8.3 Other Deep Skin and Soft Tissue Fungal Infections

Disease	Most Common Fungal Species	Remarks
Sporotrichosis	*Sporothrix schenckii*	Lymphocutaneous disease >75%, Fixed disease <25%
Chromoblastomycosis *Fonsecaea spp., Cladophialophora*	Posttraumatic	*carrionii*
Mycetoma	Aerobic filamentous bacteria	Actinomycetoma
	Madurella mycetomatis,	Eumycetoma
	M. pseudomycetomatis, M. fahalii,	
	M. tropicana, Trematosphaeria grisea,	
	Medicopsis romeroi	
Phaeohypomycosis	*Exophiala spp., Bipolaris spp.,*	Solitary skin lesions
	Curvularia spp., Pleurophomopsis spp.,	
	Phaeoacremonium spp., Alternaria spp.	
Coccidioidomycosis	*Coccidioides immitis* and *Coccidioides*	*posadasii*
Mucormycosis	Mucorales (*Rhizopus, Lichtheimia, Mucor,* and *Rhizomucor*) and *Entomophthorales* (*Basidiobolus* and *Conidiobolus*)	Potentially deadly
Lacaziosis	*Lacazia loboi*	Keloid-like lesions
Talaromycosis	*Talaromyces (Penicillium) marneffei*	Single or multiple nodules

which produce a dark pigment. The fungus penetrates the skin through a skin injury. About 4–8 weeks later, a papule develops that progresses to a slow-growing warty nodule.

Mycetoma is a chronic localized infection caused by several species of fungi and bacteria after local injury. Early lesions are painless and start from a hard nodule that spreads slowly to produce papules and sinuses that discharge fluid containing granules on to the skin surface.

Phaeohyphomycosis

Clinical presentation: This is a heterogeneous group of mycoses caused by dark-walled (dematiaceous) fungi found in organic debris. Following a local injury, patients develop a slow-growing solitary lesion such as a cyst, a nodule, a plaque, or an abscess on the extremities.

The cutaneous lesions of coccidioidomycosis can present as papules, pustules, abscesses, ulcers, and erythema nodosum among others.

Mucormycosis is caused by *Zygomycetes* in immunocompromised but sometimes even in immunocompetent patients. The most common presentation is rhinocerebral mucormycosis.

Lacaziosis (lobomycosis) is a rare chronic granulomatous fungal infection of the skin and subcutaneous tissues found in Central and South America.

Talaromycosis is endemic in tropical and subtropical regions in Southeast Asia and southern China and has become more frequent among HIV infected patients worldwide. Skin involvement with (verrucous) plaques, nodules, abscesses, and granulomas is frequent.

FINAL THOUGHT

Fungal infections are commonly seen worldwide and in all ages. They represent and important differential diagnosis to bacterial infections and chronic inflammatory dermatoses. The spectrum of fungal infections ranges from superficial cutaneous to deep skin and soft tissue infections and systemic, potentially life-threatening disorders. The knowledge of clinical presentation and laboratory diagnosis is crucial to diagnose these diseases and to initiate the appropriate treatment.

ADDITIONAL READINGS

Carrasco-Zuber JE, Navarrete-Dechent C, Bonifaz A, et al. Alarming India-wide phenomenon of antifungal resistance in dermatophytes: a multicentre study. Mycoses. 2020;10:717–728.

Carrasco-Zuber JE, Navarrete-Dechent C, Bonifaz A, et al. Cutaneous involvement in the deep mycoses: a review. Part II—systemic mycoses. Actas Dermosifiliogr. 2016;107:816–822.

Mauriziano D. Cutaneous involvement in the deep mycoses: a literature review. Part I—subcutaneous mycoses. Actas Dermosifiliogr. 2016;107:806–815.

Mayser P, Nenoff P, Reinel D, et al. S1 guidelines: tinea capitis. J Dtsch Dermatol Ges. 2020;18:161–179.

Nenoff P, Krüger C, Schaller J, et al. Mycology—an update. Part 2: dermatomycoses: clinical picture and diagnostics. J Dtsch Dermatol Ges. 2014;12:749–777.

Nenoff P, van de Sande WWJ, Fahal A, et al. Eumycetoma and actinomycetoma—an update on causative agents, epidemiology, pathogenesis, diagnostics and therapy. J Eur Acad Dermatol Venereol. 2015;29:1873–1883.

Nenoff P, Verma SB, Uhrlaß S, et al. A clarion call for preventing taxonomical errors of dermatophytes using the example of the novel Trichophyton mentagrophytes genotype VIII uniformly isolated in the Indian epidemic of superficial dermatophytosis. Mycoses. 2019;62:6–10.

Verma SB, Vasani R. Male genital dermatophytosis—clinical features and the effects of the misuse of topical steroids and steroid combinations—an alarming problem in India. Mycoses. 2016;59:606–614.

White TC, Findley K, Dawson TL Jr, et al. Fungi on the skin: dermatophytes and Malassezia. Cold Spring Harb Perspect Med. 2014;4:a019802.

Wollina U, Nenoff P, Haroske G, et al. The diagnosis and treatment of nail disorders. Dtsch Arztebl Int. 2016;113:509–518.

9 Infestations and Bites

Sam Allen

CONTENTS

Infestations and bites are common worldwide, particularly in children and areas of overcrowding. They generally cause physical nuisance, but some may even transmit serious vector-borne diseases.

SCABIES

Synonyms: Scabies mite, itch mite

Definition: The skin condition associated with scabies is caused by the reaction to fomite products of the female scabies mite or itch mite (*Sarcoptes scabiei, Acarus hominis*), as she burrows under the skin of an affected human host to lay her eggs. The hallmark of the disease is an unbearable itch.

Overview: Disease transmission is by direct and close skin-to-skin contact with an infested individual, which typically requires at least 20 minutes. The incubation period following contact is about 3 weeks, but once sensitized, subsequent infestations can cause symptoms and signs within a few days.

Clinical presentation: The clinical features of scabies infestation are an intense itch and focal patches of excoriated, eczema-like skin. Itching is typically worse at night. Scaling, oozing, and crusting are common (Figures 9.1–9.3), as is dermatitis artefacta from scratching.

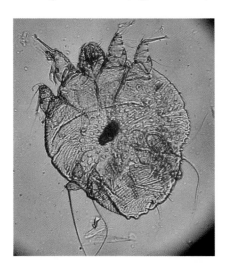

Figure 9.1 Scabies mite (*Sarcoptes scabiei*).

Source: From Wikipedia, under Creative Commons license.

DOI: 10.1201/9781003105268-9

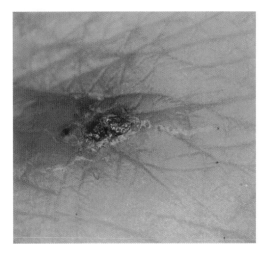

Figure 9.2 Scabies burrow and hill.

Source: From D@nDerm, used with permission.

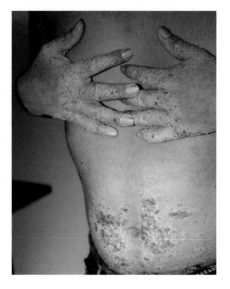

Figure 9.3 Crusted scabies.

The classic primary lesion is comprised of a whitish 2–15-mm linear or serpiginous scabies "burrow" that ends in a miniature "hill." The distribution is typically bilateral with a predilection for the palms, wrists, interdigital web spaces, under watch straps, flexural creases at the elbows and knees, axillae, areola of the breast, the lower part of the abdomen, the penis and scrotum, the buttock folds, ankles, sides of feet, and soles. Rarely, there may be bullae.

The back is usually spared. Scabies does not affect the head and neck, except in children, the elderly, or immunocompromised.

CRUSTED SCABIES

Synonym: Norwegian scabies

Overview: Scabies hyper-infection occurs in persons with impaired cell-mediated immunity, such as patients with HIV, on immunosuppressive therapy (e.g., post–organ transplant), and with Down's syndrome and in the elderly, often nursing home residents. These patients may have a very high mite load, causing widespread crusted mange-like skin, now known as crusted scabies.

Clinical presentation: Clinical suspicion is key to diagnosis, as the pathognomonic scabies burrows are not always present. Social history with an inquiry into affected family members or other residents and employees of an extended care facility are important clues.

Laboratory studies: The diagnosis is confirmed by identifying the *Sarcoptes scabiei* mite or its eggs or scabala from mineral oil skin scrapings or biopsy by using cyanoacrylate glue. Clinical response to empiric treatment suffices as indirect evidence of scabies.

Differential diagnosis: Dermatitis herpetiformis, dermatitis, ichthyosis, and contact dermatitis may be considered.

Management: Treatment of scabies requires attention to the patient, their close contacts, and any shared clothing, towels, and bedding. All family members in close contact and/or recent sexual contacts should be treated at the same time.

Topical treatments are applied to all areas of skin from the neck downward and left on as per instruction before washing off. Taking a hot bath before the application of lotion will facilitate drug delivery if the patient only bathes infrequently. Repeating the treatment after 7–10 days can ensure eradication of mites that have newly hatched. Oral antihistamines, such as hydroxyzine 25 mg every 6–8 hours, may be used to reduce intense itching.

Course and/or prognosis: To break the cycle of infection, close contacts should be treated as deemed necessary. Clothing and bedding should be machine washed using the hot cycle. Itching is gradually reduced but may not disappear until a week or longer after treatment.

Table 9.1 Treatments for Scabies

Agent	Percentage	Comments
Permethrin	5.0	first line, leave on for 8–12 hours
Malathion	0.5	second-line treatment, leave on for 8–12 hours
Crotamiton	10	leave on overnight for 2 consecutive nights, anti-pruritic effect
Monosulfiram	20	disulfiram-like reaction with alcohol
Ivermectin	12 mg	single dose, treats adult mites and eggs, necessary for crusted scabies, repeat after 7–10 days

PEDICULOSIS

Synonyms: Lice, crabs, vagabond's disease

Definition: Human lice are obligate parasites that live externally off their human hosts. Three types are affecting the head (head louse, *Pediculus humanus* var *capitis*), body (body louse, *Pediculus humanus* var *corporis*), and pubis (pubic or crab louse, *Pthirus pubis*), which are morphologically different.

Overview: Human louse-borne disease has been a scourge of humankind throughout history. It is often associated with poverty and war.

Head Lice

Synonym: pediculosis capitis

Overview: Head lice (Figure 9.4) are common in children. The female louse can live up to a month. She can lay up to 8 nits a day that are visible as 0.8- by 0.3-mm yellow-white pouches attached to the hair shaft. The nits hatch after 1 week, and after three further molts, they become adults 7–10 days later. Viable eggs are located within 6 mm of the scalp.

Clinical presentation: The most common symptom is itching of the scalp. The adult louse is about the size of a sesame seed and resembles moving dandruff. Scratching can result in excoriations and secondary infection.

Laboratory studies: Diagnosis is made by examination for identification of living lice by observation or combing with a stiff comb. Most nits can be found on the occiput or postauricular area.

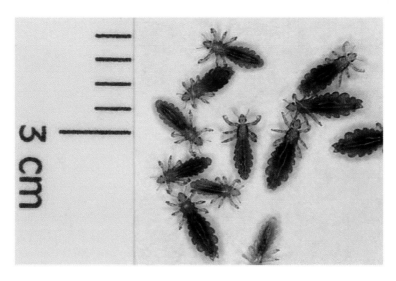

Figure 9.4   Head lice (*Pediculosis capitis*) and Nits.

Source: From D@nDerm, used with permission.

Live nits are white, while dead ones that have been treated are gray. Empty shells may remain in situ after the larvae have hatched. Careful examination is required, as 75% of infested scalps often have fewer than 10 lice.

Differential diagnosis: This condition might be called moving dandruff.

Management: Treatment is by application of a pediculicide shampoo. Siblings and playmates of children should be examined and treated. Treatment is not active against eggs and so should be repeated after 7–10 days to eradicate newly hatched nymphs. Caps and clothing coming in contact with the head should be washed in hot water.

Wet combing (i.e., passing a fine-toothed nit comb through wet hair) has gained popularity due to concerns about the chemical toxicity of pediculicidal agents.

Course: Prior exposure does not confer protective immunity. Family members and close contact should be treated at the same time, and the school notified. Some school districts insist on the child being nit-free before returning.

Final comment: The head louse is an embarrassment, but it is not associated with transmitting any disease.

Body Lice

Synonym: Pediculosis corporis

Overview: Human body louse due to *Pediculosis corporis* (Figure 9.5) is transmitted from person to person during conditions of overcrowding and poor hygiene. The adult louse is normally found in the seams of clothing and only transfer to the human body to take a blood meal, which it does several times a day. Body lice frequently lay eggs on clothing fibers on or near the seams.

The body louse is the vector for epidemic typhus (due to bacteria *Rickettsia prowazekii*), relapsing fever (due to *Borrelia recurrentis*), and trench fever (due to *Bartonella quintana*).

Clinical presentation: Itching with few skin signs is typical in the early stages. There may be minor excoriations or bluish marks (maculae cerulea), where the louse has fed. The later-stage disease is characterized by a feeling of lousiness (literally, covered in lice) and eczematous lichenification.

Laboratory studies: Body lice are 1–3 mm long, flattened dorsoventrally, and appear whitish-grey or with a reddish hue after feeding. The biology of the body louse is otherwise similar to that of the head louse.

Differential diagnosis: Scabies and scurvy may mimic excoriations caused by the body louse.

Management: Although the body louse does not live on the body, the use of a pediculicide is often recommended. Clothing and bedding should be machine washed under the hot cycle or destroyed.

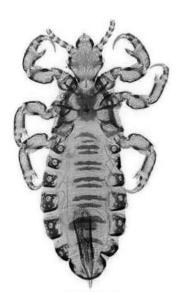

Figure 9.5 Body louse (*Pediculosis corporis*).

Source: From Vincent S Smith in Reed DL et al., Genetic Analysis of Lice Supports Direct Contact between Modern and Archaic Humans, PLoS Biology 2/11, e340, used under Creative Commons license.

Pubic Lice

Synonym: Pediculosis pubis, crabs

Overview: The crab louse (Figure 9.6) is easily differentiated by its short, broad abdomen and serrated front claws, which enable it to cling to flat, hairless surfaces and navigate over the entire skin surface, often at night and not as fast as the head louse. Crab lice are typically transmitted sexually, often in association with other sexually transmitted diseases.

Clinical presentation: Crab lice are adapted to pubic hair, but they may also be found on the beard and axillary hair. In children and less so in adults, crab louse nits are sometimes found on the eyelashes.

Management: Treatment is the same with pediculicides. Sometimes, the nits need to be manually removed, especially from the eyelids. Shaving the affected hair-bearing areas can be helpful.

Final comment: Periodically, pediculicides are said to have developed resistance, but this is usually not confirmed. Ivermectin is a viable therapeutic alternative.

MITES

Demodex Mite

Definition: Demodicosis is caused by sensitivity to the human mite *Demodex folliculorum*.

Overview: The human mite, *D. folliculorum*, can be found on nearly every adult human nose. It is often associated with folliculitis and may cause focal hair loss. Whether it is the cause of rosacea has never been proved.

Clinical presentation:*D. folliculorum* can cause folliculitis on the nose and cheeks with itching and redness. Demodicosis of the eyelids may cause congestion and lead to blepharitis.

Management: It is readily treated with topical or oral ivermectin. Metronidazole, permethrin, benzoyl benzoate, crotamiton, lindane, and sulfur creams may also be effective.

Cheyletiella Mite

Overview: Animal mange caused by Cheyletiella from dogs, cats, and rabbits may be transmitted to humans, but as humans are not a natural host, clinical manifestations will disappear within 3 weeks without treatment.

Clinical presentation: Cheyletiella dermatitis produces multiple itchy red bumps on the arms, trunk, and buttocks.

Laboratory studies: Under the microscope: Demodex mites can be seen using the 4× objective lens; however, the 10× lens enhances the ease of detection for both eggs and mites.

Differential diagnosis: Scabies, dermatitis from any cause.

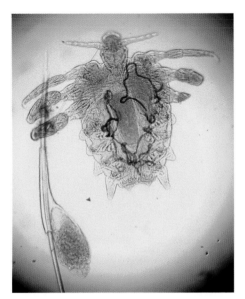

Figure 9.6 Pubic louse (*Pediculosis Pubis*).

Source: Courtesy of Michael Wunderli, from EoL.org, used under Creative Commons license.

Canine scabies infestation causes crusting and scabbing on the ears of dogs. *Sarcoptes scabiei* var. *canis* does not live on humans, but it may cause intense itching and blotchy redness where the dog has rubbed against the arms or abdomen of the owner.

Management: Pets should be treated with a suitable pesticide and kept apart. Because the mite does not live on the human, a topical steroid, such as triamcinolone 0.1% cream applied bid, should clear the skin.

Course: Demodex infestation of the eyelids can lead to chronic blepharitis. Warm eye compress, topical tea tree oil, and antibiotic ointment may be used as part of the daily eye cleansing routine.

BEDBUGS

Synonym: Cimicosis

Definition: Local skin reaction following blood meal of the common bed bug (*Cimex lectularius*).

Overview: Bedbug (*C. lectularius*) bites usually occur on the trunk or legs as pruritic, round, erythematous macules (Figure 9.7). The arthropod molts five times in its life cycle.

Clinical presentation: The groupings, often of three, are called "breakfast, lunch, and dinner." The bedbug is a nocturnal feeder and usually resides in cracks in plaster walls or elsewhere in the bedroom. It is often transmitted by suitcases or purses from one place to another.

Management: A topical steroid, such as triamcinolone 0.1% cream applied bid should clear the skin. The room and preferably the entire house should be fumigated with an insecticide. An alternative is raising the room temperature to 113°F/45°C for 1 hour.

BEE, WASP AND HORNET STING

Definition: This is the envenomation from the stinger of a flying insect into the skin.

Overview: A wasp (*synonym:* yellow jacket) and hornet sting produces an immediate, sudden, intense pain followed by a dull, throbbing pain with swelling and erythema. A larger area of swelling, erythema, and pain may remain around the bite site for up to 1 week in some individuals due to local allergic reactions. A more serious systemic reaction is anaphylaxis, which results in a shock reaction (i.e., precipitous fall in blood pressure, rapid shallow breathing, and weak pulse) that is a medical emergency. Warning signs of anaphylaxis are tingling in the throat, dizziness, respiratory difficulty, facial swelling, and syncope.

Clinical presentation: Bee stings cause pain, redness, and swelling, which often last a few hours. Localized allergic skin reactions may last for up to 1 week. Anaphylaxis may occur in some individuals, but it can be delayed for up to 20 minutes due to the time for the bee venom to reach circulation.

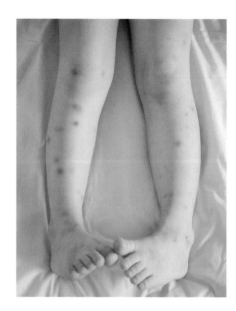

Figure 9.7 Bedbug bites.

HONEY- OR BUMBLEBEE STING

Overview: A honeybee sting is similar to a wasp sting, except the stinger, which forms part of its abdomen, is left in the victim. This will continue to pump toxin from the venom sac even after separation from the adult bee (Figure 9.8). Tearing of the stinger apparatus from the honeybee results in the sacrifice of the honeybee a few minutes after stinging.

Clinical presentation: There is an urticarial reaction in the stinger in the center of this highly painful lesion. A patient who has repeated stings may develop anaphylaxis.

Management: Removing the stinger from the stung individual as soon as possible can reduce the amount of venom injected. This can be achieved by using the edge of a plastic card. Once removed, any pain and swelling can be reduced by using a cold compress.

Honeybee stings release pheromones that signal other bees, so stings are frequently multiple. The same is true if the bee is killed. Using an upturned glass to capture the bee can prevent pheromone signaling.

Spider Bites

Synonym: Loxoscelism

Overview: Except for two species that lack a venom gland, all spiders are venomous; however, only the genus *Loxosceles* is of immense medical significance to humans. The best known of these are the black widow (*Lactrodectus mactans*) and brown recluse spider (*Loxosceles reclusa*).

Loxosceles spiders have a worldwide distribution but are most heavily concentrated in the western hemisphere, often in a domestic habitat where they hide in crevices, within cardboard, or behind furnishings. In the United States, spider bites east of the Mississippi River are not as dangerous because the destructive black widow spider resides west of the Mississippi. These spiders may be distinguished by their characteristic red or orange fiddle-back pattern displayed on their ventral (underside) surface.

Clinical presentation: The bite is often painless, but in cases of envenomation, it is followed by a sharp, penetrating pain after 2–8 hours. Paired puncta may be seen at the bite site. The bite area initially becomes pale with a penumbra of erythema (Figure 9.9). The severe pain is due to vasospasm and ischemia caused by sphingomyelinase D toxin. In severe cases, micro-hemorrhages may lead to acute renal failure.

The black widow spider bite may be serious and create large gangrenous areas that require surgical intervention. Rarely, severe cases of loxoscelism can lead to multi-organ failure, especially renal failure due to micro-hemorrhages, and even death.

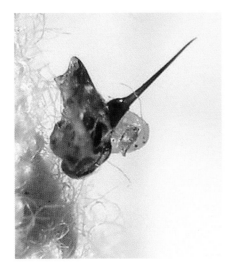

Figure 9.8 Bee sting venom sac.

Source: From Wikipedia, used under Creative Commons license.

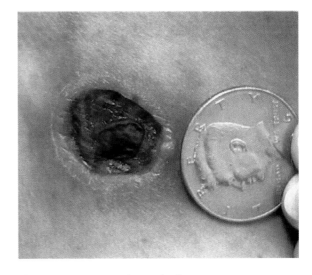

Figure 9.9 *Loxosceles* spider bite.

Source: From Swanson DL, Vetter RS. Loxoscelism. Clin Dermatol. 2006;24:213–321, used with permission.

Laboratory studies: Blood tests may show signs of hemolysis, thrombocytopenia, coagulopathy, raised d-dimer, and altered urinalysis.

Differential diagnosis: It is often difficult to distinguish between a spider bite and a bee or a hornet bite. The sting is most painful, but infrequently, a bulla may form within the red, sometimes indurated, area. With a spider bite, a blister will form over several days to leave a characteristic blue-violet sunken scar with central anesthesia. Healing gradually takes place over 8 weeks.

Management: Treatment is symptomatic with cold compresses and application of a topical steroid such as triamcinolone 0.1% cream twice daily.

FINAL THOUGHT

Infestations and bites are common skin presentations. An appropriate history and examination will usually lead to the correct diagnosis and subsequent symptomatic therapeutic relief.

ADDITIONAL READINGS

Cestari TF, Martignago BF. Scabies, pediculosis, bedbugs, and stinkbugs: uncommon presentations. Clin Dermatol. 2005;23:545–554.

Chosidow O. Scabies and pediulcosis. Lancet. 2000;355:819–826.

Coates SJ, Thomas C, Chosidow O, et al. Ectoparasites: pediculosis and tungiasis. J Am Acad Dermatol. 2020;82:551–569.

Lai O, Ho D, Glick S, et al. Bed bugs and possible transmission of human pathogens: a systematic review. Arch Dermatol Res. 2016;308:531–538.

Laing R, Gillan V, Devaney E. Ivermectin—old drug, new tricks? Trends Parasitol. 2017;33:463–472.

Laxme RRS, Suranse V, Sunagar K. Arthropod venoms: biochemistry, ecology, and evolution. Toxicon. 2019;158:84–103.

Mumcuoglu KY, Pollack RJ, Reed DL, et al. International recommendations for an effective control of head louse infestations. Int J Dermatol. 2021;60:272–280.

Swanson DL, Vetter RS. Loxoscelism. Clin Dermatol. 2006;24:213–321.

Thomas C, Coates SJ, Engelman D, et al. Ectoparasites: scabies. J Am Acad Dermatol. 2020;82:533–548.

Warrell DA. Venomous bites, stings, and poisoning: an update. Infect Dis Clin North Am. 2019;33:17–38.

10 Environmental Injuries

Soo Jung Kim and Alexander V. Nguyen

CONTENTS

The skin is the body's primary defense against environmental injuries, including light and radiation damage. The skin is also involved in thermoregulation and the prevention of mechanical damage from pressure and trauma.

LIGHT

Definition: Overexposure to sunlight can cause suntan and sunburns. Chronic light exposure leads to photoaging with the appearance of wrinkles and lentigines. Sunlight also causes photosensitivity reactions, such as polymorphous light eruption, chronic actinic dermatitis, and phototoxic and photoallergic reactions. Sunlight can also aggravate certain skin diseases.

Solar radiation encompasses a broad range of wavelengths (Figure 10.1). The biologically damaging wavelengths range from 250–400 nm and are termed ultraviolet radiation (UVR). The three subsets of UVR are UVA (320–400 nm), UVB (280–320 nm), and UVC (200–280 nm). UVC is filtered out by the ozone layer with minimal significance. Both UVA and UVB, especially UVB around 290 nm, are major damaging wavelengths to the skin.

Sunburns

Overview: Sunburns are caused by overexposure to sunlight. UVR damages keratinocytes, which leads to the release of cytokines and inflammatory mediators.

Clinical presentation: This results in the redness, swelling, blistering, and pain seen in sunburns. Severe sunburns with extensive blistering may require inpatient management. Each person's overall sensitivity to UVR is different, however, and depends largely on the inherent baseline pigmentation and the ability to produce more melanin. The Fitzpatrick scale of skin phototypes is shown in Table 10.1.

Laboratory studies: Sunburns are diagnosed clinically.

Management: These can typically be managed at home by drinking more water than usual, taking frequent cool baths or showers, and applying moisturizer. In especially irritated areas, applying over-the-counter hydrocortisone cream can be helpful. Nonsteroidal anti-inflammatory medications, such as aspirin or ibuprofen, can help to relieve redness, swelling, and pain. Blisters should not be popped due to introducing potential nidus for infection.

To prevent further sunburns, excessive UVR can be avoided by seeking shade and avoiding peak sun exposure, especially between 10 a.m. and 3 p.m.; using broad-spectrum sunscreen rated

DOI: 10.1201/9781003105268-10

VISIBLE LIGHT   ULTRAVIOLET RADIATION

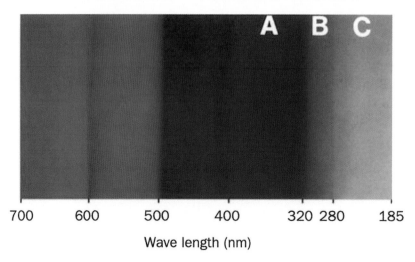

Wave length (nm)

Figure 10.1   Solar spectrum showing visible light and ultraviolet radiation: UVA (320–400 nm), UVB (280–320 nm), and UVC (200–280 nm).

Table 10.1 Fitzpatrick Classification of Skin Phototype

Phototype	Color Description	Response to UVR Burns? Tans?
I	White	Always never
II	White	Easily sometimes (with difficulty)
III	Beige	Sometimes gradually
IV	Brown	Rarely easily
V	Dark Brown	Hardly ever very easily
VI	Black	Never very easily

Source: Adapted from Bolognia J, Schaffer JV, Cerroni L, eds, Dermatology, 4th edition.

Figure 10.2   Sunburn: well-demarcated severe erythema.

Source: From Bender NR, Chiu YE. Photosensitivity, Nelson Textbook of Pediatrics, 675, 3496–3501.e1, 2020, used with permission.

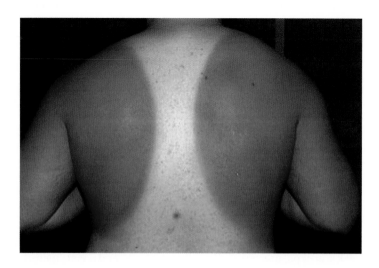

Table 10.2 Short- and Long-Term Damage by UVR Exposure

Short-Term Consequences	Long-Term Consequences
Sunburn: Erythema, blister formation	Photocarcinogenesis: development of melanoma and nonmelanoma skin cancer
Suntan: Immediate pigment darkening and delayed tanning (3 days after sun exposure)	Photoaging: atrophic, rough, wrinkled, inelastic or leathery, sallow skin
	Solar (actinic) elastosis: yellowed, thickened skin with wrinkles around eyes and mouth
	• Striated beaded lines or fibroelastolytic papulosis (small yellowish papules and plaques) along the sides of the neck
	• Actinic elastotic plaque (a translucent papule with a pearly color) on face or chest
	• Elastotic nodules (a translucent papule with a pearly color) on the ear
	• Poikiloderma of Civatte (reticulate hyperpigmentation with telangiectasia) on anterior and lateral portions of the neck
	• Cutis rhomboidalis nuchae (thickened, tough, and leathery skin with exaggerated normal skin markings) on the nape
	• Favre-Racouchot syndrome (cysts and comedones) on malar skin
	Dermatoporosis: Skin fragility due to chronic sun damage to the connective tissue of the dermis
	• Actinic purpura (purpura and ecchymoses) on extensor arms
	• Stellate pseudoscars on the forearms

at least SPF 30 (the sun protection factor, or SPF, is a measure of the fraction of UVR that reaches the skin) and applying at least every 2 hours and 30 minutes before going out; and wearing UV-protective or "opaque" clothing (the ultraviolet protective factor, or UPF, is a standardized measure of the fraction of UVR that can penetrate the fabric), wide-brimmed hats, long-sleeve shirts, and pants.

Course: Most sunburns do not cause short-term consequences, but prolonged exposure to UVR can cause long-term damage to the skin, including photoaging and increased risk of developing skin cancer (Table 10.2); therefore, sunburns should be avoided with sun avoidance and proper protective measures against UVR.

Polymorphous Light Eruption (Hutchinson's Prurigo)

Overview: Polymorphous light eruption (PMLE) is the most common dermatosis that is triggered by sunlight, and it commonly appears in patients of northern European descent. Other dermatoses aggravated by sun exposure are listed in Table 10.3.

Clinical presentation: PMLE presents as grouped, erythematous, itchy, papules on sun-exposed areas within hours to days of sun exposure. PMLE can also appear as vesicles, bullae, or papulovesicular, hence the name "polymorphous"; however, the morphology of the individual patient is usually consistent. The eruptions of PMLE occur in the spring and early summer. The regions of the body most commonly affected include the neck, outer arms, and dorsal surface of the hands in an asymmetric, patchy distribution.

Laboratory studies: PMLE can be diagnosed by history and clinical appearance. Histologically, there are variable epidermal spongiosis and perivascular infiltration of T cells in the upper and middle portions of the dermis.

Differential diagnosis: This includes lupus erythematosus, other photosensitive dermatoses, and solar urticaria.

Management: PMLE is managed by sunlight avoidance and the use of broad-spectrum sunscreen. Severely affected patients may require treatment with phototherapy, oral prednisone (30 mg daily), hydroxychloroquine (200–400 mg daily), and azathioprine (50–75 mg daily).

Course: PMLE usually begins in February or March in the northern hemisphere and disappears by July or August, only to reappear the next year. The eruptions resolve within days or weeks. Recurrences can decrease over time as PMLE demonstrates a phenomenon known as "hardening,"

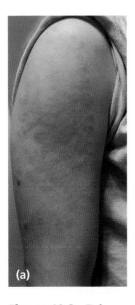
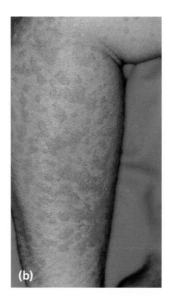
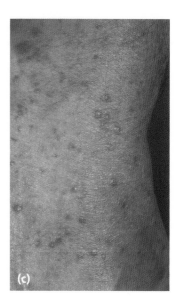

(a)   (b)   (c)

Figure 10.3 Polymorphous light eruption of the upper extremity: (a) Small pink edematous papules that are coalescing into plaques on the arm; (b) scattered discrete papulovesicular; (c) larger and more pronounced edematous erythematous papules and plaques.

Source: (a) is courtesy of Megan F. Craddock, MD. (b) and (c) are from Lim HW, Hawk JLM, Rosen CF. Photodermatologic Disorders, in Bolognia J, Schaffer JV, Cerroni L, eds, Dermatology, 4th edition, Philadelphia: Elsevier, 2018, 87:1548–1568, used with permission.

Table 10.3 Common Diseases Aggravated by Sunlight

Atopic dermatitis	Lupus erythematosus
Bullous pemphigoid	Pellagra
Cutaneous T-cell lymphoma	Pemphigus
Dermatomyositis	Rosacea
Darier disease	Seborrheic dermatitis
Lichen planus	Viral infections

wherein patients with PMLE who are chronically exposed to sunlight develop fewer eruptions over time due to the development of immunologic tolerance.

CHRONIC ACTINIC DERMATITIS

Overview: This is a severe and persistent dermatosis commonly seen in older men with a history of allergic contact dermatitis or photoallergic reactions to plants, fragrances, or topical creams. Chronic actinic dermatitis (CAD) is particularly seen in the summer.

   Clinical presentation: CAD presents as pruritic, patchy or confluent, eczematous, lichenified lesions in sun-exposed areas with well-demarcated borders at clothing lines. CAD persists despite avoidance of known triggers and sunlight. Skin folds, such as the upper eyelids and nasolabial folds, are commonly spared. In severe cases, CAD may involve areas of skin not exposed to light or triggers.

   Laboratory studies: Histologic examination demonstrates epidermal spongiosis and acanthosis as well as lymphohistiocytic infiltration of the superficial and deep dermis.

   Differential diagnosis: History, examination, photopatch testing, and histology can assist in the differential diagnosis of CAD, including cutaneous T-cell lymphoma (CTCL), photoallergic contact dermatitis, and PMLE.

   Management: Treatment of CAD requires avoidance of UVR and triggers. Topical and systemic steroids are intermittently required. Topical tacrolimus may also help. The refractory disease can

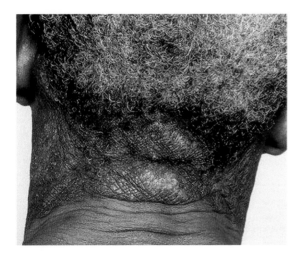

Figure 10.4 Chronic actinic dermatitis.

Source: From Lim HW, Hawk JLM, Rosen CF. Photodermatologic Disorders, in Bolognia J, Schaffer JV, Cerroni L, eds, Dermatology, 4th edition, Philadelphia: Elsevier, 2018, 87:1548–1568, used with permission.

be managed with phototherapy, cyclosporine (3.5–5 mg/kg/daily), azathioprine (1–2.5 mg/kg/daily), and mycophenolate (1–2 g daily).

Course: Erythroderma can be a rare complication of severe CAD. Some patients will have a resolution of their disease over time, in 10% over 5 years and 20% over 10 years.

HEAT

Definition: Excessive heat can overwhelm the skin's barrier function and ability to thermoregulate.

Thermal Burns

Clinical presentation: First-degree burns cause painful, erythematous skin followed by desquamation. Most sunburns are first-degree burns. Second-degree burns involve the superficial or deep dermis. Superficial second-degree burns result in the formation of vesicles and blebs with complete recovery without scarring. Deep second-degree burns are pale and anesthetic due to compromised blood flow. Third-degree burns involve the full thickness of the dermis and some subcutaneous tissues, which results in ulcerated wounds due to the destruction of skin appendages.

Management: Burn management depends on severity and location. Patients with severe burns and burns on the face, hands, and genitalia should be referred to a burn unit. Less severe burns can be managed by the immediate cold application, not opening vesicles or blebs of second-degree burns, thoroughly cleaning wounds, and keeping the area moist for optimal healing. Critical care includes evaluation of respiratory status, resuscitation with fluids, assessing for secondary infection, nutritional support, and pain control.

Course: Superficial and partial thickness burns heal within days to weeks. Third-degree burns have severe scarring and often require surgical interventions, such as grafting. Rarely, cutaneous squamous cell carcinoma (SCC) can occur at the site of an old thermal burn scar.

Miliaria

Synonyms: Heat rash, prickly heat

Overview: Miliaria occurs when sweat ducts are occluded, commonly in hot, humid climates and the neonatal period. There are three main types of miliaria (Table 10.4).

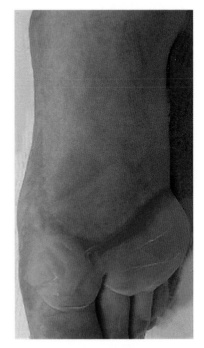

Figure 10.5 Thermal burn on the foot with blistering.

Table 10.4 Miliaria Types

Type	Presentation	Location of Sweat Gland Occlusion	Pathology
Crystallina	Small, superficial, clear, fragile blisters without inflammation	Stratum corneum	Subcorneal or intracorneal vesicles overlying an eccrine sweat duct
Rubra	Pruritic, non-follicular papules or pustules on a background of erythema	Superficial epidermis	Intraepidermal spongiosis and vesicles
Profunda	Asymptomatic skin-colored papules	Dermal-epidermal junction	Spongiosis and vesiculation of the upper aspect of the dermal portion of the sweat duct

Clinical Presentation

Laboratory studies: This is a clinical diagnosis.

Differential diagnosis: History and lack of systemic findings can assist in the differential diagnosis, including herpes simplex, acute generalized exanthematous pustulosis, and varicella.

Management: The best management is cooling with cold water compresses or air conditioning and fans. Emollients, antipyretics, and topical steroids can also be helpful. Occlusive topical formulations, such as ointments or dressings, should be avoided.

Course: Most cases resolve within a few days after leaving the hot environment.

Erythema ab Igne

Overview: Erythema ab igne (EAI) is caused by chronic or prolonged heat exposure without burning. EAI commonly occurs over the shins due to prolonged exposure to fireplaces and heaters, the lower back due to electric heating pads, and the thighs from prolonged laptop exposure and heated car seats.

Clinical presentation: EAI initially starts as mottling and reticulated erythema before progressively becoming brown-pigmented lesions.

Laboratory studies: EAI is diagnosed clinically.

Differential diagnosis: This includes livedo reticularis, cutis marmorata, and poikiloderma.

Management: EAI resolves after removal of the heat source, but more severe cases with skin atrophy and hyperpigmentation may persist.

Course. Nonhealing ulcers or skin growths in regions with prior EAI require biopsy as SCC can arise from chronic heat injury.

 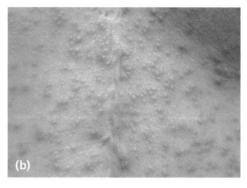

Figure 10.6 (a) Miliaria crystallina; (b) miliaria rubra.

Source: (a) Courtesy of Raegan D. Hunt, MD, Ph.D. (b) From James, WD, Elston, DM, Treat, JR, Rosenbach, MA, Neuhaus, IM. Dermatoses Resulting from Physical Factors, Andrews' Diseases of the Skin, 13th Edition, pages 13–45. 2020, used with permission.

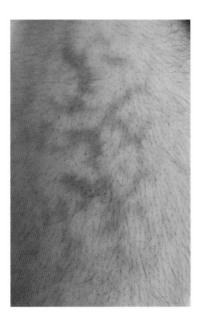

Figure 10.7 Erythema ab igne.

Source: By courtesy of Audrey J. Chan, MD.

COLD

Definition: Excessive cold can directly damage skin tissue due to reduced temperature, vaso-spasm, and vascular injury.

Frostbite

Overview: This represents acute tissue necrosis of the skin and underlying tissues due to cold exposures. Lesions commonly appear on distal and acral sites, such as the fingers, toes, nose, and ears.

Clinical presentation: Affected areas are well-demarcated and appear blanched and white before progressing to a darker or purplish hue. During rewarming, edema, blisters, and in severe cases, gangrene can appear. The severity is related to both the temperature and duration of exposure.

Laboratory studies: This is diagnosed clinically.

Management: This includes immediate rewarming with warm water baths. Fluid resuscitation, analgesics, and routine wound care are important to prevent complications. Antibiotics and

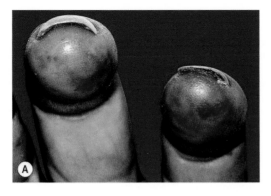
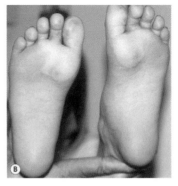

Figure 10.8 Frostbite: (a) Erythema, edema, and hemorrhage are seen on the fingertips in the first-degree frostbite; (b) bullae filled with clear fluid on the distal plantar surfaces in second-degree frostbite.

Source: From Smith ML. Environmental and Sports-Related Skin Diseases, in Bolognia J, Schaffer JV, Cerroni L, eds, Dermatology, 4th edition, Philadelphia: Elsevier, 2018; 88:1569–1594, used with permission.

a tetanus booster should be administered when warranted. If there is evidence of persisting ischemia, anticoagulation (e.g., tissue plasminogen activator, heparin) may be used.

Course: It often can take months to recover from frostbite. Patients may develop long-term sensory neuropathy and cold intolerance. Occasionally, amputation is required for severe cases.

Raynaud's Disease and Raynaud's Phenomenon

Overview: Raynaud's disease (RD) and Raynaud's phenomenon (RP) are caused by abnormal recurrent vasospasms of the digital arteries. RD is not associated with underlying disease and is more common than RP, which is caused by an underlying systemic disease. In contrast to RP, RD presents with normal capillaroscopy, no history of existing connective tissue disease, no physical findings concerning for secondary causes (e.g., sclerodactyly, calcinosis, and ulceration), and negative antinuclear antibodies (ANAs).

Clinical presentation: Raynaud's attacks lead to white (ischemic), blue (cyanotic), and then red (hyperemic) digits for minutes to hours. In RD, or primary Raynaud's, the cause of the vasospasm is unknown in the absence of associated disease, and it is mainly seen in young women. In contrast, RP, or secondary Raynaud's, is caused by an underlying disease, such as systemic sclerosis, systemic lupus erythematosus, Sjögren's syndrome, mixed connective tissue disease, and dermatomyositis. If severe, it can lead to atrophy, necrosis, and gangrene and can be complicated by infection.

Differential diagnosis: This includes thromboangiitis obliterans, cold injury, cryoglobulinemia, carcinoid syndrome, and reflex sympathetic dystrophy.

Management: RD and RP often can be managed with lifestyle modifications, including avoidance of cold exposure, smoking, and vasoconstrictive drugs as well as using hand or feet warmers. Pharmacologic therapy can be initiated if conservative measures fail and include topical nitrates or oral calcium channel blockers, pentoxifylline, phosphodiesterase type 5 (PDE5) inhibitors, and angiotensin II receptor blockers. Suggested dosing regimens are listed in Table 10.5.

Course: Patients can often attain good progress with adopted measures. Patients with RP, as opposed to RD, often may have more severe and frequent findings that require aggressive interventions.

Chilblains

Synonym: Pernio

Overview: This represents an inflammatory response arising after exposure to the cold, especially in damp climates.

Clinical presentation: Chilblains present as edematous, erythematous purple macules or papules on fingers or toes. Other locations include the nose and ears.

Laboratory studies: The diagnosis is clinical, although histopathologic examination will show papillary dermal edema and a dense lymphocytic infiltrate around blood vessels and eccrine glands.

Differential diagnosis: Pernio may be differentiated from chilblain lupus erythematosus, cryoglobulinemia, acrocyanosis, RP, cold panniculitis, leukemia cutis, and COVID-19 associated vasculitis of the digits in the right clinical context.

Management: This is primarily conservative. These patients need to avoid the cold and dampness with appropriate clothing. Smoking cessation is necessary. Topical corticosteroids and calcium channel blockers (nifedipine 20–60 mg daily) can be used.

Course: Acute pernio resolves in 1–3 weeks with the removal of the cold stimulus. Chronic pernio may continue throughout the patient's lifetime and typically worsens in colder months. If pernio is associated with systemic disease, then it is more likely to be persistent.

Table 10.5 Raynaud's Phenomenon Medication Dosing

Medication	Dosing
Calcium channel blockers	Nifedipine 30 mg daily or BID; Amlodipine 2.5–10 mg daily
Anti-inflammatory and anti-fibrinolytic agents	Pentoxifylline 400 mg TID or QID
PDE5 inhibitors	Sildenafil 20–25 mg TID
Angiotensin II receptor blockers	Losartan 25–100 mg daily

Abbreviations: TID: three times a day; QID: four times a day BID: two times a day.

RADIATION

Definition: This is caused by energetic moving waves or subatomic particles that can damage the skin through ionization and free radical generation. Radiation therapy is a common treatment for various forms of malignancies, but it is often complicated by acute or chronic radiodermatitis of the overlying skin.

Radiation Dermatitis

Synonym: Radiodermatitis

Overview: Acute radiation dermatitis is due to inflammatory changes and oxidative stress in the skin. Patients present with well-demarcated erythema, pruritus, desquamation, ulceration, and necrosis (Figure 10.9a, b). Unlike heat- or cold-induced skin damage, these findings may not be present in the hours immediately after exposure, and they tend to appear days afterward. Chronic radiodermatitis, or chronic radiation dermatitis, is skin injury months or years after exposure to radiation, which can present with fibrosis, chronic ulcerations, and secondary skin cancers. Radiation to the scalp may lead to permanent hair loss.

Laboratory studies: The diagnosis of acute and chronic radiodermatitis can be easily made clinically based on the physical examination and a history of radiation. Histopathology of acute radiodermatitis shows epidermal necrosis and sloughing, as well as dermal inflammation, vasodilation, and edema. Chronic radiodermatitis will show sclerosis of the dermal collagen, fibrosis of the vasculature, atypical fibroblasts, and absent pilosebaceous units.

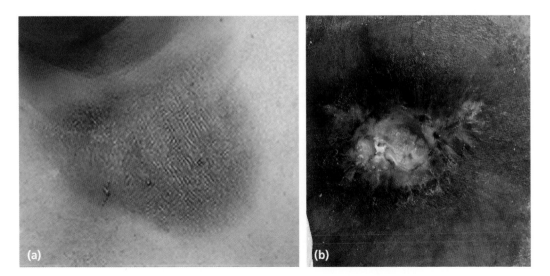

Figure 10.9 (a) Acute radiation dermatitis; (b) chronic radiation dermatitis.

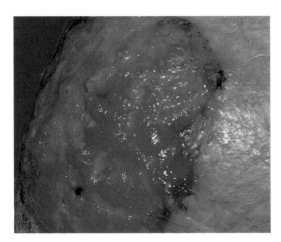

Figure 10.10 Radiation-induced basal cell carcinoma. A tumor developed on this patient's scalp 60 years after she had undergone irradiation for tinea capitis as a child. Already, she had had chronic alopecia that resulted from the x-ray therapy. The lesion was successfully excised.

Source: From Friedlander P, Hodi FS, Wick MM, Velazquez EF. Skin Cancer, Atlas of Diagnostic Oncology, 2010;13: 446–483, used with permission.

Management: This is primarily symptomatic, using topical steroids, emollients, and pain relievers to decrease the pain and discomfort. Management of chronic radiodermatitis is primarily symptomatic, as well.

Course: Radiation therapy can lead to the development of basal cell carcinoma (BCC) and SCC with a clinical latency of 20–40 years. All patients with radiation therapy require close monitoring in the years following treatment for the development of secondary skin cancers.

TRAUMA

Definition: Traumatic injury can interrupt skin integrity, and the extent of damage and healing will vary depending on the mechanism and severity of the injury.

Mechanical Trauma

Overview: This can occur through lacerations (i.e., tears of the skin due to blunt or shearing forces), abrasions (i.e., a superficial wound caused by contact with an irregular surface that does not extend to the subcutaneous tissue), and punctures (i.e., penetrating injury caused by sharp objects that can extend beyond the dermis).

Laboratory studies: The diagnosis is clinical.

Management: Gentle cleansing with soap and water and application of petroleum jelly with a bandage is recommended for the initial treatment of superficial wounds. Tetanus prophylaxis and treatment are indicated for patients with breakage of the skin and inadequate or unknown immunization history. Large lacerations and puncture wounds may require sutures and antibiotics for the prevention of infection.

Course: Superficial trauma to the skin typically leaves no long-term consequences. Deeper trauma may cause scarring.

PRURIGO NODULARIS AND LICHEN SIMPLEX CHRONICUS

Synonyms: Hyde's disease, neurodermatitis

Overview: Chronic skin damage via chronic scratching or rubbing can lead to prurigo nodularis (PN) and lichen simplex chronicus (LSC).

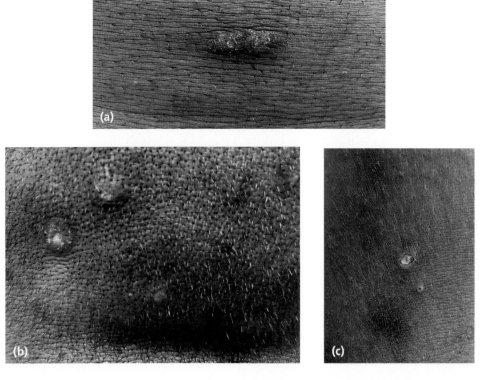

Figure 10.11 (a, b) Prurigo nodularis; (c) lichen simplex chronicus with excoriations.

Clinical presentation: PN presents as itchy, hyperpigmented, firm nodules, which are primarily distributed on the extremities and upper back. The "butterfly" sign is often present in elderly patients with itching, wherein the mid-upper areas of the back are spared due to its hard-to-reach location. LSC presents as lichenified, hyperpigmented plaques with varying degrees of overlying scale distributed on the neck, scalp, extremities, and anogenital region with a leathery appearance.

Laboratory studies: Chronic skin trauma, as well as PN and LSC, can be diagnosed clinically. A biopsy can guide the diagnosis of PN and LSC. Histologic features of PN and LSC are similar, which include marked hyperkeratosis, acanthosis with irregular rete ridges, and vertical collagen fibers in the papillary dermis.

Differential diagnosis: PN can be confused with verruca vulgaris, perforating disorders, pemphigoid nodularis, insect bites, and neoplasms, such as SCC. LSC may include lichen amyloidosis, hypertrophic lichen planus, and atopic dermatitis.

Treatment: These lesions are managed by addressing the underlying cause, which includes xerosis, atopic dermatitis, or other pruritic disorders. Topical corticosteroids and intralesional steroids are the first lines of therapies to consider. For generalized involvement, phototherapy can be helpful.

Course: PN and LSC can be difficult to treat, and a multifaceted approach is often needed.

FINAL THOUGHT

The skin provides important functions as a protective barrier for environmental insults; however, this can be overwhelmed by excessive exposure to light, heat, cold, radiation, and trauma.

ADDIONAL READINGS

Bender NR, Chiu YE. Chapter 675—Photosensitivity. In: Nelson Textbook of Pediatrics. 21st ed. Philadelphia: Elsevier; 2020. p. 3496–3501.

Calonje E, Brenn T, Lazar AJ, et al. Chapter 21—Diseases of collagen and elastic tissue. In: McKee's Pathology of the Skin. 5th ed. Philadelphia: Elsevier; 2020. p. 1015–1050.e28.

Forman SB, Roy K. Chapter 33—Vasoactive and antiplatelet agents. In: Comprehensive Dermatologic Drug Therapy. 4th ed. Philadelphia: Elsevier; 2021. p. 358–365.

Friedlander P, Hodi FS, Wick MM, et al. Chapter 13—Skin cancer. In: Atlas of Diagnostic Oncology. 4th ed. Philadelphia: Elsevier; 2010. p. 446–483.

Herrick AL. Evidence-based management of Raynaud's phenomenon. Ther Adv Musculoskelet Dis. 2017;9:317–329.

James WD, Elston DM, Treat JR, et al. Dermatoses resulting from physical factors. In: Andrews' Diseases of the Skin. 13th ed. Philadelphia: Elsevier; 2020. p. 13–45.

James WD, Elston DM, Treat JR, et al. Pruritis and neurocutaneous dermatoses. In: Andrews' Diseases of the Skin. 13th ed. Philadelphia: Elsevier; 2020. p. 46–62.

Lee RC, Teven CM. Chapter 18—Acute management of burn and electrical trauma. In: Plastic Surgery: Volume 4: Lower Extremity, Trunk, and Burns. 4th ed. Philadelphia: Elsevier; 2018. p. 392–423.

Lim HW, Hawk JLM, Rosen CF. Chapter 87—Photodermatologic disorders. In: Bolognia J, Schaffer JV, Cerroni L, eds., Dermatology. 4th ed. Philadelphia: Elsevier; 2018. p. 1548–1568.

Smith ML. Chapter 88—Environmental and sports-related skin diseases. In Bolognia J, Schaffer JV, Cerroni L, eds., Dermatology. 4th ed. Philadelphia: Elsevier; 2018. p. 1569–1594.

11 Allergic and Immunologic Reactions

Saira N. Agarwala, Aspen R. Trautz, and Sylvia Hsu

CONTENTS

Definition: The skin conditions in this chapter are related in that they occur as reactions to foreign antigens. The most common inciting factors include medications and infectious agents. Despite the similarities in the pathogenesis of these conditions, their presentations, severity, and management vary widely from acute urticaria treated with over-the-counter antihistamines to toxic epidermal necrolysis, which requires hospitalization often in the intensive care unit.

DRUG REACTIONS

Overview: Drug reactions are a common dermatologic complaint seen both in the inpatient and outpatient setting. These reactions often have overlap in their initial clinical presentation, but they have a wide spectrum of morbidity and mortality. It is therefore essential to have a high degree of suspicion for more serious drug reactions and to ensure close follow-up. The most important and first step in the treatment of all these reactions is a withdrawal of the offending medication (Table 11.1).

STEVENS-JOHNSON SYNDROME AND TOXIC EPIDERMAL NECROLYSIS

Synonym: Toxic epidermal necrolysis (TEN) is also known as Lyell syndrome.

    Definition: Considered to be a dermatologic emergency, Stevens-Johnson Syndrome (SJS)/TEN is an acute mucocutaneous reaction that is characterized by necrosis and detachment of the epidermis from the underlying dermis.

Table 11.1 Summary of Drug Reactions

Drug Reaction	Description	Common Causative Agents
Stevens-Johnson Syndrome/Toxic Epidermal Necrolysis (SJS/TEN)	Ill-defined, coalescing, erythematous macules that evolve into vesicles and bullae, leading to skin sloughing	Antibiotics (sulfamethoxazole, nevirapine), anticonvulsants (allopurinol, lamotrigine, carbamazepine, phenytoin), sulfasalazine, nonsteroidal anti-inflammatory drugs (NSAIDs), phenobarbital, etoricoxib
Morbilliform Drug Eruption	Diffuse and symmetric eruption of erythematous macules or small papules	Antibiotics (penicillins, cephalosporins, trimethoprim-sulfamethoxazole), anticonvulsants (carbamazepine, phenytoin), NSAIDs, paracetamol
Fixed Drug Eruption	Recurrent, well-demarcated, round, dusky, red to brown macules that may evolve into patches or edematous plaques	Antibiotics (trimethoprim-sulfamethoxazole, tetracyclines, penicillins, quinolones, dapsone), NSAIDs, acetaminophen, barbiturates, antimalarials (quinine), anticonvulsants (carbamazepine)
Acute Generalized Exanthematous Pustulosis (AGEP)	Numerous, non-follicular, sterile pustules with edematous erythema	Antibiotics (aminopenicillins, macrolides), antifungals, antimalarials, diltiazem

DOI: 10.1201/9781003105268-11

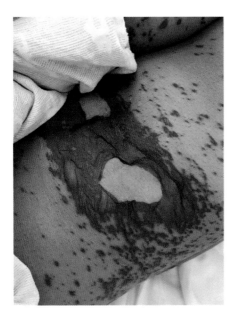

Figure 11.1   Stevens-Johnson syndrome.

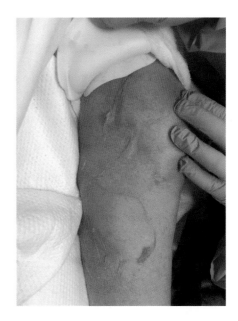

Figure 11.2   Toxic epidermal necrosis.

Overview: SJS/TEN typically occurs within the first few weeks after initiation of a culprit medication. Drugs most frequently associated with SJS/TEN include allopurinol, aromatic anticonvulsants, antibiotics (most frequently sulfonamides), and nonsteroidal anti-inflammatory drugs (NSAIDs). SJS and TEN lie on a continuum of disease based on the extent of the epidermal-dermal detachment. SJS refers to involvement of <10% total body surface area, TEN refers to >30% total body surface area, and SJS/TEN overlap is used when involvement is between 10–30%.

Clinical presentation: Patients often experience a 1–3-day prodrome of fever and flu-like symptoms before cutaneous manifestations emerge. Skin lesions generally begin centrally on the trunk and spread distally to the face, arms, and legs, including the palms and soles.

Lesions begin as ill-defined erythematous to dusky macules that coalesce (Figure 11.1). If no spontaneous sloughing of the epidermis is observed, the Nikolsky sign should be checked. To do so, a finger should be placed on an erythematous area and twisted to elicit tangential pressure. If epidermal-dermal cleavage is observed, then the test is positive. For hours to days, the epidermis necroses, and flaccid bullae form. This leads to extensive desquamation and erosions (Figure 11.2).

Painful mucosal erosions of the eyes, oral cavity, and/or genitalia are seen in 90% of cases. Involvement of the epithelium of the respiratory and/or gastro-intestinal tracts can also be seen in a smaller percentage of patients. Other systemic manifestations include lymphadenopathy, cytopenias, hepatitis, and cholestasis.

Laboratory studies: Histopathology can help to confirm the diagnosis of SJS/TEN as well as exclude similarly presenting conditions. Early lesions of SJS and TEN exhibit basilar apoptotic keratinocytes, whereas later disease is characterized by necrosis of the entire epidermis, often with overlying blister and sparse lymphocytic perivascular infiltrate. Direct immunofluorescence is negative.

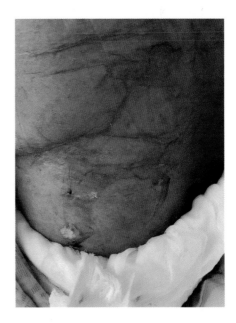

Figure 11.3   Toxic epidermal necrosis.

Due to the propensity for SJS/TEN patients to become critically ill, a complete blood count with differential and the complete metabolic panel should be obtained on all patients. Additionally, these patients are at high risk for bacterial and fungal superinfection of their lesions with subsequent sepsis; therefore, they should undergo cultures of blood, wounds, and mucosal lesions throughout their hospitalization course.

Differential diagnosis: This includes erythema multiforme, autoimmune bullous dermatoses, fixed drug eruption, morbilliform drug reaction, and staphylococcal scalded skin syndrome.

Management: The first step of management is the prompt cessation of the offending drug. Supportive care remains the foundation of treatment. Removal of the offending drug is estimated to reduce the risk of death by about 30% per day. Patients with severe disease covering greater than 10–20% total body surface area can benefit from placement in an intensive care unit, such as a burn unit. Much like burn patients, loss of epithelium leaves SJS/TEN patients extremely susceptible to the environment, and patients require intensive supportive treatment to prevent and manage electrolyte abnormalities, hypovolemia, hypothermia, and infection.

To date, there have been no randomized controlled clinical trials showing the efficacy of specific therapies. Effective supportive care may often be adequate. In clinical practice, a variety of therapies have been used including systemic corticosteroids, intravenous immune globulin, cyclosporine, and antitumor necrosis factor monoclonal antibodies.

Course: There is no evidence to date that can be used to predict the extent to which epidermal detachment will occur in a given patient; however, most patients will reach the maximum distribution of their disease between 2–15 days after onset. SJS/TEN is a deadly disease, with 6-week mortality of approximately 25% and 1-year mortality reaching 34%.

As would be expected, patients with larger body surface area involvement have higher mortality. Additionally, patients with total body surface area involvement of >30% have a significantly increased risk of developing bloodstream infections from *Staphylococcus aureus* and *Pseudomonas aeruginosa*.

Approximately one-quarter of patients with SJS/TEN will require mechanical intubation. Of those who survive, many patients are left with permanent scarring, especially in areas that became infected or required surgical debridement and/or grafting. Numerous long-term complications secondary to mucous membrane involvement can also occur.

Final comment: SJS/TEN is an extremely serious dermatologic condition with high morbidity and mortality. Prompt recognition, diagnosis, and treatment—namely, cessation of the offending medication—are critical when managing patients with this condition.

Morbilliform Drug Eruption

Synonyms: Exanthematous drug eruption, maculopapular drug eruption, measles-like drug eruption

Definition: Morbilliform drug eruptions are the most common type of drug hypersensitivity reaction. The word *morbilliform* stems from the measles-like macules and papules that characterize the drug reaction.

Overview: Morbilliform drug eruption is synonymous with exanthematous reaction, which means a sudden, widespread eruption that spares the mucous membranes. Although it can be caused by any medication, antibiotics are the most commonly implicated culprit. Morbilliform drug eruption represents the most common type of drug hypersensitivity reaction. It is self-limited and resolves with the withdrawal of the offending medication.

Clinical presentation: Morbilliform drug eruptions present as a sudden, symmetric, widespread eruption of erythematous macules and papules, which are primarily located on the trunk and proximal arms and legs; however, the face, palms, and soles can be involved. Rarely, pustules and bullae may form. This widespread rash closely resembles viral exanthems, and the two are often clinically indistinguishable; therefore, a careful history and medication review are required.

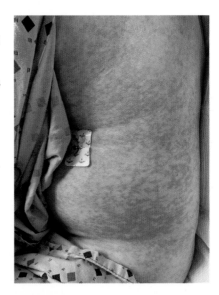

Figure 11.4 Morbilliform drug eruption.

Morbilliform drug reactions are exanthems rather than anthems; thus, they usually do not involve mucosal surfaces. If mucosal involvement is evident, there should be high clinical suspicion for a more serious drug reaction, such as SJS/TEN. This drug reaction typically occurs 1 week after the initiation of a new medication but may appear as early as 2 days in sensitized individuals. The rash may appear even after cessation of the medication, as drug half-lives can vary.

Laboratory studies: Morbilliform drug eruption is a clinical diagnosis and does not require laboratory studies. Should studies have already been ordered, a complete blood count may show eosinophilia, which is also seen in drug reaction with eosinophilia and systemic symptoms (DRESS) and acute generalized exanthematous pustulosis (AGEP). Besides, a complete metabolic panel should be normal in patients with a morbilliform drug eruption.

Histopathology shows a superficial perivascular and interstitial infiltrate containing eosinophils and sometimes neutrophils. Vacuolar interface changes and/or spongiosis can be present.

Differential diagnosis: Possible diagnoses include viral exanthem, DRESS, AGEP, and SJS/TEN. Morbilliform drug eruption is very difficult to distinguish from a viral exanthem based on clinical presentation alone. As a result, careful history taking is necessary to determine the etiology. Medications do not need to be new to the patient to cause a morbilliform drug eruption.

Management: As is the case in the management of many drug reactions, the most important step is the removal of the offending agent; however, if the culprit drug is necessary and there are no other alternatives, then the patient can finish the course of the culprit drug. For example, if the medication is for chemotherapy and the patient is responding well to treatment, then the drug can be continued if the reaction is mild and there is close monitoring.

Further management can include symptomatic treatment with antihistamines and topical steroids. The use of systemic corticosteroids is generally not recommended.

Course: Morbilliform drug eruptions are self-limited and resolve with withdrawal of the offending medication. Patients should have full resolution of the eruption within 2–4 weeks.

Final comment: Morbilliform drug eruption is not a dangerous drug eruption. It does not evolve into SJS/TEN.

Fixed Drug Eruption

Definition: Fixed drug eruption (FDE) is a type of predictable and recurrent cutaneous drug reaction that appears in the same location(s) following the administration or reexposure to a medication.

Overview: FDE is a type of drug hypersensitivity reaction with a predictable and recurrent pattern. This fixed, recurrent reaction typically manifests as round, hyperpigmented lesions that are sometimes pruritic. The most commonly implicated medications include NSAIDs, acetaminophen, antimicrobials, barbiturates, antimalarials, and anticonvulsants.

Clinical presentation: FDE presents as well-demarcated round dusky red to brown macules, which may evolve into patches or edematous plaques that are often pruritic or painful (Figures 11.5 and 11.6). They typically appear within hours at the same site each time the drug

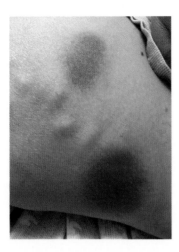

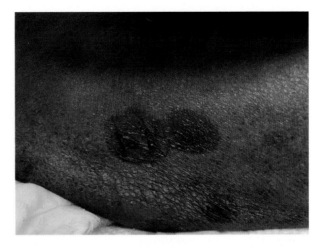

Figure 11.5 Fixed drug eruption.

Figure 11.6 Fixed drug eruption.

is administered, but they may also appear on additional areas of the body with each subsequent exposure to the medication. The areas become inflamed and may even blister, leaving evidence of post-inflammatory hyperpigmentation.

Lesions may occur anywhere, but they most commonly appear on the lips, genitalia, hands, and feet. There is generally an absence of systemic signs, such as fever. Although the patches typically appear within hours, they may take up to 2 weeks to develop.

FDE can rarely present as more generalized or atypical lesions that mimic other, sometimes more serious, skin diseases, such as SJS/TEN. Known variants of FDE include generalized FDE, generalized bullous FDE, erythema multiforme-like FDE, and non-pigmenting FDE. Classic FDE has a typical history and a clear absence of systemic signs.

Laboratory studies: FDE is a clinical diagnosis, but provocation tests or biopsy may be obtained if the diagnosis is unclear or if there is suspicion of a more serious drug reaction. To confirm the diagnosis, provocation tests may be conducted, which include patch testing or oral provocation when the patient takes their medication and is observed for a reaction.

Histopathology findings depend on the stage of the lesions when the biopsy is obtained. In general, there is hydropic degeneration of basal keratinocytes, necrotic cells in the epidermis, lymphocytic infiltration of the dermis, and dermal melanophages.

Differential diagnosis: This may include erythema multiforme, SJS/TEN (especially for generalized bullous FDE), DRESS, and bullous pemphigoid.

Management: Clinicians should promptly remove the offending drug and provide symptomatic treatment, such as topical corticosteroids and oral antihistamines, to relieve associated pain or pruritus.

Course: FDE resolves following cessation of the offending medication. Post-inflammatory hyperpigmentation is common. Patients should be advised to avoid the offending medication.

Final comment: FDE can typically be diagnosed based on clinical appearance in conjunction with a characteristic history. FDE is a non-dangerous skin eruption.

Acute Generalized Exanthematous Pustulosis

Definition: Acute generalized exanthematous pustulosis (AGEP) is a febrile drug reaction that typically starts a few days after the initiation of a new medication.

Overview: AGEP is a systemic drug reaction that results in a widespread eruption of pustules that rapidly resolve with the removal of the offending drug. Antimicrobials, antifungals, antimalarials, and diltiazem are the most common offending agents.

Clinical presentation: In the acute phase, AGEP manifests as an eruption of hundreds of sterile, non-follicular pustules (Figure 11.7). The pustules typically arise on the face or intertriginous areas and spread rapidly to involve the trunk, arms, and legs. AGEP does not typically involve mucosal sites. Resolving AGEP may appear as widespread superficial desquamation.

Systemic organ dysfunction is uncommon in AGEP; however, constitutional signs and symptoms may be present. Patients often have a high fever and lab abnormalities, such as neutrophilia, eosinophilia, and elevated liver enzymes. The majority of cases are caused by medications (90%) and generally occur within 48 hours of administering the suspected medication.

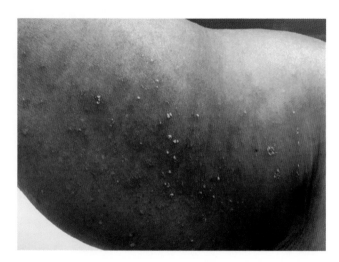

Figure 11.7 Acute generalized exanthematous pustulosis.

Laboratory studies: Clinical presentation and laboratory findings are often adequate to suggest the diagnosis. Histopathologic findings show a spongiotic pattern with subcorneal and/or intraepidermal pustules with eosinophils in the pustules or dermis. Superficial, interstitial, and mid-dermal infiltrate rich in neutrophils may also be seen as well as necrotic keratinocytes.

Differential diagnosis: These include generalized acute pustular psoriasis (von Zumbusch type), SJS/TEN, DRESS, and staphylococcal scalded skin syndrome

Management: Clinicians should promptly remove the offending drug and provide symptomatic treatment with topical corticosteroids and/or systemic steroids.

Course: AGEP is a self-limited disease with a favorable prognosis and a mortality rate of less than 5%. Removal of the offending drug will result in rapid resolution.

Final comment: AGEP is often seen in the inpatient setting as a resolving desquamating eruption.

ERYTHEMA MULTIFORME

Definition: Erythema multiforme (EM) is an acute, relatively short-lived, immune-mediated reaction of the skin, occurring in response to a variety of antigenic stimuli.

Overview: The majority of EM cases are associated with occult or overt infection with herpes simplex virus (HSV). Additional precipitating factors for EM include *Mycoplasma pneumoniae*, parapoxvirus (orf), and *Histoplasma capsulatum* (Table 11.2). Some infections have a high incidence of subsequent EM, particularly following recurrent infection.

There are two forms of EM: EM major and EM minor. Although both forms are characterized by the same primary lesions, the presence of severe mucosal involvement and systemic symptoms, such as fever and arthralgias, differentiate EM major from EM minor. To avoid confusion, it should be noted that EM major previously included SJS; however, it is now understood that EM major and SJS are two distinct diseases. Although medications, such as NSAIDs, sulfonamides, antiepileptics, and antibiotics, have been associated with EM in the literature, the interpretation of these associations is complicated by the previous grouping of EM major and SJS.

Clinical presentation: Classically, the eruption of EM is characterized by targetoid lesions; however, these lesions may not be seen in all patients presenting with EM, and, if present, they are often indicative of later stages of the disease process. The targetoid lesions of EM are typically less than 3 cm in diameter, well circumscribed, and display three zones of color. Early lesions can display two colors. The central zone can be crusted or contain a bulla. Lesions often begin as erythematous papules.

In terms of distribution, the face and arms, especially the extensor surfaces, are preferentially involved. Involvement tends to be symmetrically distributed. It has been reported that approximately 70% of patients with EM will develop mucosal involvement. The oral mucosa is most often affected, but the involvement of the anogenital mucosa and conjunctiva has been reported. Although

Table 11.2 Common Causes of Erythema Multiforme

Infectious—Viral
Herpes simplex virus (HSV)
Parapoxvirus (orf)
Adenovirus
Hepatitis viruses
Cytomegalovirus
Human immunodeficiency virus (HIV)
Varicella zoster virus
Infectious—Bacterial and Fungal
Mycoplasma pneumoniae
Histoplasma capsulatum
Dermatophyte infection (tinea)
Miscellaneous
Exposure to poison ivy
Inflammatory bowel disease

mucosal involvement can be seen in both EM minor and EM major, it is much more severe and symptomatic in those with EM major. These patients can develop blisters of the lips and buccal mucosa, which lead to painful erosions and often significant crusting. Patients with EM major suffer from nonspecific systemic symptoms, including fever, malaise, myalgia, and arthralgia.

Laboratory studies: Laboratory testing in EM is generally not required. The biopsy can be utilized when the diagnosis is unclear. Patients presenting with EM and concurrent respiratory complaints can undergo workup for possible *Mycoplasma pneumoniae* as the underlying cause of their EM. Recurrent cases can involve workup for HSV.

Differential diagnosis: In the early stages of EM, insect bites and papular urticaria should be considered. The differential also includes urticaria multiforme, SJS, FDE, bullous pemphigoid, Kawasaki disease, small vessel vasculitis, and Rowell syndrome. Polymorphous light eruption and juvenile spring eruption can mimic recurrent EM.

Management: Symptomatic treatment is the mainstay of management. To alleviate cutaneous pruritus, burning, and generalized skin discomfort, oral antihistamines, and topical corticosteroids can be used. To alleviate pain from nondisabling oral involvement, high-potency topical steroid gel, such as fluocinonide 0.05%, can be applied 2–3 times daily, or mouthwashes with equal parts of viscous lidocaine (2%), diphenhydramine (12.5 mg/5 mL), and antacids can be used to swish-and-spit up to four times daily.

EM major with functional impairment or significant oral involvement can be treated with systemic corticosteroids, such as prednisone 0.5–1 mg/kg/day for 3–5 days. If oral involvement prohibits the ability to maintain adequate oral intake, then hospitalization may be necessary to control pain and hydration status.

Patients with recurrent episodes secondary to HSV infection can be started on prophylactic antiviral therapy. Prophylaxis should be continued for at least 6 months to assess efficacy. It should be noted that only acyclovir prophylaxis has undergone double-blind, placebo-controlled study for its efficacy in preventing EM recurrence. For adults, prophylactic regimens include oral acyclovir 10 mg/kg/day in divided doses, valacyclovir 500–1000 mg twice daily, and famciclovir 250–500 mg twice daily. In the acute setting, treatment with antivirals has not been shown to reduce symptom severity or duration.

Course: EM lesions tend to erupt acutely, and patients develop crops of new lesions over a 3–5-day period. The time from symptom onset to clearance is typically less than 2 weeks but no longer than 4 weeks. A subset of patients can experience recurrence of EM over 6–10 years. Studies have shown these patients to have between 2–6 recurrences per year, but recurrences can be more frequent and last longer in immunosuppressed patients.

The vast majority of patients do not experience any long-term sequelae; however, EM major with involvement of the conjunctiva can infrequently lead to ocular tissues, such as keratitis, conjunctival scarring, and vision impairment, if not appropriately managed.

Final comment: EM is a largely self-limited condition that occurs in response to infection, such as HSV. Symptomatic treatment is often all that is required, but patients with frequent recurrence may benefit from antiviral prophylaxis.

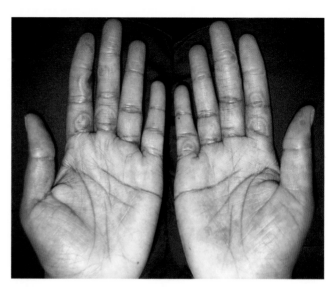

Figure 11.8 Erythema multiforme.

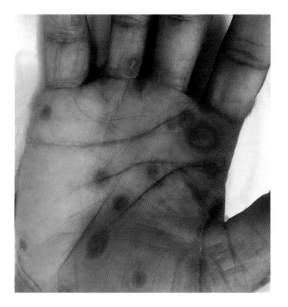

Figure 11.9 Erythema multiforme.

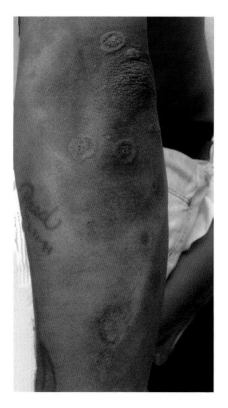

Figure 11.10 Erythema multiforme.

URTICARIA AND ANGIOEDEMA

Definition: Urticaria is extremely common and can affect about one-fifth of all people at some point in their lives. The condition is mediated by histamine release from cutaneous mast cells, which is most frequently secondary to an allergic process, but it can also be autoimmune, infectious, pharmacologic, or physical in nature.

Overview: In some patients, the etiology of urticaria is never determined. The release of histamine causes pruritus, while the release of other vasodilatory mediators causes localized swelling. When the process occurs deeper in the dermis and subcutaneous tissue, it is termed angioedema.

Urticaria can be classified temporally; acute urticaria is considered when the condition has been present for less than 6 weeks, while chronic urticaria is used to describe the condition lasting longer. Urticaria can also be classified as either spontaneous or physical/inducible.

Angioedema is most often seen as a component of urticaria. When angioedema occurs in the absence of wheals, other etiologies should be considered, such as hereditary angioedema, acquired C1 esterase inhibitor deficiency, and reaction to angiotensin-converting enzyme (ACE) inhibitors.

Clinical presentation: Urticaria presents as wheals with or without angioedema. Wheals are well-circumscribed pruritic plaques of variable size and shape. Wheals arise suddenly, and, by definition, individual lesions last less than 24 hours. They may assume odd, polycyclic, annular, and geographical forms. Angioedema occurs deep in the dermis and subcutaneous tissue. It can also affect submucosal areas and, more rarely, the gastrointestinal tract. Cutaneous involvement can present with large areas of ill-defined swelling that lasts for up to 72 hours. The overlying skin is often normal in color or may present with slight erythema. Involved areas tend to be more painful and less pruritic than wheals.

Acute urticaria can be seen in patients of all ages, but there tends to be a higher prevalence in children with atopic dermatitis. Although the etiology of acute urticaria is most often unable to be determined, a significant percentage of cases, especially in children, are associated with common bacterial and viral infections. Various parasitic infections, the prodromal phase of viral hepatitides, and human immunodeficiency virus (HIV) have been reported to cause acute urticaria. Type

I, IgE mediated allergic reactions, such as those to beta-lactam antibiotics, stinging and biting insects, foods, latex, and animal saliva, are also associated with acute urticaria. Although urticaria can be the only presenting complaint in these allergic reactions, it exists on a spectrum with anaphylaxis, which holds significant morbidity and mortality.

Another etiology of acute urticaria occurs when particular substances induce direct mast cell activation. Medications, such as opioid narcotics, muscle relaxants, and vancomycin, in addition to foods, such as tomatoes and strawberries, and environmental exposure to the nettle plant can induce urticaria in this manner.

Chronic spontaneous urticaria (CSU) is more common in adults and exhibits a female predominance. The urticarial lesions present identically to those of acute urticaria with individual wheals lasting less than 24 hours; however, CSU differs from acute urticaria in that urticarial lesions recur for more than 6 consecutive weeks. Additionally, the etiology of CSU differs. Approximately 30% of patients with CSU have autoantibodies against the high-affinity IgE receptor (FcεRI) or against the Fc portion of IgE. In terms of symptomatology, a subset of patients with CSU experience systemic symptoms, including fatigue, arthralgias, gastrointestinal upset, headache, palpitations, and wheezing. CSU has been associated with autoimmune conditions, most often autoimmune thyroid disease, but also rheumatoid arthritis, type I diabetes mellitus, Sjögren syndrome, celiac disease, and systemic lupus erythematosus.

Urticaria can also be induced by physical phenomena. These are termed the physical or inducible urticarias. Physical urticarias tend to develop minutes after a stimulus is experienced, resolve in about 2 hours, and occur at the site of exposure. Following is a list of common physical urticarias and their triggers:

- Dermatographism: This is the most common physical urticaria. Patients develop linear wheals in areas where skin experiences shearing forces from scratching or tight clothing. Simple dermatographism, that is dermatographism without pruritus, is estimated to occur in 5% of the population. Symptomatic dermatographism presents with wheals and pruritus, is less common than simple dermatographism, and tends to be more distressing for patients.

- Cold urticaria: Wheals, burning, and pruritus develop after exposure to cold temperatures followed by rewarming. The reaction can be elicited by placing an ice block on the skin.

- Delayed pressure urticaria: Urticarial lesions develop some time (on average 4–6 hours) after pressure on the skin, which can be from belts or other tight clothing. Patients may experience a reaction on the posterior thighs after prolonged sitting or on the soles from prolonged standing. Pain and burning at the site are often more prominent than pruritus. There is an association with chronic spontaneous urticaria.

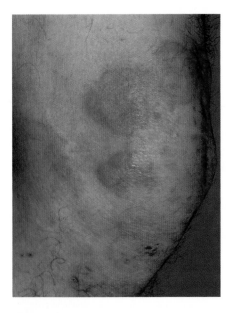

Figure 11.11 Urticaria.

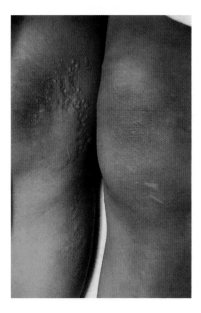

Figure 11.12 Urticaria.

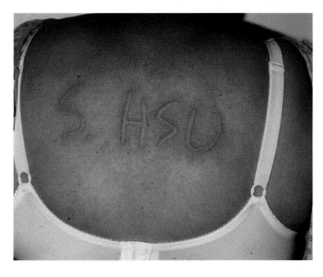

Figure 11.13 Dermatographism.

- Solar urticaria: Urticarial lesions develop on exposed skin a few minutes following exposure to the sun. Various wavelengths of light may also be responsible. When unrecognized, solar urticaria may cause an acute collapse in sunbathers.

- Cholinergic urticaria: Multiple small, pruritic, urticarial papules develop after exercise or hot baths, which can stimulate the postganglionic cholinergically innervated sweat glands. This disorder can be very disabling when severe since it can effectively prevent patients from participating in any kind of physical activity.

Laboratory studies: Acute urticaria generally does not require a diagnostic workup. In cases where there is suspected type I allergy to food or environmental factors, allergy testing can be pursued. If the initial trial of antihistamines does not provide relief, CSU should be evaluated with limited bloodwork, including a complete blood count with differential and erythrocyte sedimentation rate and/or C-reactive protein.

Table 11.3 **Types of urticaria and common causes.**

	Classification	Causes
Acute Urticaria	Urticaria lasting <6 weeks	• Most often an unknown trigger • Common bacterial and viral infections • Parasitic infections • The prodromal phase of viral hepatitides • Human immunodeficiency virus (HIV) • Type I, IgE mediated allergic reactions • Direct mast cell activation
Chronic Spontaneous Urticaria	Urticarial lesions recur for at least 6 weeks or longer	• Most frequently idiopathic • Autoantibodies against high-affinity IgE receptor (FcεRI) or Fc portion of IgE
Physical Urticaria	Urticaria that is induced by physical phenomenon	• Shearing forces on the skin (dermatographism) • Cold temperatures (cold urticaria) • Pressure on the skin (delayed pressure urticaria) • Sun exposure (solar urticaria) • Exercise or hot baths (cholinergic urticaria)

Table 11.4 American and International Clinical Guidelines for Urticaria

American Guidelines	International Guidelines
Step 1:	*Step 1:*
Second-generation antihistamines as earlier.	Second-generation antihistamines as earlier.
Assess for patient tolerance and efficacy before advancing.	Can advance if inadequate control: 2–4 weeks or earlier if symptoms are intolerable.
Step 2:	*Step 2:*
• Dose advancement of second-generation antihistamines from Step 1 (up to 4 times daily dose)	Increase the dose of second-generation antihistamine up to four times the daily dose.
• Add another second-generation antihistamine	Can advance if inadequate control: 2–4 weeks or earlier if symptoms are intolerable.
• Add an H2 antagonist	
• Add leukotriene receptor antagonist	
• Add the first-generation antihistamine to be taken at bedtime	
Assess for patient tolerance and efficacy before advancing.	
Step 3:	*Step 3:*
Dose advancement of potent antihistamines (e.g., hydroxyzine or doxepin)	Add omalizumab on to second-generation antihistamine therapy.
Assess for patient tolerance and efficacy before advancing.	Can advance if inadequate control within six months or earlier if symptoms are intolerable.
Step 4:	*Step 4:*
Addition of an alternative agent:	Add cyclosporine on to second-generation antihistamine therapy.
• Omalizumab or cyclosporine	
• Use of other anti-inflammatory agents, immunosuppressives, or biologic	

Testing for autoimmune thyroid disease can be warranted if there is supporting clinical suspicion. The physical urticaria can be provoked in a clinical setting by using standardized provocation tests.

Differential diagnosis: Urticarial vasculitis is often indistinguishable from urticaria, but lesions last greater than 24 hours. The differential includes urticaria pigmentosa, familial cold urticaria, bradykinin-mediated angioedema (e.g., hereditary angioedema), and urticarial pemphigoid.

Management: Careful patient history taking is useful in determining aggravating factors of urticaria. It may be helpful to ask the patient to keep a diary of symptoms to identify possible precipitants. If a precipitating factor is identified, then avoidance of the trigger is the hallmark of management.

Treatment of urticaria follows a stepwise approach. Although both international and American guidelines begin with the same first step in treatment, subsequent advancements in treatment differ as noted. Short courses of oral corticosteroids, such as prednisone 30–50 mg daily, can be used to treat severe urticaria. These agents should not be used as maintenance therapy.

• Step 1: Symptomatic treatment with second-generation antihistamines (e.g., cetirizine 10 mg daily, levocetirizine 5 mg daily, fexofenadine 180 mg daily, loratadine, 10 mg daily)

Course: The course for urticaria varies greatly from patient to patient. Although some patients will experience near-total control of symptoms with daily oral second-generation antihistamines, sometimes obtaining symptom resolution within a year, others will continue to experience symptoms for decades.

Final comment: Urticaria is an extremely common skin disorder that presents with significant clinical variability. Special attention should be given to patient history, since this can often help determine the etiology.

ERYTHEMA NODOSUM

Definition: Erythema nodosum (EN) is a common form of panniculitis, in which there is inflammation within the subcutaneous fat. It is a delayed hypersensitivity reaction in which crops of tender subcutaneous nodules can develop in response to antigenic stimuli.

Overview: Although approximately 30–50% of cases have no identifiable underlying cause, EN is known to occur secondary to a variety of conditions. The most common causes of secondary EN include streptococcal infections, viral upper respiratory tract infections, bacterial gastroenteritis, coccidiomycosis, medications, and systemic diseases, such as sarcoidosis, tuberculosis, and inflammatory bowel disease. EN is more prevalent in women who are 20–40 years old. Additionally, it is more often seen in areas where certain predisposing infections, such as *Coccidioides immitis*, are more commonly encountered.

Clinical presentation: EN classically presents with the acute development of crops of tender, erythematous, slightly raised, subcutaneous nodules on the bilateral legs, most notably the shins. The nodules range in size from 1–5 cm in diameter. Less commonly, lesions can present on the thighs and forearms. With gentle palpation, the deep nature of the nodules can be appreciated. Nonspecific systemic symptoms, such as malaise, fever, and arthralgias, may accompany.

Laboratory studies: A skin biopsy can be performed in atypical cases. The histology classically depicts a septal panniculitis. Laboratory abnormalities can assist in the diagnosis of an underlying cause. A complete blood count can help to assess for infection or malignancy. Erythrocyte sedimentation rate and/or C-reactive protein can indicate widespread inflammation and possible systemic disease. Antistreptolysin O titers and rapid streptococcal tests can evaluate for possible strep infection as the precipitating factor. A chest x-ray can assess for sarcoidosis and tuberculosis.

Differential diagnosis: This includes erythema induratum (nodular vasculitis), pancreatic panniculitis, subcutaneous bacterial or fungal infections, malignant subcutaneous infiltrates (lymphoma), and cutaneous polyarteritis nodosa.

Management: Treatment includes bed rest and leg elevation, NSAIDs, salicylates, and saturated solution of potassium iodide (450–1500 mg/day) if indicated. In resistant or recurrent cases, other systemic immunosuppressants can be considered. When determined, the management of the underlying condition is key.

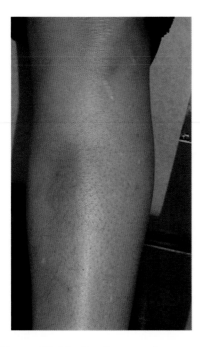

Figure 11.14 Erythema nodosum.

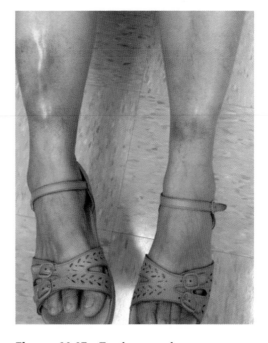

Figure 11.15 Erythema nodosum.

Table 11.5 Common Causes of Erythema Nodosum

Drugs
　Penicillin
　Sulfonamides
　Oral contraceptives

Infections
　Streptococcal infection
　Tuberculosis
　Leprosy
　Coccidioidomycosis
　Histoplasmosis
　Blastomycosis
　Hepatitis B
　Mononucleosis

Malignancy
　Lymphoma
　Leukemia

Miscellaneous
　Crohn's disease
　Ulcerative colitis
　Sarcoidosis
　Pregnancy
　Sweet syndrome
　Behçet's disease

Course: The lesions tend to last from a few days to a few weeks, with the majority of cases resolving by 8 weeks. As the lesions resolve, they can leave an ecchymotic appearance on the affected areas. EN nodules do not ulcerate and do not scar, but pigmentary changes caused by the lesions can persist for up to one year.

Final comment: EN is largely a self-limited condition. Special attention must be paid to rule out associated conditions, such as sarcoidosis, tuberculosis, and inflammatory bowel disease.

ERYTHEMA INDURATUM

Synonyms: Nodular vasculitis, erythema induratum of Bazin

Definition: Erythema induratum (EI), or nodular vasculitis, is a form of panniculitis. It is a relatively uncommon finding most classically associated with latent or active tuberculosis (TB) infection but may also be medication-induced or, rarely, idiopathic.

Overview: EI is a panniculitis that occurs as a hypersensitivity reaction, most commonly to an underlying TB infection. EI associated with TB is considered a tuberculid. Historically, EI, or EI of Bazin, has been used to describe TB-associated nodular vasculitis, but some clinicians use these phrases interchangeably.

Despite its potential association with TB, it is considered a hypersensitivity reaction rather than an infectious process. Medications implicated in drug-induced EI include etanercept and propyl-thiouracil. EI may occasionally be associated with a variety of autoimmune diseases, but this is considered rare and only documented in various case reports. EI most commonly occurs in adult women.

Clinical presentation: EI classically presents as tender, violaceous, subcutaneous, 1–2-cm nodules on the calf. They are often erythematous with occasional ulceration. Rarely, EI may arise elsewhere on the body, including the anterior shin, trunk, arms, or face. Healing lesions often scar with variable post-inflammatory hyperpigmentation. Patients with EI not associated with the underlying disease typically do not have fever, chills, or other constitutional symptoms.

Laboratory studies: The diagnosis of EI typically requires a biopsy. The histology of EI has two components: panniculitis and vasculitis. The panniculitis affects the lobules of fat rather than the septae. There is a mixed inflammatory infiltrate and granuloma formation. The vasculitis component can include different-sized vessels but most commonly the septal veins in the involved fat.

Interferon-gamma release assay or tuberculin skin test can evaluate for underlying tuberculosis. A chest x-ray may also be ordered to evaluate for possible tuberculosis.

Differential diagnosis: This includes EN and polyarteritis nodosa. Other panniculitides can be considered.

Management: EI is generally managed by controlling the underlying cause. In the case of TB-associated EI, patients should be started on standard TB treatment for either latent or active disease. In drug-associated EI, withdrawal of the medication can lead to resolution. Supportive care for the lesions can be provided with mild pain medications and other treatments to support healing, such as leg elevation.

Steroids may be considered if underlying TB infection has been excluded. In some cases, the identifiable cause of EI is unclear, and treatment can be difficult. In these patients, or patients with non-resolving nodular vasculitis with associated underlying disease, oral potassium iodide is effective.

Course: EI is non-life-threatening and typically resolves after treatment of the underlying cause. If there is no identifiable cause or if the patient has relapsing EI, treatment with systemic steroid or potassium iodide may be effective.

Final comment: EI is classically described as a tuberculid affecting the subcutaneous fat on the calves; however, it may also be associated with other underlying disease and drugs, or it may be idiopathic.

PRURITUS

Synonym: Itching

Definition: Pruritus is a common symptom, rather than a disease entity, with a multitude of possible causes. It is an uncomfortable sensation in the skin, which is mediated by various neuro-humoral pathways and can be relieved by rubbing or scratching.

Overview: Pruritus is a symptom that can have a variety of possible causes. Underlying etiologies of pruritus can include dermatologic diseases (e.g., atopic dermatitis, xerosis, scabies), systemic diseases (e.g., diseases of pregnancy, drug-induced pruritus), neurologic and psychiatric diseases, or internal malignancy (e.g., Hodgkin lymphoma). Chronic pruritus can have a significant impact on quality of life.

Clinical presentation: Clinical signs of long-standing pruritus include excoriations, ecchymoses, lichen simplex chronicus, or prurigo nodularis. The exact clinical presentation of pruritus depends on its etiology. Three different clinical groups of pruritus have been proposed: pruritus on diseased or inflamed skin, pruritus on nondiseased skin, and pruritus with secondary scratch lesions.

Laboratory studies: Biopsy may be helpful in patients who present with obvious signs of primary skin involvement. Histology findings will depend on the underlying cause. Blood work and other studies (MRI, CT, etc.) may be useful if a systemic cause is suspected.

Differential diagnosis: Pruritus on inflamed skin is predominantly due to dermatologic disease. The possible list of etiologies is quite broad but includes inflammatory, infectious, auto-immune, and neoplastic causes. Common inflammatory dermatoses include atopic dermatitis, psoriasis, contact dermatitis, xerosis, drug reactions, and scars. Infectious dermatoses include mycotic, bacterial, or viral infections, folliculitis, scabies, and arthropod bites. Autoimmune dermatoses include bullous dermatoses, particularly, dermatitis herpetiformis, as well as bullous pemphigoid. Neoplastic causes are typically related to cutaneous lymphomas and leukemias including cutaneous T-cell-lymphoma, cutaneous B-cell lymphoma, and leukemic infiltrates of the skin.

Pruritus on noninflamed skin may be due to systemic, neurologic, or psychiatric causes. These secondary causes can be due to almost any etiology, and these patients often present with the classic signs of long-standing pruritus. A good first approach is to review the patient's medications as several common medications have been linked to pruritus (e.g., opioids, ACE inhibitors, amiodarone, hydrochlorothiazide, estrogens, simvastatin, allopurinol). Common systemic diseases to consider include chronic renal failure, liver diseases, hyperthyroidism, malabsorption, and perimenopausal pruritus. Certain infectious diseases may also cause chronic pruritus such as HIV infection, helminths, or parasites. Malignancy is again a consideration in systemic disease usually of hematologic origin. Etiologies include polycythemia vera, Hodgkin lymphoma, and non-Hodgkin lymphoma. Pregnancy is also associated with certain systemic causes of pruritus including cholestasis of pregnancy, polymorphic eruption of pregnancy, pemphigoid gestationis, and prurigo gestationis.

Management: This is dependent upon the underlying cause. Treatment can include a combination of antipruritic medications, such as pramoxine, antihistamines, and topical corticosteroids, and behavioral therapy.

FINAL THOUGHT

Pruritus is a common finding in many cutaneous diseases. Common causes include mockenhaupxerosis, atopic dermatitis, and urticaria.

ADDITIONAL READINGS

Antia C, Baquerizo K, Korman A, et al. Urticaria: a comprehensive review: epidemiology, diagnosis, and work-up. J Am Acad Dermatol. 2018;79:599–614.

Magerl M, Altrichter S, Borzova E, et al. The definition, diagnostic testing, and management of chronic inducible urticarias—the EAACI/GA(2) LEN/EDF/UNEV consensus recommendations 2016 update and revision. Allergy. 2016;71:780–802.

Miliszewski MA, Kirchhof MG, Sikora S, et al. Stevens-Johnson syndrome and toxic epidermal necrolysis: an analysis of triggers and implications for improving prevention. Am J Med. 2016;129:1221–1225.

Mockenhaupt M, Viboud C, Dunant A, et al. Stevens-Johnson syndrome and toxic epidermal necrolysis: assessment of medication risks with emphasis on recently marketed drugs. The EuroSCAR-study. J Invest Dermatol. 2008;128:35–44.

Sekula P, Dunant A, Mockenhaupt M, et al. Comprehensive survival analysis of a cohort of patients with Stevens-Johnson syndrome and toxic epidermal necrolysis. J Invest Dermatol. 2013;133:1197–1204.

Sidoroff A, Dunant A, Viboud C, et al. Risk factors for acute generalized exanthematous pustulosis (AGEP)-results of a multinational case-control study (EuroSCAR). Br J Dermatol. 2007;157:989–996.

Ständer S, Weisshaar E, Mettang T, et al. Clinical classification of itch: a position paper of the International Forum for the Study of Itch. Acta Derm Venereol. 2007;87:291–294.

Wetter DA, Davis MD. Recurrent erythema multiforme: clinical characteristics, etiologic associations, and treatment in a series of 48 patients at Mayo Clinic, 2000 to 2007. J Am Acad Dermatol. 2010;62:45–53.

Yosipovitch G, Rosen JD, Hashimoto T. Itch: from mechanism to (novel) therapeutic approaches. J Allergy Clin Immunol. 2018;142:1375–1390.

Zuberbier T, Aberer W, Asero R, et al. The EAACI/GA²LEN/EDF/WAO guideline for the definition, classification, diagnosis and management of urticaria. Allergy. 2018;73:1393–1414.

12 Connective Tissue Disorders

Laura Atzori, Caterina Ferreli, and Franco Rongioletti

CONTENTS

Synonym: Collagen diseases

Definition: Connective tissue disorders (CTDs) are a heterogeneous group of conditions that share autoimmune pathogenesis associated with an abnormal function or structure of the elements of the connective tissue. Major CTDs include lupus erythematosus, scleroderma, dermatomyositis, and Sjogren syndrome.

LUPUS ERYTHEMATOSUS

Overview: Lupus erythematosus is a complex autoimmune systemic disease with variable clinical features. Skin involvement is common in systemic lupus erythematosus (SLE) and is divided into specific skin lesions with typical histopathology and non-specific skin manifestations (Table 12.1).

Table 12.1 Classification of Cutaneous Manifestations in Systemic Lupus Erythematosus (LE)

Specific Lesions		
Acute cutaneous LE	**Subacute cutaneous LE**	**Chronic cutaneous LE**
• Localized (malar or butterfly eruption)	• Annular	• Classic DLE
• Generalized:	• Papulo-squamous or psoriasiform lesions	• Hypertrophic (verrucous) DLE
Maculo-papular eruption	• Symmetric, widespread, superficial non- scarring lesions	• Lupus panniculitis
Bullous lupus		• Lupus tumidus
Toxic epidermal necrolysis variant of SLE	• Photoexposed areas	• Chilblain lupus
		• Discoid/lichen planus overlap

LE-Nonspecifc Lesions	
Skin vascular lesions	**Nonvascular lesions**
• Leukocytoclastic vasculitis	• Papulonodular mucinosis
• Raynaud's phenomenon	• Anetoderma/cutis laxa
• Urticarial vasculitis	• Erythema multiforme
• Polyarteritis nodosa-like	• Nonscarring alopecia
• Degos's disease like	• Urticaria
• Atrophie blanche-like	• Aseptic pustulosis
• Livedo reticularis	• Calcinosis
• Periungual teleangectasias	
• Thrombophlebitis	
• Leg ulcers	

DOI: 10.1201/9781003105268-12

DISCOID LUPUS ERYTHEMATOSUS

Definition: Chronic cutaneous lupus erythematosus (CCLE) includes discoid lupus erythematosus (DLE), lupus tumidus, chilblain lupus, and lupus panniculitis. The most common type is DLE, which accounts for 80% of CCLE. Less than 5% of patients develop the systemic disease.

Clinical presentation: DLE is more common in women in the fourth decade and skin of color. It is characterized by sharply demarcated, raised figurate, erythematous-violaceous, disk-like plaques (Figure 12.1) with deep follicular keratotic plugs that leave behind hypo- and hyperpigmented scars. DLE lesions can be localized to the head and neck or disseminated to the trunk and extremities. Scalp lesions are found in 60% of patients, which can cause cicatricial alopecia (Figure 12.2). Hypertrophic lupus is an uncommon variant of DLE that is characterized by the development of hyperkeratotic, verrucous plaques.

Laboratory studies: Serologic examination is usually not decisive with a low incidence of ANA positivity. The gold standard for the diagnosis is histopathology, which is prototypic of an interface dermatitis of the vacuolar type (Figures 12.3 and 12.4). Direct immunofluorescence shows linear or granular immunoglobulin (IgG, or less IgM) and/or complement deposition at the dermo-epidermal junction in 80–90% of cases.

Management: Essential preventive measures include sun avoidance and the use of sunscreen. Topical treatment with corticosteroids represents the first line of treatment. Intralesional steroid injections are useful in individually resistant lesions. Topical calcineurin inhibitors, especially tacrolimus ointment, have been proven to be effective, especially for facial involvement. For widespread disease, hydroxychloroquine remains a cornerstone of treatment. Systemic corticosteroids can be evaluated in highly active diseases when antimalarials are either contraindicated or

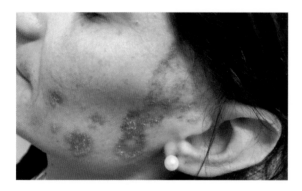

Figure 12.1 Discoid lupus erythematosus.

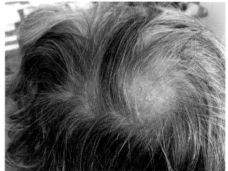

Figure 12.2 Discoid lupus erythematosus with scalp involvement.

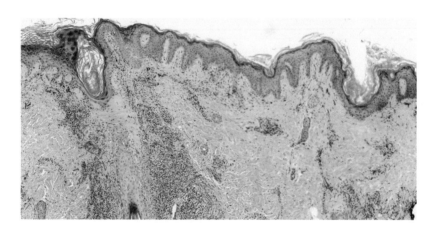

Figure 12.3 Discoid lupus erythematosus histology.

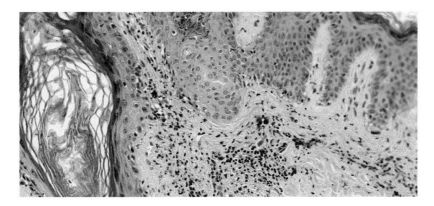

Figure 12.4   Discoid lupus erythematosus histology.

ineffective. Dapsone is an alternative option as well as thalidomide in some European countries. The refractory disease has been treated with retinoids, methotrexate, mofetil or mycophenolate acid, cyclosporine, and azathioprine with variable results. Give suggested doses.

Course: Lesions of DLE leave behind scars, which can often be disfiguring. Scarring alopecia is another frequent and severe complication. The disease course is unpredictable with spontaneous healing in about 50% of patients. There are also frequent relapses, especially after sun exposure, and sudden widespread disease (5–10% of patients), which should always be evaluated for SLE.

Final comment: CCLE may occur in the setting of systemic LE or as an independent disorder. DLE is the most common form. Confirmatory histopathology is indicated.

SYSTEMIC LUPUS ERYTHEMATOSUS

Definition: Systemic lupus erythematosus (SLE) can affect virtually any organ of the body. The generation of numerous types of autoantibodies causes several combinations of clinical signs and laboratory abnormalities.

Clinical presentation: SLE is more common in women in their 30's with a predilection for darker-skinned patients. The new classification of SLE diagnostic criteria following the European League Against Rheumatism (EULAR) and the American College of Rheumatology (ACR) is presented in Table 12.2. Skin manifestations are present in 80% of cases, and specific acute lesions can be associated with overt systemic symptoms. A typical sign is the malar or butterfly eruption, which presents with erythema that crosses both cheeks but spares the nasolabial folds (Figure 12.5).

A generalized photosensitive, pruritic maculopapular eruption is another specific manifestation, characterized by widespread dermatitis on photo exposed areas and above the waistline. A nonscarring form of alopecia, very similar to telogen effluvium is seen during exacerbations of SLE with an excessive shedding of thin and brittle hairs that are referred to as "lupus hairs." Acral lesions resembling erythema multiforme in patients with LE (discoid or systemic), associated with immunological changes including positive tests for rheumatoid factor, speckled antinuclear antibody, positive anti-Ro or anti-La antibodies have been named Rowell's syndrome. Rarely, a severe acute form can resemble toxic epidermal necrolysis. Occasionally, blistering may complicate very acute forms with bullous lesions (bullous LE).

Laboratory studies: Investigation for signs of systemic disease is always mandatory, especially for renal involvement. Antibody testing is critical and should begin with an ANA screen followed by a specific autoantibody profile (Table 12.3).

The cornerstone of diagnosis is the histopathology showing an interface dermatitis, which is typically less pronounced when compared to DLE subtypes. Direct immunofluorescence (DIF) of involved skin and possibly non-involved skin shows granular or linear immunoglobulins and complement deposition at the dermal-epidermal junction (lupus band test).

Management: Among systemic agents, antimalarials (e.g., hydroxychloroquine 400 mg/daily) remain a first-line treatment. Short courses of corticosteroids are sometimes necessary to control flares. Oral retinoids and some immunosuppressive treatments, including methotrexate, cyclophosphamide, azathioprine, and mycophenolate mofetil, are alternative therapies. Anti-BlyS antibody belimumab has demonstrated a good responder index and has recently been approved

Table 12.2 New Classification Criteria of the European League Against Rheumatism and the American College of Rheumatology for Systemic Lupus Erythematosus (SLE; 2019)

Entry criterion: Presence of antinuclear antibodies at a titer of ?1:80 on Hep-2 cells or an equivalent positive test.

Additive criteria: Do not count a criterion if there is a more likely explanation than SLE; occurrence of a criterion on at least one occasion is sufficient; criteria need not to occur simultaneously; at least one clinical criterion and ?10 points are required: within each domain only the highest weighted criterion is countered towards the total score.

Clinical Domains and Criteria	Weight	Immunology Domains and Criteria	Weight
Constitutional		*Antiphospholipid antibodies*	
Fever	2	Anti-cardiolipin antibodies or	2
Hematologic		Anti-beta2GP1 antibodies or	
Leukopenia	3	Lupus anticoagulant	
Thrombocytopenia	4		
Autoimmune hemolysis	4		
Neuropsychiatric		*Complement proteins*	
Delirium	2	Low C3 or low C4	3
Psychosis	3	Low C3 and low C4	4
Seizure	5		
Mucocutaneous		*SLE-specific antibodies*	
Nonscarring alopecia	2	Anti-dsDNA antibodies or	6
Oral ulcers	2	Anti-Smith antibodies	
Subacute cutaneous or discoid lupus	4		
Acute cutaneous lupus	6		
Serosal			
Pleural or pericardial effusion	5		
Acute pericarditis	6		
Musculoskeletal			
Join involvement	6		
Renal			
Proteinuria >0.5 g/24h			
Renal biopsy Class II or V lupus nephritis			
Renal biopsy Class III or IV lupus nephritis			
TOTAL SCORE:			

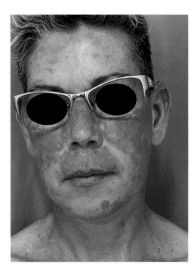

Figure 12.5 Systemic lupus erythematosus.

Table 12.3 Autoantibody Tests for Systemic Lupus Erythematosus assessment.

Test	Abbreviation	Clinical Significance
Antinuclear antibodies (on HEp-2 cells)*	ANA	Screening for autoimmunity
Extractable nuclear antigens (ENA)	ENA	Screening for autoimmunity
Native-DNA or double strains-DNA antibodies	n-DNA or ds-DNA	Marker for systemic lupus erythematosus
Deoxyribonuclear protein	DNP	Marker for systemic lupus erythematosus
Histone antibodies	AHIST	Drug-induced lupus erythematosus
Anti- Smith antibodies	Sm	Marker for systemic lupus erythematosus
Ribonuclear protein	RPN	Systemic lupus erythematosus, mixed connective tissue disease, scleroderma
SS-A (Ro) antibodies	SS-A (Ro)	Lupus erythematosus (photosensitivity); Sjögren's disease; dermatomyositis
SS-B (La) antibodies	SS-B (La)	Subacute cutaneous lupus erythematosus (SCLE), neonatal lupus erythematosus
Proliferating cell nuclear antigen	PCNA	Systemic lupus erythematosus with proliferative glomerulonephritis
Anti-Ku (Ki) antibodies	Ku (Ki)	Systemic lupus erythematosus; polymyositis/scleroderma overlap
Phospholipid antibodies (Lupus anticoagulant)	LAC	Systemic lupus erythematosus with thrombosis

Note: *HEp-2: human epithelial cell tissue substrate.

in SLE. Topical treatment with corticosteroids or calcineurin inhibitors is considered adjuvant treatment.

Because photosensitivity is a common denominator of all skin manifestations, patient education on proper sun protection is a crucial measure in SLE.

Course: About 10–20% of patients do not respond adequately to the immunosuppressive treatment, and a mean of 0.5 flares per year has been estimated. An analysis of causes of death and timing showed that active SLE and infections prevailed during the first 5 years of disease, while thromboses are the most common cause of death in the long-term.

Final comment: Cutaneous involvement in SLE comprises a wide range of dermatologic manifestations, and diagnosis requires proper clinical and histopathologic classification of the subtypes.

SCLERODERMA

Definition: Scleroderma refers to an autoimmune fibrosing disorder, which can be divided into localized (LSc) and systemic (SSc) forms.

LOCALIZED SCLERODERMA (LSC)

Synonym: Morphea

Overview: Localized scleroderma (LSc) is characterized primarily by the thickening and hardening of the skin. This is typically in the absence of systemic involvement. It is a rare, idiopathic disease that occurs in children and adults with an incidence of about 3 per 100,000 people and is three times more common in women.

Clinical presentation: Morphea presents with single or multiple variably sized inflammatory or thickened sclerotic plaques over the trunk or extremities. These lesions eventually resolve and often leave behind permanent atrophy and dyspigmentation depending on the disease course and level of involvement (Figure 12.6). Morphea has a variety of clinical presentations that are illustrated in Table 12.4.

Laboratory studies: Diagnosis is typically made clinically. Some patients have elevated ANA levels. Histopathology can be helpful in doubtful cases by showing sclerosis of the reticular dermis with progressive loss of appendages and vessels, which often replaces subcutaneous tissue (Figure 12.7).

Differential diagnosis: Systemic sclerosis and several scleroderma-like conditions should be excluded (Table 12.5).

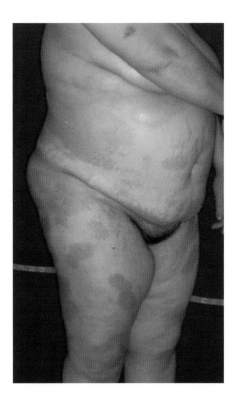

Figure 12.6 Morphea.

Table 12.4 Clinical presentation of localized scleroderma (Lsc)

Type of LSc	Clinical Presentation
Limited type	
Plaque-morphea (classical plaque type)	• Oval-shaped lesions surrounded by an erythematous border ("lilac ring") • In later stages, sclerotic in the center with a whitish or ivory color; old lesions may become atrophic and dyspigmented • May lead to hair loss and loss of the skin appendages • Predominantly located on the trunk
Guttate morphea	• Multiple small yellowish or whitish sclerotic lesions with a shiny surface • Early inflammatory lesions may present as erythematous macules • Predominantly located on the trunk
Atrophoderma of Pierini and Pasini (superficial morphea)	• Symmetrical, single or multiple, sharply demarcated, hyperpigmented, non-indurated patches • Located on the trunk or extremities
Generalized type	
Generalized LSc/morphea	• Four or more indurated plaques of more than 3 cm in diameter, involving two or more of seven anatomical sites (head-neck, each extremity, anterior and posterior trunk) • Often distributed symmetrically and tend to coalesce
Disabling pansclerotic morphea	• Extensive involvement of the skin, fat tissue, fascia, muscle, and bone • Fibrosis often results in severe contractures and poorly healing, large ulcerations and necroses • Absence of systemic involvement

Table 12.4 (Continued)

Linear type

Linear LSc/morphea of the extremities	• Longitudinally arranged linear, band-like lesions that may follow the lines of Blaschko • May heal with residual hyperpigmentation • May cause severe growth retardation, muscle atrophy, flexion contractures, myositis, arthritis, and psychological disability
Linear LSc/morphea "en coup de sabre"	• Typically located on the frontoparietal region, ranging paramedian from the eyebrows into the hair-bearing scalp • May be accompanied by scarring alopecia, seizures, migraine, headache, and eye involvement
Progressive facial hemiatrophy (Parry Romberg syndrome)	• Progressive facial hemiatrophy with involvement of the subcutaneous tissue, muscle, and bone but usually not the skin • May result in severe facial asymmetry • Concomitance with linear LSc "en coup de sabre" in up to 40%
Deep type (deep morphea)	• Fibrotic process mainly affecting the deeper layers (subcutaneous fat tissue, fascia, and underlying muscle) • Typically arranged symmetrically on the extremities
Mixed type	• Combined linear and plaque type or linear and generalized LSc; predominant in children
Eosinophilic fasciitis (Shulman syndrome)	• Rapid onset with symmetrical swelling of the extremities sparing hands and feet • Indurated and fibrotic lesions with typical "peau d'orange"–like appearance • Cutaneous veins appear as depressed compared to the surrounding tissue ("negative vein sign")

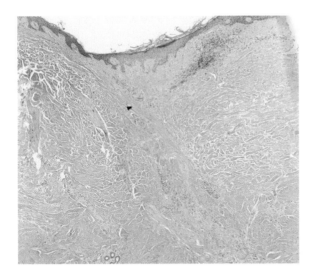

Figure 12.7 Morphea histology.

Management: There is no single evidence-based treatment regimen that is superior for all cases. Topical corticosteroids are the main treatment for plaque-like morphea. Topical tacrolimus 0.1% or calcipotriene are alternative choices. Active extensive morphea or generalized morphea are treated with methotrexate, combination therapy of systemic steroids and methotrexate, or with phototherapy with ultraviolet A1 (UVA1) or narrowband UVB. Linear scleroderma of the face or extremities generally requires the combination of systemic corticosteroids and methotrexate to limit functional disability and/or aesthetic outcomes.

Course: Disease activity typically continues for 3–6 years, but some patients develop longer periods of activity or recurrences. Self-healing is possible. Tissue sclerosis may cause joint contractures and other functional impairments.

Table 12.5 Differential Diagnosis of Scleroderma

LS Subtype	Differential Diagnoses
Limited local scleroderma (LSc; morphea)—initial inflammatory phase	Lichen sclerosus
	Erythema chronicum migrans
	Cutaneous mastocytosis
	Granuloma annulare
	Mycosis fungoides
	Drug-related reactions
	Chronic radiation dermatitis
	Porokeratosis Mibelli
Limited LSc (morphea)—late stage mainly with hyperpigmentation	Postinflammatory hyperpigmentation
	Lichen planus actinicus
	Cafe au lait spots
	Erythema dyschromicum perstans
Limited LSc (morphea)—late stage mainly with atrophy	Acrodermatitis chronica atrophicans
	Lipodystrophy
	Lichen sclerosus
	Scarring
Limited LSc (morphea)—late stage mainly with sclerosis	Necrobiosis lipoidica
	Pretibial myxedema
Generalized LSc	Systemic sclerosis
	Mixed connective tissue disease
	Pseudoscleroderma
	Scleredema adultorum
	Scleromyxedema
	Chronic graft-vs.-host disease
	Nephrogenic systemic fibrosis
	Porphyria cutanea tarda
Linear LSc en coup de sabre	Panniculitis
	Lupus erythematosus profundus
	Progressive lipodystrophy
	Localized lipodystrophy
	Focal dermal hypoplasia
	Steroid atrophy

SYSTEMIC SCLERODERMA

Synonym: Systemic sclerosis (SSc)

Definition: This is a generalized connective tissue disorder that is characterized by microvascular damage, autoimmunity, and excessive fibrosis of the skin and various internal organs. Skin thickening of the fingers of both hands, which extend proximal to the metacarpophalangeal joints, is the main diagnostic criterion.

Overview: The majority of patients are women. Young African American patients tend to have an earlier onset of disease and a more severe course. SSc can be divided into limited cutaneous systemic scleroderma (lcSSc), formerly known as the CREST syndrome (Calcinosis, Raynaud's phenomenon, Esophageal dysmotility, Sclerodactyly, and Telangiectasia), and a diffuse cutaneous systemic scleroderma (dcSSc). There are different autoantibody profiles, patterns of organ involvement, and prognosis. In systemic scleroderma, there is the involvement of the internal organs, such as the digestive tract, heart, lungs, and kidneys.

Clinical presentation: Raynaud's phenomenon is often the first manifestation of the disease. In lcSSc, the characteristic fibrotic skin changes are limited to fingers, hands (Figure 12.8), and face. Internal organ involvement occurs in the later stages of the disease process. On the upper portion of the trunk, some areas of depigmentation, the so-called "salt and pepper" sign, can be present.

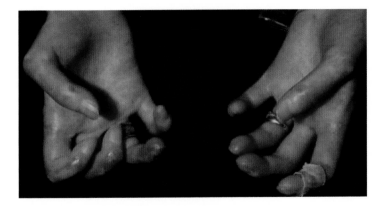

Figure 12.8 Systemic sclerosis affecting the hands

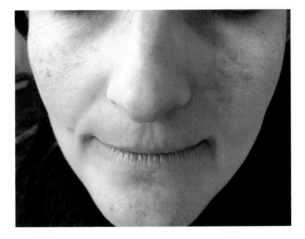

Figure 12.9 Systemic sclerosis affecting the face.

In dcSSc, the induration involves the distal and proximal portions of the extremities, face, and trunk. Systemic involvement occurs in the early stages of the disease. Typical facial features include microstomia, beaked nose, telangiectasias, and perioral furrows (Figure 12.9). The main differences between lcSSc and dcSSc are outlined in Table 12.6.

Laboratory studies: ANA test is positive in approximately 95% of patients with SSc. Anti-topoisomerase I (anti-Scl-70) antibodies are associated with dcSSc and a higher risk of severe interstitial lung disease. Anti-centromere antibody is typically associated with limited cutaneous lcSSc. Antibodies to RNA polymerase III are found in patients with dcSSc and are generally associated with rapidly progressive skin involvement, as well as an increased risk for a renal crisis.

Table 12.6 Clinical Difference between Limited and Diffuse Systemic Sclerosis (SSc)

SSc Limited Form	SSc Diffuse Form
• Long duration of Raynaud's phenomenon • Acral sclerosis limited to hands, forearms, feet • Possible involvement of the face • Skin calcinosis, teleangiectasias, esophageal involvement • Late pulmonary arterial hypertension • Anti-centromere antibody positive in 70–80%	• Early onset of Raynaud's phenomenon (within 1 year of skin changes) • Rapid involvement of the trunk, face, and extremities • Early and significant incidence of lung fibrosis, gastrointestinal, myocardial, and renal disease • Anti-Scl-70 (topoisomerase-1) positive in 30%

Capillary abnormalities of the proximal nail fold of the hands can be visualized with derma-toscopy or capilleroscopy. Histologically, cutaneous involvement is characterized by excessive deposition of compact and organized bundles of collagen in the dermis and subcutis, which can be similar appearing to morphea.

Differential diagnosis: Apart from the distinction from localized scleroderma, the differential diagnosis includes other systemic conditions that can mimic scleroderma. This includes scler-edema, nephrogenic systemic fibrosis, and scleromyxedema (Table 12.5).

Management: No effective therapy for SSc has been developed, and the risk of mortality remains high. At present, several immunosuppressants, including methotrexate (skin, inflamma-tory arthritis, myositis), cyclophosphamide, and mycophenolate mofetil (lung, skin), and azathio-prine (skin, lung, myositis) are being used for treatment.

Corticosteroids should be generally avoided, and high-dose or even long-term use of low to moderate doses of corticosteroids have been associated with precipitation of scleroderma renal cri-sis. Corticosteroids should be used only in cases of inflammatory myositis, inflammatory arthritis, and/or active inflammatory alveolitis.

The treatment of Raynaud's phenomenon includes calcium channel blockers coupled with pro-tection against cold and smoking cessation. In severe forms with trophic disorders, intravenous iloprost and bosentan are possible therapeutic options. Bosentan has demonstrated efficacy in the secondary prevention of digital ulcers.

Course: SSc is associated with high mortality with life expectancy dependent on the extent and severity of internal organ involvement. The most common cause of mortality in the past was scleroderma renal crisis, which can often be reduced with the advent of ACE inhibitors. Currently, the pulmonary disease is the most common cause of mortality. Prognosis in SSc has improved over the past 30 years with 5-year survival rates of up to 80%; however, patients with advanced pulmonary arterial hypertension have a less than 50% 2-year survival rate.

Final comment: While morphea is confined to the skin and/or underlying tissues, systemic sclerosis has the highest cause-specific mortality of all connective tissue diseases. Therapy is often difficult and not curative. Treatments for specific skin and systemic complications targeting vascu-lopathy, immune inflammation, and fibrosis have emerged.

DERMATOMYOSITIS

Definition: Dermatomyositis (DM) is an autoimmune disease characterized by the distinctive association of skin manifestations with muscle weakness; however, cases without muscle weak-ness can occasionally be diagnosed.

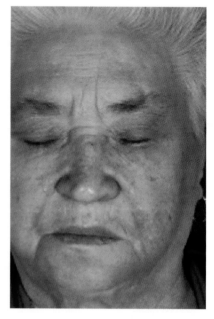

Overview: DM affects patients of any age with two incidence peaks between 5–15 years and 40–60 years of age. Women are more affected than men. A genetic predis-position, environmental factors, including viral infections, smoking, and sun exposure, malignant neoplasms of the internal organs, and drug intake, may trigger activation of the immune system.

Clinical presentation: Characteristic findings include a violet to dusky erythematous-edematous eruption on the face (heliotrope eruption; Figure 12.10), especially superior eyelids, chest (V sign), and back (shawl sign) as well as the presence of flat-topped, lichenoid violaceous papules and plaques overlying the hands, including the knuckles and metacarpophalangeal and interpha-langeal joints (Gottron's papules; Figure 12.11). Other findings include erythematous to violaceous macules and plaques on the elbows and knees (Gottron's sign; Figure 12.12) and nail folds.

Another peculiar manifestation is the mechanic hands, which refer to hyperkeratotic, scaly plaques on radial and ulnar aspects of the first three fingers. Less common skin changes include calcinosis cutis (more often associated with juvenile DM) and bullous and necrotic lesions. There is proximal myositis, which causes pain and tenderness, as well as profound weakness. Amyopathic dermatomyositis

Figure 12.10 Dermatomyositis affecting the face.

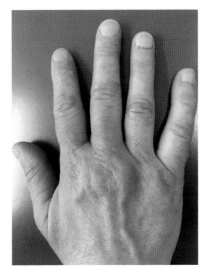

Figure 12.11 Dermatomyositis: Gottron's papules.

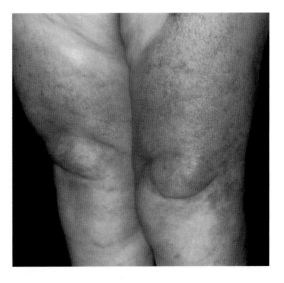

Figure 12.12 Dermatomyositis: Gottron's sign.

is a cutaneous form that occurs without muscle involvement. A constellation of visceral organ involvement includes interstitial lung disease, arthritis, myocarditis, and dysphagia.

Laboratory studies: LSc is characterized primarily by the thickening and hardening of the skin. This is typically in the absence of systemic involvement.

Blood chemistry and myositis autoantibodies that not only are highly disease-specific but also associated with distinct clinical features are reported in Table 12.7. Anti-MDA5 should be checked since this has been linked to rapidly progressing interstitial lung disease, which is typically fatal.

Table 12.7 Laboratory Assessment in Dermatomyositis

Test	Typical Findings
• Serum CK	• Elevated in 90% of patients; most specific enzyme
• Aldolase, transaminases, lactate dehydrogenase	• Useful to a smaller extent than CK
• Creatinine	• Decreased levels in long-standing myositis
• Myoglobin in serum or urine	• Indicative of muscle inflammation, predictive of clinical relapse
• Rheumatoid factor	• Elevated in 10–20% of the patients, often in those with overlap syndrome
• Anti-aminoacyl tRNA synthetase (anti-ARS) antibodies • (Jo-1, PL-7, PL-12, EJ, OJ, KS, Ha, Zo)	• Specific of polymyositis, associated with the antisynthetase syndrome (clinical triad of arthritis, myositis, and interstitial lung disease)
• Anti-Mi-2 (nuclear antigen)	• Classic DM, photosensitivity
• Anti-Transcriptional intermediary factor 1-γ (TIF1-γ) antibodies	• Suggestive of cancer-associated myositis, and severe cutaneous findings
• Melanoma differentiation-associated gene 5 (MDA5)	• Correlates with disease activity and rapidly progressive interstitial lung disease
• Anti-small ubiquitin-like modifier-1 activating enzyme (anti-SAE) antibody,	• Adult DM, dysphagia
• Antinuclear matrix protein 2 (NXP-2 or MJ, antip140)	• Juvenile DM, calcinosis
• Anti-signal recognition particle (Anti-SRP)	• Adult DM, acute onset necrotizing myopathy
• Anti-HMGCR	• Necrotizing myopathy, statin use

Abbreviations: CK, creatine phosphokinase; DM, dermatomyositis; HMGCR, 3-hydroxy-3-methylglutaryl coenzyme A reductase.

Nailfold capillaroscopy is a useful diagnostic tool, which demonstrates a "scleroderma-like" pattern. Histopathology of the skin reveals an interface dermatitis of a vacuolar-type similar to LE. The gold standard assessment for muscle involvement is electromyography, but a muscle biopsy is showing an inflammatory myositis can also be diagnostic.

Management: Systemic corticosteroids are the first line of therapy, which can be given as monotherapy or in combination with steroid-sparing immunosuppressive agents. These include azathioprine, methotrexate, mycophenolate mofetil, or high-dose intravenous immunoglobulins.

Course: Periods of spontaneous symptomatic relief are reported. Overall, prognosis has improved since the use of high-dose corticosteroids, which have a 50–90% response rate. Importantly, especially in refractory disease, a paraneoplastic phenomenon should be considered. Skin necrosis, cutaneous vasculitis, vesiculobullous lesions, and pruritus or a burning skin sensation in older patients are all cutaneous signs that can strongly suggest malignancy.

Final comment: Patients with a peculiar history of skin and muscular symptoms should provide clinical suspicion for DM, which can be easily confirmed by laboratory findings. Early recognition of potential systemic involvement, as well as potential paraneoplastic conditions, can allow for prompt and appropriate disease management.

SJÖGREN'S SYNDROME

Definition: Sjörgren's syndrome (SjS) is an autoimmune disease that can affect the exocrine glands. It is characterized by lacrimal and salivary gland inflammation with resultant dysfunction.

Overview: With an estimated prevalence of 0.5% in the general population, SjS has a strong predilection for Caucasian women.

Clinical presentation: The main clinical findings are decreases in tears (xeropthalmia) and salivary secretion (xerostomia). Widespread skin xerosis is reported in about 50% of patients, and frequent transient eczematous skin eruptions can mimic atopic dermatitis. There may be a history of photosensitivity with annular erythema or polycyclic erythematous, papulosquamous eruptions resembling subacute cutaneous LE, which is found mainly in patients of Asian ancestry. Oral candidosis and dental carries are chronic complications. SjS may occur alone (primary disease) or in association with a secondary disease, especially rheumatoid arthritis, SLE, and SSc. Clinical findings of SjS are summarized in Table 12.8.

Table 12.8 Clinical Findings in Sjögren's Syndrome (SjS)

Primary SjS	• Dry eye: Keratoconjunctivitis
	• Dry mouth: cracked lips and tongue; sore throat; difficult swallowing, chewing dry food, talking; taste/smell changes
	• Swollen parotid glands
	• Skin xerosis (23–67%)
	• Purpura (10–15%); livedo reticularis
	• Vasculitis (10%)
	• Skin ulcers (8%)
	• Photosensitive erythematous annular lesions (5–10%)
	• Vaginal dryness
	• Raynaud's phenomenon (18–37%)
	• Joints: nonerosive symmetrical arthritis (15–30%)
	• Chronic obstructive lung disease (10%); bronchiectasis (8%); interstitial lung disease (5%)
	• Pericarditis
	• Renal tubular acidosis (11%), glomerulonephritis, interstitial cystitis, nephrolithiasis
	• Muscle weakness or pain, fatigue
	• Neuropathy
	• Other symptoms: low-grade fever, dizziness, esophageal reflux

Table 12.8 (Continued)

Secondary SjS	• Systemic lupus erythematosus
	• Systemic sclerosis
	• Rheumatoid arthritis
	• Still's disease
	• Sarcoidosis
	• Inflammatory myopathies
	• Primary biliary cirrhosis
	• Autoimmune hepatitis
	• Autoimmune thyroiditis
	• Celiac disease
	• Multiple sclerosis
	• Infections: chronic hepatitis C; HTLV-1; HIV
	• Drugs: anticholinergics (atropine, scopolamine), sympathomimetic (ephedrine); benzodiazepines; selective serotonin reuptake inhibitors; tricyclic antidepressant; phenothiazines, antihistamines; nicotine; opioids; beta-blockers (atenolol, propranolol); diuretics.

Table 12.9 American College of Rheumatology/ European League Against Rheumatism Classification Criteria for Sjögren's Syndrome

Criterion	Score
Labial salivary gland with focal lymphocytic sialadenitis and focus score of ≥1 foci/4 mm	3
Anti-Ro/SSA positive	3
Ocular staining score ≥5 (or van Bijsterveld score ≥4) in at least one eye	1
Schirmer test ≤5 mm/5 minutes in at least one eye	1
Unstimulated whole saliva flow rate ≤0.1 mL/minute	1
Total score equal or >4 for the diagnosis of primary Sjögren's Syndrome	

Laboratory studies: Criteria for diagnosis are reported in Table 12.9.

Management: No specific cure has been established. Symptomatic treatment is generally provided to relieve mucosal and skin xerosis. Patients with more severe involvement require the use of oral steroids and steroid-sparing immunosuppressive agents, such as methotrexate, azathioprine, mycophenolate mofetil, leflunomide, and cyclophosphamide. Limited experience with the TNF-α inhibitor infliximab and with rituximab have shown some benefits.

Course: A very slow progression is characteristic of primary SjS. There is often a prominent impact on patient quality of life, but the disease is not life-threatening. When internal organ involvement occurs, morbidity and mortality become relevant, especially for the high incidence of non-Hodgkin B-cell lymphoma. Poor prognostic factors include severe parotid involvement, vasculitis/purpura, and hypocomplementemia.

FINAL THOUGHT

Patients with SjS present with variable and insidious symptoms of difficult classification. These can overlap with other autoimmune conditions, which requires referral to the appropriate specialist, including the ophthalmologist. Cutaneous manifestations often precede systemic findings and may be important for early diagnosis.

ADDITIONAL READINGS

Bogdanov I, Kazandjieva J, Darlenski R, et al. Dermatomyositis: current concepts. Clin Dermatol. 2018;36:450–445.

Callen JP. Cutaneous lupus erythematosus: reflecting on practice-changing observations over the past 50 years. Clin Dermatol. 2018;36:442–449.

Fanouriakis A, Kostopoulou M, Alunno A, et al. 2019 update of the EULAR recommendations for the management of systemic lupus erythematosus. Ann Rheum Dis. 2019;78:736–745.

Ferreli C, Gasparini G, Parodi A, et al. Cutaneous manifestations of scleroderma and scleroderma-like disorders: a comprehensive review. Clin Rev Allergy Immunol. 2017;53:306–336.

Knobler R, Moinzadeh P, Hunzelmann N, et al. European Dermatology Forum S1-guideline on the diagnosis and treatment of sclerosing diseases of the skin, Part 1: localized scleroderma, systemic sclerosis and overlap syndromes. J Eur Acad Dermatol Venereol. 2017;31:1401–1424.

Kowal-Bielecka O, Fransen J, Avouac J, et al. Update of EULAR recommendations for the treatment of systemic sclerosis. Ann Rheum Dis. 2017;76:1327–1339.

Kuhn A, Aberer E, Bata-Csörgő Z, et al. S2k guideline for the treatment of cutaneous lupus erythematosus—guided by the European Dermatology Forum (EDF) in cooperation with the European Academy of Dermatology and Venereology (EADV). J Eur Acad Dermatol Venereol. 2017;31:389–404.

Lipsker D, Lenormand C, Rongioletti F. Skin and autoimmune rheumatic diseases. In: Bijlsma WJ, Hachulla E, editors. EULAR. Textbook on Rheumatic Diseases. 3rd ed. London: BMJ; 2018.

Shiboski CH, Shiboski SC, Seror R, et al. 2016 American College of Rheumatology/European League Against Rheumatism classification criteria for primary Sjögren's syndrome. Ann Rheum Dis. 2017;76:9–16.

Thorar P, Torre K, Lu J. Cutaneous features and diagnosis of primary Sjögren syndrome: an update and review. J Am Acad Dermatol. 2018;79:736–745.

13 Vasculitides

Ivy M. Obonyo, Virginia A. Jones, Kayla A. Clark, and Maria M. Tsoukas

CONTENTS

Definition: The vasculitides are a heterogeneous group of clinicopathologic disorders, which involve inflammation of blood vessels (vasculitis) and variable ischemia, necrosis, and tissue damage. Vasculitis may be primary or a secondary manifestation of underlying systemic disease. These diseases are classified based on the size of the vessel affected (i.e., small, medium, or large vessel; Table 13.1). While the inflammatory response of some vasculitides may be confined to a single organ, others may involve several organs.

COVID-19 VASCULOPATHY

Overview: COVID-19-associated vasculitis/vasculopathy is a group of vasculitides caused by the severe acute respiratory syndrome coronavirus 2 (SARS-CoV-2). The etiology of COVID-19 vasculitis is not well elucidated and continues to evolve. Studies to date show that SARS-CoV-2 infects its host via the angiotensin-converting-enzyme 2 receptor on endothelial cells. These same findings have proposed that SARS-CoV-2 infection and subsequent host inflammatory response enable the initiation of endotheliitis. Ultimately, the outcome of this response may lead to widespread endothelial dysfunction and apoptosis.

    Clinical presentation: This can vary and present with systemic manifestations, such as fever and cough, in addition to symptoms of diseases listed in the differential diagnosis section.

    Laboratory studies: To date, there is no standardized method of detecting COVID-19 vasculitis. Typically, a combination of clinical, radiologic, and histopathologic findings is used. Histology of postmortem biopsies of patients with COVID-19 have demonstrated macro- and microvascular thrombosis in the arteries, veins, arterioles, capillaries, and venules in all major organs.

    Differential diagnosis: The following list is not exhaustive and is developing as our knowledge of the virus evolves. Other diagnoses to consider include urticarial vasculitis, lymphocytic vasculitis, Kawasaki disease, Kawasaki-like disease, and multiple inflammatory syndrome.

    Management: No defined management exists. Interventions listed in case reports include IV corticosteroids, intravenous immune globulin, aspirin, and supportive therapy.

    Course: As this is a novel disease, long-term conclusions regarding the course and prognosis disease remain to be determined.

    Final comment: COVID-19 can involve all organs, including the circulatory system. The associated pathologies induced by COVID-19 will evolve with our knowledge of the virus.

IMMUNE COMPLEX SMALL-VESSEL VASCULITIS

Overview: Small-vessel vasculitides are a group of disorders that primarily affect small vessels (i.e., small intraparenchymal arteries, arterioles, capillaries, and venules). In the following, we describe leukocytoclastic vasculitis (LCV), IgA vasculitis, urticarial vasculitis, and cryoglobulinemic vasculitis.

DOI: 10.1201/9781003105268-13

Table 13.1 Vasculitis Classification Compiled From to the 2012 Revised International Chapel Hill Consensus Conference

Type	Name
Large-Vessel Vasculitis	Giant Cell Arteritis
	Takayasu Arteritis
Medium-Vessel Vasculitis	Polyarteritis Nodosa
	Kawasaki disease
Small-Vessel Vasculitis	**ANCA-Associated Vasculitis**
	• Granulomatosis with Polyangiitis (Wegner's)
	• Eosinophilic Granulomatosis with Polyangiitis (Churg-Strauss)
	• Microscopic Polyangiitis
	Immune-Complex Small-Vessel Vasculitis
	• Cryoglobulinemic Vasculitis
	• Hypocomplementemic Urticarial Vasculitis (Anti-C1q Vasculitis)
	• IgA Vasculitis (Henoch-Schönlein)
	• Anti-glomerular basement membrane disease
Variable Vessel Vasculitis	Behçet's disease
	Cogan's syndrome
Single-Organ Vasculitis	Cutaneous leukocytoclastic angiitis
	Cutaneous arteritis
	Primary central nervous system vasculitis
	Isolated Aortitis
	Others
Vasculitis associated systemic disease	Lupus vasculitis
	Rheumatoid vasculitis
	Sarcoid vasculitis
	Others
Vasculitis associated with probable etiology	Hepatitis C virus–associated cryoglobulinemic vasculitis
	Hepatitis B virus–associated vasculitis
	Syphilis-associated aortitis
	Drug-associated immune complex vasculitis
	Drug-associated ANCA-associated vasculitis
	Cancer-associated vasculitis
	Others

Abbreviations: ANCA, antineutrophil cytoplasmic antibody.

Leukocytoclastic Vasculitis

Synonym: Hypersensitivity vasculitis

Definition: This is a small-vessel, immune complex-mediated vasculitis of the dermal capillaries and venules. LCV is idiopathic in nearly half of cases, and secondary LCV has been linked to underlying systemic autoimmune diseases, chronic infections, malignancies, and drugs.

Clinical presentation: The major cutaneous clinical findings of LCV include erythematous macules, nonblanching petechiae, and bilateral, palpable purpura commonly on the lower extremities and buttocks (Figures 13.1 and 13.2). Lesions range in size between 1 mm to 1 cm. In extremely rare instances, the presentation can be unilateral and localized. Clinical findings include hemorrhagic vesicles and bullae, pustules, nodules, crusted ulcers, and livedo reticularis. Systemic symptoms may comprise low-grade fevers, general malaise, myalgias, and arthralgias.

Laboratory studies: The gold standard for diagnosis of LCV is skin biopsy with direct immunofluorescence. Baseline labs (e.g., complete blood counts, liver function test, and renal function tests) may also be considered. Additional workup to rule out an underlying disease may be conducted in the setting of high clinical suspicion.

Histologic features depict infiltration with polymorphonuclear neutrophils in and around the vessel walls, signs of activation, degranulation, and neutrophilic death as portrayed by leukocytoclasis, with evidence of tissue damage and fibrinoid necrosis (Figures 13.3 and 13.4).

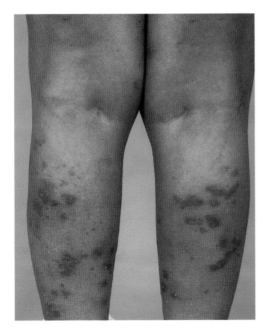

Figure 13.1 Purpuric papules and plaques, some annular, on the flexor aspects of the legs in a skin of color patient with leukocytoclastic vasculitis.

Source: From Visualdx (www.visualdx.com), used with permission.

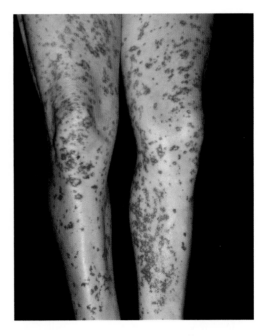

Figure 13.2 Purpuric papules and plaques, some annular, on the extensor aspects of the legs in a patient with leukocytoclastic vasculitis.

Source: From Visualdx (www.visualdx.com), used with permission.

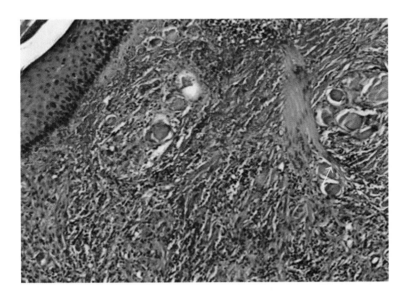

Figure 13.3 Leukocytoclastic vasculitis of thin walled, papillary dermal vessels characterized by mural fibrinoid necrosis and nuclear dust (arrow). A marked perivascular neutrophilic infiltrate and many extravasated red blood cells are present (hematoxylin and eosin stain; 100×).

Source: From Liu PY, Prete PE, Kukes G. Leukocytoclastic Vasculitis in a Patient with Type 1Cryoglobulinemia. Case Reports in Rheumatology. 2011; 2011:124940, used under Creative Commons License.

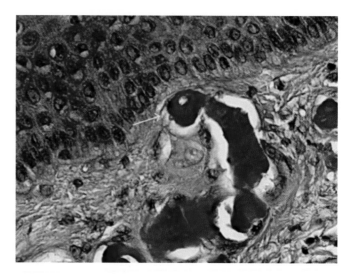

Figure 13.4 Intraluminal monoclonal immunoglobulin casts in superficial papillary dermal vessels. Note the swollen endothelial cells (arrow; periodic acid-Schiff stain, 400×).

Source: From Liu PY, Prete PE, Kukes G. Leukocytoclastic Vasculitis in a Patient with Type 1 Cryoglobulinemia. Case Reports in Rheumatology. 2011; 2011:124940, used under Creative Commons license.

Differential diagnosis: This includes thrombocytopenic purpura, benign pigmented purpura, Schamberg disease, systemic vasculitides, and polyarteritis nodosa.

Management: The treatment for mild idiopathic LCV includes supportive measures, such as leg elevation, rest, compression stockings, and antihistamines. Dapsone or colchicine are useful for generalized disease. In the chronic or resistant forms, a 4–6-week course of tapering corticosteroid dose, commonly prednisone administered at a dose of 0.5 mg/kg per day of ideal body weight until new lesion formation ceases, is the standard of treatment. If the cause of LCV is believed to be drug-induced, then the offending agent should be withdrawn. In cases of secondary LCV, the underlying infection, systemic disease, or malignancy should be treated if discovered.

Course: Nearly 90% of patients undergo spontaneous resolution of LCV within weeks to months. The remaining cases progress to chronic disease varying from 2 to 4 years in duration. The mortality due to LCV is low and is usually caused by systemic involvement.

Final comment: LCV is associated with a low mortality index. Detailed history and physical examination are requisite to determine if LCV is limited to cutaneous involvement and to rule out systemic disease.

Henoch-Schönlein Purpura

Synonym: IgA vasculitis

Overview: This is the most common vasculitis seen in pediatric patients, particularly in children under the age of 10 years. Henoch-Schönlein purpura (HSP) is a small-vessel vasculitis alongside granulomatosis with polyangiitis, eosinophilic granulomatosis with polyangiitis, and microscopic polyangiitis. Due to HSP's leukocytoclastic nature, the disease process manifests as a multisystem clinical presentation involving the skin, joints, kidneys, and gastrointestinal tract. HSP has been linked to malignancy, medications, and most notably upper respiratory tract infections, explaining its tendency to present in the winter months.

Clinical presentation: About 95% of patients with HSP present with a cutaneous eruption, most often manifesting as palpable petechiae or purpura on the buttocks and legs. (Figure 13.5) In addition to skin findings, 70–90% of patients present acutely with musculoskeletal involvement, including arthralgias and arthritis. Up to 72% of patients present symptomatically with abdominal pain and potentially life-threatening gastrointestinal bleeds, which can present with hematemesis or melena.

Renal involvement is also classically associated with HSP in 20–55% of patients and commonly presents as microscopic hematuria. When left untreated, renal involvement can progress to nephrotic syndrome and less commonly glomerulonephritis. It is important to note that in up to 14% of men with HSP, orchitis with the risk of testicular torsion can occur.

Laboratory studies: Histopathologically, HSP resembles LCV but affects smaller blood vessels. Neutrophil infiltration, with areas of necrosis and fibrin, contributes extensively to the inflammatory process in the dermis.

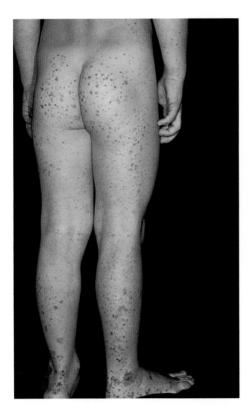

Figure 13.5 Palpable purpura on the proximal lower extremity.

Source: Courtesy of Thomas Habif, www.dermnet. com/images/Henoch-Schonlein-Purpura/ picture/14796, used under Creative Commons license.

Differential diagnosis: This may include other presentations of vasculitis, such as microscopic polyangiitis (MPA) and granulomatosis with polyangiitis (GPA). Systemic lupus erythematosus (SLE), sepsis, clotting disorders and thrombocytopenia should be considered.

Management: HSP, without renal involvement, is self-limited, and therefore, only supportive care is offered to improve comfort. If severe, treatment is geared toward the involved organ system. When arthralgias and arthritis is present, consider nonsteroidal anti-inflammatory drug (NSAID) therapy for symptomatic relief. Prednisone at 40 mg daily for several days may be used when abdominal pain is present. Immunosuppressive therapies, such as dapsone, rituximab, and cyclophosphamide, are generally reserved for complicated and severe cases. Additional interventions, such as anticoagulation, plasmapheresis, and tonsillectomy have also been tried, but a unanimous treatment plan has yet to be determined.

Course: HSP in children has an excellent prognosis with complete resolution in most patients. HSP has the ability to recur in some patients, with milder manifestations seen in comparison to the initial presentation. Morbidity is associated with renal involvement.

Final comment: HSP is well characterized due to its unique presentation and established diagnostic criteria. Although HSP is most often seen in children, adults with HSP can be screened for malignancy. Clinically, HSP presents characteristically with skin, joint, gastrointestinal, and kidney involvement but is self-limited in nature unless severe. Although well studied, a definitive treatment plan is still needed.

Urticarial Vasculitis

Overview: This is a rare and often misdiagnosed entity that presents similarly to acute and chronic urticaria. Most cases are idiopathic, but associations with autoimmune diseases and infections, including the novel COVID-19 virus, have been drawn. There is a female predominance, particularly for patients in their 40s. Clinically and histopathologically, urticarial vasculitis is varied and can share clinical presentation with other diseases.

Clinical presentation: Urticarial vasculitis can present cutaneously (Figure 13.6) with or without systemic findings. Tender and pruritic skin lesions, central clearing, and palpable purpura

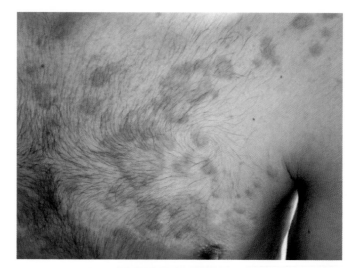

Figure 13.6 Vasculitic urticaria with pruritic hives located in the anterior thorax.

Source: From González A, Velásquez-Franco C, Pinto L et al. (2009). Urticarial Vasculitis. Revista Colombiana de Reumatología. 16. 154–166, used under Creative Commons license.

can be found on physical examination. Some of these lesions may persist for longer than 24 hours, resulting in scarring and hyperpigmentation.

Extracutaneous findings are common yet varied. Gastrointestinal and musculoskeletal manifestations have been reported, with renal and pulmonary symptoms presenting later on in the disease course. Less commonly, ophthalmologic complications have been reported.

Laboratory studies: Due to the extensive differential diagnosis list, urticarial vasculitis is confirmed by skin biopsy. Laboratory studies may show elevated erythrocyte sedimentation rate (ESR), hypocomplementemia, circulating immune complexes, autoantibodies, and anemia of chronic disease.

Microscopically, LCV can be seen as well as inflammation, predominantly neutrophils with some eosinophils and lymphocytes, of the capillary and postcapillary venule. Extravasated erythrocytes found perivascularly and in the interstitium with fibrin deposition may also be seen. On immunofluorescence, immunoglobulins, complement, and/or fibrinogen may be seen in a granular pattern. These findings help differentiate urticarial vasculitis from chronic allergic urticaria, which is characterized by lymphohistiocytic perivascular cuffing without extravasated erythrocytes.

Differential diagnosis: This includes acute and chronic urticaria, hypereosinophilic syndrome, mast cell disorders, polymorphous eruption of pregnancy, pemphigoid, systemic lupus erythematosus, and additional autoinflammatory diseases.

Management: The severity of the disease course determines the treatment plan. If pruritic in nature, administer antihistamines for symptom relief. If purely cutaneous, therapeutic agents, such as dapsone, colchicine, hydroxychloroquine, and indomethacin, may be used. When extracutaneous manifestations are found, then corticosteroids, such as oral prednisone may be tried. In severe cases, azathioprine, mycophenolate mofetil, cyclophosphamide, and cyclosporine are treatment options.

Course: Primarily idiopathic in nature, urticarial vasculitis may also be due to drug reactions, infections, autoimmune disorders, and paraneoplastic syndromes. Patients with hypocomplementemia may have systemic findings and worse prognosis.

Final comment: Urticarial vasculitis is a disease process that is predominately idiopathic and requires a skin biopsy to diagnose. The disease presents cutaneously with or without extracutaneous manifestations.

Cryoglobulinemic Vasculitis

Overview: Cryoglobulins stem from B cells in the context of infection, autoimmune disorders, or lymphoproliferative disorders. Cryoglobulinemias are categorized by clonality into three types: type I, type II, and type III. Type I is monoclonal and has the potential to be malignant, whereas types II and III are polyclonal and frequently present simultaneously. The release of cryoglobulins

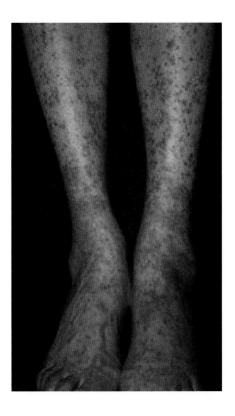

Figure 13.7 Classic cryoglobulinemia-related small-vessel vasculitis of lower extremities characterized by erythematous palpable maculopapular rash in an HCV-positive patient.

Source: From Hayat A, Mitwalli A. Hepatitis C and kidney disease. Hepat Res Treat. 2010;2010:534327, used under Creative Commons license.

into circulation can result in cutaneous and extracutaneous deposition presenting clinically as cryoglobulinemic vasculitis.

Clinical presentation: Cryoglobulinemic vasculitis may present cutaneously with or without systemic symptoms. Mild fever, purpura, and arthralgias may be seen on physical examination, whereas severe cases may involve the kidneys and central nervous system. Although rare, gastrointestinal and cardiopulmonary signs and symptoms may arise. Cryoglobulinemic vasculitis is most often seen in the context of hepatitis C virus (Figure 13.7), and its disease course and management are varied.

Laboratory studies: Cryoglobulins precipitate when cooled below core body temperature and dissolve when brought back to 37°F and can be used as a diagnostic tool in the context of cryoglobulinemic vasculitis. Immunoblotting is the most sensitive and specific test, but immunofixation and immunoelectrophoresis have also been used. Cryoglobulins may be measured indirectly by assessing levels of serum complement, monoclonal immunoglobulin, or rheumatoid factor.

Differential diagnosis: This would include infectious endocarditis, hyperviscosity syndrome, and the small-vessel vasculitides, GPA, eosinophilic granulomatosis with polyangiitis (EGPA), and MPA.

Management: Cryoglobulinemic vasculitis is most often due to an underlying lymphoproliferative (type I), infectious (type II/III) or autoimmune cause (type II/III). When lymphoproliferative, treatment can include plasmapheresis, rituximab, or corticosteroids. When infectious in nature, usually due to Hepatitis C Virus (HCV), treatment includes antiviral therapies (PegIFN/ribivarin) when mild, and rituximab ± plasmapheresis prior to antiviral therapeutics when severe. When due to an underlying autoimmune disease, such as Sjogren's, treatment includes immunosuppressives, such as high-dose corticosteroids, rituximab, cyclophosphamide, and mycophenolate mofetil, or plasmapheresis.

Course: When left untreated, cryoglobulinemic vasculitis can progress to renal failure, multifocal neuropathy, and worsening cutaneous manifestations. When HCV positive, viral load is monitored over time as this reflects long-term complications. There is a 35 times greater risk of B-cell non-Hodgkin lymphoma in HCV-positive patients and 4 times greater risk in HCV-negative patients. HCV-negative patients also have increased risk of death by sepsis when left untreated.

Morbidity and mortality rates have been associated with cryoglobulinemic vasculitis with survival rates varying depending on the type and HCV status. The lymphoproliferative presentation (type I) has the highest survival rate, whereas mixed cryoglobulinemic vasculitis (type II/III) depends on HCV status. Noninfectious mixed cryoglobulinemic vasculitis has the second-highest survival rate, whereas infectious mixed cryoglobulinemic vasculitis has the lowest survival rate.

Final comment: Cryoglobulinemic vasculitis has varied etiologies but is most commonly caused by infection. HCV is the most common infectious agent followed by HIV and Hepatitis B. Clinicians should be aware that therapies are dependent on HCV status and severity of vasculitis.

ANCA-Associated Vasculitis

Overview: Antineutrophil cytoplasmic antibody (ANCA)–associated vasculitis (AAV) is an umbrella term used to classify three small-vessel vasculitis diagnoses as follows: GPA, EGPA, and MPA (Table 13.2). Due to significant overlap in clinical presentation, a positive ANCA can be used to further differentiate these diagnoses. ANCA autoantibodies can be differentiated by patterns found on immunofluorescence (IF). Cytoplasmic patterns found on IF are classified as cANCA, or PR3-ANCA, whereas perinuclear patterns are classified as pANCA, or MPO (myeloperoxidase)-ANCA. MPA and EGPA are likely to stain pANCA positive, whereas GPA is likely to stain cANCA positive. Although not diagnostic, the staining patterns of ANCA help guide clinicians when narrowing the differential diagnosis.

Granulomatosis with Polyangiitis (Wegener's Granulomatosis)

Overview: GPA is a systemic disorder that is characterized by necrotizing vasculitis of the small arteries and veins. Classically, GPA is characterized by a triad of necrotizing granulomas of the upper and lower respiratory system, systemic vasculitis, and necrotizing glomerulonephritis. While the etiology is unclear, the pathogenesis may involve ANCA. Infections (e.g., *Staphylococcus aureus*, HCV, cytomegalovirus, Epstein-Barr virus, and parvovirus) and medications (e.g., hydralazine, phenytoin, antithyroid medications, sulfasalazine, allopurinol) have also been linked to the clinical phenotype of the disease. Genetic associations in GPA have been elucidated and include defective alpha 1 antitrypsin allele, CTLA-4, involved in activation of T cells, *PRTN3* gene, and the HLA-DP gene.

Clinical presentation: Common skin manifestations include palpable purpura and nodules. Necrotic ulcers, vesicles, bullae, urticarial plaques, petechiae, and subcutaneous nodules may also be present (Figures 13.8 and 13.9). Ocular involvement is common, as are oral manifestations (e.g., petechial hemorrhages), myalgias and arthralgias, rhinorrhea, and saddle-nose deformity due to granulomatous involvement of the nasal septum. Pulmonary signs, such as cough and hemoptysis, and renal signs, including hematuria and proteinemia, are also common.

Laboratory studies: Several diagnostic criteria have been proposed to aid in the diagnosis of GPA and to differentiate it from other vasculitides. Two widely used criteria are the American College of Rheumatology (ACR) criteria and the ear, nose, lung, and kidney (ELK) criteria.

The ACR criteria delineate a urinary sediment depicting red blood cell casts or >5 red blood cells per high-power field, abnormal findings on chest x-ray, oral ulcer or nasal discharge, and the

Table 13.2 Antineutrophil cytoplasmic antibody (ANCA)–associated vasculitis (AAV) classification.

Granulomatosis with Polyangiitis (Wegner's)	PR3-ANCA (c-ANCA) 75% of the time on immunofluorescence.
Eosinophilic Granulomatosis with Polyangiitis (Churg-Strauss)	MPO-ANCA (p-ANCA) positive 45% of the time on immunofluorescence. ANCA negative in 50% of cases.
Microscopic Polyangiitis	MPO-ANCA (p-ANCA) positive 60% of the time on immunofluorescence.

Abbreviations: ANCA, antineutrophil cytoplasmic antibody; AAV, ANCA-associated vasculitis; PR3, proteinase 3 antibodies; MPO, myeloperoxidase antibodies

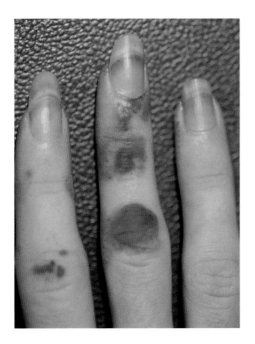

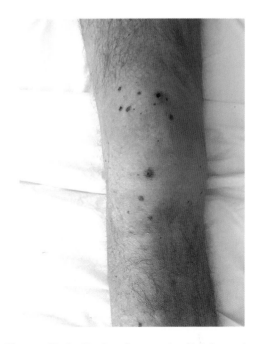

Figure 13.8 Purpuric papules and patches and some hemorrhagic vesicles and bullae on the fingers. Splinter hemorrhages are also present in this patient with GPA.

Source: From Visualdx (www.visualdx. com), used with permission.

Figure 13.9 Dark red, necrotic, slightly tender lesions developed symmetrically on joints and knees of a patient with GPA.

Source: From Sibille A, Alfieri R, Malaise O, et al. Granulomatosis With Polyangiitis in a Patient on Programmed Death-1 Inhibitor for Advanced Non-small-cell Lung Cancer. Front Oncol. 2019; 9:478, used under Creative Commons license.

presence of granulomatous inflammation as per biopsy. The presence of two or more criteria was associated with 92% specificity and 88% sensitivity.

The ELK criteria include ELK manifestations in addition to a positive c-ANCA or typical histopathologic finding qualifies for a diagnosis of GPA. Histologically, pauci-immune necrotizing granulomas are typically visualized in small and medium-sized blood vessels. When purely cutaneous in presentation, the histology may show a neutrophilic infiltrate (Figure 13.10). On immunofluorescence, c-ANCA stains are localized to the cytoplasm whereas multiplied nuclei are non-reactive. Antibodies are directed against PR3.

Differential diagnosis: GPA is a multisystemic disease associated with a broad list of differential diagnoses, which may include other AAVs, autoimmune disorders (e.g., systemic lupus erythematosus), sarcoidosis, amyloidosis, infections, and malignancies. Drug toxicities, such as levamisole, amphetamines, and cocaine, may also be considered.

Management: Treatment is based on disease involvement and is classified into two phases: induction phase and maintenance phase. A combination of immunosuppressive agents, such as cyclophosphamide, glucocorticoids, rituximab, azathioprine, and methotrexate, are the mainstay of induction therapy, whereas a single immunosuppressive agent is typically used in the maintenance phase. Dosing and regimen vary. Alternatively, plasmapheresis may be considered.

Course: GPA is associated with significant morbidity and mortality, which is caused by organ dysfunction or the adverse effects associated with prolonged use of glucocorticoids or immunosuppressive agents. On average, a patient with GPA without clinical intervention has a life expectancy of about 5 months, with 1-year survival rate less than 30%. Currently, a majority of patients who receive clinical intervention have a life expectancy of 8–9 years.

Final comment: GPA is a disease with significant morbidity and mortality in which relapses are common. Consultation with rheumatology, and possibly ophthalmology, pulmonology, or nephrology depending on end organ involvement, is recommended for long-term management.

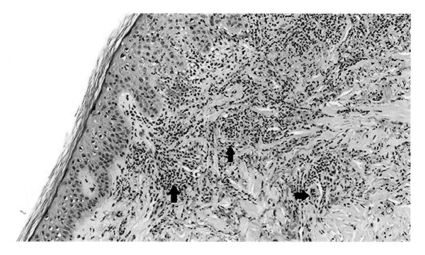

Figure 13.10 Hematoxylin and eosin (HE) staining shows blood vessels (white areas) with surrounding neutrophilic inflammatory aggregates (arrows), establishing the diagnosis of neutrophilic vasculitis. Picture magnification: 20×; scale bar: 50 μ.

Source: From Sibille A, Alfieri R, Malaise O, et al. Granulomatosis With Polyangiitis in a Patient on Programmed Death-1 Inhibitor for Advanced Non-small-cell Lung Cancer. Front Oncol. 2019; 9:478, used under Creative Commons License.

Eosinophilic Granulomatosis with Polyangiitis

Synonym: Churg-Strauss syndrome

Overview: This is a rare presentation of necrotizing vasculitis characteristically seen in patients with asthma. EGPA affects the small vasculature and is a part of the ANCA family, similar to GPA and MPA.

Clinical presentation: EGPA is known to present sequentially, characterized by 3 phases: prodromal, eosinophilic, and vasculitic. The prodromal phase presents with long-standing asthma and can last anywhere from a few months to several years. Rhinitis, upper respiratory symptoms, fever, weight loss, and arthralgias may be seen. The eosinophilic phase presents with eosinophilia >10% and causes lung damage in the majority of cases. Extrapulmonary involvement may also be seen manifesting as cardiomyopathy and gastrointestinal symptoms. The eosinophilic phase is followed by the vasculitic phase, which causes inflammation of the small vasculature. EGPA varies in severity, and clinical presentations differ.

Laboratory studies: Histologic study will show eosinophilia in the tissues (>10%), disseminated small vessel vasculitis, extravascular granulomatous change, and fibrinoid necrosis (Figure 13.11). When active, C-reactive protein (CRP) and ESR may be elevated. IgE is also elevated in patients with EGPA, but this is not specific. Elevated IgG4 levels are more specific and should be measured. Up to 90% of EGPA patients are positive for p-ANCA, but this is not diagnostic. Eotaxin-3, a chemokine that attracts eosinophils, is both sensitive and specific to EGPA when active.

Differential diagnosis: This includes the other AAV, GPA and MPA. Although similar in presentation, a history of asthma may suggest EGPA. Idiopathic hyper-eosinophilic syndrome, allergic bronchopulmonary aspergillosis, and parasitic infection should be considered until a biopsy is obtained.

To aid in obtaining the diagnosis, the ACR criteria are used, including asthma, eosinophilia, neuropathy, pulmonary infiltration, paranasal sinus pathology, and extravascular eosinophils infiltration. Patients must present with four of the six characteristics to make the diagnosis.

Management: This is case dependent and based on the prognosis. Oral prednisone can be used initially as first-line treatment, ± intravenous methylprednisolone when severe. If the patient improves, then the steroid may be tapered. If the condition worsens, a biologic, such as rituximab and mepolizumab, may be used.

Course: Prognosis is determined using the 5-factors scoring system or FFS founded by the French Vasculitis Study Group. This includes elevated creatinine >1.58 mg/dl, proteinuria >1 g per day, cardiomyopathy, and gastrointestinal and central nervous system involvement. Patients with

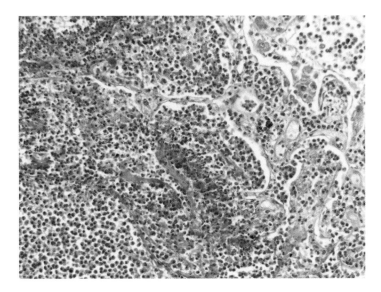

Figure 13.11 Churg-Strauss syndrome is a rare systemic vasculitis that is accompanied by peripheral eosinophilia and asthma. In the center of the image, there is a blood vessel exhibiting fibrinoid necrosis. It is surrounded by a dense mixed inflammatory infiltrate containing a large number of eosinophils.

Source: Courtesy of Yale Rosen, https://commons.wikimedia.org/w/index.php?curid=82802159, used under Creative Commons license.

an FFS of 0 demonstrate higher survival rates in comparison to patients with an FFS ≥ 1. Overall, EGPA is a mild form of vasculitis in comparison to GPA and, therefore, has lower mortality rates.

Final comment: EGPA is a part of the AAV family and is exclusively seen in asthma patients. Although rare, patients can present with disseminated disease, prompting clinicians to follow the disease course closely. Treatment is case dependent and based on diagnostic criteria and prognostic factors.

Microscopic Polyangiitis

Overview: MPA is an autoimmune disease that is idiopathic in nature and part of the AAV family. Most patients are between the age of 50–60 years with a slight male predominance. MPA damages the small vessels systemically marking the potential of affecting multiple organ systems.

Clinical presentation: The disease process of MPA can present clinically with cutaneous, renal, pulmonary, gastrointestinal, and neurologic manifestations. Up to 60% of patients present cutaneously with palpable purpura and petechiae. Rapidly progressive glomerulonephritis is seen in more than 80% of patients with MPA prompting urine studies. Up to 55% of patients with MPA may present with pulmonary findings, such as alveolar hemorrhage due to vascular inflammation of the pulmonary capillaries. Patients may present clinically with hemoptysis, dyspnea, and pleuritic chest pain. Abdominal pain, gastrointestinal bleeding, and neuropathy may also be obtained from the history and physical examination.

Laboratory studies: When suspicious of MPA, a renal and pulmonary biopsy are indicated to observe inflammatory changes of the vasculature. A chest x-ray may show alveolar hemorrhage as a part of the disease process due to inflammatory infiltrates. ANCAs can be assessed, but only 50–75% of patients with MPA are MPO-AAV positive (Figure 13.12), and a negative finding still requires a diagnostic workup.

Differential diagnosis: This includes the other AAV, EGPA, and GPA. EGPA presents exclusively in asthma patients, and without this history, the differential can be narrowed to MPA and GPA. Clinically, it may be difficult to differentiate between these two. MPA is an MPO-AAV (p-ANCA), whereas GPA is a PR3-AAV (c-ANCA) and, by ANCA analysis alone, us different. Additionally, granulomatous change is seen in GPA but not MPA.

Management: Prognosis of MPA is poor without therapeutic intervention due to systemic involvement. Mortality rates are high, especially in patients with pulmonary and renal

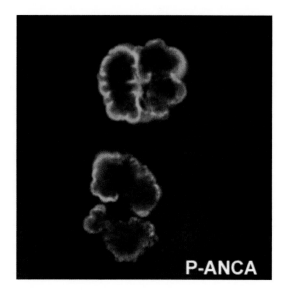

Figure 13.12 Immunofluorescence pattern produced by binding of serum from a patient with microscopic polyangiitis to ethanol-fixed neutrophils.

Source: Courtesy of Malittle, https://en.wikipedia.org/wiki/P-ANCA#/media/File:P_anca.jpg, in the public domain.

involvement, and therefore, pharmacotherapy is indicated. Immunosuppressives may be initiated, particularly oral or intravenous cyclophosphamide and oral prednisone in combination. If severe, intravenous methylprednisolone or plasmapheresis may be considered in addition to immunosuppressants.

Course: As with other systemic diseases, MPA varies in its disease course. Some cases present acutely, while others demonstrate a chronic presentation of nonspecific symptoms for years prior to making a definitive diagnosis of MPA. Without proper treatment, there is a 90% mortality rate within one year of diagnosis.

Final comment: MPA is a systemic vasculitis that is idiopathic in nature with characteristics of an autoimmune disease. As a part of the AAV family, studies suggest that the MPO-AAV (p-ANCA) associated with MPA plays an important role in the pathogenesis of the disease course but is not diagnostic. Clinicians should be wary of renal and pulmonary involvement, which can pose a threat to life if therapeutic interventions are not implemented.

Cutaneous Polyarteritis Nodosa

Overview: Cutaneous polyarteritis nodosa (CPAN) is a rare form of vasculitis that affects small to medium sized vessels. Although predominantly idiopathic in nature, CPAN is best characterized as an immune complex-mediated disease and varies in clinical presentation. Unlike systemic polyarteritis nodosa, the cutaneous form lacks visceral involvement but may still include extracutaneous findings.

Clinical presentation: CPAN most commonly presents as livedo reticularis, ulcerations, and subcutaneous nodules (Figure 13.13) that are tender in nature. These findings are most often found on the legs, but they may also be found elsewhere prompting a thorough skin examination. Tender subcutaneous nodules present initially, in most cases, followed by ulcerations and livedo reticularis. Edema may accompany these findings, particularly of the lower extremities. Extracutaneous findings may occur in some patients and include nonspecific findings, such as neuropathy, myalgias, and arthralgias.

Laboratory studies: Tender subcutaneous nodules and livedo reticularis with central ulceration, with or without extracutaneous symptoms, should prompt a skin biopsy to confirm CPAN. A deep incisional biopsy alongside a normal skin sample is recommended when ulcerations are found. The following should be obtained to differentiate between CPAN systemic polyarteritis nodosa and other vasculitides: complete blood count, ESR, liver and renal studies, cryoglobulins, ANA, rheumatoid factor, ANCA, and complement levels. Antistreptolysin-O titer may also be obtained if suspicious of a streptococcal infection.

Differential diagnosis: This includes erythema nodosum, systemic polyarteritis nodosa, MPA, EPGA, GPA, urticarial vasculitis, and erythema induratum.

Management: CPAN is chronic and may have a remitting and relapsing pattern. Therapeutic options are dependent on disease severity. Consider topical steroids, such as mometasone, when

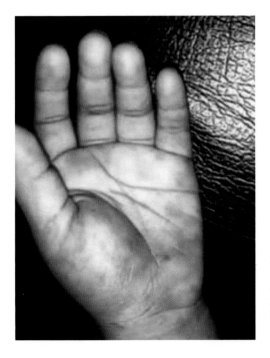

Figure 13.13 Multiple tender subcutaneous nodules in the palm.

Source: From Kumar K, Ramaswamy S, Saldana K. (2016). Cutaneous Polyarteritis Nodosa Presenting with Digital Gangrene. J Nepal Paediatric Soc. 36. 82. 10.3126/jnps.v36i1.1448, used under Creative Commons License.

mild with erythema only. NSAIDs or colchicine may be used in mild cases that present with livedo reticularis and nodules. Oral prednisolone can be efficacious when severe. If CPAN is due to group A beta hemolytic streptococcal infection, then treat with penicillin.

Course: CPAN is a chronic cutaneous disease that has the ability to spontaneously occur and resolve. Although predominantly idiopathic, other causes have been identified, including HCV and group A beta hemolytic streptococcus. CPAN can present across all ages without gender predominance, and the mortality rate is extremely low prompting a favorable prognosis.

Final comment: CPAN is predominately idiopathic, but it has been seen with group A beta hemolytic streptococcus, inflammatory bowel disease, HCV, parvovirus B-19, and mycobacterium tuberculosis. Systemic polyarteritis nodosa is a feared complication, but an association has yet to be found. Due to the varied etiology and clinical presentations, investigation is required.

Kawasaki Disease

Definition: Kawasaki disease (KD) is an acute febrile generalized vasculitis that most commonly affects children younger the age of 5 years. The exact origin is unknown, and in developed countries, KD is the primary cause of pediatric acquired heart disease.

Overview: In the United States, KD affects individuals of all races and ethnicities, but in many cases, it is diagnosed in those of Asian ancestry. There have been documented cases of KD internationally.

Clinical Presentation: Two types are known.

I. Classic Kawasaki Disease

KD is a clinical diagnosis; classic KD is defined as having a fever for minimum of 5 days with 4 of the 5 following findings:

1. Erythematous fissured lips, "strawberry tongue" (Figure 13.14), erythematous oropharyngeal mucosa

2. Bilateral nonexudative conjunctivitis (Figure 13.15)

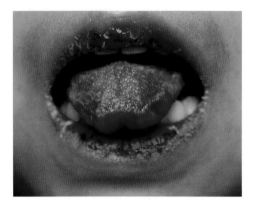

Figure 13.14 Hemorrhagic crusting of the lips and "strawberry tongue" in a patient with Kawasaki disease.

Source: Courtesy of Kawasaki Disease Foundation, Inc.

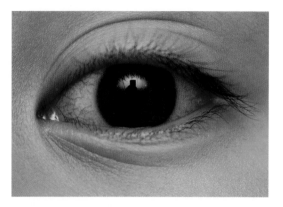

Figure 13.15 Nonexudative conjunctivitis in a patient with Kawasaki disease.

Source: Courtesy of Kawasaki Disease Foundation, Inc.

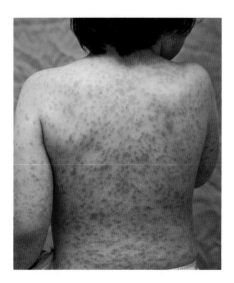

Figure 13.16 Widespread eruption of confluent and discrete erythematous macules and papules on the trunk and arms of a patient with Kawasaki disease.

Source: Courtesy of Kawasaki Disease Foundation, Inc.

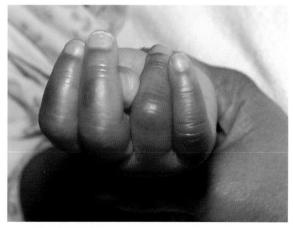

Figure 13.17 Edema and erythema of fingers in a patient with Kawasaki disease.

Source: From VisualDx (www.visualdx.com), used with permission.

3. Polymorphous eruption (Figure 13.16) that can be morbilliform, scarlatiniform, or erythema multiforme-like

4. Erythematous, edematous hands or feet during acute illness (Figure 13.17), periungual desquamation during weeks 2–3 of illness

5. Cervical lymphadenopathy (often unilateral, ³1.5-cm diameter)

II. Incomplete Kawasaki Disease

1. Children or infants with an extended fever without an alternative explanation

2. Having than four principal clinical findings

3. Having supportive echocardiographic or laboratory studies.

Laboratory studies: Although laboratory studies are not requisite for classic KD diagnosis, the algorithm for incomplete KD includes several laboratory studies. Compatible laboratory studies include normal or elevated white blood count (WBC) with neutrophilic predominance, thrombocytosis (in second week of illness), anemia (normochromic and normocytic), elevated CRP and ESR, hypoalbuminemia, hyponatremia, elevated GGT and ALT, and sterile pyuria.

When KD is suspected, echocardiography should be performed at diagnosis as well as 1–2 and 4–6 weeks after treatment in uncomplicated patients. Patients with coronary artery abnormalities during acute illness should have echocardiography repeated more often.

Differential diagnosis: This includes multisystem inflammatory syndrome in children (potentially linked to SARS-CoV-2), drug hypersensitivity reactions, scarlet fever, measles, Rocky Mountain spotted fever, leptospirosis, and toxic shock syndrome. Other causes include juvenile idiopathic arthritis, adenovirus, and enterovirus.

Management: Treatment should be initiated within the first 10 days of diagnosis of classic and incomplete KD. Administer IVIG (2 g/kg) as a single infusion with aspirin. Aspirin should be administered 4 times daily, total daily cumulative dose of 80–100 mg/kg/d until afebrile for 48–72 hours. Next, give aspirin 3–5 mg/kg/d until there are no signs of coronary changes 6–8 weeks after presentation of illness. Aspirin may be administered indefinitely in patients with coronary abnormalities.

Some therapeutic options for patients with recrudescent or persistent fever 36 hours post-IVIG include a second dose of IVIG (2 g/kg), IVIG 2 g/kg + IV prednisolone 2 mg/kg/d in three doses until afebrile, next orally until CRP normalizes, then taper for 2–3 weeks, or infliximab 5 mg/kg IV as a single infusion for 2 hours. Patients nonresponsive to a second dose of IVIG or corticosteroids necessitate additional treatment.

Course: Acute and long-term outcomes of KD are related to the extent of cardiac pathology. Coronary artery involvement is particularly important for long-term outcomes.

FINAL THOUGHT

Morbidity and mortality of patients with KD are most often caused by cardiovascular complications, making early diagnosis and prompt intervention necessary.

ADDITIONAL READINGS

Baigrie D, Bansal P, Goyal A, et al. Leukocytoclastic Vasculitis (Hypersensitivity Vasculitis). In: StatPearls [Internet]. Treasure Island, FL: StatPearls Publishing; 2020.

Cacoub P, Comarmond C, Domont F, et al. Cryoglobulinemia vasculitis. Am J Med. 2015;128:950–955.

Cartin-Ceba R, Peikert T, Specks U. Pathogenesis of ANCA-associated vasculitis. Curr Rheumatol Rep. 2012;14:481–493.

Davis MDP, van der Hilst JCH. Mimickers of urticaria: urticarial vasculitis and autoinflammatory diseases. J Allergy Clin Immunol Pract. 2018;6:1162–1170.

Garlapati P, Qurie A. Granulomatosis with Polyangiitis (GPA, Wegener Granulomatosis). In: StatPearls [Internet]. Treasure Island, FL: StatPearls Publishing; 2020.

Hetland LE, Susrud KS, Lindahl KH, et al. Henoch-Schonlein purpura: a literature review. Acta Derm Venereol. 2017;97:1160–1166.

Kubaisi B, Abu Samra K, Foster CS. Granulomatosis with polyangiitis (Wegener's disease): an updated review of ocular disease manifestations. Intractable Rare Dis Res. 2016;5:61–69.

Roncati L, Ligabue G, Fabbiani L, et al. Type 3 hypersensitivity in COVID-19 vasculitis. Clin Immunol. 2020;217:108487.

Sunderkotter CH, Zelger B, Chen KR, et al. Nomenclature of cutaneous vasculitis: dermatologic addendum to the 2012 revised International Chapel Hill Consensus Conference Nomenclature of Vasculitides. Arthritis Rheumatol. 2018;70:171–184.

Younger DS. Overview of the vasculitides. Neurol Clin. 2019;37:171–200.

14 Vesiculobullous Diseases

Snejina Vassileva and Kossara Drenovska

CONTENTS

Overview: A variety of skin diseases may present with the temporary appearance of blisters under the influence of either external (physical, chemical, biologic) or internal metabolic factors, or due to severe inflammatory changes in the epidermis or at the dermal-epidermal junction (DEJ). In the group of vesiculobullous dermatoses, blistering is the major clinical feature, which results from genetically determined or autoimmune loss of basic structural elements in the skin that maintain cohesion between keratinocytes or between the epidermal layer and the dermis within the basement membrane zone (BMZ). Vesiculobullous diseases can be classified histologically based on the level of the skin at which the cleft occurs and the mechanism of the blistering process.

The majority of vesiculobullous dermatoses are acquired organ-specific autoimmune diseases in which the autoantibodies target structural proteins in the skin, and their diagnosis relies on the application of specialized immunopathology techniques that reveal the presence of in vivo deposited or circulating autoantibodies against various structural proteins (Tables 14.1 and 14.2).

Either hereditary or acquired, vesiculobullous diseases constitute one of the major sources of morbidity and mortality in dermatology.

PEMPHIGUS

Definition: Pemphigus (from *pemphix*, Greek for "blister") is a group of rare autoimmune blistering diseases (AIBDs) that are mediated by autoantibodies against epidermal desmosomal antigens and are clinically characterized by the formation of flaccid bullae and subsequent erosions on normally appearing skin and/or mucosa in young adults, usually in their 30–40 s.

Overview: Pemphigus is mediated by IgG autoantibodies, which are directed against epidermal cell adhesion proteins, the desmogleins, and cause loosening of the links between epidermal cells (acantholysis) with further intraepidermal blister formation. Both desmogleins 1 and 3 with molecular weight 160 kDa and 130 kDa, respectively, are targeted in pemphigus vulgaris, while desmoglein 1 alone is the antigen of superficial pemphigus. Pemphigus shows irregular geographic distribution with a higher incidence reported from Mediterranean countries, North Africa, Iran, Japan, Brazil, and among Ashkenazi Jews, where it reaches 1.6–3.2/100000.

Clinical presentation: There are two main clinical variants of pemphigus, which differ in severity and prognosis: pemphigus vulgaris and pemphigus foliaceus.

Pemphigus vulgaris (PV) is the most common clinical form that usually presents with mucocutaneous lesions. In more than 50% of patients, the oral cavity is initially affected by persisting, painful erosions, which negatively affect eating (Figure 14.1a). The nasopharynx, larynx, esophagus, conjunctiva, or genital mucosa may also be involved. Cutaneous lesions are characterized by flaccid bullae on clinically normal skin, which are quickly ruptured and followed by painful erosions covered with crusts (Figure 14.1b). Nikolsky's sign is positive, which is lateral pressure on normal-appearing skin near a lesion that results in the splitting of the epidermis. A rare subtype of PV, pemphigus vegetans, presents with papillomatous and vegetating lesions that develop from previous erosions in intertriginous areas (periorificial, axillar, or inguinal folds).

DOI: 10.1201/9781003105268-14

Table 14.1 Summary of the Autoantigens Involved in the Autoimmune Blistering Diseases

Blistering Disease	Target Antigen		
	Type	Ultrastructural location	Molecular weight
Intraepidermal AIBDs			
P. vulgaris, P. vegetans	Dsg 3, Dsg 1	Desmosome, extracellular	130 kDa, 160 kDa
P. foliaceus, SUS, Endemic *P. foliaceus*	Dsg 1	Desmosome, extracellular	160 kDa
P. herpetiformis	Dsg 3, Dsg 1	Desmosome, extracellular	130 kDa, 160 kDa
IgA pemphigus/SPD type	Desmocollin 1	Desmosome, extracellular	105 kDa
IgA pemphigus/IEN type	Desmocollin 2	Desmosome, extracellular	115 kDa
	Dsg 3, Dsg 1	Desmosome, extracellular	130 kDa, 160 kDa
Paraneoplastic pemphigus	Desmoplakin 1	Desmosome, intracellular	250 kDa
Paraneoplastic autoimmune multiorgan syndrome	Desmoplakin 2	Desmosome, intracellular	210 kDa
	Envoplakin	Desmosome, intracellular	210 kDa
	Periplakin	Desmosome, intracellular	190 kDa
	Epiplakin	Desmosome, intracellular	>700 kDa
	Plectin	Hemidesmosome, intracellular	500 kDa
	BPAG1 (BP230)	Hemidesmosome, intracellular	230 kDa
	A2ML1	Protease inhibitor	170 kDa
	Dsg 3, Dsg 1	Desmosome, extracellular	130 kDa, 160 kDa
	Desmocollin 1–3	Desmosome, extracellular	105, 115 kDa
Subepidermal AIBDs			
Bullous pemphigoid	BPAG1 (BP230)	Hemidesmosome, intracellular	230 kDa
	BPAG2 (BP180)	Hemidesmosome/extracellular	180 kDa
Pemphigoid gestationis	BPAG1 (BP230)	Hemidesmosome, intracellular	230 kDa
	BPAG2 (BP180)	Hemidesmosome, extracellular	180 kDa
Lichen planus pemphigoides	BPAG1 (BP230)	Hemidesmosome, intracellular	230 kDa
	BPAG2 (BP180)	Hemidesmosome, extracellular	180 kDa
	Collagen VII	Sub-lamina densa/AFs	290 kDa, 145 kDa
Mucous membrane pemphigoid	BPAG1 (BP230)	Hemidesmosome, intracellular	230 kDa
	BPAG2 (BP180)	Hemidesmosome, extracellular	180 kDa
	α6β4 integrin	Hemidesmosome	120 kDa
	• α6 subunit	• extracellular	200 kDa
	• β4 subunit	• intracellular	165, 135, 105 kDa
	Laminin 332 (α3β3γ2)	Lower lamina lucida	600 kDa
	Laminin 311 (α3β1γ1)	Lower lamina lucida	
Linear IgA disease	LAD1	Anchoring filaments	97/120 kDa
	Collagen VII	Sub-lamina densa/AFs	290 kDa, 145 kDa
Anti-laminin γ1 (anti p-200) pemphigoid	Laminin γ1	Lower lamina lucida	200 kDa
Epidermolysis bullosa acquisita	Collagen VII	Sub-lamina densa/AFs	290 kDa, 145 kDa
Bullous systemic LE	Collagen VII	Sub-lamina densa/AFs	290 kDa, 145 kDa
Dermatitis herpetiformis	eTG (TG3)	Papillary dermis*	

Abbreviations: AIBDs, autoimmune bistering diseases; P, pemphigus; Dsg, desmoglein; kDa, kilodaltons; SUS, Senear-Usher syndrome (Pemphigus erythematosus); SPD, subcorneal pustular dermatosis; IEN, intraepithelial neutrophilic; BPAG, bullous pemphigoid antigen; A2ML1, Alpha-2-macroglobulin 1-like antigen; AFs, anchoring fibrils; LE, lupus erythematosus; eTG, epidermal transglutaminase.

Note: * Location of eTG/IgA immune aggregates in the skin.

Table 14.2 Clinical Presentation, Histology, and Immunofluorescence Findings of Autoimmune Blistering Diseases

Disease	Clinical Presentation	Histology	DIF	IIF
Intraepidermal AIBDs				
Pemphigus vulgaris	Flaccid blisters and erosions on mucous membranes and skin	Suprabasal acantholysis and blister formation	Intercellular IgG and C3 in the epidermis/ epithelium	Circulating IgG anti-ECS antibodies (ME or HS substrate)
P. vegetans	Vegetating and pustular lesions in intertriginous areas	Suprabasal acantholysis and clefts, hyperkeratosis; pseudoepitheliomatous hyperplasia, and papillomatosis	Intercellular IgG and C3 in the epidermis/ epithelium	Circulating IgG anti-ECS antibodies (ME or HS substrate)
P. foliaceus	Flaccid bullae and erosions healing with crusting and scaling in seborrheic areas; sometimes erythroderma; no mucosal involvement	Acantholysis and blister formation in the superficial epidermis	Intercellular IgG and C3 in the epidermis/ epithelium	Circulating IgG anti-ECS antibodies (ME or HS substrate)
P. erythematosus	Flaccid bullae and erosions healing with crusting and scaling in seborrheic areas; no mucosal involvement	Acantholysis and blister formation in the superficial epidermis	Intercellular IgG and C3 in the epidermis/ epithelium; band of IgM at BMZ	Circulating IgG anti-ECS antibodies (ME or HS substrate)
P. herpetiformis	Grouped vesicles and erosions on erythematous skin (DH-like); pruritus	Subcorneal pustules, eosinophilic spongiosis, acantholysis may be minimal or absent	Intercellular IgG and C3 in the epidermis/ epithelium	Circulating IgG anti-ECS antibodies (ME or HS substrate)
IgA pemphigus	SPD type: flaccid pustules with annular or circinate pattern; IEN type: pustules with a "sunflower" configuration on the trunk	Subcorneal acantholytic blister (SPD type); Suprabasal acantholytic blister with inflammatory neutrophil-predominant infiltrate (IEN type)	Intercellular IgA in the upper epidermis (SPD type), or throughout the whole epidermis (IEN type)	Circulating IgA (±IgG) anti-ECS antibodies (ME or HS substrate)
Paraneoplastic pemphigus	Severe mucositis; polymorphic skin lesions (similar to PV, BP, EM, GVHD, or LP); pulmonary involvement; underlying hematopoietic malignancy	Suprabasal acantholysis, keratinocyte necrosis and dyskeratosis, interface dermatitis, lichenoid band-like infiltrate into the upper dermis	Intercellular IgG in the epidermis ± linear IgG and/or C3 along the BMZ	Circulating IgG anti-ECS antibodies (ME or HS, and rat bladder substrate)
Subepidermal AIBDs				
Bullous pemphigoid	Elderly affected; intense pruritus, tense blisters, and erosions on inflamed or normal background; rare mucosal involvement	Subepidermal blister with inflammatory eosinophil-predominant infiltrate	Linear IgG (±IgA) and/or C3 along the BMZ (n-serrated)	Circulating IgG anti-BMZ antibodies— epidermal pattern (SSS substrate)
Pemphigoid gestationis	Occurs during pregnancy or post-partum period; intense pruritus, urticarial plaques and/or blisters on the abdomen, trunk, and extremities	Subepidermal blister with inflammatory eosinophil-predominant infiltrate	Linear C3 and/ or IgG along the BMZ	Circulating complement-fixing IgG1 anti-BMZ antibodies ("herpes gestationis" factor)—epidermal pattern (SSS substrate)
Lichen planus pemphigoides	Middle-aged patients with LP; tense blisters on both LP lesions and normal skin, predominantly on extremities	Subepidermal blister with eosinophilic infiltrate; lichenoid lesions show the typical features of LP	Linear IgG and/ or C3 along the BMZ; lichenoid lesions show both linear IgG and "ovoid" bodies in the papillary dermis	Circulating IgG anti-BMZ antibodies— epidermal or mixed epidermal and dermal pattern (SSS substrate)

Table 14.2 (Continued)

Disease	Clinical Presentation	Histology	DIF	IIF
Mucous membrane pemphigoid	Recurrent blistering and erosions of the mucous membranes and rarely the skin, healing with adhesions, scarring and strictures	Subepithelial blister with or without inflammatory infiltrate	Linear IgG (or IgA) and C3 along the BMZ	Circulating IgG anti-BMZ antibodies—epidermal or mixed epidermal and dermal pattern (SSS substrate)
Linear IgA disease	Children or adults affected; tense blisters and erosions with annular ("string of pearls") configuration; typically on flexor surfaces, trunk, perineum, face; oral mucosa often involved	Subepidermal blister with inflammatory, neutrophil- or eosinophil predominant infiltrate.	Linear IgA and C3 along the BMZ	Circulating IgA anti-BMZ antibodies—epidermal, dermal, or mixed pattern (SSS substrate)
Anti-laminin γ1 pemphigoid	Tense blisters and erosions, erythematous plaques	Subepidermal blister with neutrophils predominant infiltrate in the upper dermis	Linear IgG and/or C3 along the BMZ (n-serrated)	Circulating IgG anti-BMZ antibodies—dermal pattern (SSS substrate)
Epidermolysis bullosa acquisita	Mechanobullous type: trauma-induced blisters healing with scarring and milia on extensor surfaces Inflammatory type: similar to BP, MMP, or LAD	Subepidermal blister with or without inflammatory infiltrate	Linear IgG (or IgA) and C3 along the BMZ (u-serrated)	Circulating IgG anti-BMZ antibodies—dermal pattern (SSS substrate)
Bullous systemic lupus erythematosus?	Occurs in patients with SLE; tense blisters and erosions with or without pruritus; predilection for face and upper trunk	DH-like: subepidermal blister with neutrophil-predominant dermal infiltrate (papillary neutrophil microabscesses); leukocytoclasia	Linear or granular IgG (or IgA, IgM) along the BMZ (u-serrated)	Circulating IgG anti-BMZ antibodies—dermal pattern (SSS substrate)
Dermatitis herpetiformis	Intense pruritus; grouped prurigo-papules, vesicles, excoriations, and crusts, typically on extensor surfaces of upper and lower extremities; associated GSE (may be asymptomatic)	Subepidermal blister with neutrophil-predominant dermal infiltrate (papillary neutrophil microabscesses)	Granular deposits of IgA and C3 at the tips of the dermal papillae	Circulating IgA endomysial antibodies (ME substrate)

Abbreviations: AIBDs, autoimmune blistering diseases; DIF, direct immunofluorescence; IIF, indirect immunofluorescence; ECS, epithelial cell surface; ME, monkey esophagus; HS, human skin; SSS, salt split skin; DH, dermatitis herpetiformis; P, pemphigus; SPD, subcorneal pustular dermatosis; IEN, intraepithelial neutrophilic; PV, pemphigus vulgaris; BP, bullous pemphigoid; EM, erythema multiforme; GVHD, graft-versus-host disease; LP, lichen planus; BMZ, basement membrane zone; MMP, mucous membrane pemphigoid; LAD, linear IgA disease; SLE, systemic lupus erythematosus; GSE, gluten-sensitive entheropathy.

Pemphigus foliaceus (PF) is a superficial form of the disease, which is characterized by transient, flaccid bullae, puff pastry–like exfoliation, and superficial, crusted erosions on the chest, scalp, face, or interscapular area in the absence of mucosal involvement (Figure 14.2a). PF demonstrates a mild course, but rarely, severe erythrodermic forms may be observed. Endemic PF has been reported from Tunisia, Brazil, and Colombia, where the disease is also called by the Amazon population Fogo Selvagem (port-*wild fire*).

Another rare form of superficial pemphigus, called pemphigus erythematosus (PE; Senear-Usher syndrome), manifests with clinical and immunologic features of both pemphigus and discoid lupus erythematosus (LE; Figure 14.2b). It affects photo-exposed areas, predominantly the scalp, face, and upper trunk.

Other rare varieties include pemphigus herpetiformis, which combines features of dermatitis herpetiformis and pemphigus, and IgA pemphigus, which is mediated by IgA autoantibodies.

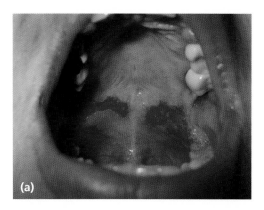

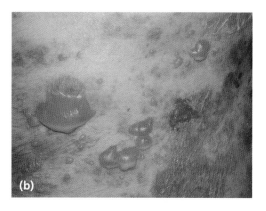

Figure 14.1 Pemphigus vulgaris: (a) Painful persisting erosions of the soft palate and (b) cutaneous involvement in pemphigus—flaccid vesicles and bullae with hypopion; the surrounding epidermis is slouging (positive Nikolsky sign).

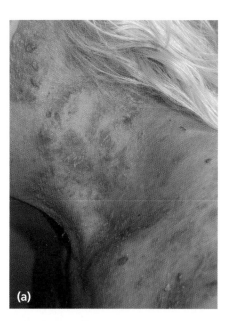

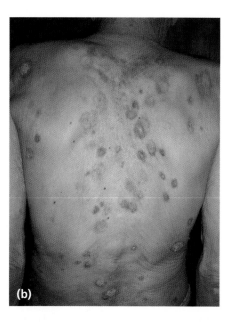

Figure 14.2 Pemphigus foliaceus: (a) Transient, flaccid bullae, puff pastry–like exfoliation and superficial crusty erosions on the face, neck, and upper trunk; (b) superficial bullae, scaling and crusting leisons suggestive of chronic cutaneous lupus or a papulosquamous disorder in a patient with *P. erythematosus*.

There are also drug-induced pemphigus and contact pemphigus related to numerous medications (D-penicillamine, penicillin, angiotensin-converting-enzyme inhibitors—e.g., captopril, enalapril, nifedipine, beta-blockers) and skin contact with pesticides or other chemical substances, respectively.

Patients with occult or diagnosed neoplasia, such as lymphoma, leukemia, thymoma, Castleman disease, and less frequently, solid tumors of the internal organs, may develop paraneoplastic pemphigus/paraneoplastic autoimmune multiorgan syndrome (PNP/PAMS). The presentation includes severe mucositis (Figure 14.3a), polymorphic skin lesions resembling bullous pemphigoid, erythema multiforme, lichen planus, or graft-versus-host disease, palmoplantar involvement (Figure 14.3b), and systemic findings, including obliterative bronchiolitis.

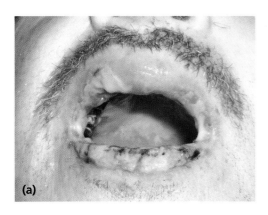

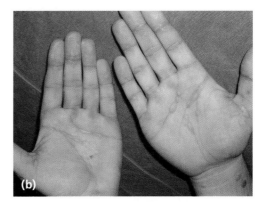

Figure 14.3 Paraneoplastc pemphigus: (a) Severe mucositis extending to the lip vermilion; (b) palmo-plantar involvement is one of the clinical criteria.

Additionally, pemphigus may be associated with other autoimmune diseases, such as thymoma, myasthenia gravis, rheumatoid arthritis, systemic LE, systemic scleroderma, and pernicious anemia.

Laboratory studies: The diagnosis of pemphigus requires histologic, immunofluorescent (IF), and immunoserologic tests.

Routine histology of skin or mucosal biopsy was taken from a fresh blister reveals intraepidermal suprabasal acantholytic bullae in PV or subcorneal clefting in PF. Single and groups of acantholytic cells may be observed in the blister fluid (Figure 14.4a). Direct immunofluorescence (DIF) performed on perilesional skin reveals intercellular IgG and complement (C) 3 deposits in the epidermis, resembling "chicken wire," "honeycomb," or "fishnet" (Figure 14.4b). Indirect immunofluorescence (IIF) detects circulating pemphigus IgG autoantibodies directed against the surface proteins of epidermal keratinocytes. IIF is performed on the epithelial substrate, most commonly monkey esophagus. The titer of pemphigus autoantibodies corresponds to disease severity. Positive IIF on rat bladder substrate is a specific diagnostic clue for PNP/PAMS.

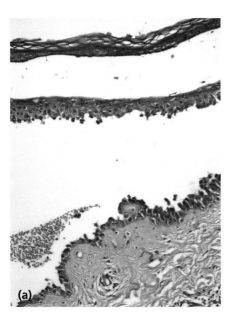

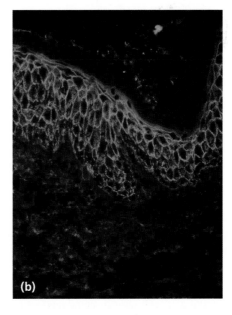

Figure 14.4 Pemphigus vulgaris: (a) Histology—intraepidermal suprabasal acantholytic blister is found; (b) direct immunofluorescence microscopy—intercellular deposits of IgG and C3 in the epidermis.

Autoantibodies against desmogleins 1 and 3, or envoplakin, the latter being specific for PNP/PAMS, may be detected by commercially available enzyme-linked immunosorbent assays (ELISAs). Other tools for determining the specificity of circulating antibodies against desmogleins 1 and 3, desmoplakins, envoplakin, and periplakin include immunoprecipitation or immunoblotting (IB).

Abnormalities are rarely detectable through routine laboratory work up in mild to moderate pemphigus. On the contrary, severe forms with extensive mucocutaneous involvement may present with leukocytosis, increase ESR, hypoalbuminemia, electrolyte imbalance, hypo- or hyperglycemia, and hypercoagulation. In PNP/PAMS, additional diagnostic methods may be involved in the search of accompanying malignancy, such as MRI and CT imaging.

Differential diagnosis: Oral PV may resemble mucous membrane pemphigoid, oral lichen planus, aphthae or Behçet's disease, *Herpes simplex* virus infection, erythema multiforme, and Stevens-Johnson syndrome. Skin lesions should be differentiated from bullous pemphigoid, impetigo, varicella-zoster virus infection, Grover's disease, and bullous drug eruptions, including toxic epidermal necrolysis (TEN). PF manifests with erosions and scaling rather than blistering and can be mistaken for seborrheic dermatitis. In pemphigus vegetans, Hailey-Hailey disease (benign chronic familial pemphigus) or vegetating pyoderma should be ruled out.

Management: Systemic steroids, such as prednisone (0.5 to 1.5 mg/kg/day), are the treatment of choice in pemphigus. Once control of the disease is achieved, dose tapering is undertaken followed by long-term maintenance therapy. The use of steroid-sparing immunomodulatory agents, such as azathioprine (1–2.5 mg/kg/day), mycophenolate mofetil (2 g/day) or mycophenolic acid (1440 mg/day), or cyclophosphamide (50 mg/d p.o. or 500–750 mg/month i.v.), helps to diminish the steroid side effects. Dapsone (100–300 mg/day) may be useful in PH, while retinoids or synthetic antimalarials are to be considered in pemphigus vegetans or some cases of superficial pemphigus. In severe or corticosteroid-resistant disease, high doses of intravenous immunoglobulins (IVIG; 2 g/kg per cycle of 2–5 days) or rituximab (2 infusions of 1000 mg two weeks apart, with maintenance treatment of one infusion of 500 mg at month 12 and 18), may be taken into consideration. Recently, rituximab alone or in combination with systemic steroids was suggested as first-line treatment in pemphigus. Recalcitrant cases may also be treated by plasmapheresis, immunoadsorption, or extracorporeal photochemotherapy (photopheresis). Extensive mucocutaneous lesions require the topical application of antiseptic solutions, antibiotics, and corticosteroid creams, as well as treatment of any superimposed candidosis.

Course: Until the 1950s, 60–90% of patients died from the disease. The introduction of steroids significantly improved its prognosis, but at the expense of introducing steroid-related complications, such as systemic infections, sepsis, and thromboembolism. Despite the introduction of new therapies, pemphigus, especially severe PV or PNP/PAMS, continues to have a chronic relapsing course and life-threatening potential.

Final comment: The pemphigus group of diseases is characterized by common pathogenetic mechanisms and clinical presentations but varies significantly in their treatment modalities and prognosis.

PEMPHIGOID

Definition: The term *pemphigoid* encompasses a group of AIBDs characterized by the production of autoantibodies directed against different structural components of the DEJ, which result in subepidermal blistering. The pemphigoid group of bullous dermatoses comprises bullous pemphigoid, mucous membrane (cicatricial) pemphigoid, pemphigoid gestationis, and lichen planus pemphigoides. Other rare forms include anti-laminin γ1 pemphigoid and anti-laminin 332 pemphigoid.

Bullous Pemphigoid

Definition: Bullous pemphigoid (BP) is a common subepidermal AIBD typically affecting elderly individuals and characterized by a pruritic, polymorphic blistering eruption that mainly involves the skin and rarely the mucous membranes.

Overview: BP is mediated by autoantibodies that recognize two hemidesmosomal proteins, the transmembrane BP antigen 180 (BP180, BPAG2, collagen XVII) and the intracellular BP antigen 230 (BP230, BPAG1). Antibodies directed against BP180 are of primary pathogenic importance. The binding of autoantibodies to their target antigens results in complement activation, accumulation of inflammatory cells, and release of enzymes (proteases and elastases) that induce dermal-epidermal splitting.

Clinical presentation: BP is characterized by a polymorphic, intensely pruritic eruption consisting of tense blisters on inflamed, urticaria-like, or normal-appearing skin. The skin lesions are usually widespread and symmetric, favoring the flexural surfaces of the extremities, abdomen, and lateral parts of the trunk. The blisters are filled with clear or hemorrhagic fluid and rupture to leave moist erosions and crusts that heal without scarring (Figure 14.5a). During a prodromal phase that may last for weeks or even months, blisters may not be present, and skin lesions may look more like eczema or urticaria (Figure 14.5b). Mucous membranes are only rarely involved.

Atypical clinical variants of BP include vesicular, polymorphic, prurigo nodularis-like, vegetating, erythrodermic, seborrheic, erosive, dyshidrosiform (palmoplantar), pediatric childhood, and drug-induced pemphigoid. Localized forms can be observed confined to the legs (pretibial pemphigoid) or the vulvar region in young girls (vulvar pemphigoid).

A rare variant of BP referred to as pemphigoid gestationis (PG; formerly called herpes gestationis), exclusively affects pregnant women or women with a trophoblastic tumor (choriocarcinoma or hydatiform mole). PG usually begins during the second or third trimester of pregnancy or after delivery with pruritic urticarial plaques and blisters around the umbilicus that spread to the trunk, back, buttocks, and extremities. Relapses may occur with subsequent pregnancies.

A distinct form of BP occurring in patients with concomitant lichen planus (LP) is lichen planus pemphigoides (LPP). Blisters occur on both normal skin and the LP lesions, which is in contrast to bullous LP, where blistering is confined to the lichenoid changes.

BP patients show a higher prevalence of neurologic diseases, in particular multiple sclerosis, stroke, and dementia, in addition to other associated autoimmune and malignant diseases, which are most likely related to their older age. Recent studies suggest that dipeptidyl peptidase 4 (DPP-4) inhibitors (gliptins) are associated with an increased risk of inducing BP in patients with diabetes.

A recently described variant of BP with autoantibodies that recognize a 200-kDa protein of the DEJ (laminin γ1 chain), referred to as anti-laminin γ1 pemphigoid (formerly anti-p200 pemphigoid), is characterized by a pruritic vesiculobullous eruption mimicking BP but in a younger age group and frequent association with psoriasis.

Laboratory studies: The diagnosis of BP relies on the histologic findings of subepidermal blistering with an eosinophil-rich inflammatory infiltrate, and on the results of immunopathologic

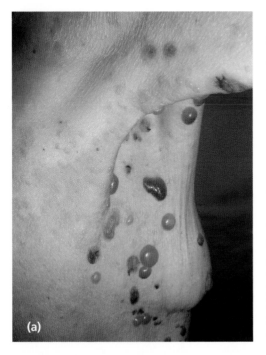 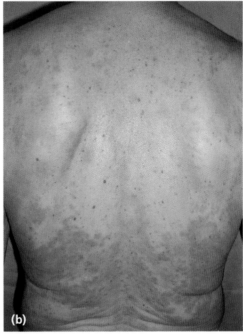

Figure 14.5 Bullous pemphigoid: (a) Tense blisters filled on normal appearing and inflamed background; (b) prebullous Bullous pemphigoid—only pruritic urticaria-like and eczematous lesions are present.

testing. DIF microscopy on perilesional skin reveals linear deposits of IgG and C3 along the BMZ (Figure 14.6a). A so-called n-serration pattern of the immune deposits has been described as characteristic for BP in contrast to the "u"-serration pattern in epidermolysis bullosa acquisita (EBA).

IIF reveals circulating IgG anti-BMZ antibodies in patient's sera, which react with the epidermal side (roof) of 1M NaCl-split normal human skin (salt-split skin, SSS) substrate (Figure 14.6b); this differentiates BP from EBA and anti-laminin γ1 pemphigoid, where the binding occurs at the floor of the blister (Figure 14.6c).

Antibodies to BP230 and immunodominant NC16A portion of BP180 are detected in patient sera using commercially available ELISAs. Other diagnostic modalities to determine the immune reactivity of the circulating BMZ antibodies are immunoblotting and immunoprecipitation techniques.

Differential diagnosis: BP may resemble a variety of dermatoses, including other subepidermal AIBDs, drug reactions, neurodermatitis, urticaria, prurigo, vasculitis, erythema multiforme, Sweet syndrome, TEN, bullous impetigo/tinea, arthropod reaction, and vesicular scabies. PG requires differentiation from other pruritic dermatoses of pregnancy (e.g., polymorphic eruption of pregnancy, erythema multiforme, atopic dermatitis of pregnancy). Localized vulvar pemphigoid might be misdiagnosed as child abuse.

Management: Treatment has to take into account the patient's general condition, disease severity, and comorbidities. High-potency topical steroids (clobetasol propionate cream) and systemic steroids (0.5–0.75 mg/kg/day) are recommended in both extensive and localized/limited or mild BP. The use of a steroid-sparing adjuvant, such as doxycycline (200 mg/day) and dapsone (1.5 mg/kg/day), and immunosuppressants, including azathioprine (1–3 mg/kg/day), cyclosporine (3–5 mg/kg/day), mycophenolate mofetil (2 g/day), and methotrexate (15 mg/week), are reserved

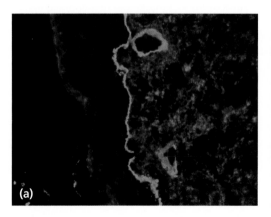

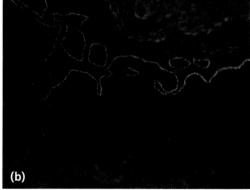

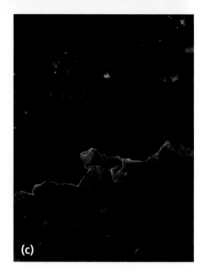

Figure 14.6 Immunopathologic diagnosis of bullous pemphigoid: (a) The direct immunofluorescence reveals linear deposition of IgG along the dermal-epidermal junctio; (b) indirect immunofluorescence on salt-split skin substrate—fluorescence at the roof of the blister diagnostic of bullous pemphigoid; (c) fluorescence at the floor of the blister is found in epidermolysis bullosa acquisita.

to cases unresponsive to corticosteroids. Alternatively, IVIG, rituximab, omalizumab, immunoadsorbtion, and plasma exchange may be considered in severe or recalcitrant cases.

Course: BP has a chronic course, which is usually self-limited over a 5–6-year period. It is traditionally thought to have a better prognosis than pemphigus, but increasing evidence suggests higher mortality, which may be related to the older age group and associated medical comorbidities, including neurologic, cardiac, and renal diseases.

Final comment: BP is the most frequent AIBD in the elderly population. It classically manifests with an intensely pruritic, generalized vesiculobullous eruption, but several atypical variants exist, whose differentiation from other causes of skin blistering relies on the combination of clinical, histologic, immunofluorescent, and immunoserologic findings.

Mucous Membrane Pemphigoid

Synonyms: Cicatricial pemphigoid, scarring pemphigoid, benign mucous membrane pemphigoid, benign pemphigus, ocular pemphigus

Definition: Mucous membrane pemphigoid (MMP) encompasses a group of AIBDs with a similar phenotype characterized by subepithelial blisters, erosions, and scarring of mucous membranes or less frequently the skin.

Overview: Blistering in MMP results from the reactivity of IgG and/or IgA autoantibodies directed against heterogeneous structural components of the DEJ, including BP180 and/or BP230, 97/120 kDa LABD antigen, laminin-332 (formerly laminin 5, epiligrin), laminin-6, α6-integrin, β4-integrin, and collagen VII of the BMZ.

Clinical presentation: MMP may affect any mucous membrane lined by Malpighian epithelium. The average age of onset is 65 years, but it can occur in children and young adults. The most common sites of involvement are the oral and ocular mucosa, where blisters and erosions may heal with scarring and cause significant disability. The ocular disease can progressively lead to symblepharon, entropion, trichiasis, and blindness (Figure 14.7a). Other sites include the pharynx, nose, larynx, esophagus, anus, and genitals, where the scarring process and adhesions can lead to stenosis, strictures, and atresia.

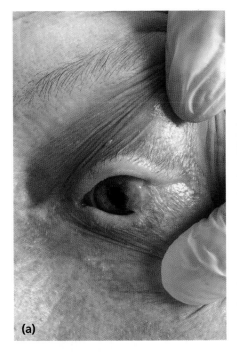

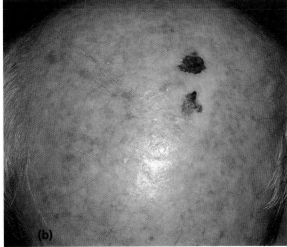

Figure 14.7 (a) Mucous membrane pemphigoid: adhesions, scarring and symblepharon in the ocular variant; (b) Brunsting-Perry cicatricial pemphigoid with blisters healing with atrophy in the head and neck area.

A rare variant of MMP characterized by the presence of autoantibodies directed against laminin 332, known as anti-laminin 332/anti-epiligrin cicatricial pemphigoid, is associated with an increased relative risk for solid cancer, such as adenocarcinoma.

Skin lesions are rare and present as mild, generalized, or localized blisters healing with milia and atrophic scarring. A rare type of localized disease, referred to as Brunsting-Perry cicatricial pemphigoid, is more common in elderly men and usually occurs on the head and neck (Figure 14.7b).

Laboratory studies: Similar to BP, the diagnosis is confirmed through histology and DIF microscopy. IIF can be negative in approximately 70% of cases. Antigen specificity of circulating antibodies may be defined using immunoblotting and immunoprecipitation and ELISA.

Differential diagnosis: BP, PV, PNP, erythema multiforme, linear IgA dermatosis, EBA, erosive LP, lichen sclerosis (when genitals are involved), and fibrosing/cicatrizing conjunctivitis should be considered.

Management: The therapy of MMP depends on disease severity, sites of involvement, and degree of progression. In patients with more severe, rapidly progressing disease, systemic steroids (prednisone 1–1.5 mg/kg/day) are first-choice treatment in combination with dapsone (50–200 mg/day), azathioprine (1–2 mg/kg/day), or oral or intravenous pulse cyclophosphamide (1–2 mg/kg/day PO; or 0.5–1 g/m² monthly IV). Alternatively, rituximab can be successfully used. Surgical interventions should be avoided until disease activity has been suppressed, because more severe adhesions and scar formation may result. There may be beneficial effects from antimicrobials (e.g., tetracyclines), mycophenolate mofetil, or IVIG (2–3 g/kg/cycle).

Course: MMP has a chronic but progressive course and extremely variable prognosis. Limited oral or combined oral and skin involvement considered being of "low risk," shows a tendency for spontaneous healing and less pronounced scarring. The overall evolution of MMP, however, is associated with high morbidity and mortality, especially if left without treatment. A multidisciplinary approach is required to minimize the risk of diverse late complications, including esophageal and laryngeal stenosis, strictures, airway constriction, dysphagia, urinary and sexual dysfunction, and blindness.

Final comment: MMP is a group of immunologically different but phenotypically similar chronic disorders, which predominantly affect the mucous membranes. They can cause significant morbidity due to chronic mucosal blistering, inflammation, pain, and scarring.

OTHER VESICULOBULLOUS DISEASES

Linear IgA Disease

Synonyms: Linear IgA bullous disease, chronic bullous dermatosis of childhood

Definition: Linear IgA dermatosis (LAD) is a rare subepidermal mucocutaneous AIBD of children and adults, which is characterized by linear deposition of IgA along the BMZ.

Overview: LAD is mediated by IgA autoantibodies directed against heterogeneous antigen targets of the BMZ, ultrastructurally localized to lamina lucida or the sub-lamina densa. The two most characteristic target antigens are the 97 kDa protein (LABD97) and 120 kDa protein (LAD-1), which corresponds to the cleaved portion of the extracellular domain of BP180. Other identified LAD target antigens include the full-length BP180, BP180 noncollagenous (NC)16A, BP230, laminin-332, laminin-γ1, α6β4 integrin, and type VII collagen (255 kDa and 290 kDa).

Clinical presentation: The skin lesions consist of vesicular papules and blisters that tend to be arranged in an arcuate or annular pattern with a tendency to heal in the center. This forms the so-called cluster-of-jewels or string-of-pearls grouping of blisters at the periphery of urticarial plaques.

The childhood-onset form of LAD, known also as the chronic bullous disease of childhood, is characterized by involvement of the lower part of the abdomen, thighs, genital area, buttocks, wrists, and ankles (Figure 14.8a). In contrast, adulthood LAD has a slightly different, polymorphic presentation with lesions on the trunk and occasionally the head and extremities (Figure 14.8b).

Involvement of the mucous membranes (oral, ocular) is not unusual and ranges in severity from mild to severe oral or conjunctival cicatricial lesions indistinguishable from MMP.

The onset of LAD may be spontaneous or triggered by skin trauma, ultraviolet radiation exposure, infections, and a wide range of drugs, including antibiotics (e.g., vancomycin), analgesics, nonsteroidal anti-inflammatories, antihypertensives, antiepileptics, vaccines, or immunosuppressants. Drug-induced LAD tends to present with positive Nikolsky signs and large erosions and is more severe than the spontaneous form.

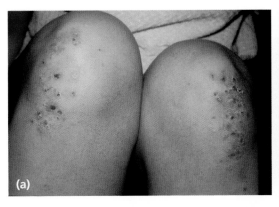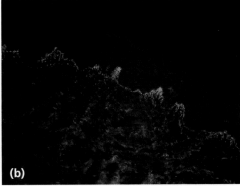

Figure 14.8 Clinical manifestations of linear IgA disease: (a) Tense blisters with annular arrangement (string-of-pearls sign) on the inner thighs of a 4-year-old girl; (b) widespread targetoid lesions with peripheral blistering over the trunk in an adult patient.

There is a well-documented association of LAD with other autoimmune disorders, especially inflammatory bowel disease, and various lymphoid and nonlymphoid malignant diseases.

Laboratory studies: The diagnosis of LAD is based on histology, which invariably shows a subepidermal blister with a superficial predominantly polymorphonuclear dermal infiltrate, and on the detection of linear IgA along the BMZ upon DIF microscopy of perilesional skin. IIF studies reveal circulating low-titer IgA (and sometimes IgG) antibodies directed against the epidermal (lamina lucida type) or less commonly dermal side (sub-lamina densa type) of SSS substrate.

Differential diagnosis: LAD is often mistaken for other bullous diseases, such as impetigo, tinea, or varicella in children and BP, DH, or PH in adults. Some cases mimicking erythema multi-forme, Stevens-Johnson syndrome, and TEN have to be differentiated.

Management: Skin lesions respond rapidly to highly potent topical steroids alone or combined with sulfones (dapsone or sulfapyridine) and/or low-dose prednisone. Immunosuppressants, rituximab, IVIG, and antitumor necrosis factor-α can be used in patients unresponsive to other treatments. In drug-induced cases, withdrawal of the suspected drug is essential.

Course: The natural disease course is variable with spontaneous remission between 3–6 years after the onset in the majority of patients and chronic relapsing disease in others, mainly those aged <70 years and with mucosal involvement. Childhood LAD usually remits before puberty.

Final comment: Due to the heterogeneity of its clinical presentation, overlapping with BP, MMP, and EBA, LAD can be considered as a group of subepidermal blistering disorders rather than a single nosologic entity.

Dermatitis Herpetiformis

Synonyms: Duhring's disease

Definition: Dermatitis herpetiformis (DH) is a chronic subepidermal AIBD that is characterized by an intensely pruritic cutaneous eruption, typical immunofluorescence findings, and association with gluten-sensitive enteropathy (GSE) identical to that seen in celiac disease (CD).

Overview: DH is currently regarded as a special, distinct form of a CD with combined intestinal and cutaneous manifestations. Both CD and DH are induced by gluten ingested from wheat, rye, and barley in genetically (mainly HLA) susceptible individuals and are characterized by the presence of a variable combination of gluten-dependent clinical manifestations, celiac-specific antibodies, and HLA-DQ2 or DQ8 haplotypes. Tissue transglutaminase (TG2) and epidermal transglutaminase (TG3) are identified as the major autoantigens in CD and DH, respectively.

Clinical presentation: DH is clinically manifested by a polymorphic symmetrical eruption that classically involves the bilateral extensor surfaces of the upper and lower extremities, elbows, knees, scalp, nuchal area, and buttocks (Figure 14.9a). Primary lesions are erythematous papules surmounted by vesicles that are grouped together in a herpetiform fashion. Due to the intense pruritus associated with the eruption, excoriations and erosions covered by hemorrhagic crust may predominate. Malabsorption, iron deficiency, and growth retardation in children, as well as other extraintestinal manifestations of CD (e.g., infertility, liver disease, nephropathy, neuropathy, cerebellar ataxia), may also occur.

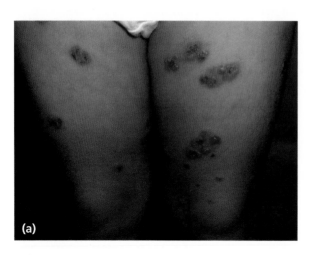 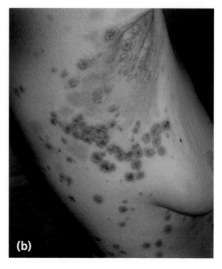

Figure 14.9 Dermatitis herpetiformis: (a) A symmetrical polymorphic eruption with classic predilection for the knees, elbows, and extensor surfaces; (b) direct immunofluorescent shows granular deposits of IgA at the dermal-epidermal junction, predominantly at the tips of dermal papillae.

Similar to those with CD, patients with DH have a higher incidence of associated other auto-immune disorders, including thyroiditis, diabetes type I, Addison disease, vitiligo, and alopecia areata, plus an increased risk for developing enteropathy-associated T-cell lymphomas. Examination for possible signs and symptoms of these associations is necessary.

Laboratory studies: The diagnosis of DH is based on clinical, histologic, and IF criteria. Histologically, subepidermal splitting and infiltration of dermal papillary tips with neutrophils (neutrophillic microabscesses) are seen.

The gold standard for the diagnosis of DH is the DIF microscopy of uninvolved perilesional skin revealing pathognomonic granular IgA deposits along the DEJ, which is mostly confined to the dermal papillary tips (Figure 14.9b). IIF microscopy and ELISAs reveal the presence of circulating IgA anti-TG2 and -TG3 antibodies in the serum of patients.

Small-bowel mucosal biopsy reveals partial villous atrophy in 70–80% of patients with DH.

Differential diagnosis: DH should be differentiated from other AIBDs, such as BP, LAD, and herpetiform pemphigus. Other pruritic dermatoses, such as papular urticaria, atopic, nummular, or contact dermatitis, and scabies, should be considered in the differential. Bullous systemic LE (BSLE) can clinically and histologically resemble DH but is immunopathological similar to EBA.

Management: The cornerstone of treatment of DH is the gluten-free diet for a lifetime and administration of sulfones, such as dapsone 50–100 mg/daily. In patients who are intolerant to dapsone due to side effects (e.g., hemolysis, methemoglobinemia, agranulocytosis) or glucose-6-phosphate dehydrogenase (G6PD) deficiency, sulfapyridine 0.5–2.0 g daily (to a maximum dose of 4.0 g/daily) is an alternative. Strict adherence to a gluten-free diet may result in remission of both cutaneous and gastrointestinal symptoms.

Course: The eruption runs a chronic course with flares and remissions, especially if unrecognized or left untreated.

Final comment: DH represents the cutaneous manifestation of CD. It characteristically presents with an intensely pruritic cutaneous eruption, which dramatically improves with a gluten-free diet and sulfones.

Epidermolysis Bullosa

Definition: Epidermolysis bullosa (EB) is a heterogeneous group of rare hereditary or acquired (EBA) disorders characterized by extreme fragility of the skin, and sometimes mucous membranes, to minimal mechanical trauma, which results in blisters and erosions.

Overview: The loss of integrity of the epidermis is due to mutations in the genes encoding for various BMZ structural proteins (hereditary EB) or to autoimmunity towards those proteins

(EBA), which results in their absence or aberrant expression and subsequent disruption of the DEJ. The affected individuals may have inherited the mutated gene from an affected parent (autosomal-dominant or recessive mode of inheritance) or have the mutated gene as the result of a de novo gene mutation.

Based on the ultrastructural level of blister formation, four major types of hereditary EB are currently distinguished: EB simplex (EBS), junctional EB (JEB), dystrophic EB (DEB), and Kindler syndrome (KS); each one is further subdivided into subtypes (Table 14.3).

Table 14.3 Major Types and Subtypes of Hereditary Epidermolysis Bullosa

EB type	EB Subtype	Inheritance Pattern	Level of Cleavage	Affected Proteins
EBS	Localized (previously Weber-Cockayne)	AD	Basal keratinocytes	Keratin 5, keratin 14
	Intermediate (previously Koebner)	AD	Basal keratinocytes	Keratin 5, keratin 14
	Severe (previously Dowling-Meara)	AD	Basal keratinocytes	Keratin 5, keratin 14
	Other rare subtypes: EBS-MP[a], EBS-migr[a], Intermediate (previously Ogna)[a], autosomal recessive intermediate, EBS-AR BP230[b], EBS-AR exophilin 5[b], EBS-MD[b], EBS-PA[b], localized with nephropathy CD151[b]	AD[a] or AR[b]	Basal keratinocytes	Keratin 5/14, plectin, BP230, exophilin-5, integrin α6β4, CD151 antigen
JEB	Severe JEB (previously Herlitz)	AR	Lamina lucida	Laminin-332
	Intermediate JEB (previously non-Herlitz)	AR	Lamina lucida	Laminin-332 or collagen XVII (BP180)
	JEB with pyloric atresia	AR	Lamina lucida	Integrin α6β4
	Other rare subtypes: JEB-loc, JEB-inv, JEB-LO, JEB-LOC s-me, JEB-RR	AR	Lamina lucida	Laminin-332, collagen XVII, integrin α6β4, laminin α3, integrin α3
DEB	DDEB (previously Pasini or Cockayne-Touraine) • Intermediate • Localized • Pruriginosa • Self-improving	AD	Sub-lamina densa, AF	Collagen VII
	RDEB • Intermediate (previously non-Hallopeau-Siemens) • Severe (previously Hallopeau-Siemens) • Inversa • Localized • Pruriginosa • Self-improving	AR	Sub-lamina densa, AF	Collagen VII
	DEB severe	Compound heterozygosity	Sub-lamina densa, AF	Collagen VII
Kindler syndrome	Kindler syndrome	AR	Multiple cleavage planes	Kindlin-1

Abbreviations: EB, epidermolysis bullosa; EBS, Epidermolysis bullosa simplex; AD, autosomal dominant; AR, autosomal recessive; EBS-MP, EBS with mottled pigmentation; EBS-migr, EBS with migratory circinate erythema; EBS-AR BP230, localized or intermediate with BP230 deficiency; EBS-AR exophilin 5, localized or intermediate with exophilin-5 deficiency; EBS-MD, intermediate with muscular dystrophy; EBS-PA, Severe with pyloric atresia; JEB, junctional EB; JEB-loc, JEB localized; JEB-inv, JEB inversa; JEB-LO, JEB late onset; LOC s-me, laryngo-onycho-cutaneous syndrome; JEB-RR, JEB with respiratory and renal involvement (JEB with interstitial lung disease and nephrotic syndrome); DEB, dystrophic EB; DDEB, dominant DEB; AF, anchoring fibrils; RDEB, recessive DEB.

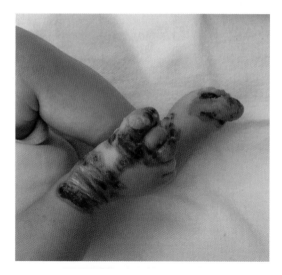

Figure 14.10 Epidermolysis bullosa simplex: multiple mechanobullous lesions with herpetiform configuration on the feet of a 3-month-old baby.

EBA is the rare acquired autoimmune form of EB that is mediated by antibodies against type VII collagen, which is the major component of anchoring fibrils in the DEJ; EBA, therefore, belongs to the group of subepidermal AIBDs.

Clinical presentation: The onset of hereditary EB is usually at birth or early childhood except for some subtypes of JEB. The clinical presentations are highly variable, and the severity correlates with the level of the skin at which blisters form.

In EBS, the blisters occur in the basal layer of the epidermis, and the disease is usually milder and confined to the palms and soles, with erosions healing without scars (Figure 14.10).

When the separation takes place within the lamina lucida of the BMZ as in JEB, affected patients have lesions with atrophy and/or exuberant granulation tissue formation along with severe mucosal involvement (gastrointestinal, respiratory, genitourinary tracts, and the eyes) severe anemia, and marked growth retardation. Patients may die early in life or may have prolonged debilitating disease.

In DEB, the blisters occur within the sublamina densa region at the uppermost dermis. The clinical picture ranges from mild (Figure 14.11a) to severe, depending on the subtype and inheritance mode (dominant DEB or recessive DEB), but the healing of blisters with considerable scarring and milia formation is a characteristic sign that usually leads to mutilating deformities, especially of the hands and feet (Figure 14.11b). There is also marked scarring of the mucosae, which affects the pharynx and esophagus, eyes, and genitourinary tract. DEB patients are at a higher risk of occurrence of squamous cell carcinomas (SCC; Figure 14.11c).

In KS, where blisters occur at multiple cleavage planes due to loss-of-function mutation in the kindlin-1 gene, early childhood blistering resolves with cutaneous atrophy, progressive poikiloderma, and pronounced photosensitivity.

Acquired EB is clinically heterogeneous. Although all patients have marked skin fragility and blisters occurring at sites of minor trauma, there is an inflammatory phenotype of the disease that manifests with widespread blistering eruption resembling BP, MMP, or LAD. The classic variant of EBA shows features reminiscent of hereditary DEB with localized, noninflammatory blisters, scarring, and milia formation limited to trauma-prone skin surfaces (Figure 14.12).

Laboratory studies: Distinguishing the major types of hereditary EB in the neonatal period based on clinical features is unreliable. The accurate laboratory diagnosis is based on the identification of the level of skin cleavage via immunofluorescence antigen mapping (IFM) and/or transmission electron microscopy (TEM) on a skin biopsy sample from a spontaneous or induced blister. Subtypes are then defined based on the mode of transmission, IFM and TEM, and clinical presentation.

The diagnosis of EBA relies on the same diagnostic algorithm as the other subepidermal AIBDs. The histology invariably reveals a subepidermal blister, and the DIF on perilesional skin shows linear deposits of IgG (or IgA) and C3 at the BMZ with a "u"-serration pattern. Serum IgG (or IgA) anti-BMZ antibodies bind to the dermal side of a SSS substrate (Figure 14.6c). Circulating autoantibodies to type VII collagen are detected by ELISA, IIF on BIOCHIP with Col7-NC1 transfected human cells, and IB.

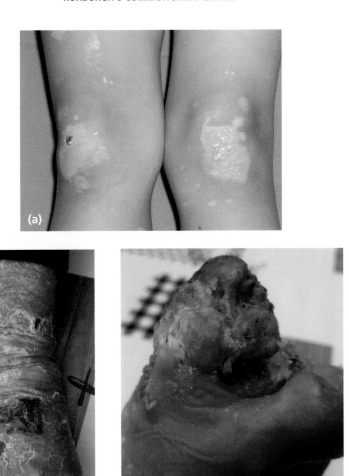

Figure 14.11 Dystrophic epidermolysis bullosa (DEB): (a) Blisters confined to the knees and lower legs, healing with atrophic scars and milia in a child with the dominant DEB; (b) in RDEB, severe blistering leads to atrophy, scarring and mutilating deformities of the hands and feet; (c) squamous cell carcinoma is a frequent complication of RDEB.

Differential diagnosis: The differential diagnosis of hereditary EB includes any cause of blistering in the neonatal period, including incontinentia pigmenti, bullous ichthyosiform erythroderma, bullous impetigo, diffuse cutaneous mastocytosis, staphylococcal scalded skin syndrome, *Herpes simplex* infection, neonatal or congenital varicella, neonatal pemphigus, and pemphigoid.

EBA requires differentiation from porphyria cutanea tarda/pseudoporphyria, BP, MMP, LAD, and BSLE, the latter being the other AIBD due to autoimmunity to type VII collagen.

Management: In the absence of specific therapy for inherited EB, management focuses on the avoidance of trauma, prevention of blistering and secondary infection, skincare measures, including wound care (use of nonadhesive dressings), prevention and treatment of complications, pain control, monitoring of the water–electrolyte balance, nutritional support when necessary, and early diagnosis of SCC.

EBA treatment is challenging and often unsatisfactory. Systemic corticosteroids in combination with immunosuppressants may be ineffective in some cases. Some therapeutic success has been reported with colchicine, dapsone, photopheresis, infliximab, or high-dose intravenous immunoglobulin.

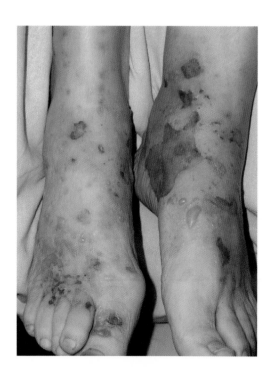

Figure 14.12 Epidermolysis bullosa acquisita: The inflammatory phenotype resembles bullous pemphigoid, but mechanobullous involvement on trauma-prone sites as the feet is suggestive of the diagnosis.

Course: The various subtypes of hereditary EB have varying prognoses based on the mode of transmission and a combination of phenotypic, immunofluorescence, ultrastructural, and molecular findings. In some subtypes, disease manifestations are limited and life expectancy is normal, whereas other subtypes can be fatal in infancy (particularly subtypes of JEB) or may be associated with severe lifelong disfiguring disease and even death.

Mild cases of EBA follow a chronic course, whereas aggressive disease is often difficult to control and is associated with a significant mortality rate.

FINAL THOUGHT

Disorders in the group of EB represent a spectrum of blistering and scarring conditions that range from being mild with some inconvenience to life-threatening.

ADDITIONAL READINGS

Amber KT, Murrell DF, Schmidt E, et al. Autoimmune subepidermal bullous diseases of the skin and mucosae: clinical features, diagnosis, and management. Clin Rev Allergy Immunol. 2018;54:26–51.

Feliciani C, Joly P, Jonkman MF, et al. Management of bullous pemphigoid: the European Dermatology Forum consensus in collaboration with the European Academy of Dermatology and Venereology. Br J Dermatol. 2015;172:867–877.

Fine JD, Bruckner-Tuderman L, Eady RA, et al. Inherited epidermolysis bullosa: updated recommendations on diagnosis and classification. J Am Acad Dermatol. 2014;70:1103–1126.

Gottlieb J, Ingen-Housz-Oro S, Alexandre M, et al. Prost-Squarcioni C. Idiopathic linear IgA bullous dermatosis: prognostic factors based on a case series of 72 adults. Br J Dermatol. 2017;177:212–222.

Has C, Bauer JW, Bodemer C, et al. Consensus reclassification of inherited epidermolysis bullosa and other disorders with skin fragility. Br J Dermatol. 2020;183:614–627.

Joly P, Horwath B, Patsatsi K, et al. Updated GUIDELINES on the management of Pemphigus vulgaris and foliaceus initiated by the European Academy of Dermatology and Venereology (EADV). J Eur Acad Dermatol Venereol. 2020 (in press).

Neff AG, Turner M, Mutasim DF. Treatment strategies in mucous membrane pemphigoid. Ther Clin Risk Manag. 2008;4:617–626.

Schmidt E, Kasperkiewicz M, Joly P. Pemphigus. Lancet. 2019;394:882–894.

Schmidt E, Zillikens D. Pemphigoid diseases. Lancet. 2013;381:320–332.

Vassileva S, Drenovska K, Manuelyan K. Autoimmune blistering dermatoses as systemic diseases. Clin Dermatol. 2014;32:364–375.

15 Disorders of Keratinization and Other Genodermatoses

Roselyn Stanger and Nanette Silverberg

CONTENTS

Overview: The differentiation process in which basal epidermal cells gradually mature and transform into stratum corneum cells is known as keratinization. In this process, which takes about 14 days, plump, cuboidal or spheroidal, hydrated, highly metabolically active cells gradually become tough, hardened, biochemically inactive, thin, shield-like structures that are programmed to desquamate off the skin surface. This process is biochemically complex; therefore, it is not surprising that it is subject to genetically determined errors. During keratinization, a tough, chemically resistant, cross-linked protein band is laid down just inside the plasma membrane, and the whole cell flattens to a thin disc, or corneocyte. The corneocyte's water content is reduced from the usual 70% to 30%, and most of the cellular organelles, including its nucleus, are eliminated. The keratinous tonofilaments become organized in bundles and are spatially oriented. A further characteristic feature of the normal stratum corneum is the presence of an intercellular cement material that contains non-polar lipid and glycoprotein.

The stratum corneum is the major barrier to water loss and penetration of chemical agents that come into contact with the skin. It also provides some mechanical protection and prevents penetration by microbes, ultraviolet light, and allergens. A scale is merely an aggregate of horn cells that have failed to separate from each other in desquamation, and the condition known as hyperkeratosis is an exaggeration of this problem. Regardless of the particular fault ultimately responsible, the final common pathogenic pathway is a failure in the normal loss of intercorneocyte binding force (cohesion) in the superficial stratum corneum.

Skin disease can be extremely disabling. There is a primitive revulsion at a disordered skin surface, which results in significant isolation and social and emotional deprivation. Patients with chronic skin disorders often become severely depressed. It is not often appreciated just how severely physically disabled some patients with skin disease are. The abnormal scaling and hyperkeratotic skin do not have the normally excellent extensibility and compliance, so movements can be limited.

DOI: 10.1201/9781003105268-15

XERODERMA

Synonyms: Xerosis cutis, asteatotic dermatitis, winter itch (Figure 15.1)

Definition: The term derives from the Greek xeros, meaning dry, and xeroderma just means dry skin. The skin can appear dry, cracked, or scaly and may have signs of inflammation.

Overview: Xeroderma does not represent a single disease process. In fact, xeroderma is used to describe scaliness rather than water content. Individuals will have reduced lipids in the stratum corneum. Xeroderma or xerosis is exceptionally common in certain conditions and populations. Patients may suffer from associated pruritus, termed eczema craquale. There are some normal individuals who tend to have "dry" skin, and they are more susceptible to stimuli that provoke scaling. Aging tends to make the surface of the skin feel "drier," and this can be associated with pruritus. A low relative humidity aggravates the problem, as does repeated vigorous washing, especially in hot water with soaps and cleansing agents. Xeroderma tends to be worse in the wintertime. Xeroderma is seen in many patients with atopic dermatitis. Xeroderma is also seen during the course of severe wasting disease, such as carcinomatosis, intestinal malabsorption, and chronic renal failure, but it should not be confused with acquired ichthyosis.

Clinical presentation: Because the appearance of scaling transiently disappears if the abnormal skin is hydrated, it has mistakenly been believed that scaling is the manifestation of water deficiency. Enhanced appearance of skin lines, dullness of the skin, and increased prominence on dermatoscopy of the intercellular space are noted.

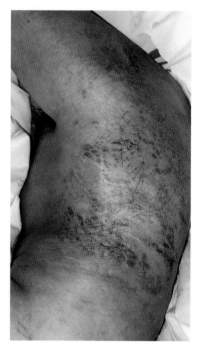

Figure 15.1 Xerosis of the skin demonstrating dry scales and hyperlinearity

Laboratory studies: A biopsy of the skin can be performed for intractable locations. Histopathologic study may reveal spongiotic dermatitis with intracellular edema, acanthosis, hyperkeratosis, and varying degrees of inflammatory infiltrate. Patients with xerosis of recent and rapid onset should be considered for a workup, including complete blood count, complete metabolic panel, LDH, 25 OH vitamin D, and vitamins B6, B12, E. Should there be any abnormality, consider consultations with a gastroenterologist and other specialists to rule out malabsorption or other pathologies.

Differential diagnosis: Ichthyosis and atopic dermatitis should be considered.

Management: Xerosis is very common and can be generally addressed with improvements in skincare, including reduction in usage of sodium laurel sulfate, reduced bathing times (under 15 minutes), and application of emollients directly after bathing. Emollients with specialized ingredients, such as ammonium lactate, urea, or ceramides, can enhance hydration of the skin as hygroscopic agents. Topical corticosteroids or nonsteroidal agents can also be prescribed for the associated pruritus.

Course and prognosis: Xerosis is commonly seasonal. Most xerosis is chronic, so ongoing management is usually needed; however, there are situations in which the underlying condition improves, and the associated xerosis will improve.

Final comment: Xerosis is a very common condition that is usually easily managed.

ICHTHYOSIS

Definition: Ichthyosis is a form of dryness and scaling that can occur in specific patterns and/or distributions. (Figures 15.2–15.4)

Overview: The term *ichthyosis* (meaning fish) is unfortunate, as the scale of "modern" fish is, in fact, mesodermal rather than ectodermal in origin. The term *ichthyosis* is used to describe generalized, noninflammatory disorders of keratinization and implies a congenital origin.

Clinical presentation: There are more than 20 conditions that are caused by inborn errors of development in the skin causing genetic ichthyosis (Table 15.1). Ichthyosis can also be acquired (Table 15.2).

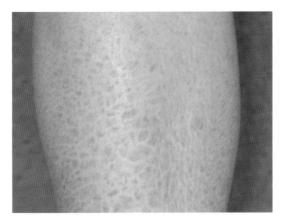

Figure 15.2 Dry scales of the anterior shins demonstrating exaggerated skin lines and dry scales in a Hispanic patient with ichthyosis vulgaris.

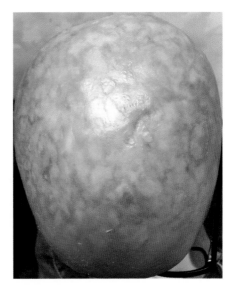

Figure 15.3 Alopecia of the scalp in a Pakistani preteen currently with lamellar ichthyosis phenotype who was born with a harlequin ichthyosis phenotype.

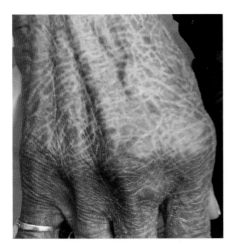

Figure 15.4 Acquired ichthyosis presenting with xerosis of the extensor extremities, chest, back and abdomen in an Afro-Caribbean woman with monoclonal gammopathy.

Laboratory studies: Histopathology can be used for diagnosis in some settings, particularly to improve diagnosis in genetic ichthyoses (see Table 15.1). Laboratory testing should be performed when ichthyosis occurs as a new onset condition in adulthood, including complete blood count, complete metabolic panel, 25 OH vitamin D, lactate dehydrogenase (LDH), serum protein electrophoresis (SPEP), urine protein electrophoresis (UPEP), and vitamins B6, B12, and E. Evaluations for infections, including HIV and HTLV1, should be considered. Chest x-ray and CT scan of the chest may be needed to rule out Hodgkin's disease. For genetic or congenital ichthyosis, specialized ichthyosis whole exome screens (e.g., Congenital Ichthyosis XomeDx®*Slice*, GeneDX) can be performed to identify the genetic locus and confirm the subtype.

Differential diagnosis: This includes atopic dermatitis, genetic syndromes, and xerosis.

Management: Patients with ichthyosis vulgaris or other conditions associated with having "dry" or "sensitive" skin should be diligent about establishing good skin care routines. This means showering or bathing only once a day, for 5–10 minutes, with lukewarm water. This can be challenging in the summertime when patients are often taking multiple showers a day. Bath products should be fragrance free and designed for sensitive skin. Harsh soaps should be avoided. After the bath or shower, patients should pat dry with a towel, as opposed to harsh scrubbing or rubbing of the skin, and apply moisturizer right away. In general, patients should try to apply moisturizers twice a day. The "greasier" moisturizers, such as petrolatum, are typically the most effective, but

Table 15.1 Selected Types of Genetic Ichthyosis

Name of Ichthyosis	Mutation	Genetic Inheritance Type	Cutaneous Features	Other Features of the Genetic Syndrome	Testing Other than Whole Exome Sequencing
Netherton's Syndrome	SPINK5	AR	Congenital erythroderma and scaling, annular plaques with doubled edged scale, abnormal "bamboo" hair	Food and other allergies, high IgE, failure to thrive, temperature and electrolyte imbalances, recurrent infections	Genetic testing
X-Linked Recessive ichthyosis	STS	XR	Large, dark brown scales on neck, trunk, extremities that spares flexures, palms, soles, face	Corneal opacities, cryptorchidism, increased risk testicular cancer, hypogonadism	Lipoprotein electrophoresis, increased plasma cholesterol sulfate levels. Maternal carriers may have decreased serum estradiol
Congenital Ichthyosiform Erythroderma	KRT1,KRT1-	AR	Erythroderma, erosions, and blistering at birth. Later, hyperkeratosis over joints with a cobblestone pattern.		Genetic testing
Ichthyosis Vulgaris	FLG	AD	Fine scale on extremities and trunk that spraes flexures, hyperlinear palms/soles	Associated with keratosis pilaris and atopic dermatitis	Genetic testing β
Lamellar ichthyosis	TGM1 > ABCA12	AR	Collodion membrane at birth with ectropion; then large, thick, plate-like brown scales involving flexures	Scarring alopecia, heat intoleranace	Genetic testing
Harlequin Ichthyosis	ABCA12	AR	Thick, yellow-brown scale with fissures, severe ectropion, eclabium, ear deformities	Temperature and electrolyte instability in neonates, high risk death from sepsis or respiratory failure	Genetic testing

Abbreviations: AD, autosomal dominant; AR, autosomal recessive; XR, x linked recessive.

Table 15.2 Precipitating Causes of Acquired Ichthyosis

Precipitating Causes	Comments
• Hodgkin's disease and other reticuloses	• Rarely, other neoplastic diseases
• Essential fatty acid deficiency	• Due to dietary deficiency, blind loop syndrome, or intestinal bypass operation
• Serum lipid-lowering drugs	• For example, nicotinamide, butyrophenones
• Leprosy	• Usually subsequent to treatment
• AIDS	• Accompanied by severe pruritus

the "best" are the ones that patients will actually comply with using. Creams can be lighter and easier to apply in the summer. Lotions can be more comfortable for areas with lots of terminal hairs, such as the chest of men. If the patient lives in centrally heated rooms, then humidifiers can raise the relative humidity. There are some current data supporting the use of biologic agents in the setting of ichthyosis, specifically secukinumab, which has been described as having beneficial effects on symptoms and appearance.

Course: Course of genetic ichthyoses is often chronic and unremitting; however, newer therapeutics exist that may benefit such patients.

Final comment: Ichthyoses are a complex series of acquired or genetic conditions requiring specialized care.

NETHERTON SYNDROME

Definition: Netherton syndrome is a rare, autosomal recessive, genetic ichthyosis that presents in the neonatal period with erythroderma and scaling (ichthyosiform erythroderma; Figure 15.5).

Overview: The disease is caused by a mutation in the gene *SPINK5*, which encodes the protein LEKT1, a serine protease inhibitor.

Clinical presentation: The classic Netherton syndrome includes fragile, short, and brittle hair, known as bamboo hair (trichorrhexis invaginata), and a tendency to develop other atopic tendencies, such as food allergies. The classic clinical presentation is known as ichthyosis linearis circumflexa, which are annular plaques with a classic double-edged scale. Patients may also experience blistering, erosions, and pruritus.

Laboratory studies: Histopathologic study will demonstrate psoriasiform changes and usually is not required to make the diagnosis. Immunohistochemical staining can show diminished expression of *SPINK5*.

Patients should be monitored for temperature and electrolyte instability, especially hypernatremic dehydration. Patients are at a high risk for skin and respiratory infection and may suffer from recurrent infections. There is a low threshold to pan-culture in the setting of suspected infections. Patients may demonstrate increased levels of IgE as well as eosinophilia.

Genetic testing is required. Light microscopy of the hair can reveal the typical bamboo-shaped hair shafts, which resembles a ball-and-socket-joint appearance of the connection of two neighboring hair shafts. Such hair findings are often easier to find on the eyebrow hair.

Differential diagnosis: Many of the skin diseases that present with erythroderma and ichthyosis can have overlapping clinical presentations. Genetic testing, with or without a skin biopsy, is often required to help make the diagnosis. The differential diagnosis can include congenital ichthyosiform erythroderma, Omenn syndrome, erythrokeratoderma variabilis, hyper-IgE syndrome, and psoriasis, among others.

Management: Neonates require care in the neonatal intensive care unit, as they are at high risk of temperature and electrolyte dysregulation, skin and respiratory infections, sepsis, and fluid loss. Several topical agents can be used to help heal the skin, including emollients, gentle exfoliants, and topical steroids; however, topical tacrolimus should be avoided due to increased

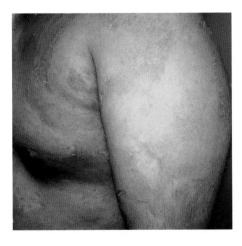

Figure 15.5 Icthyosis linearis circumflexa in a 16-year-old Middle Eastern boy with Netherton syndrome demonstrating double-edged scale.

absorption leading to potentially toxic systemic levels. Topical keratolytics may be too irritating. Patients with pruritus may be given antihistamines. Nutrition is essential to help mitigate the effects of failure to thrive, and patients may benefit from the help of a professional nutritionist. Patients with anaphylaxis or other atopic tendencies can be referred to an allergist and/or pulmonologist. Biologic agents that have recently been described to improve clinical features include secukinumab and dupilumab.

Course: In general, the skin condition tends to improve with age; however, ichthyosiform erythroderma tends to persist, with many patients experiencing flares during their lifetime.

Roughly three-quarters of patients will develop other atopic disorders and, in particular, anaphylaxis to food and other allergies. Patients may initially suffer from failure to thrive.

Final comment: Netherton syndrome combines genetic ichthyosis with distinctive dermatologic features and immune defects.

VOGT-KOYANAGI-HARADA SYNDROME

Definition: The Vogt-Koyanagi-Harada syndrome (VKHS) is a rare, multisystem autoimmune disease that mostly affects the skin, eyes, and central nervous system with vitiligo, chronic panuveitis, and sensorineural hearing loss.

Overview: This syndrome is a constellation of findings, including vitiligo and ocular problems, such as panuveitis. The syndrome affects tissues with melanocytes and is more common in individuals of Hispanic/Latinx, Asian, Native American, and Middle Eastern descent. The disease is thought to be a result of immune response to melanocyte-specific proteins.

Clinical presentation: In addition to generalized vitiligo, which may have been present for a while, inflammation of tissues with melanocytes can occur, including panuveitis, sensorineural hearing loss, vertigo, and tinnitus. The standard VKHS begins with headaches, malaise, and eye pain for a few days accompanied by acute neurologic symptoms, such as transverse myelitis, cranial nerve palsies, hemiparesis, and optic neuritis. The second stage involves acute uveitis, the third stage involves extensive depigmentation that is rapid in onset and spread, and the fourth stage involves chronic relapsing uveitis in which retinal fibrosis can occur. Alopecia and poliosis can also be noted.

Laboratory studies: Laboratory studies appropriate to vitiligo patients, including complete blood count with differential, thyroid studies, and 25 OH vitamin D levels, are recommended. Histopathologic study would be consistent with vitiligo in the skin. Other studies may include ophthalmologic examination, audiology examination, and neurology referrals and evaluations. CT/MRI can delineate some changes in the white matter.

Differential diagnosis: A syndrome similar to VKHS has been reported after therapy for melanoma with immune checkpoint inhibitor therapy.

Management: Systemic corticosteroids are the usual standard of care; however, recently adalimumab and janus kinase (JAK) inhibitors have been described as beneficial for the ocular disease, with the latter having an additional benefit on vitiligo.

Course: Early institution of systemic agents is very beneficial in controlling disease. Reversal of vitiligo has been described as a positive prognostic factor.

Final comment: VKHS is a syndrome associated with vitiligo, which requiring emergent intervention for best outcomes in vision and hearing.

KERATOSIS PILARIS

Synonym: Chicken skin (Figure 15.6)

Definition: This extremely common condition presents as monomorphic rough skin-colored follicular papules surrounding the hair follicles of the outer aspect of the upper arms and thighs, sometimes with background erythema (see Figure 15.3).

Overview: This is commonly seen in children and young adults, and children often have an involvement

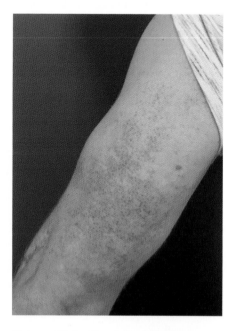

Figure 15.6 Keratotic follicular papules of the arms with associated erythema.

of their cheeks. In young children, background erythema of the cheeks can be noted, termed keratosis pilaris rubra faceii. Keratosis pilaris can be an isolated diagnosis and can also be seen in patients with underlying skin disorders, such as atopic dermatitis and ichthyosis vulgaris, among others. There is often a positive family history.

Clinical presentation: The most common presentation are follicular papules of the cheeks, upper arms, and thighs, beginning in the toddler years and showing facial improvement in teen years. Background erythema and associated pruritus is often noted. Severe disease can cause loss of the eyebrows, termed ulerythema ophyrogenes, which can be seen in syndromes, such as cardiofaciocutaneous syndrome.

Laboratory studies: A skin biopsy can confirm the diagnosis but is not required and is rarely performed to make the diagnosis. If a syndrome is suspected based on associated features, then a genetic evaluation may be needed. As keratosis pilaris is sometimes noted with obesity, studies related to metabolic syndrome may be needed in some patients. Recently, altered *ABCA12* expression has been demonstrated in keratosis pilaris skin.

Differential diagnosis: This may include for folliculitis, atopic dermatitis, lichen spinulosis, and lichen nitidus, among others. It can be an isolated finding, or it can be associated with underlying skin disorders. By itself, keratosis pilaris cannot point to one specific diagnosis over the other, and the overall clinical picture must be used to make the broader diagnosis.

Management: Patients should be educated that this is chronic. Although topical agents can help to improve the texture and roughness of the skin, as well as treat any itching or redness, it will likely remain with them throughout their lifetime. Patients should be instructed to follow a gentle skincare routine. Keratolytic agents (containing urea or lactic acid used twice a day) are routinely prescribed to help exfoliate plugs from the hair follicles. While patients are often asymptomatic, low- to mid-potency topical steroids (e.g., hydrocortisone 2.5% cream or triamcinolone 0.1% cream used twice a day for 1–2 weeks) can be used if erythema is present. Topical retinoids may help to reduce roughness (e.g., tretinoin); however, they can be irritating, which can further worsen the condition. Chemical peels can be used in some adults to smooth the skin more rapidly. When keratosis pilaris rubra faceii is present, vascular wavelength lasers can be used to reduce facial erythema.

Course: While the rough texture of the skin tends to persist, there tends to be general improvement over time. Facial disease remits in most individuals during adolescence.

Final comment: It is important to explain to patients that there is no cream that will make their skin completely smooth and that treatments are supportive.

ICHTHYOSIS VULGARIS

Definition: Ichthyosis vulgaris is the most common form of ichthyosis presenting with dry scales of the shins most commonly (see Figure 15.2).

Overview: Ichthyosis vulgaris is autosomal semi-dominant in inheritance and caused by a mutation in the gene filaggrin. Filaggrin is important in the aggregation of keratin filaments, and this defect results in abnormal skin barrier function.

Clinical presentation: It is characterized by fine scaling of the extremities, typically the extensor surfaces of the lower legs. This often spares the flexural surfaces. It is associated with both atopic dermatitis and keratosis pilaris. Patients may also have prominent creases on the palms and soles—a finding also associated with atopy. The onset is typically in early childhood.

Laboratory studies: A skin biopsy is often not required for the diagnosis but will show a diminished granular layer and overlying orthohyperkeratosis. Immunohistochemistry can show decreased filaggrin expression. When a family history is positive, then genetic testing can be helpful if the differential diagnosis includes other hereditary forms of ichthyosis.

Differential diagnosis: There are many ichthyoses, and there can be overlapping clinical presentations. These include lamellar ichthyosis, X-linked ichthyosis, xerosis, atopic dermatitis, and acquired ichthyosis.

Management: Emollients and a gentle skin care routine are the cornerstones of treatment. Emollients should be applied twice a day. Gentle exfoliating agents containing urea or lactic acid can be used focally to improve the appearance of scales; however, these cannot be used over a large body surface area because of the increased absorption in a setting of impaired skin barrier function. Topical retinoids (e.g., tretinoin, tazarotene) can also be used but as with keratosis pilaris, may be too irritating for certain patients. Systemic retinoids can be considered for severe cases. Low- to mid-potency topical steroids (e.g., triamcinolone 0.1% cream or ointment) can be used for short durations for significant erythema and pruritus.

Course: Typically, the scaling diminishes with age. Patients may develop other atopic disorders, such as atopic dermatitis and keratosis pilaris.

Final comment: Ichthyosis vulgaris is a common dry skin condition linked as well to atopic dermatitis. Emollients and keratolytics are the mainstay of therapy.

DARIER'S DISEASE

Synonyms: Keratosis follicularis, Darier-White disease.

Definition: This disorder is characterized by the presence of warty, brown, crusted papules on the chest or other seborrheic areas, classically in middle-aged and older men (Figure 15.7). Segmental variants can occur.

Overview: This autosomal dominant disorder is caused by mutations in the *ATP2A2* gene, which encodes the sarcoplasmic/endoplasmic reticulum Ca2+ ATPase isoform 2 protein (SERCA2), resulting in acantholysis and dyskeratosis.

Clinical presentation: This condition usually appears after adolescence with papules and plaques in a seborrheic distribution. Nail abnormalities, such as white and red linear alternating longitudinal bands, and mucosal changes, such as white cobblestone papules, are also noted. Superinfection with *Staphylococcus* and *Candida* may occur. Quality of life can be impaired.

Laboratory studies: Histopathology shows focal acantholytic dyskeratosis with 2 kinds of cells: (1) "corps ronds," which are eosinophilic bodies that are round, large, acantholytic keratinocytes in stratum spinosum and stratum granulosum and (2) "grains," which are small, dense, basophilic bodies of acantholytic cells stratum corneum.

Differential diagnosis: Seborrheic dermatitis and Hailey-Hailey are similar in appearance at times. Grover's disease can have some similarities.

Management: Topical treatment with mild keratolytics, such as salicylic acid 2% or tretinoin 0.025–0.05% may be helpful. Oral retinoids, including isotretinoin, can be beneficial. Bacterial and fungal cultures can be considered, as superinfection is common. A new agent, DX314, is being investigated for Darier's disease, which has enhanced selectivity for RA-metabolizing enzyme CYP26B1, causing increased retinoid activity endogenously but maintaining the integrity of the skin barrier.

Course: Spontaneous remission is not typical; therefore, long-term management is needed.

Final comment: Darier's disease is a condition associated with papules and plaques in the seborrheic distribution with superinfection commonly complicating lesions.

PALMOPLANTAR KERATODERMA

Definition: Palmoplantar keratoderma (PPK) describes a group of disorders in which there is marked thickening of palmar and plantar skin due to a localized abnormality of keratinization.

Overview: The disorder is very heterogeneous, with autosomal dominant, autosomal recessive, and sex-linked recessive types being described. There is also a wide range of clinical features, with involvement of the dorsal hands and feet in some patients and an odd "punctate" palmar pattern

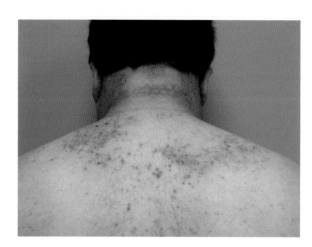

Figure 15.7 Darier's disease: Greasy scaling plaques on the neck and upper portion of the back.

in others. In one inherited variety, there is a close association with the development of esophageal carcinoma. Some cases are hereditary, while others are acquired due to internal conditions.

Clinical presentation: Thickening or hyperkeratosis of the palms and soles is typical with extension onto the dorsal hands or over the wrist in some patients, termed transgrediens. Aggravation with age is termed progrediens. Hyperhidrosis and erythema are often associated features. Fingernail changes can also be noted. Hyperkeratotic lesions and plaques in additional locations can be hallmarks of specific syndromes. Hereditary variants can be associated with other conditions (e.g., keratitis or esophageal cancers). A careful personal and family history are needed. New-onset lesions in adults can be a part of an internal syndrome, such as that associated with an internal malignancy.

Laboratory studies: Histopathologic study of a biopsy from the hyperkeratosis of the palms may confirm the thickening. Some PPK cases have additional histopathologic features, such as epidermolytic hyperkeratosis.

Differential diagnosis: Diseases to be considered are psoriasis, collagen vascular diseases, hand eczema, pityriasis rubra pilaris, and contact dermatitis.

Management: Topical emollients, keratolytics, and topical retinoids are first-line therapy. Oral retinoids can be used in more severe cases. Erythema and pruritus can be managed with topical corticosteroids. Botulinum neurotoxin injections have been used to manage associated hyperhidrosis and sometimes improve the appearance of PPK in pachyonychia congenita.

Course: Fortunately, most patients are not as disabled as may be thought from the clinical appearance. As long as they keep their skin surface flexible and smooth with emollients and keratolytics, they can manage everyday activities quite well.

Final comment: Palmoplantar keratoderma has to be evaluated based on clinical features, associated health findings, and histopathology.

TUBEROUS SCLEROSIS

Definition: This is a neurocutaneous illness with associated typical skin and neurologic findings.

Overview: Tuberous sclerosis (TS) is a rare, autosomal dominant, neurocutaneous syndrome that is caused by mutations in hamartin (*TSC1*) or tuberin (*TSC2*), which results in hamartomas involving almost every organ system. Although a family history can be helpful, many patients have a sporadic mutation prompting the disease.

Clinical presentation: Major skin abnormalities include early-onset hypopigmented macules, which can be leaf-shaped (ash-leaf macules), confetti, or thumbprint like. Pink-red papules may appear around the nose and cheeks, which increase in number during adolescence and are known, inappropriately, as adenoma sebaceum. Firm whitish plaques (shagreen patches) with a cobblestone surface and subungual fibromata are other skin findings. Cerebral malformations often result in epilepsy, infantile spasms, and developmental delays; complications related to seizures are a leading cause of mortality. Renal hamartomas occur in 50% of patients; complications relating to renal dysfunction are the second-leading cause of mortality. Unfortunately, almost every organ system is involved in these patients, and multidisciplinary care from a young age is of the utmost importance.

To confirm the diagnosis, patients must have the *TSC1* or *TSC2* mutation or meet two major criteria or one major criterion and two minor criteria, which are made widely available. Skin findings are particularly helpful in this disorder, as they are often the earliest presenting signs. For example, the ash-leaf spots are the first of the skin findings to be present and can be seen as early as infancy. The typical facial angiofibromas tend to appear around puberty.

Laboratory studies: Skin biopsies can confirm the findings of the ash-leaf spots, adenoma sebaceum, and shagreen patches, which are part of the major diagnostic criteria. Genetic testing can be used to help make the diagnosis.

Differential diagnosis: Due to the wide variety of clinical presentations, there is an extensive list. Each of the typical skin findings (e.g., ash-leaf spots, facial angiofibromas, shagreen patches, periungual fibromas) carries its own extensive list of differential diagnoses. The suspicion for tuberous sclerosis should arise in an infant with light-colored skin patches, the presence of seizures or spasms, and developmental delay, along with other internal organ findings that can accompany this disorder.

Management: Patients require multidisciplinary care, including dermatology, neurology, nephrology, ophthalmology, cardiology, gastroenterology, pulmonology, and good dental hygiene. Early identification of seizure activity and adequate seizure control have been demonstrated to help improve long-term intellectual development. As for the skin manifestations, there is evidence that topical rapamycin may be helpful for treating the facial angiofibromas, but lasers and other destructive measures have also been used either alone or in combination.

Course: Early management has been beneficial in the control of infantile spasms resulting in improved intellectual quotient. It has not yet been shown that early skin management produces long-term results; however, photodynamic therapy, topical rapamycin, topical everolimus, and topical sirolimus have been beneficial in reducing the appearance of facial lesions.

Final comment: TS is a neurocutaneous disorder requiring multidisciplinary management and ongoing surveillance.

INCONTINENTIA PIGMENTI

Synonym: Bloch Sulzberger disease

Definition: Incontinentia pigmenti (IP) is an X-linked dominant disorder that is lethal in boys and therefore seen in girls and boys with Klinefelter's syndrome. It was originally described by Marion Sulberger (1895–1983) and Bruno Bloch (1878–1933).

Overview: This neuroectodermal disorder affects the skin, hair, teeth, eyes, and central nervous system. The condition results from a mutation of the X-chromosome gene NEMO/IKK -gamma gene, which is located on chromosome Xq28. The X-chromosome is inactivated selectively in girls, such that only one is active in any cell; therefore, there can be mosaic involvement of the skin and tissues. Patients can suffer from seizures, developmental delays, and visual impairment.

Clinical presentation: This disorder has four stages of clinical findings. Figure 15.8. In the first 2 weeks of life, neonates will have linear or whorled streaks of vesicles in a Blaschkoid distribution typically along the extremities, believed to be caused by cellular apoptosis. This is followed by a verrucous appearance of the lesions, darkening of the affected areas with a flattened appearance (hyperpigmentation), and then lightening of the affected areas (hypopigmentation). Retinal and neurologic changes should be screened for in infancy. Dental anomalies occur in two-thirds of patients with conical incisors, canines, and bicuspids.

Laboratory studies: A biopsy taken in the early stages shows eosinophilic spongiosis. The verrucous stage shows hyperkeratosis and acanthosis with dyskeratotic cells. Eosinophils will usually be noted in the skin. Melanophages in a thickened papillary dermis are seen in the hyper-pigmented stage. Colloid bodies and apoptotic cells may be seen in the hypopigmented phase. Laboratory studies may show eosinophilia.

Karyotype analysis should be performed in males with suspected IP to rule out Klinefelter's syndrome (XXY karyotype). Evaluation by an ophthalmologist and neurologist are required. Genetic referral is ideal. A head CT scan and an MRI are usually performed in conjunction with a neurologic evaluation.

Differential diagnosis: Birthmarks that follow the lines of Blaschko can often have similarity to IP, particularly the stages involving linear pigmentation.

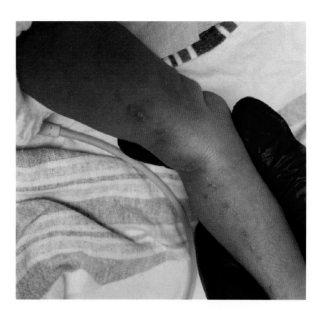

Figure 15.8 A Hispanic infant girl with linear blisters consistent with incontinentia pigmenti, confirmed by biopsy demonstrating eosinophilic spongiosis.

Management: There has been some discussion of topical tacrolimus being helpful in the early lesions, while systemic steroids may be used for neurologic disease.

Course: Lesions improve with age as they trend toward hypopigmentation.

Final comment: IP is a multisystem disorder, largely manifesting with skin lesions. Cosmetic outcomes are usually good with improvement over time.

RASOPATHIES

The following disorders can be classified as RASopathies: Neurofibromatosis Type 1 (NF1), Noonan, Costello, LEOPARD, cardio-facio-cutaneous syndrome. NF1 (and, briefly, Costello syndrome) are described. RASopathies are genodermatoses with origins in the RAS pathways.

Neurofibromatosis Type 1

Synonym: Von Recklinghausen's disease

Definition: This is an autosomal dominant multisystem disorder, yet about half of patients with this disorder have sporadic mutations, so there is not always a positive family history. It was originally described by Friedrich von Recklinghausen (1833–1910).

Overview: This condition presents in early childhood with café au lait macules. Seizure disorder and associated tumors in the eye, skin, and central nervous system can cause morbidity and mortality.

Clinical presentation: Patients present with brown café au lait macules that vary in size; the appearance of such freckle-like lesions in the axillae is diagnostic of the disorder (Figures 15.9–15.11). In addition, patients can have skin-colored to pink, compressible soft skin tumors called neurofibromas, some of which are pedunculated. These may be present in large numbers, which can cause considerable cosmetic disability. Patients can also develop larger plexiform neuromas, which may have a risk (~10%) of transforming into malignant peripheral nerve sheath tumors. Patients are also subject to the development of a wide range of neoplastic lesions, including pheochromocytoma and fibrosarcoma, among others. It is crucial that these patients have follow-up with ophthalmology, as they may develop optic gliomas, which can lead to blindness. In addition, slit lamp examination may reveal the presence of Lisch nodules, which are a major diagnostic criterion for this disorder and can help confirm the diagnosis.

Laboratory studies: Biopsies can help to identify malignant changes in plexiform neuromas. However, most of the cutaneous lesions are clinical. Ophthalmology and neurology consultations are needed. Genetic screening can be performed. Other studies include CT and MRI, which can be used to identify intracranial features of NF1.

Differential diagnosis: There are many other syndromes associated with café au lait spots including Legius syndrome, which can mimic NF1 in the skin but lacks the neurological changes. NF-1, McCune Albright syndrome, and Legius syndrome are all associated with café au lait macules.

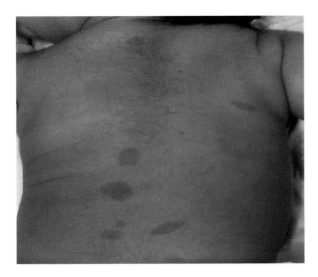

Figure 15.9 Latin X infant with early presentation of multiple cafe au lait macules.

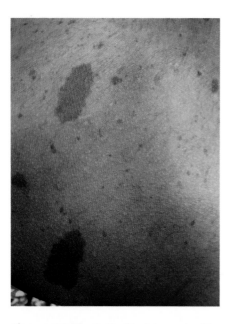

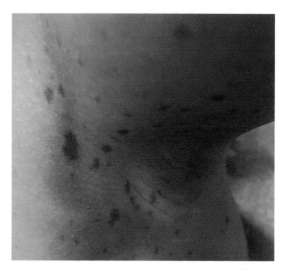

Figure 15.11 African American 9-year-old girl with axillary freckling (Crowe's sign).

Figure 15.10 Latin X adolescent with mixed axillary freckling (Crowe's sign) and cafe au lait macules.

Management: Multidisciplinary management includes dermatology, ophthalmology, neurology, radiology, genetics, orthopedics, and potentially other practitioners. Newer therapeutics are under evaluation, including MEK inhibitors for plexiform neuromas that are not amenable to surgery.

Course and/or Prognosis: When the seizures are well-managed from an early age, neurologic prognosis is improved long term. Cutaneous lesions, such as neurofibromas, can be surgically removed to reduce cosmetic burden.

Final comment: NF1 is an autosomal dominant multisystem disorder that requires careful monitoring, which can improve long-term morbidity and mortality.

Costello Syndrome

Definition: This is a very rare autosomal dominant RASopathy characterized by lax (or redundant) skin (especially over the neck, hands, and feet), internal organ involvement (primarily cardiac), increased risk of malignancies, and severe feeding difficulties. Most patients have *de novo* mutations.

Overview: The characteristic findings are lax skin on the hands and feet, pulmonic stenosis, cardiac abnormalities, and increased risk of malignancies, such as transitional cell bladder cancer and rhabdomyosarcoma.

Clinical presentation: Costello syndrome is the result of a heterozygous germline mutation in the *HRAS* gene. Patients with Costello syndrome can have extremely variable phenotypic presentations. Cutaneous findings include lax skin of the hands and feet, deep palmar and plantar creases, curly hair, acanthosis nigricans or even generalized hyperpigmentation, low-set ears, periorificial papillomata, and coarse facial features. Cardiac abnormalities include hypertrophic cardiomyopathy, arrhythmias (e.g., supraventricular tachycardia), and congenital heart defects (e.g., valvar pulmonic stenosis). Patients can also have macrocephaly, hydrocephalus, or cerebellar abnormalities (e.g., Chiari malformations); diffuse hypotonia; and joint laxity. Infants can suffer from failure to thrive, and as they get older, children may have developmental delays, intellectual disabilities, and short stature. As mentioned earlier, patients are at increased risk for malignancies, in particular rhabdomyosarcoma and neuroblastoma in children and transitional cell carcinoma of the bladder in adolescents and young adults.

Laboratory studies: While a biopsy of lax skin can confirm the presence of lax skin, it is not the most crucial aspect of diagnosis. As this is a multidisciplinary disease, blood tests should be ordered based on a multidisciplinary approach. The diagnosis of Costello syndrome is clinical together with genetic testing, as the majority of patients will have evidence of *HRAS* mutation.

MRI and CT scan may be needed, as well as genetic testing to identify the *HRAS* mutation. Other studies can be performed in accordance with a multidisciplinary approach.

Differential diagnosis: Cutis laxa is another inherited disorder that can present with lax skin and multi-organ involvement, yet it is due to mutations in either *FBLN5* or Elastin or *ATP7A*. Noonan syndrome, another RASopathy, can have similar clinical features, such as short stature, developmental delay, macrocephaly, curly hair, low-set ears, and cardiac abnormalities.

Management: Patients should be managed with a multidisciplinary team, including cardiologists, gastroenterologists (as supplemental feeding is often required and feeding abnormalities can be severe), orthopedic surgery (for joint deviation or tendon abnormalities), neurologists, neurosurgeons, oncologists, and early intervention childhood specialists (to address developmental delays). The facial papillomata can be removed with destructive measures. Patients also need close follow-up for malignancy screening. Finally, genetic counseling should be offered to every patient.

Course: Patients with Costello syndrome can have a wide variety of clinical presentations, ranging from a mild phenotype to early death. Close follow-up with a multidisciplinary team is essential.

Final comment: Costello syndrome is a very rare autosomal dominant RASopathy, and patients must be managed by a multidisciplinary team.

McCune Albright Syndrome

Definition: This a neurocutaneous/osteo-hormonal disorder, having a typical café au lait macule with jagged edges and associated with bony and endocrine disorders.

Overview: McCune Albright syndrome is a disorder of hypopigmentation caused by a postzygotic somatic activating mutation in *GNAS1* in the affected tissues; this is a mosaic condition.

Clinical presentation: There are three key features associated with this disorder. Patients have café au lait macules, such as those found in patients with neurofibromatosis. Classically, the borders of the lesions are jagged, and their appearance has been referred to as the "coast of Maine." Second, patients have abnormal skeletal findings, including polyostotic fibrous dysplasia, which can lead to fractures, bone pain, gait abnormalities, skeletal deformities, and malignant degeneration. Third, patients have endocrinologic abnormalities, such as precocious puberty, hypophosphatemic rickets, and Cushing syndrome.

Laboratory studies: A biopsy is not needed to identify the café au lait. Laboratory studies for calcium and phosphorus may be helpful. Genetic testing will usually confirm GNAS gene mutations with mosaic gene expression in the tissues. Endocrinopathies, such as neonatal Cushing's syndrome, may occur for which an endocrinologic referral may be beneficial. X-rays may confirm clinical features.

Differential diagnosis: Isolated café au lait macules, NF1, and Legius syndrome all present with cafe au lait macules.

Management: When a "coast of Maine" macule is identified, a referral to endocrine, orthopedics, and genetics may help to confirm the condition. Laser of cafe au lait macules has variable efficacy.

Course: Cafe au lait macule(s) is the first manifestation, and other features may manifest over time.

Final comment: McCune Albright is a multisystem mosaic skin and systemic disorder, which can affect the bones and endocrine system.

Legius Syndrome

Definition: This is an autosomal dominant disorder caused by mutations in *SPRED1*.

Overview: The disease is characterized by ≥6 café au lait macules and intertriginous freckling. Neurologic changes and bony changes of neurofibromatosis are absent.

Clinical presentation: Multiple café au lait macules, axillary freckling, and macrocephaly are found. Patients can also have learning disabilities. Although this disorder is a so-called RASopathy like neurofibromatosis, patients do not have neurofibromas, Lisch nodules, or optic gliomas.

Laboratory studies: Ruling out of NF1 can include genetic testing, ophthalmologic examination, and careful full-body skin examinations for at least the first 6 years of life.

Differential diagnosis: This includes NF1 and McCune Albright syndrome.

Management: Ophthalmology, genetics, and neurology examinations can help to rule out NF1, as can frequent skin examinations.

Course: As learning disabilities can be noted, neurologic and neurodevelopmental evaluation can aid in support of the patient's growth and intellectual development.

Final comment: Legius syndrome should be suspected in children with café au lait macules who do not manifest second clinical criterion to make the diagnosis of NF1.

OTHER GENODERMATOSES

PTEN Syndromes

Definition: The following two disorders are characterized by mutations in the phosphatase and tensin homolog (PTEN) tumor suppressor gene. PTEN negatively regulates the AKT/mTOR pathway, which is involved in cell growth and survival.

Clinical presentation: Cowden syndrome (also called multiple hamartoma syndrome) is an autosomal dominant disorder. The clinical findings include several notable skin findings (e.g., sclerotic fibromas, facial tricholemmomas, palmoplantar keratoses, lipomas, skin tags), macrocephaly, overgrowth of several tissues, and most importantly an increased risk of several cancers. Bannayan-Riley-Ruvalcaba syndrome (BRRS) has overlap with the clinical findings of Cowden syndrome, but in addition, patients have pigmented macules on the penis, lipomas, hemangiomas, macrocephaly, and mental retardation.

Laboratory studies: Bloodwork should be performed based on a multidisciplinary approach. While a biopsy can help to confirm the diagnosis of cutaneous findings, such as a lentigo or lipoma, genetic testing is required for diagnosis. The skin findings are not pathognomonic for BRRS. Genetic screening can show germline *PTEN* mutations, which can be identified in about 60–70% of patients with BRRS. Long-term cancer screening should include breast, thyroid, and renal cancers in confirmed patients, as well as an MRI or CT scan.

Differential diagnosis: Cowden syndrome and BRRS can have many overlapping clinical features, and both share *PTEN* mutations.

Management: A multidisciplinary approach including gastroenterology (to identify polyps and rule out malignancy), neurologists (as patients may have macrocephaly, hypotonia, muscle weakness, and seizures), oncologists (as patients may have an increased risk for the solid tumors associated with Cowden syndrome, including thyroid, breast, endometrial, and renal cancers), orthopedic surgeons (as patients may have joint hyperextensibility and scoliosis, among other findings), early childhood specialists (to help with developmental delay), and genetic counseling. Skin findings can be removed with destructive measures, such as with lasers.

Course: Patients require multidisciplinary care and must be closely monitored for the development of malignancies. As BRRS can have overlap with Cowden syndrome, patients need close follow-up.

Final comment: Cowden Syndrome and BRRS are multisystem diseases that require multidisciplinary care and close follow-up for the development of malignancies.

DISORDERS OF HAIR AND NAILS

Pachyonychia Congenita

Definition: Pachyonychia congenita (PC), of which there are two main types, Type I and Type 2, are autosomal dominant disorders involving mutations in various keratins; however, approximately one-third of patients can have *de novo* mutations.

Overview: PC is a condition associated with plantar keratoderma and associated cutaneous features.

Clinical presentation: The three key features found in both types of PC are onychodystrophy (abnormal appearance of the nails), plantar keratoderma (thickening of the skin on the soles of the feet), and plantar pain. Type 1 involves mutations in *KRT6A* and *KRT16*. In addition to three main features described earlier, it is also characterized by benign (as opposed to premalignant) oral leukoplakia and follicular hyperkeratosis of the extensors, such as the knees and elbows, and paronychia. Type 2, caused by mutations in *KRT6B* and *KRT17*, is characterized by the presence of natal/prenatal teeth and steatocystomas/vellus hair cysts.

Laboratory studies: A skin biopsy can help to confirm the diagnosis of steatocystomas, which are classically associated with PC. Other studies, including an MRI or CT scan may be required. Diagnosis is made based on clinical grounds or genetic testing that reveals a heterozygous mutation in one of the five keratin genes associated with PC (i.e., *KRT6A*, *KRT6B*, *KRT6C*, *KRT16*, and *KRT17*).

Differential diagnosis: There are several other genetic disorders that fall under the category of ectodermal dysplasias, including hypohidrotic ectodermal dysplasia, hidrotic ectodermal dysplasia, Rubinstein-Taybi syndrome, and the p63-associated dysplasias. While there may be some overlap in the clinical findings, combination of a physical examination and genetic testing can help confirm the correct diagnosis. There are also many diseases that can be associated with palmoplantar hyperkeratosis.

Management: Management of painful keratoderma on the soles should be addressed, and patients must be encouraged to minimize friction and trauma to the feet; wear proper-fitting, comfortable shoes (possibly with special orthotics); and utilize socks that minimize retention of sweat in the feet. Hyperkeratotic areas can be managed with physical paring and/or emollients or oral retinoids, such as acitretin. Topical keratolytics are only minimally effective. Patients must also have good nail hygiene and may require periodic nail avulsion for cosmetic benefit. Patients need to have good oral hygiene to manage any oral leukoplakia. The cysts themselves are benign but can be removed with destructive measures, such as excisions, lasers, or draining (temporary measure if infected or painful). Areas of skin with hyperkeratosis can be prone to secondary infections, and regular scheduled bleach baths may be helpful for prevention. There are case reports of the use of oral statins, injectable botulinum toxin for painful hyperkeratosis of the soles, and oral and topical sirolimus to improve the pain associated with plantar hyperkeratosis.

Babies with natal teeth should be referred to a dentist. PC may be aggravated by high humidity and temperatures. Genetic counseling should also be provided.

Course: PC generally lacks association with systemic diseases that require frequent follow-up.

Final comment: There are two types of PC that should be distinguished from each other either based on clinical findings or genetic screening.

EPIDERMAL NEVUS SYNDROMES

Definition: Epidermal nevi are streak-like, verrucous, typically hyperpigmented skin markings along Blaschko's lines.

Overview: Epidermal nevus syndrome is an umbrella term for a variety of neurocutaneous syndromes. There are many congenital disorders that present with epidermal nevi in conjunction with various systemic manifestations, and multiple genes have been implicated, including *FGFR3*, *HRAS*, *PIK3CA*, *PTEN*, and *AKT1*, among others.

Clinical presentation: While epidermal nevi can be an isolated finding, patients can also have a range of extracutaneous finings, with neurologic symptoms being the most common and prominent. Such patients require a thorough history, physical examination, and a meticulous skin examination. For example, Apert syndrome is caused by a mutation in *FGFR2* and presents with nevus comedonicus or acneiform nevi, severe and early-onset acne, and skeletal and central nervous system abnormalities.

Laboratory studies: Although a skin biopsy can confirm the diagnosis of an epidermal nevus, it is not the most important aspect of the diagnosis, as the underlying systemic manifestations are the causes of morbidity and mortality for these patients. Bloodwork should be guided by a multidisciplinary approach. Other studies may include an MRI and CT scan. Genetic testing should be performed to clarify which epidermal nevus syndrome is affecting a particular patient; however, not all the gene mutations are known.

Differential diagnosis: This list is already vast as this is merely an umbrella term. Patients need a full systemic workup and genetic testing to help confirm the specific diagnosis affecting them.

Management: Genetics, ophthalmology, neurology, and nephrology are among the specialties sometimes required to manage patients with epidermal nevus syndrome. The epidermal nevi themselves are generally benign, but they can be removed surgically or with lasers for cosmetic improvement.

Course: The prognosis is based on the extent of extracutaneous findings. Unfortunately, neurologic complications can be a source of morbidity and mortality.

FINAL THOUGHT

The presence of epidermal nevi can be an isolated finding or merely a marker of an underlying syndrome, of which there are many epidermal nevi syndromes. Patients should receive a thorough examination and multidisciplinary care to ensure that any underlying systemic manifestations are managed appropriately and from an early age.

ADDITIONAL READINGS

Hagelstein-Rotman M, Meier ME, Majoor BCJ, et al. Increased prevalence of malignancies in fibrous dysplasia/McCune-Albright Syndrome (FD/MAS): data from a National Referral Center and the Dutch National Pathology Registry (PALGA). Calcif Tissue Int. 2020. https://doi.org/10.1007/s00223-020-00780-6.

Lalor L, Davies OMT, Basel D, et al. Café au lait spots: when and how to pursue their genetic origins. Clin Dermatol. 2020;38:421–431.

Laura FS. Epidermal nevus syndrome. Handb Clin Neurol. 2013;111:349–368.

Mazereeuw-Hautier J, Hernández-Martín A, O'Toole EA, et al. Management of congenital ichthyoses: European guidelines of care, part two. Br J Dermatol. 2019;180:484–495.

Paller AS. Profiling immune expression to consider repurposing therapeutics for the ichthyoses. J Invest Dermatol. 2019;139:535–540.

Patil YB, Garg R, Rajguru JP, et al. Vogt-Koyanagi-Harada (VKH) syndrome: a new perspective for healthcare professionals. Family Med Prim Care. 2020;28(9):31–35.

Silverberg NB. A pilot trial of dermoscopy as a rapid assessment tool in pediatric dermatoses. Cutis. 2011;87:148–154.

Specht S, Persaud Y. Asteatotic Eczema. 2020 Jul 10. In: StatPearls [Internet]. Treasure Island, FL: StatPearls Publishing; 2020 Jan. PMID: 31747214.

Teng JM, Cowen EW, Wataya-Kaneda M, et al. Dermatologic and dental aspects of the 2012 International Tuberous Sclerosis Complex Consensus Statements. JAMA Dermatol. 2014;150:1095–1101.

Tolliver S, Smith ZI, Silverberg NB. The genetics and diagnosis of pediatric neurocutaneous disorders: neurofibromatosis and tuberous sclerosis complex. Clin Dermatol. In press.

Veit JGS, De Glas V, Balau B, et al. Characterization of CYP26B1-Selective inhibitor, DX314, as a potential therapeutic for keratinization disorders. J Invest Dermatol. 2021;141:72–83.

16 Oral Diseases

Marcia Ramos-e-Silva, José Wilson Accioly Filho,
Sueli Carneiro, and Nurimar Conceição Fernandes

CONTENTS

Overview: Oral lesions are more difficult to diagnose than those on the skin because the color contrast is lower and the presentation of secondary factors, such as maceration, abrasion, and infection, are greater. The grouping and distribution of the lesions are not always distinct, and it is not uncommon for the diagnosis to be obtained by observing the presence of associated skin lesions or by changes in the original lesion.

MOUTH

Alterations of the Tongue

Glossodynia

Synonym: Stomatodynia

   Definition: The term *stomatodynia* indicates a burning or stinging sensation in the entire mouth without an apparent lesion or cause. Glossodynia is limited to the tongue.

   Differential diagnosis: Because these are diagnoses of exclusion, it is necessary to rule out, before making this diagnosis, possible causes of burning and stinging on the oral mucosa, which may include contact stomatitis, candidosis, anemia, dyspepsia, and drug reaction. The process seems to have an emotional overlay.

   Management: The patients, often women, may benefit from antidepressants and even psychotherapy.

DOI: 10.1201/9781003105268-16

Rhomboid Median Glossitis

Overview: This appears as an area without any papilla on the dorsal surface of the tongue, in its posterior and middle portion, and just in front of the sulcus terminalis.

Clinical presentation: It is usually rhomboid-, lozenge-, or diamond-shaped. The cause is still unknown, representing a developmental change or chronic focal candidosis. It occurs more frequently in diabetics, smokers, denture users, and HIV-positive patients. It is often asymptomatic, but there can be a burning sensation.

Benign Migratory Glossitis

Synonym: Geographic tongue, exfoliative glossitis areata

Overview: This alteration of the tongue, especially its dorsal aspect, is of unknown cause. There is a possible hereditary pattern and affects 1–2% of the population, regardless of age and predominantly occurring in women.

Clinical presentation: There are several erythematous plaques, depilated, curved, circinate, and usually painless, with a whitish and slightly elevated border (Figure 16.1). While the fungiform papilla remains intact and prominent, the filiform papilla peels off. The atrophic appearance is due to the loss of filiform papilla. The migratory aspect of the condition predominates, showing erythematous plaques that disappear from one place on the tongue, only to reappear in another. It may represent an atopic background, psoriasis, vitamin deficiencies, or hereditary factors. Occasionally, it is associated with glossodynia.

Management: Although there is no recommendation for treatment, sometimes applications of 7% salicylic acid in an alcoholic vehicle or 0.1% tretinoin solution, four times a day, lead to a rapid resolution.

Fissured Tongue

Synonym: Scrotal tongue, plicate tongue

Overview: It can be congenital and, sometimes, familial with a polygenic inheritance pattern It is seen in Down and Melkersson-Rosenthal syndromes, and in some patients, there is an association with geographic tongue.

Clinical presentation: The tongue shows longitudinal, transverse, or oblique fissures in part or on its entire dorsal surface. Food debris can be lodged in these fissures, causing or contributing to inflammation and a feeling of discomfort.

Management: Treatment is not necessary; however, instructions on local hygiene through the use of mouthwash and brushing of the tongue should be emphasized (Figure 16.2).

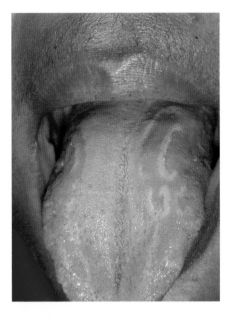

Figure 16.1 Benign migratory glossitis.

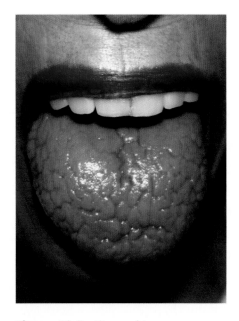

Figure 16.2 Fissured tongue.

Hairy Black Tongue

Overview: It is a reactive process due to several predisposing factors, including radiotherapy for cancer of the head or neck, prolonged antimicrobial therapy, poor oral hygiene, oral antibiotics, and abuse of tobacco. Unfortunately, very little is known about this condition.

Clinical presentation: It represents benign hyperplasia of the filiform papilla found in the anterior two-thirds of the tongue. The dorsal surface becomes velvety and black as a result of the growth and elongation of the filiform papilla and their colonization by chromogenic bacteria, which give the dark color (Figure 16.3). Hairy black tongue is, in general, asymptomatic, although in some patients it can cause halitosis, changes in taste, and vomiting.

Management: In most cases, no specific treatment is necessary, it is only advisable to improve oral hygiene by brushing the tongue, moving back and forth, at least twice a day, and using a mouthwash. Clinical manifestations usually disappear within a few weeks. If it does not disappear, it is best to seek and identify a specific cause, such as a medication, in which case it is necessary to change that agent or, at least, adjust the dose. In addition, an antifungal or antibiotic can be prescribed to try to eliminate the microorganisms more quickly and speed up the treatment. There is anecdotal use of antimicrobials, topical triamcinolone acetonide, salicylic acid, gentian violet, vitamin B complex, thymol, topical or oral retinoids, and topical keratinolytics, such as 20% podophyllin, 30% urea solution, and trichloroacetic acid, although local irritation and possible systemic absorption are important potential side effects to be considered. Dental evaluation by a dentist may be necessary in challenging cases, although this is rarely needed. Resistant cases may improve with light electrodessication or us of the carbon dioxide laser.

Oral Hairy Leukoplakia

Overview: First described by David Grinspan (1911–2003) in 1984, it appears almost exclusively in HIV-infected individuals and seems to be related to infection by the Epstein-Barr virus. Occasionally, it can be identified in other immunosuppressed patients and rarely in healthy people. It has no malignant potential.

Clinical presentation: It appears as a whitish lesion with wrinkled plaques, being flat and smooth and later becoming elevated, with a wrinkled, irregular, or linear surface. It particularly affects the lateral and ventral sides of the tongue, and its size varies from a few millimeters to several centimeters.

Differential diagnosis: These include candidosis, oral leukoplakia, white sponge nevus, oral frictional keratosis, smoker's keratosis, proliferative verrucous leukoplakia, lichen planus, lichenoid reactions, and condyloma acuminatum, among others.

Management: As it is generally asymptomatic, it requires treatment only, when there is discomfort. There may be a candidal or bacterial infection, so antifungal and/or antimicrobials may be helpful. It has no premalignant potential and can improve spontaneously or with zidovudine; there are still patients who benefit from acyclovir. A few applications 25% podophyllin can be helpful. Topical tretinoin can also be applied two or three times a day until the lesions disappear. Cryotherapy is an alternative, but it is not widely used. Unfortunately, recurrence is a problem.

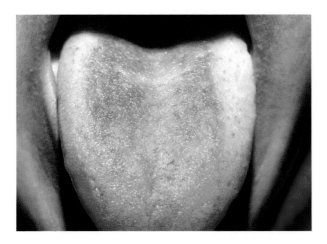

Figure 16.3 Hairy black tongue.

Eosinophilic Ulcer of the Tongue

Overview: Its greatest importance lies in the possible presence or subsequent development of an underlying disorder, such as sarcoidosis, Melkersson-Rosenthal syndrome, or Crohn's disease.

Clinical presentation: It presents as an ulcerated lesion of the tongue (Figure 16.4) often covered by a pseudomembrane. It is probably triggered by trauma.

Differential diagnosis: It resembles a syphilitic chancre and sometimes squamous cell carcinoma.

Laboratory studies: Histopathologic examination shows a dense infiltrate of eosinophils in the chorion, accompanied by some histiocytes and neutrophils.

Management: It tends to regress spontaneously so that no intervention is needed.

ALTERATIONS OF THE LIPS

Actinic Cheilitis

Overview: This is an inflammatory reaction of the lips, resulting from excessive exposure to the sun for many years. It usually affects the lower lip of elderly patients with a history of prolonged exposure to the sun.

Clinical presentation: It begins with edema and mild erythema, dryness, and fine desquamation. Subsequently, there is much more intense dryness and desquamation with erosions. There is a high risk of leukoplakia and cancer in this type of cheilitis. (Figure 16.5).

Laboratory studies: Histopathologic examination will show.

Management: It is most important to avoid excessive sun exposure and to use lip sunscreens. It is impossible to know when actinic cheilitis will develop into neoplasia, so all cases must be treated, if they did not disappear with less sun exposure and use of sunscreens. Topical medications, such as 5-fluorouracil, usually prescribed for 2–3 weeks, may be applied without affecting normal skin. Side effects, such as pain, burning, and swelling, may occur. Complete removal of the lesions can be achieved by cryotherapy, electrosurgery, or surgery as vermilionectomy.

Angular Cheilitis

Synonym: Perleche

Overview: It usually occurs in elderly individuals who wear dentures, but it can develop from simple overlapping of the upper lip and chin due to atrophy of the dental alveoli or dental arch in older patients, creating an environment favorable to microbial opportunism (*Candida albicans*, staphylococci, streptococci). It can present in children who have the habit of sucking their fingers or lollipops.

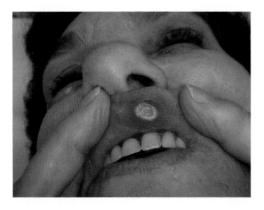

Figure 16.4   Eosinophilic ulcer of the tongue.

Source: From Gurfinkel PCM, Gurfinkel ACM, Tullia Cuzzi, Ramos-e-Silva M. Eosinophylic ulcer of the oral mucosa: case report. SkinMed 2012;10(4):228–231, used with permission.

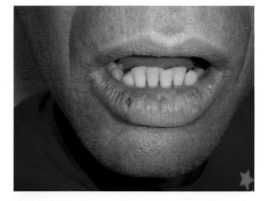

Figure 16.5   Actinic cheilitis.

Clinical presentation: This is a nonspecific maceration with cracking and erythema, superficial ulceration, and crusting at the angles of the mouth, which may extend to the skin. Additional associated factors include riboflavin deficiency, intraoral candidosis, occurring in patients with diabetes, AIDS, or chronic mucocutaneous candidosis.

Management: Adjustment of predisposing factors, such as the use of suitable dental prostheses and surgical correction of the lip angles, changing the configuration of the corner of the mouth that promotes the accumulation of saliva and food, use of antibiotics or nystatin, preferably associated with topical corticosteroids, are usually effective.

Glandular Cheilitis

Overview: It is a rare condition characterized by hypertrophic, inflammatory swelling of the lower salivary glands of the lower lip, producing labial ectropion and making glandular ductal orifices visible. Of these, it is possible to express a thick mucous secretion by expression.

Clinical presentation: Two basic types of glandular cheilitis are described: simple (Puente and Acevedo) and deep or apostematous suppurative (Volkmann; Figures 16.6 and 16.7). The latter is the result of secondary bacterial infection in the former, with the elimination of purulent secretion through the ductal orifices. It is believed to be a consequence of chronic irritation, atopy, excessive sun exposure, or factitious dermatitis. Rarely, it may develop into squamous cell carcinoma.

Management: Intralesional corticosteroids may reduce the problem. Occasionally, vermilionectomy may be necessary.

Granulomatous Cheilitis

Overview: It can occur as an isolated phenomenon or as a simultaneous manifestation of other illnesses.

Clinical presentation: It is characterized by diffuse and progressive swelling of the lips, with the surrounding skin being normal or erythematous. The lower lip is most frequently affected.

Its greatest importance lies in the possible presence or subsequent development of an underlying disorder such as sarcoidosis, Melkersson-Rosenthal syndrome, or Crohn's disease.

Laboratory studies: Histopathologic changes, as the term implies, consist of chronic inflammation with the formation of focal granulomas with epithelioid and giant cells. No caseosis is observed, and there is no evidence of an infectious etiology or foreign body reaction.

Melkersson-Rosenthal Syndrome

Overview: It represents a triad, consisting of recurrent facial paralysis or paresis, non-depressible edema of the lips, and scrotal tongue (macroglossia; Figure 16.8).

Clinical presentation: The outbreaks usually start during adolescence, with paralysis of one or both facial nerves and with edema of the upper lip, chin, and occasionally of the lower lip and perioral tissues. The etiology is unknown, but there may be a genetic predisposition.

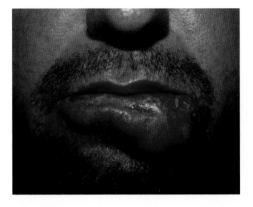

Figure 16.6 Apostematous suppurative of Volkmann (outside view).

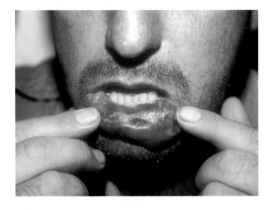

Figure 16.7 Apostematous suppurative of Volkmann (inner view).

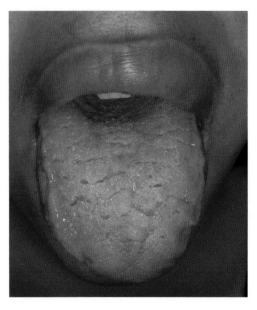

Figure 16.8 Melkersson-Rosenthal syndrome (lip and tongue).

Laboratory studies: Histopathologic examination usually shows a non-necrotizing tuberculoid or sarcoid granulomatous inflammation with B lymphocytes predominating in the center of the granuloma and T cells in the surrounding area. The inflammatory cells can sometimes be dispersed into the connective tissue without granulomatous formation.

Management: There is no satisfactory treatment. Any intervention should be to the prevention of lip deformities and facial paralysis. Local measures, such as cold compresses, may reduce the edema, and Vaseline® or other lip moisturizers to prevent lip fissures. Sometimes, intralesional injections of corticosteroids, alone or in combination with cheiloplasty, a surgical procedure, may show more favorable results, especially in severe cases. Clofazimine has been used successfully in some cases, in a regimen of 100 mg per day with reduction after 10 days to 200–400 mg weekly for 3–6 months. Skin color change, nausea, and vomiting are frequent adverse reactions, and the patient should be informed.

ORAL CHANGES IN ETIOLOGY POSSIBLY AUTOIMMUNE

Recurrent Aphthous Stomatitis

Synonym: Aphthae

Overview: This represents one or multiple painful ulcers of the mucosa, especially oral, of a recurrent, nontraumatic, nonvesicobullous nature that is sometimes familial. Its etiology is very controversial and is undoubtedly multiple. Infectious, psychologic, gastrointestinal (or psychosomatic?), hematologic, endocrine (or psychosomatic?), nutritional, allergic, hereditary, and/or autoimmune etiologies have all been proposed. Currently, recurrent aphthous stomatitis is considered an immunopathologic process that involves cell-mediated cytolytic activity in response to human leucocyte antigen (HLA) or external antigens, ultimately destroying the basal cell layer.

Clinical presentation: The lesion begins with vague discomfort for up to 48 hours, and then a small, circumscribed reddish lesion appears. The pain is intense and the ulcer, usually round, well defined, and ranging from 2–5 mm in diameter. It is, in general, deep with a yellowish base. Its edges are hardened, and the area around the ulceration is erythematous (Figure 16.9). It may

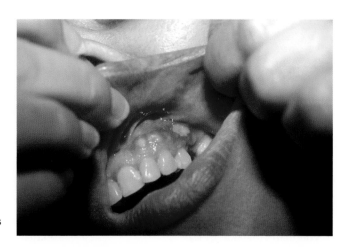

Figure 16.9 Recurrent aphthous stomatitis.

last from 5–7 days, with complete disappearance in up to 14 days. In severe cases, they may have a larger diameter and last longer.

Two variants are considered according to severity, the *minor,* a less severe form and with fewer attacks of this disease; and *major,* with several large and painful ulcers at the same time and very frequent eruptions, including the picture called "recurrent necrotic mucous periadenitis," which evolves with the appearance of one or more ulcers of greater size and depth, usually over a mucoid gland.

Management: This is very controversial, and the result is quite individual. In the outbreak, antiseptics, protective agents (milk of magnesia and cyanoacrylates), antibiotics in mouthwash (tetracycline and doxycycline), topical anesthetics, or topical and intralesional corticosteroids can be used. In more severe cases, systemic corticosteroid therapy (0.5–1 mg per kilo), colchicine (0.5–2 mg/day), retinoids (20–40 mg/day), dapsone (100 mg/day) or even intramuscular gamma globulin are recommended; while to prevent relapses, avoiding certain foods, such as citric fruits, chocolate, and eggs, injecting subcutaneously gamma globulin in small doses, or taking colchicine, chloroquine, and oral metronidazole have been suggested. Thalidomide and pentoxifylline, acting as immunomodulators, have already showed effectiveness in severe cases and relapses.

Behçet's Disease

This is a chronic inflammatory disease of uncertain cause and prognosis that has the name of the Turkish dermatologist (Hulusi Behçet [1889–1948]), who described it in 1937. With a predominance among men, in the age group between 20–30 years, Behçet's disease has an immunologic nature, probably due to association with complement activation and formation of immune complexes (see Chapter 11). Its immunogenetic basis has already been demonstrated, with an increase in HLA-B5, B27, and B12.

It is defined clinically utilizing major criteria as recurrent oral ulcers or aphthae being the most frequent (90–100% of cases), uveitis or iridocyclitis (30–90%), genital ulcers (60–80%), and skin lesions (50–80%; Figures 16.10, 16.11, and 16.12) The minor criteria are fever, asthenia, painful arthritis, enterocolitis, epididymitis, recurrent thrombophlebitis, arteritis, central nervous system manifestations, and family history.

Therapy should only be symptomatic and, in severe cases, systemic corticosteroids, immunosuppressors, colchicine, or dapsone may be tried.

Oral Lichen Planus

Overview: It frequently appears in association with the characteristic erythematous-violaceous skin lesions, and there may be remissions and recurrences. When it is exclusively oral, the incidence of malignancy varies from 0.4–2.5%, and erosive and hypertrophic forms appear to be in higher danger for malignant transformation.

Clinical presentation: Among the oral forms are reticular (Figure 16.13), which is the most frequent, atrophic, erosive or ulcerated, linear or annular, hypertrophic or leukoplastic (Figure 16.14), bullous, and pigmented. There may also be desquamative gingivitis (Figure 16.15) that causes

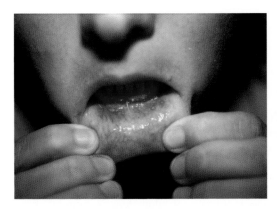

Figure 16.10 Behçet's disease.

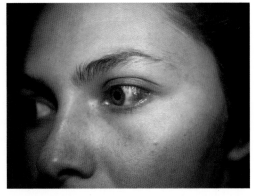

Figure 16.11 Behçet's disease (same patient as Figure 16.10 and 16.12).

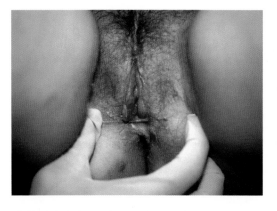

Figure 16.12 Behçet's disease (same patient as Figure 16.10 and 16.11).

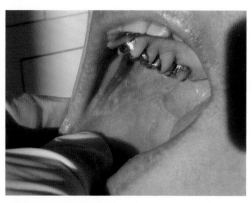

Figure 16.13 Reticular form of oral lichen planus.

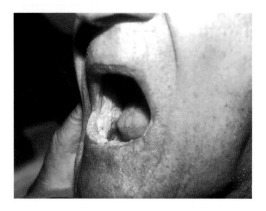

Figure 16.14 Hypertrophic form of oral lichen planus.

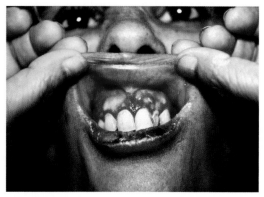

Figure 16.15 Desquamative gingivitis in oral lichen planus.

erosion, atrophy, and scaling of the gums. Oral lesions predominate on the cheek mucosa, tongue, and gums, and it appears that the erosive and atrophic forms have a higher risk of malignancy.

Differential diagnosis: This depends on the form are leukoplakia and erythroplakia, aphthae, lupus erythematosus, squamous cell carcinoma, and others. The dryness, scaling, and ulcerations of desquamative gingivitis, seen in lichen planus, can also be a manifestation of pemphigoid or pemphigus vulgaris.

Management: Pure and asymptomatic oral lichen planus, in general, does not need treatment. For the more severe and/or symptomatic cases, triamcinolone in Orabase®, applied four or more times a day may be helpful. Rinsing the mouth with doxycycline or tetracycline dissolved in water may reduce the symptoms. Oral steroids are sometimes necessary. Clofazimine and colchicine have also been used. Cryosurgery is an option for treating the hypertrophic form.

ORAL INFECTIONS

Candidosis

Synonym: Thrush, monilial infection of the mouth

Overview: Intra-oral infection by yeasts of the genus *Candida*, almost always of the albicans species, can have varied manifestations

Clinical presentation: These include pseudomembranous candidosis, with low elevated whitish and easily detachable plaques; acute atrophic, characterized by erythematous areas and a few white lesions, especially on the back of the tongue; chronic granulomatous or candidal leukoplakia, possibly precancerous, present as whitish plaques but not detachable; and chronic mucocutaneous, which occurs in immunocompromised children, and affects the skin, mucous membranes, and nails.

There may be mild to severe burning, often exaggerated in HIV-positive patients receiving immunosuppressive therapies, patients wearing dental prostheses, and diabetics.

Laboratory studies: Mycologic examination and sometimes a biopsy are needed for confirmation.

Management: Treatment is similar to that used for candidosis of the skin with nystatin, clotrimazole, and miconazole in mouthwash or oral gel, or oral ketoconazole (200–400 mg/day), fluconazole (200 mg on the first day, then 100 mg per day), and itraconazole (100–200 mg per day for 1 to 2 weeks). In the most persistent leukoplastic lesions, surgical excision of the lesions may be necessary.

PREMALIGNANT AND MALIGNANT PROCESSES OF THE ORAL MUCOSA

Overview: Oral cancer is responsible for 3–4% of all malignancies and has a mortality rate of 50% in 5 years, and in the United States, about 30 thousand new cases are diagnosed per year, with recent annual increases. See Table 16.1.

The assessment of any alteration of the oral mucosa is of the utmost importance, because up to 20% of the leukoplakia, 40% of the floor lesions of the mouth, and 80% of the persistent erythematous lesions erythroplasia are already premalignant or malignant. The detection of precancer and oral cancer still in its early stages allows the total eradication of the tumor.

As irritating and predisposing factors in the genesis of precancerous alterations and oral cancer, smoking, repeated trauma due to ill-fitting dental prostheses, chronic infection by *Candida albicans*, and even viruses, alcohol, and atrophic lesions of the oral mucosa, such as may occur with atrophic glossitis associated with tertiary syphilis and pernicious anemia, which make the mucosa more vulnerable to carcinogens.

PRECANCEROUS CONDITIONS

Leukoplakia

Overview: This is the most common oral precancer, affecting 0.1–5% of the population.

Clinical presentation: It appears as a whitish or grayish plaque. It may be asymptomatic, persistent, and adherent to the mucosa. It is often a diagnosis of exclusion, mainly seen in men between 40–60 years old. Any location of the oral mucosa can be affected; however, it is more frequent in the buccal mucosa and the internal area of the labial commissures. The rate of malignant transformation has been estimated at 3–6%, but it is probably higher (Figure 16.16).

Laboratory studies: The histopathology is often inconsistent; there may be hypertrophic- or hyperkeratosis acanthosis, sometimes with numerous mitoses.

Differential diagnosis: Hypertrophic lichen planus and granulomatous candidosis are among the most important to be excluded.

Management: For leukoplakia, it is essential to remove the irritating factor, if any, such as restriction of smoking, alcohol, and other agents. Curettage and electrocoagulation, cryotherapy, or total surgical excision of the lesion can be performed.

Erythroplasia

Overview: Oral erythroplasia is rare and can affect both sexes, usually between 50–70 years of age. It appears as a nonspecific erythematous plaque without any other cause and asymptomatic, especially on the floor of the mouth, retro-molar, or mandibular alveolar region.

Table 16.1 Premalignant Conditions, Oral Cancer, and Their Predisposing Factors

Premalignant Conditions and Oral Cancer		Predisposing Factors
Premailgnant lesions	Leukoplakia	Smoking, repeated trauma by dentures, chronic *Candida* infection, viruses, alcohol, and atrophic lesions, such as atrophic glossitis tertiary syphilis, pernicious anemia, which make the oral mucosa vulnerable to carcinogens
	Erythroplakia	
Malignant lesions	Squamous cell carcinoma	
	Melanoma	Genetics

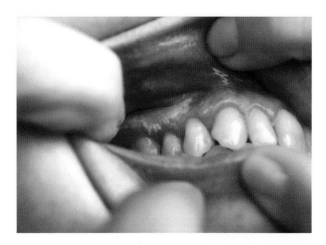

Figure 16.16 Leukoplakia.

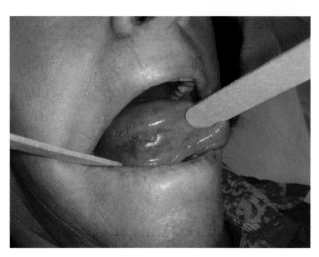

Figure 16.17 Erythroplakia.

Clinical presentation: It can manifest as a flat or slightly elevated erythematous plaque, with a velvety and smooth surface and well-marked edges, or as a macula or erythematous plaque, whitish on the periphery and with an irregular surface. Severe epithelial dysplasia, carcinoma, being *in situ* or invasive, is already present in 91% of oral erythroplasia, demonstrating the severity and importance of this type of lesion (Figure 16.17).

Laboratory studies: Erythroplakia shows features of reactive/regenerative epithelium and some degree of epithelial dysplasia. It may be invasive squamous cell carcinoma, carcinoma *in situ* or moderate to severe epithelial dysplasia, dysplasia.

Differential diagnosis: Any erythematous lesions of the oral mucosa should be differentiated form erythroplakia. These include candidosis, burns, and traumatic lesions.

Management: Due to its high incidence of malignancy, erythroplakia should be treated as such, and it should always completely excised by surgery.

MALIGNANT TUMORS

Squamous Cell Carcinoma

Synonym: Verrucous carcinoma

Overview: This is responsible for 90% of malignant neoplasms of the mouth and, inside the mouth, 50% occur on the tongue; among the extraoral ones, the most frequent is located on the lower lip, which shows the importance of this diagnosis concerning the mouth (Figures 16.18–16.20).

In addition to preventing caries and removing trauma caused by fractured teeth or unfitted dentures, one of the most important reasons for periodic examination of the mouth in the early

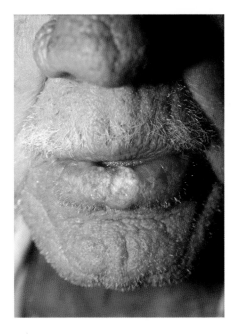

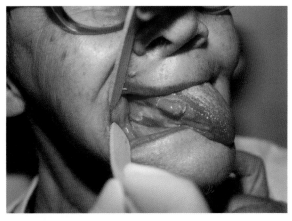

Figure 16.19 Squamous cell carcinoma.

Figure 16.18 Squamous cell carcinoma.

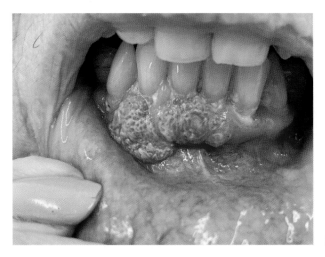

Figure 16.20 Verrucous carcinoma.

detection of precancer, as well as cancer. Clinical diagnosis by the specialist, aided by the 1% toluidine blue technique, which stains the dysplastic and malignant cells, and by biopsy, sometimes requiring immunohistochemical techniques, must be mandatory in all suspected cases.

Clinical presentation: The onset of the lesion is quite varied, ranging from an erythematous or whitish plaque lesion to a tumor that rapidly enlarges. The most frequent locations are the lateral border of the tongue, lower lip, and floor of the mouth and often have varied appearances. Such lesions can be white to red, ulcerated or not, and smooth, papular or vegetating, appearing in the later decades.

Verrucous carcinoma, considered a less severe variant of squamous cell carcinoma, translates clinically to a white exophytic mass, with a verrucous surface, with slow growth and rare metastases. Eighty to 90% of verrucous carcinomas affect the buccal, alveolar, or gingival mucosa.

Laboratory studies: A biopsy of these suspected lesions should always be performed in suspicious lesions, already malignant lesions, or even premalignant for exclusion or confirmation, so

197

early therapy can be prescribed, which substantially improves the prognosis. Depending on the stages, an oncologist must be involved in the treatment of these patients.

Differential diagnosis: Leukoplakia, erythroplakia, lichen planus, oral viral papilomas, and condyloma lata may show similar presentations.

Management: The therapy of squamous cell carcinomas depends on each case, that is, its location, size, whether it is well differentiated or not in histology and whether there are regional metastases, which are very frequent. Only 50% of the lesions are painful, which delays the patient's early search for medical care. Sometimes, the lesions have enlarged so much that they are untreatable. Total surgical removal of the tumor is the ideal therapy, but chemotherapy, immunotherapy, and/or radiotherapy may be employed.

Melanoma

Overview: This is rare on the oral mucosa and accounts for about 1.5% of malignant cases.

Clinical presentation: It is initially a brownish-black, macular lesion evolving into an ulcerative nodule that bleeds easily (Figures 16.21 and 16.22) and evolves to heterogeneous blue, gray, red, or purplish shades of colors and depigmented areas. It is frequently located on the palate and gums. The prognosis is poor because the diagnosis is often made late. This is not a common diagnosis, and even more rarely, there may be amelanotic melanoma.

Laboratory studies: Histopathology is characteristic and remains the gold standard for the diagnosis. As in the skin, oral lesions show atypical melanocytes with mitotic figures, initially in a radial (horizontal) growth on the epidermis and later forming dermal nests of variable sizes and shapes in a vertical growth.

Differential diagnosis: Melanocytic nevus and all types of oral melanosis must be differentiated from melanoma.

Management: Therapy will depend on the phase when it is diagnosed. When there is early detection, only excision with posterior extension of the surgical margins is usually enough. For more long-lasting lesions, deeper tumors, when there is no possibility of surgical removal, and for metastatic melanoma, chemotherapy may be needed with interleukins 2 (IL-2). The new biologics, including ipilimumab, pembrolizumab, or nivolumab, are added to the therapeutic regimen, providing a better prognosis of lesions that did not show any improvement with other therapies.

FINAL THOUGHT

Oral mucosal and semi-mucosal diseases are frequently observed disorders. While they may be isolated findings, sometimes, they reflect a systemic disease. It is very important to maintain good oral health. Periodic examination of the mouth should be mandatory at least at 6-month intervals.

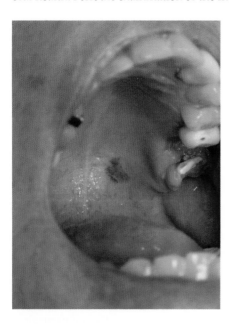

Figure 16.21 Melanoma.

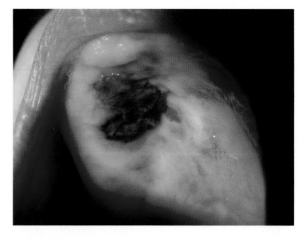

Figure 16.22 Melanoma.

Source: Courtesy of Drs. Roberto Resende and Flávio Monteiro, Porto Alegre, Brazil.

ADDITIONAL READINGS

Allen CM, Camisa C, McNamara KK. Oral diseases. In: Bolognia JL, Schaffer JV, Cerroni L, editors. Dermatology. 4th ed. Philadelphia: Elsevier; 2018. p. 1220–1242.

Alrashdan MS, Cirillo N, McCullough M. Oral lichen planus: a literature review and update. Arch Dermatol Res. 2016;308:539–551.

de Azevedo AB, Dos Santos TCRB, Lopes MA, et al. Oral leukoplakia, leukoerythroplakia, erythroplakia and actinic cheilitis: analysis of 953 patients focusing on oral epithelial dysplasia. Oral Pathol Med. 2021 Online ahead of print.

Fitzpatrick SG, Cohen DM, Clark AN. Ulcerated lesions of the oral mucosa: clinical and histologic review. Head Neck Pathol. 2019;13:91–102.

Harte MC, Saunsbury TA, Hodgson TA. Thalidomide use in the management of oromucosal disease: a 10-year review of safety and efficacy in 12 patients. Oral Surg Oral Med Oral Pathol Oral Radiol. 2020;130:398–401.

Holmstrup P. Oral erythroplakia—what is it? Oral Dis. 2018;24:138–143.

Lambertini M, Patrizi A, Fanti PA, et al. Oral melanoma and other pigmentations: when to biopsy? J Eur Acad Dermatol Venereol. 2018;32:209–214.

Pires FR, Barreto ME, Nunes JG, et al. Oral potentially malignant disorders: clinical-pathological study of 684 cases diagnosed in a Brazilian population. Med Oral Patol Oral Cir Bucal. 2020;1(25):e84–e88.

Plewa MC, Chatterjee K. Aphthous stomatitis. 2021 Feb 3. In: StatPearls [Internet]. Treasure Island, FL: StatPearls Publishing; 2021 Jan. Last viewed May 09, 2021.

Villa A, Sonis S. Oral leukoplakia remains a challenging condition. Oral Dis. 2018;24:179–183.

17 Wound Healing, Ulcers, and Scars

Saloni Shah, Christian Albornoz, and Sherry Yang

CONTENTS

PRINCIPLES OF WOUND HEALING

Definition: Wound healing is a fundamental process that is triggered by acute tissue injury to the epidermal or dermal layers.

  Overview: The wound healing process can be divided into three main phases:

1. A coagulation phase in which platelets are initially recruited to form a hemostatic plug. This phase also includes an inflammatory process involving the recruitment of immune cells, such as neutrophils, monocytes, and/or macrophages, to the site of injury.

2. A migratory or re-epithelialization stage occurs early in the wound healing process.

3. A dermal repair and remodeling phase occurs within months of the initial wound event.

Any aberrations during these stages of wound healing can lead to chronic wound complications, as well as nonhealing ulcers.

FACTORS CONTRIBUTING TO POOR WOUND HEALING

Various conditions are necessary for adequate and proper wound healing. The absence or disruption of the following factors may contribute to poor wound healing.

1. **Chronic corticosteroid use:** Beginning with the coagulative and inflammatory phase, chronic corticosteroid use can lead to downregulation of the immune system and decreased recruitment of inflammatory cells, including lymphocytes, macrophages, and neutrophils. This may delay the inflammatory response and future stages of wound healing.

2. **Nutritional deficiencies:** Deficiencies in vitamin C can delay the immune response and prevent collagen synthesis, which is necessary for re-epithelialization. Zinc and protein are needed during the re-epithelization and dermal repair processes; deficiencies may affect cellular proliferation and impair re-epithelialization.

3. **Poor tissue oxygenation:** Hypoxia due to decreased blood flow can significantly delay all stages of the wound healing process and increase the likelihood of complications.

DOI: 10.1201/9781003105268-17

4. **Superinfection:** Biofilms, a common cause of microbial superinfections, can prevent re-epithelialization and increase the likelihood of complications in chronic wounds. If superinfection is identified, debridement and antimicrobial therapy can help facilitate wound healing.

VENOUS INSUFFICIENCY

Definition: Venous insufficiency is defined as an impediment to flow within the venous circulation, resulting in dilation of venules and increased pressure. This ultimately results in capillary leakage and extravasation into surrounding soft tissue. This most commonly affects lower leg veins.

Pathophysiology: The development of venous insufficiency begins with obstruction, valve incompetence, and/or elevated hydrostatic pressures within the calves. This results in venous hypertension and dilation of postcapillary venules, which compromises endothelial function. Venous insufficiency creates an environment for transudation, fibrin deposition in perivascular vessels, and extravasation of red blood cells causing hemosiderin deposition. Risk factors include the history of venous thrombosis, phlebitis, leg injury, congestive heart failure, pregnancy, prolonged standing, and varicose veins.

Epidemiology: In the United States and Europe, the prevalence of venous ulceration is 1–3% in those older than 65 years old. Epidemiologic studies have demonstrated that women are preferentially affected.

Clinical presentation: Venous insufficiency typically occurs in the lower extremities and around bony prominences.

Acute venous insufficiency may present as venous stasis dermatitis, which manifests as pruritic erythematous to hyperpigmented, thin, scaly plaques or patches, with or without associated leg pain or cramps (Figure 17.1). There is typically a background of pitting edema and brown hemosiderin deposition.

Chronic venous disease can lead to three main dermatologic manifestations:

1. Lipodermatosclerosis: A panniculitis characterized by inflammation of the subcutaneous fat, which causes painful hardening of the skin and an "inverted champagne bottle" appearance of the lower legs.

2. Elephantiasis nostra verrucosa: Chronic venous insufficiency leading to dilation of superficial lower leg veins. With time, this leads to superimposed hyperkeratotic papulonodules and cutaneous hypertrophy (Figure 17.2). If left untreated, enlargement of the extremity may occur, which may lead to functional impairment.

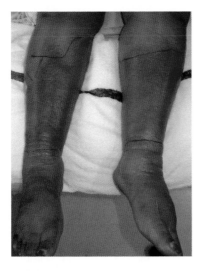

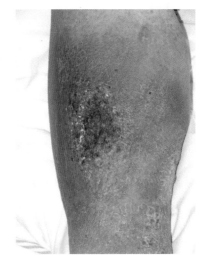

Figure 17.1 Acute venous stasis dermatitis with brightly erythematous, well-defined plaques symmetrically distributed on edematous lower extremities.

Figure 17.2 Elephantiasis nostra verrucosa with marked lymphedema, surrounding erythema, and thick, adherent, hyperkeratotic plaques on the shin.

3. Venous stasis ulcers: Single or multiple shallow ulcers characterized by well-defined, irregularly shaped borders. Lesions most commonly occur around the medial calf or malleolus. Rarely, squamous cell carcinoma (SCC) can develop in long-standing ulcers.

Laboratory studies: No laboratory studies are required to diagnose venous insufficiency or ulcerations. Duplex ultrasonography can assess the degree of venous insufficiency, show perforating veins, and rule out potential complications, such as deep vein thrombosis. Phlebography may also be performed in conjunction with x-ray, CT, or MRI. If the diagnosis remains uncertain, a skin biopsy can be performed for histologic examination.

Differential diagnosis: Neuropathic and arterial ulcers and lymphedema should be considered in the differential. Clinical history, imaging, and histologic techniques may help differentiate these diagnoses.

Management: Improving venous drainage through compression therapy, Unna boots, and leg elevation is the mainstay of therapy. Unna boots may be left on for up to 2 weeks until the ulcer heals. Leg elevation can minimize edema and is recommended for approximately 1.5–2 hours per day in 30-minute intervals.

Proper wound care is essential for timely healing. A dressing should be applied underneath the compression bandage or stocking, which should have antimicrobial properties and be partially absorptive to provide high humidity at the wound interface to facilitate re-epithelialization. Studies have found similar efficacy among alginate, hydrocolloid, and plain dressings.

Topical steroids may be used in patients with venous stasis dermatitis to treat inflammation and associated irritation. Keratolytics can help exfoliate chronic cutaneous manifestations of venous insufficiency, including elephantiasis nostra verrucosa and lipodermatosclerosis.

Minimally invasive vascular surgeries, including laser or radiofrequency ablation and foam sclerotherapy, may be considered in patients who are less responsive to compression therapy. This can prevent recurrence but will not expedite the healing of existing ulcers.

Prognosis: The outcome of venous ulcers largely depends on the ability to correct underlying contributing factors. Unfortunately, venous ulcers have a high recurrence rate with 50–70% of patients presenting with a second ulcer.

Final comment: Venous insufficiency has multiple causes that are related to decreased blood flow through the venous circulation. Venous ulcers can present with edema and brown discoloration. Additional manifestations include venous stasis dermatitis, lipodermatosclerosis, and elephantiasis nostra verrucosa. The aim of management is to facilitate wound healing through adequate dressing and improvement in the venous circulation.

ARTERIAL AND ISCHEMIC ULCERATIONS

Definition: Arterial insufficiency, most commonly caused by atherosclerosis, can lead to poor perfusion and decreased oxygen delivery to the lower extremities. Arterial insufficiency can clinically present as an arterial ulcer.

Pathophysiology: Arterial ulceration begins with an inciting trauma or breaks in the skin that leads to a small ulceration exposed to oxygen and bacteria. In patients without comorbid conditions, ulcers typically heal in 1–2 weeks; however, in patients who have peripheral arterial disease, narrowing of the arterial lumen leads to impaired blood flow to the lower extremities, which results in chronic ischemia and poor healing. In time, these ulcers can enlarge and demonstrate hemorrhage, calcification, and necrosis.

Epidemiology: Arterial ulcers are generally less common than their venous counterparts. The likelihood of an arterial ulcer developing is largely based on patient risk factors.

Risk factors: The major risk factor for arterial ulcers is atherosclerosis. Several modifiable risk factors can contribute, including hyperlipidemia, hypertension, diabetes mellitus, tobacco use, and obesity. Genetic factors may cause a hypercoagulable state. Hypercoagulable conditions include the presence of Factor V Leiden and prothrombin gene mutations and deficiencies in protein S or C. Family history of peripheral arterial disease or arterial ulcers. in the absence of an identified genetic etiology, may predispose patients to develop arterial ulcers.

Clinical presentation: Signs of chronic arterial insufficiency include thin, shiny atrophic skin with loss of hair over the lower extremities and toes. The skin may be cool to touch and appear pale with leg elevation and cyanotic with lowering of the leg. Pulses and capillary refill will be greatly diminished. There may be intermittent claudication that worsens with elevation and ultimately progresses to chronic pain.

Laboratory studies: To assess for comorbidities that may increase a patient's likelihood of developing an arterial ulcer, laboratory studies should include tests for hyperlipidemia (e.g., total cholesterol,

HDL, LDL, triglycerides), diabetes mellitus (e.g., glucose, hemoglobin A1c), and hypercoagulable state. Doppler ultrasonography can be performed to obtain an ankle-brachial pressure index (ABPI). To visualize arterial blood flow and any indications of arterial stenosis or plaques, three imaging techniques can be utilized: ultrasound and doppler (noninvasive), CT angiography, and invasive arteriography.

Differential diagnosis: Possible diagnoses, when assessing for an arterial ulcer, may include small- to medium-vessel vasculitis; vasculopathy, including hyperviscosity syndrome, disseminated intravascular coagulation (DIC), and cryoglobulinemia; emboli (e.g., postcatheterization, septic, cardiac); thromboangiitis obliterans; drug-induced necrosis due to coumadin, heparin, cocaine, or vasopressors; and vasospastic processes, including Raynaud's disease. Laboratory studies, imaging, and histology may be used to differentiate among these diagnoses.

Management

Upon diagnosis of an arterial ulcer, wound care should immediately be initiated. The TIME principle can be followed (Table 17.1).

Once the wound healing process has been initiated, the source of arterial insufficiency must be identified. Most commonly, cases arise due to atherosclerosis and may be initially managed with antiplatelet regimens and lifestyle modifications; however, revascularization through surgical or endovascular intervention may be necessary.

Prognosis: Arterial insufficiency is slowly progressive and may take months to years to manifest as an ulcer or other cutaneous finding. If arterial insufficiency is not identified and addressed promptly, patients may present with dry gangrene. Infection of the affected foot can occur, which may require amputation if not a candidate for surgical revascularization.

Final comment: Arterial insufficiency leads to decreased arterial blood flow. If not diagnosed, the dermatologic manifestation may occur. Management of these ulcers includes proper wound care as well as addressing the underlying contributing mechanisms.

DECUBITUS ULCERS

Synonyms: Pressure ulcer, pressure sores, bedsores

Definition: Decubitus ulcers (DUs) form due to prolonged pressure placed on bony areas of the body, which result in local tissue ischemia.

Overview: DUs commonly occur in patients who have impaired mental status, because they may not be able to sense prolonged pressure on bony surfaces of their skin. The inciting factor is often constant external pressure that exceeds the pressures within the arterial and venous systems, which leads to impaired blood flow and reduced oxygenation. Poor tissue perfusion results in ischemia and necrosis of the overlying skin. Additional factors that may lead to ischemia include friction due to movement of underlying soft tissue that may decrease blood flow to the skin and excess moisture that can cause progressive thinning and breakdown of skin.

Clinical presentation: DUs may be classified into four distinct stages (Table 17.2).

Table 17.1 The TIME Principle

- Tissue debridement
- Infection control
- Moisture balance
- Epidermal advancement of the edges of the wound

Table 17.2 Classification of Decubitus Ulcers

Stage I:	The epidermis remains intact, appearing erythematous and warm without blanching. Patients may report pain.
Stage II:	The epidermis begins to break down and form an overlying ulcer with subsequent involvement of the dermal layer. Patients may continue to report pain and tenderness. Exudate begins to appear to cover the open wound.
Stage III:	The ulcer progresses through the dermis and begins to involve subcutaneous tissue (Figure 17.3). Patients may not report any pain during this stage due to significant tissue damage. Adipose tissue may be visible, but muscle, tendon, or bone are not. Exudate formation will begin to increase.
Stage IV:	The ulcer extends deeper to involve muscle, tendon, and bone. Patients are not likely to report pain during this stage. Exudate is often greatest.

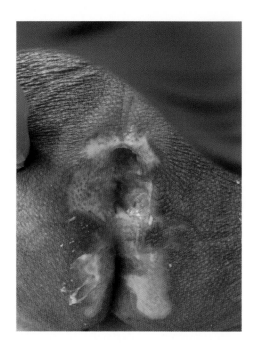

Figure 17.3 Decubitus ulcer, stage III, with sharply demarcated borders and a fibrinous base extending from the intergluteal cleft to the medial buttocks.

The most common bony locations for DU formation include the occiput, scapula, elbow, sacrum and ischial tuberosity, heel, lateral malleolus, greater trochanter, shoulder, and ear. If the ulcer is not addressed promptly, significant complications, including osteomyelitis and sepsis, may occur.

Laboratory studies: Complete blood count (CBC) may show an elevation in white blood cells (WBCs) due to inflammation and possible infection. Patients may have a low hemoglobin and mean corpuscular volume in the setting of anemia of chronic disease. Nutritional studies, including albumin, prealbumin, transferrin, and serum protein levels, should be obtained to assess the likelihood of complications during the wound healing process. Blood cultures can help to rule out infection. An erythrocyte sedimentation rate (ESR) can help to identify underlying osteomyelitis in addition to imaging studies, including x-ray, CT, and MRI.

Differential diagnosis: Arterial, venous, and neuropathic ulcers should be included in the differential. Cellulitis and pyoderma gangrenosum should also be considered since they may appear similar to early decubitus ulcers.

Management: This is largely dependent on the stage of the ulcer. The main objectives are to reduce excessive external pressure that produced the lesion and to perform appropriate wound care to ensure adequate healing. If a DU at any stage presents with underlying local or systemic infection, antibiotics should be started. Any lesion with necrotic tissue (stage III or IV), should be debrided before performing proper wound care.

For an ulcer that has only extended through the epidermis or superficial dermis (stage I or II), a moist dressing may be applied after cleansing. For stage III or IV ulcers, which have a deeper extension, extra care must be taken by applying an absorbent dressing. If no improvement is seen, surgery may be considered to help relieve external pressure.

Consideration should be given to using pressure-relieving beds, such as the Clinatron® bed. Turning the bedridden patient should be done frequently, but there is no magic to a 2-hour turn schedule. Use of irritants, such as Betadine® or Daikin's solution, should not be employed.

Prognosis: With appropriate treatment and wound care, early-stage ulcers have a high likelihood of healing within 6 months of presentation. As ulcers begin to involve deeper structures, the rate of complication and infection is greatly increased.

Final comment: DUs commonly present in inpatient settings and in patients who have impaired mental status. The underlying pathophysiology includes prolonged external pressure on a bony surface of the body, which leads to tissue ischemia. Management includes relieving excessive external pressure and performing proper wound care. Prognosis is largely stage-dependent and equally dependent on the patient's physiologic status.

NEUROPATHIC ULCERS

Definition: Neuropathic ulcers are related to underlying peripheral neuropathy, which involves loss of sensation and autonomic response to painful stimuli or injury. This can lead to an increased likelihood of painless ulcer formation, most commonly of the foot. Additional underlying comorbidities that can result in lower extremity ischemia can contribute to chronic wounds.

Overview: The underlying pathophysiology of neuropathic ulcers involves two main mechanisms:

1. Peripheral neuropathy, often caused by diabetes mellitus or vitamin B12 deficiency, classically results in loss of sensation of the distal extremities in a so-called glove and stocking distribution.

2. Peripheral vascular disease due to an underlying comorbidity can result in poor blood flow and ischemia of the lower extremities, which can interfere with wound healing.

The most common example of neuropathic ulcers is the diabetic foot. Patients with diabetes mellitus are most commonly impacted due to nonenzymatic glycation of large vessels. This can lead to peripheral vascular disease and sorbitol accumulation in Schwann cells of the peripheral nervous system, which causes autonomic neuropathy and loss of sensation. These compounded effects contribute to ischemia, wound formation, decreased sensation, and delayed wound healing.

Clinical presentation: Neuropathic ulcers typically present as punched-out lesions in regions of the foot that receive extended pressure. These include the hallux or metatarsophalangeal joints on the planter surface. The epidermis of the lower foot may become dehydrated and cracked. Patients will likely exhibit a "glove and stocking" pattern of sensation loss; however, the lower extremities will often maintain a strong pulse and warm skin unless comorbid arterial insufficiency exists.

Laboratory studies: Patients should be checked for diabetes mellitus (e.g., hemoglobin A1c), which is the most common underlying pathophysiology of neuropathic ulcers. CBC can determine if a concurrent infection is present. Nutritional studies (e.g., vitamin B12) can rule out an underlying deficiency that can contribute to peripheral neuropathy. ABPI should be obtained to assess for comorbid arterial insufficiency. The Ipswich Touch Test can assess the degree of peripheral neuropathy in patients with diabetes mellitus and the likelihood of concurrent ulceration formation.

Differential diagnosis: Arterial and venous insufficiency should be considered. Cutaneous infections or burns may be included in the differential. Besides, the presence of underlying comorbidities, including atherosclerosis, obesity, and hypertension, should be evaluated since their presence can greatly impact outcomes and treatment course.

Management: Treatment of the ulcer is the first step. If necrotic tissue is present, debridement or irrigation should be performed. Patients should be assessed for underlying cutaneous infections or osteomyelitis. Once complications have been ruled out, proper wound care should be performed. Patients may be given a cast or boot to prevent direct pressure on the ulcer and facilitate healing.

Management of the underlying disease is key to preventing future ulcerations. The most common causes include diabetes mellitus and vitamin B12 deficiency; however, any pathologic disease that includes loss of sensation and proprioception of the lower extremities may lead to neuropathic ulcers and must be identified. These include autoimmune diseases, systemic infections (e.g., Lyme disease, syphilis, HIV), and inherited disorders.

Prognosis: Likelihood of recurrence is largely based on control of underlying disease, length of presentation of the initial ulceration, and the number of ulcers with which the patient first presented. Complications, including underlying infection, can interfere with healing and increase the likelihood of future ulcer formation. Studies have shown that about one-third of patients with a neuropathic ulcer from diabetic complications are likely to require future amputation.

Final comment: Neuropathic ulcers typically present in patients with diabetes mellitus or vitamin B12 deficiency due to underlying peripheral neuropathy. These ulcers present as punched-out lesions, and patients will often maintain a strong pulse and warm skin. Management involves treating the ulcer as well as underlying pathophysiology. There is a high risk of recurrence and future amputation in diabetic patients.

LESS COMMON CAUSES OF ULCERATION

Pyoderma Gangrenosum

Overview: Pyoderma gangrenosum typically starts as inflammatory pustules that quickly transform into larger painful ulcerations. Ulcers can be single or multiple, and they are classically described as having a cribriform base with undermined gunmetal gray borders.

Clinical presentation: Lesions often worsen or develop at the site of skin trauma. The underlying pathophysiology is believed to be due to uncontrolled neutrophilic inflammation (Figure 17.4). Approximately 50% of patients will have associated systemic diseases, including inflammatory bowel disease, rheumatoid arthritis (RA), and hematologic conditions.

Laboratory studies: Diagnosis is based on the exclusion of infection, other underlying inflammatory conditions, and malignancies because pyoderma gangrenosum is rather non-specific.

Management: Small, isolated ulcers may be managed with topical corticosteroids, but severe cases may require systemic treatment. Immunomodulatory therapy, including cyclosporine, dapsone, minocycline, prednisone, and infliximab, is effective. Due to pathergy, it is important to avoid surgical debridement and minimize skin trauma.

Vasculitis

Definition: Cutaneous vasculitis is characterized by inflammation of small or medium-sized vessels that can lead to compromised circulation and vascular destruction.

Overview: Various types of vasculitides exist, and their underlying pathophysiology may begin in the arterioles, capillaries, or postcapillary venules. Risk factors include smoking, hepatitis B, hepatitis C, and various autoimmune conditions, such as RA, lupus erythematosus, and scleroderma.

Clinical presentation: Ulcers that develop from vasculitis may present as highly vascularized small lesions that slowly increase in size, erythema, and necrotic tissue formation. These lesions are often painful at rest and are most commonly located on the lower extremities.

Laboratory studies: Diagnosis may be confirmed by skin biopsy and should involve laboratory investigation of associated conditions.

Management: This includes wound care, topical and/or systemic immunosuppressants, and management of underlying risk factors.

Vasculopathy

Definition: Vasculopathy is a broad term for compromised circulation due to a primary obstructive process in the vessel lumen.

Overview: The underlying pathophysiology varies and includes hypercoagulable states, microangiopathic hemolytic anemias, emboli, calcium or oxalate crystal deposition, and antiphospholipid antibodies.

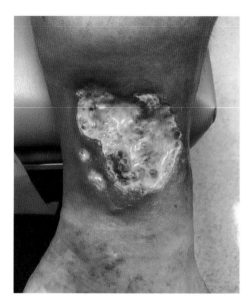

Figure 17.4 Pyoderma gangrenosum with undermined border and gunmetal gray coloration at the ulcer margin.

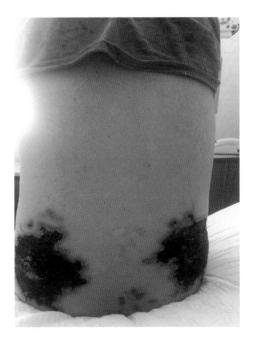

Figure 17.5 Occlusive vasculopathy with large, retiform necrotic eschars symmetrically distributed on the lateral flanks with dull surrounding erythema.

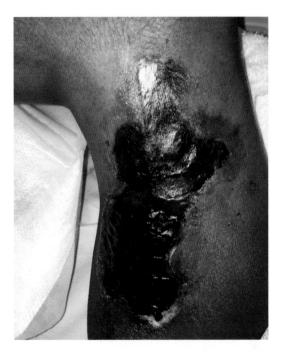

Figure 17.6 Calciphylaxis with large angulated necrotic eschar with surrounding purpura.

Clinical presentation: The classic vasculopathy is fixed retiform or stellate purpura with ulceration due to ischemic tissue necrosis (Figure 17.5).

Laboratory studies: Diagnosis includes clinical evaluation and biopsy to rule out primary vasculitis.

Management: This consists of treating the underlying cause, anticoagulation, proper wound care, and adequate elevation to facilitate circulation.

Calciphylaxis

Definition: This specific form of vasculopathy is defined by excessive deposition of calcium in the arterioles and capillaries, which results in diminished blood flow and poor oxygenation of tissue.

Clinical presentation: Patients present with painful necrotic ulcerations that can extend into the epidermal, dermal, and subcutaneous adipose tissue layers (Figure 17.6). The pathophysiology is not well understood; however, previous epidemiologic studies have found that calciphylaxis is more prevalent in those who are on dialysis for end-stage renal disease. The incidence of uremic calciphylaxis is relatively low, but it is often rapidly progressive and carries high morbidity and mortality rates.

Laboratory studies: Diagnosis is largely based on clinical presentation and past medical history, including laboratory studies that assess for renal dysfunction. Confirmation can be made by visualization of calcifications, thrombosis, and hyperplasia of the small arteries and capillaries within the dermal and subcutaneous layers.

Management: Immediate management involves proper wound care to prevent further necrosis and infection. Intravenous sodium thiosulfate, low calcium hemodialysis, phosphate binders, bisphosphonates, and calcined may help correct calcium metabolism. Unfortunately, there is a relatively poor prognosis.

Infection

Definition: In patients who are immunocompromised, various systemic and opportunistic mycoses can lead to cutaneous manifestations through hematogenous dissemination.

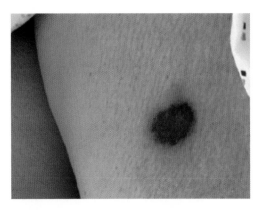

Figure 17.7 Mucormycosis with a solitary round necrotic plaque surrounded by a thin erythematous halo.

Clinical presentation: Skin findings are often widespread and may include papules, abscesses, plaques, purpura, and ulcers. Causal species include *Aspergillus, Cryptococcus, Histoplasma, Blastomyces, Coccidioides, Paracoccidioides, Rhizopus,* and *Mucor* (Figure 17.7).

Acid-fast bacilli are a less common cause of skin ulcerations and generally develop 1–2 months after the onset of the bacterial infection. These lesions begin as small nodules and progress to large, necrotic ulcerations that can spread to subcutaneous tissue and bone. The underlying infection is generally due to the *Mycobacterium* genus.

Ecthyma gangrenosum is associated with *Pseudomonas aeruginosa* infection and generally develops in immunocompromised patients. These lesions are rapidly progressive, beginning as small, painless macules and becoming large necrotic ulcers with pustules and surrounding erythema. The most common location is the axillary and anogenital regions.

Laboratory studies: Appropriate bacterial and fungal cultures are needed, along with a skin biopsy for histologic studies, including additional stains.

Management: Treatment of all ulcers with underlying infection requires appropriate antimicrobials, debridement of necrotic tissue, and proper wound dressing.

Malignancy

Overview: Cutaneous carcinomas that commonly ulcerate include SCC (Figure 17.8) and basal cell carcinoma (BCC). Metastases of various tumors to the skin can also manifest as ulcerating tumors. Rarely, a chronic, nonhealing ulcer can lead to secondary malignant transformation with SCC, which is known as a Marjolin ulcer. This process takes many years to develop and is most commonly seen in men between the ages of 40–60 years.

Factitial/Self-Induced Ulcers

Overview: These ulcers often develop due to underlying psychologic conditions that cause patients to manually self-induce skin lesions.

Clinical findings: These lesions are prone to developing infections as patients are introducing foreign bacteria when physically breaking the skin barrier. Diagnosis should be suspected, when ulcers are localized to reachable areas and have a "gouged out" or geometric shape (Figure 17.9).

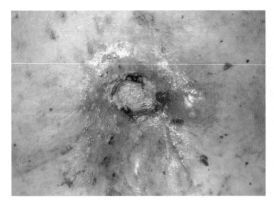

Figure 17.8 Invasive squamous cell cancer with large erythematous, focally hyperkeratotic, and poorly defined plaque on the chest.

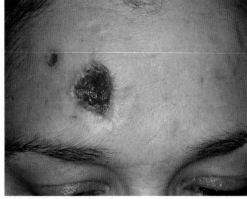

Figure 17.9 Factitious disorder with geometric-shaped ulcers on the forehead.

Table 17.3 Wound Care

A. Nutritional Status

Deficiencies in any of the following nutrients can result in chronic wounds that have increased risk of infection and complication:

1. Vitamin A and C deficiencies increase the likelihood of a suboptimal immune response and risk of infection.
2. Anemia decreases the transport of oxygen to the wound site resulting in decreased collagen formation and impaired wound closure.
3. Zinc or copper deficiency interrupts collagen synthesis and overall tensile strength of the skin.
4. Protein deficiency prolongs the wound repair process since essential enzymes that are required in healing are deficient.
5. Poor volume status increases the risk of complications. Patients should be monitored for symptoms and signs of volume depletion, including hypotension, poor skin turgor, and decreased urine output.

B. Wound Debridement

Four main types:

1. Surgical debridement is the most invasive and often requires local or general anesthesia. The necrotic or infected tissue is removed through surgery, and the wound is disinfected to eliminate microbes.
2. Mechanical debridement involves hydrotherapy and irrigation to remove nonviable tissue with the use of water.
3. Enzymatic debridement involves the use of chemical enzymes to digest necrotic tissue. These enzymes include streptokinase, collagenase, and DNAse. Hypertonic saline may also be used, as well as fluorouracil 5% cream or solution.
4. Autolytic debridement utilizes occlusive dressings to provide an environment that facilitates intrinsic debridement processes of phagocytic cells and proteolytic enzymes for wound healing. These dressings include hydrocolloids, hydrogel, and transparent films. This method may only be used if blood supply is preserved within the dermal layer and minimal necrosis is present.

Management: This includes wound care and psychiatric intervention (Table 17.3)

Infection control: All patients should be evaluated for infection in the context of skin ulcerations. Signs of local infection include erythema, warmth, pain, and purulent exudate. If the infection is not managed promptly, there is potential for systemic spread, which can manifest as fever, chills, and sweating. Management of local infection includes topical antimicrobials specific to the infectious agent. If systemic infection is severe, then broad-spectrum intravenous antibiotics should be initiated immediately or, in less severe cases, once a culture has been performed.

Optimization of blood flow: Blood flow is crucial in facilitating the wound healing process. In patients who have slow-healing lesions, poor blood flow must be considered. Initial management includes maximizing warmth, hydration, edema control, and pain control. If this does not adequately address poor perfusion, then revascularization procedures may be performed to restore blood flow.

Wound Dressings

Selection of the type of wound dressing is largely based on the characteristics of the presenting wound. Moist dressings are now standard of care over wet-to-dry or dry dressings. Moist dressings foster an ideal healing environment during the initial inflammatory phase and later re-epithelization phase. Table 17.4 provides an outline of the various types of wound dressings.

Hyperbaric oxygen therapy (HBOT) may be supplemented in patients who have slow-healing ulcers. Management involves placing a patient in a pressurized chamber that is 2–3 times greater than atmospheric pressure. This creates an oxygen-rich environment that facilitates fibroblast and collagen proliferation, increased angiogenesis, and expanded antimicrobial activity, which leads to enhanced wound healing. Previous studies have confirmed the efficacy of HBOT therapy in diabetic and venous insufficiency ulcers.

A growing body of evidence has confirmed great potential in using stem cell therapy to facilitate wound healing for ulcers. Multipotent adult stem cells, including mesenchymal stromal cells and endothelial progenitor cells, may aid in the upregulation of helpful cytokines and growth factors that can improve healing in patients with impaired intrinsic mechanisms.

Table 17.4 Various Types of Wound Dressings and Indications

Type	Properties	Indication	Exudate Level	Necrotic Tissue Level	Moist vs. Dry	Maximum Time Left in Place
Gauze			Low	Low	Dry	
Films	Polyurethane sheets with hypoallergenic acrylic adhesive Impermeable to bacteria/water; permeable to air/water vapor	Anatomical sites that require constant movement	Low	Low	Moist	24–72 hours
Hydrogels	Insoluble polymers with high water content Permeable to air/water vapor	Facilitates intrinsic autolytic debridement for wounds that have necrotic tissue present	Low	High	Moist	24–72 hours
Hydrocolloids	Cross-linked matrix gelatin, pectin, and carboxymethyl-cellulose Impermeable to air/water vapor	Rehydrate dried, necrotic tissue Autolytic debridement Wounds in cavities/sinuses	Low	High	Moist	24–72 hours
Foams	Polyurethane or silicone foam	Contains excess exudate in wound	Moderate	Moderate	Moist	1–7 days
Calcium Alginates	Calcium/sodium salt of alginic acid from brown seaweed	Wounds in cavities/sinuses	High	Low	Moist	24 hours

KELOIDS AND HYPERTROPHIC SCARS

Definition: Aberrant processes in wound healing and excessive collagen synthesis may lead to the formation of keloids and hypertrophic scars following skin trauma.

Clinical findings: Keloids will specifically grow beyond the border of the initial wound and will typically present with similar pigmentation of the patient's skin (Figure 17.10). In contrast, hypertrophic scars are always confined to the region of the presenting wound and will typically present as erythematous lesions with variable pigmentation.

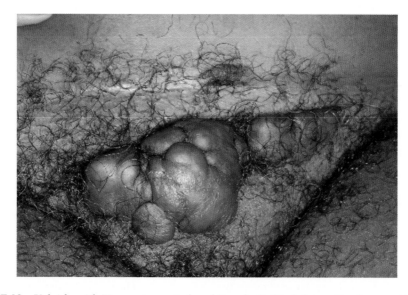

Figure 17.10 Keloids with Hyperpigmented and Exophytic Nodules on the Suprapubic Area.

Management: often involves intralesional steroids to break down excess collagen within the dermis. Multiple injections are needed depending on lesion severity, and combination treatments with 5-fluorouracil can be helpful. Silicone elastomer sheets can reduce the production of collagen by creating an environment within the epidermis that tightly controls fibroblast functioning. Pressure dressings may be used to relax the surrounding tissue leading to reduction of keloid or hypertrophic scar formation. Surgical excision or laser treatment can be helpful. The recurrence rate is high.

Oftentimes, these management options are combined to achieve optimal outcomes. For example, surgical excision may be followed by intralesional steroids or silicone elastomer sheets to reduce the risk of recurrence.

FINAL THOUGHT

Keloids and hypertrophic scars involve issues with proper wound healing and collagen synthesis. Prevention of lesions in at-risk individuals is difficult, and even successful management of lesions is often met with high recurrence rates.

ADDITIONAL READINGS

Braswell SF, Kostopoulos TC, Ortega-Loayza AG. Pathophysiology of pyoderma gangrenosum (PG): an updated review. J Am Acad Dermatol. 2015;73:691–698.

Brooklyn T, Dunnill G, Probert C. Diagnosis and treatment of pyoderma gangrenosum. BMJ. 2006;333:181–184.

George C, Deroide F, Rustin M. Pyoderma gangrenosum—a guide to diagnosis and management. Clin Med. 2019;19:224–228.

Grey JE, Harding KG, Enoch S. Venous and arterial leg ulcers. BMJ. 2006;332:347–350.

Jones V, Grey JE, Harding KG. Wound dressings. BMJ. 2006;332:777–780.

Juckett G, Hartman-Adams H. Management of keloids and hypertrophic scars. Am Fam Physician. 2009;80:253–260.

Mervis JS, Phillips TJ. Pressure ulcers: pathophysiology, epidemiology, risk factors, and presentation. J Am Acad Dermatol. 2019;81:881–890.

Singer AJ, Tassiopoulos A, Kirsner RS. Evaluation and management of lower-extremity ulcers. N Engl J Med. 2018;378:302–303.

Sundaresan S, Migden MR, Silapunt S. Stasis Dermatitis: pathophysiology, Evaluation, and Management. Am J Clin Dermatol. 2017;18:383–390.

Xie T, Ye J, Rerkasem K, et al. The venous ulcer continues to be a clinical challenge: an update. Burns Trauma. 2018;6:18. https://doi.org/10.1186/s41038-018-0119-y. eCollection 2018.

18 Granulomatous Diseases

Albert Alhatem, Robert A. Schwartz, Muriel W. Lambert, and W. Clark Lambert

CONTENTS

SARCOIDOSIS

Name: *Sarco–* means "flesh"; the suffix *–(e)ido–* means "type," "resembles," or "like"; and *–sis–* means "condition." The whole word means "a condition that resembles crude flesh" (Figure 18.1).

Definition: It is a multisystem inflammatory granulomatous disorder. The lesions consist of *naked granulomas* devoid of peripheral lymphocytes and that are noncaseating (Figure 18.2).

Overview: Sarcoidosis is a moderately uncommon disease with a predilection for individuals of African American and Caucasian descent. It is characterized by epithelioid granulomas. The affected organs include, lungs, skin, lymph nodes, eyes, and bone. Cutaneous lesions comprise about 20% of the presenting signs, especially in African American women.

Clinical presentation: General findings include weight loss, loss of appetite, fatigue, fever, chills, and night sweats. Erythema nodosum is the most common initial nonspecific sign. Alternatively, there can be a wide variety of histologically specific cutaneous findings. Cutaneous lesions can arise anywhere with facial lesions being the most common. They characteristically consist of collections of histiocytes devoid of areas of central necrosis and, in at least some places, of a rim of lymphocytes (Figure 18.2); this feature is considered diagnostic and such granulomas are known as *naked granulomas*. A similar pathology may be seen very uncommonly, however, in cutaneous reactions to a variety of noninfectious stimuli, including some ingredients in cosmetics and deodorants. A diagnosis of *sarcoidosis* should, therefore, not be rendered pathologically, only granulomatous dermatitis, consistent with sarcoidosis.

The skin manifestations include scattered reddish-brown to yellow-brown *apple jelly* macules, papules, and plaques and nodules, which are commonly on the face and extremities. Variants include nodular type, subcutaneous variant, angiolymphoid sarcoidosis, lupus pernio, lichenoid variant, and miliary types.

Papular sarcoidosis: many papules of various colors. It is commonly acute. The most frequent location is the face, especially the eyelids and nasolabial folds. It can develop into coalescent plaques with coalescent lesions plus atrophy and hypopigmentation in the healed sites.

Nodular sarcoidosis: granulomas in the dermis or subcutaneous tissue. It may form nodules, which should be differentiated from foreign body reactions, granuloma annulare, rheumatoid nodules, and mycobacterial infections.

DOI: 10.1201/9781003105268-18

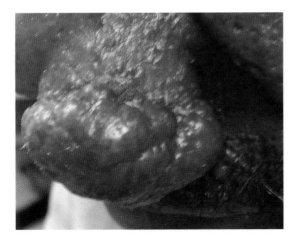

Figure 18.1 Sarcoidosis on the nose.

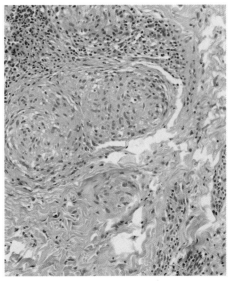

Figure 18.2 Sarcoidal granulomas without central necrosis.

Subcutaneous sarcoidosis: commonly found in middle-aged women as erythematous hyperpigmented nodules with a linear distribution on the forearms. It is usually associated with an autoimmune disease.

Maculopapular sarcoidosis: Acute asymptomatic or pruritic hyperpigmented patches, commonly on the eyelids and may also affect the neck, trunk, extremities, or mucous membranes.

Plaque sarcoidosis: Erythematous or brown discrete plaques on shoulders, arms, back, or buttocks. Less common variants of plaque sarcoidosis include the following:

Lupus pernio: Infiltrative plaques primarily found on the central portion of the face in African Americans women. Less commonly, the lesions may affect the extremities and are usually more resistant to treatment than other sarcoidosis lesions. If left untreated, the lesions may cause destruction and disfigurement from the erosion of cartilage and bone.

Hypopigmented sarcoidosis: Hypopigmented round to oval patches or barely raised plaques. The classic finding is the fried egg appearance due to papules found in the center of some lesion.

Atrophic and ulcerative sarcoidosis: Depressed plaques with ulceration and coexistent mucocutaneous and systemic manifestations, often afflicting African American women.

Morphea form: Initially, sclerotic plaques that evolve into depressed lesions more often afflicting the legs.

Cutaneous sarcoid granulomata and chronic facial lesions are associated with a poor prognosis due to the pulmonary fibrosis and uveitis. Lupus pernio is often associated with advanced lung fibrosis, bone cysts, and eye disease.

Laboratory studies: The histopathology consists of granuloma formation without central necrosis with rare focal caseation. These granulomas are formed by epithelioid cells (histiocytes), located in the dermis and sometimes in the subcutaneous fat. Langshan's type multinucleated cells and sometimes asteroid (eosinophilic star-shaped inclusion) and Schaumann (basophilic, laminated calcified whorls) bodies may be seen.

Diagnostic serum biomarkers include angiotensin-converting enzyme and serum soluble IL2 receptor that can also be non-specific.

Management: Although the lesions may disappear spontaneously, prednisone 40–60 mg daily, methotrexate 10–25 mg weekly, minocycline 100 mg bid, doxycycline 100 mg bid, or hydroxychloroquine 200–400 mg daily may be used. Facial lesions often respond to topical steroids or intralesional triamcinolone.

In widespread disease, treatments can include hydroxychloroquine 200–400 mg per day or chloroquine 250 mg per day, methotrexate 10–25 mg given once weekly for adults, or minocycline 100 mg twice daily, or doxycycline 100 mg twice daily.

GRANULOMA ANNULARE

Synonym: Necrobiotic papulosis.

Definition: Granuloma annulare (GA) is an inflammatory condition characterized by grouped, smooth, reddish-brown or discolored papules and plaques and necrobiotic granulomas on histology. The disease was first described in 1895 by Thomas Colcott Fox (1849–1916) and was named *granuloma annulare* by Henry Radcliffe Crocker (1846–1909) in 1902.

Overview: It is a moderately common entity usually found on the extremities, but it may occur on any part of the body. It has two forms: localized and generalized. The most commonly affected age groups include children, teenagers, or young adults. The generalized form is more likely to be found in older adults with a mean age of 50 years. There is a female predominance of 2:1. The etiology is unknown, but several hypotheses have been proposed, including a delayed hypersensitivity reaction to infections or trauma, which is mediated by tumor necrosis factor-alpha (TNF-α). Whether this is an autoimmune condition or paraneoplastic is speculative.

Clinical presentation: There are small, grouped, reddish-brown or discolored papules, which tend to be in an arcuate or circular distribution, and plaques with a broad spectrum of clinical variants: localized, generalized, atypical, subcutaneous, perforating, and patch-type (Figure 18.3). GA profundis is a rare variant with larger, deeper lesions with predilection for the trunk.

Laboratory studies: Histopathologic study reveals zones of degenerated collagen (necrobiosis) surrounded by epithelioid histiocytes and lymphocytes in a palisaded array (Figure 18.4). The central area contains mucin (Figure 18.5). Multinucleated giant cells may sometimes be present.

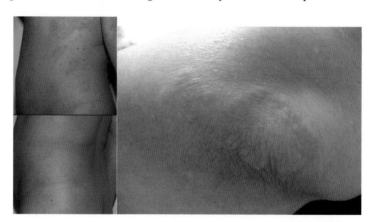

Figure 18.3 Granuloma annulare. Lesions may range from small grouped papules to papules in an arcuate or annular shape to (uncommonly) plaques.

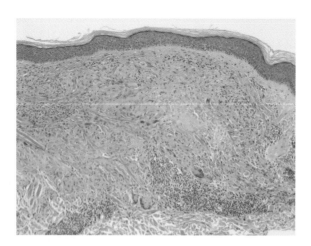

Figure 18.4 Granuloma annulare. Palisading granulomatous pattern with thick, free collagen bundles ("floating" sign).

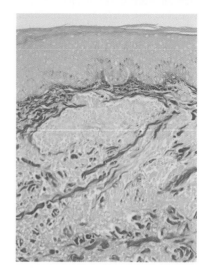

Figure 18.5 Granuloma annulare. Colloidal iron staining showing dermal mucin deposition (×80: ×180)

Eosinophils can be observed. Mucin deposition in large quantity is found in the interstitium, which may be stained with an Alcian blue or colloidal iron stain.

A KOH scraping or fungal culture will rule out candidosis or dermatophytosis.

Differential diagnosis: This may include tinea corporis, actinic granuloma, annular lichen planus, erythema annulare centrifugum, or sarcoidosis.

Management: Topical corticosteroids or intralesional steroids can be helpful. Pentoxifylline, 400 mg three times daily, can be considered but is usually unnecessary.

Course: GA may spontaneously resolve within a few weeks or months, but it can also become chronic.

NECROBIOSIS LIPOIDICA

Synonym: Necrobiosis lipoidica diabeticorum

Definition: Necrobiosis lipoidica (NL) is a moderately uncommon granulomatous necrotizing skin disorder of unknown etiology. It can affect the lower extremities of diabetics; however, it may occur in nondiabetic patients. There may also be an association with obesity, hypertension, dyslipidemia, and thyroid disease.

Overview: NL has a predilection for women and is often found on the legs following trauma. There is no relationship between the severity or control of diabetes mellitus and the incidence of NL or the recovery of either.

Clinical presentation: NL most frequently appears as plaques on the legs and arms, but it can affect the trunk, nipples, or penis. The plaques may vary between being asymptomatic or tender. Initially, it may be a yellowish plaque like *apple jelly* with an atrophic center becoming erythematous and even ulcerating.

Laboratory studies: Histologically, there is a large area of necrobiosis (partial necrosis of the dermis) surrounded by a superficial and deep perivascular and interstitial mixed inflammatory cell infiltrate, including lymphocytes, plasma cells, mononucleated and multinucleated histiocytes, and eosinophils in the dermis and subcutis. There may also be necrotizing vasculitis with adjacent necrobiosis and necrosis of adnexal structures (Figure 18.6). The lesion forms a palisading granuloma, but in contrast to granuloma annulare, the granuloma is quite large, and contents are necrobiotic collagen instead of mucin.

Differential diagnosis: It can be difficult to distinguish NL from GA or a rheumatoid nodule, but NL is usually much larger and does not contain dermal mucin.

Management: Topical and intralesional corticosteroids may be helpful, as can the use of an occlusive dressing. Other therapies for nonulcerated lesions, which cannot be managed adequately with local corticosteroids, include topical tacrolimus (0.1% ointment twice daily for 8 weeks), topical psoralen plus ultraviolet A (PUVA) photochemotherapy, twice weekly until improvement, and systemic medications, such as chloroquine 200 mg per day or hydroxychloroquine 400 mg per day for 2–12 months. In the diabetic patient, appropriate use of oral hypoglycemic agents or insulin is often helpful.

Course: The course of NL is usually chronic with slow progression over years to eventual stabilization. The area of necrobiosis may become much smaller (Figure 18.7). Uncommonly, a secondary skin cancer may arise. The development of new nodules in sites of long-standing NL or ulcers should raise suspicion for squamous cell carcinoma, and a skin biopsy may be indicated.

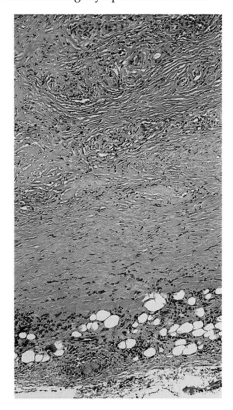

Figure 18.6 Necrobiosis lipoidica. Early stage. Superficial and deep perivascular/periadnexal and interstitial inflammation (hematoxylin and eosin stain ×120).

Source: Courtesy of David Suster, MD Pathology Department, Rutgers University.

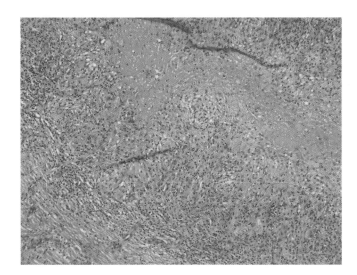

Figure 18.7 Necrobiosis lipoidica, late stage. Note the reduction in central contents (hematoxylin and eosin ×220).

NEUTROPHILIC DERMATOSES

Overview: These are a group of cutaneous disorders sharing histologic evidence of intense epidermal, dermal, or hypodermal neutrophilic infiltrates without infection or true vasculitis. The clinical and pathologic characteristics along with the associated diseases dictates the classification of the neutrophilic dermatoses Table 18.1).

SWEET SYNDROME

Synonym: Acute febrile neutrophilic dermatosis, Gomm-Button disease

Definition: Sweet syndrome (SS) is a cutaneous eruption consisting of erythematous papules and plaques, seen as a dermal nonvasculitic neutrophilic infiltration on biopsy, with fever and peripheral neutrophilia. The syndrome was named after Robert Douglas Sweet (1917–2001) who

Table 18.1 Summary of the Neutrophilic Dermatoses

Affecting the Epidermis
- Pustular psoriasis
- Drug-induced/acute generalized exanthematous pustulosis
- Keratoderma blennorrhagicum
- Sneddon-Wilkinson disease (subcorneal pustulosis)
- IgA pemphigus (subcorneal pustular dermatosis type, intraepidermal neutrophilic IgA dermatosis type)
- Amicrobial pustulosis of the folds
- Infantile acropustulosis
- Transient neonatal pustulosis

Affecting the Dermis
- Sweet syndrome
- Pyoderma gangrenosum
- Behçet's disease
- Bowel-associated dermatosis-arthritis syndrome
- Inflammatory bowel disease (may also have small-vessel vasculitis)
- Neutrophilic eccrine hidradenitis
- Rheumatoid neutrophilic dermatitis
- Neutrophilic urticaria
- Still's disease
- Erythema marginatum
- Hereditary periodic fever syndrome

first reported it in 1964. It is also known as Gomm-Button disease in honor of the first two patients Sweet diagnosed with the condition.

Overview: SS is moderately uncommon and can arise without predilection for sex or age. SS has two main features: (1) Abrupt onset of papules and painful erythematous plaques and (2) predominately neutrophilic infiltrate without signs of leukocytoclastic vasculitis on histologic examination. Minor criteria include prior fever or infection, fever, arthralgia, conjunctivitis, concurrent malignancy, leukocytosis, and rapid response to corticosteroid therapy. The diagnosis is based on clinical-pathologic correlation.

The condition is subdivided based on the clinical features into classic or idiopathic SS, malignancy-associated SS, and drug-induced SS. SS is considered a cutaneous marker of systemic disease. SS is often associated with hematologic disease, like leukemia, and immunologic diseases, including rheumatoid arthritis, inflammatory bowel disease, or Behçet syndrome. Some pregnant patients are affected in the first and second trimester without risk to the fetus. The pathogenesis has been proposed to be linked to hypersensitivity reaction, cytokine dysregulation, and genetic susceptibility.

Clinical presentation: These include acute, tender, edematous, erythematous, asymmetric plaques, and nodules. Bullae can occur on the head, neck, and extremities, especially ton he dorsal aspect of the hands and fingers. Less frequently, SS presents as bullous SS, subcutaneous SS, or a neutrophilic dermatosis of the dorsal hands.

Systemic features include fever, arthralgia, conjunctivitis, iridocyclitis, and aphthae. SS can also affect other systems causing encephalitis, aseptic meningitis, myocarditis, aortitis and aortic stenosis, coronary artery occlusion, neutrophilic alveolitis, pleural effusions, airway obstruction, hepatitis, hepatomegaly, neutrophilic inflammation of the intestines, splenomegaly, mesangial glomerulonephritis, hematuria, proteinuria, and sterile osteomyelitis.

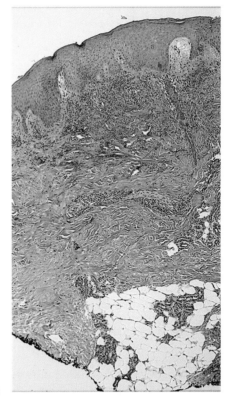

Figure 18.8 Sweet syndrome. Prominent edema in the superficial dermis and dense infiltrate of neutrophils in the upper and mid-dermis with sparing of the epidermis (hematoxylin and eosin ×40).

Laboratory studies: There may be neutrophilia in 50% of patients, elevated ESR >30 mm/h in 90%, and a slight increase in alkaline phosphatase (83%), along with proteinuria. Histologic examination shows prominent edema in the superficial dermis, dense infiltrate of neutrophils in the upper and mid-dermis with sparing of the epidermis (Figure 18.8), limited or no leukocytoclasis, and endothelial swelling with absence of vasculitis. A few eosinophils may also be present.

Management: The gold standard treatment is prednisone, 0.5–1 mg/kg per day for 1–2 weeks or until resolution of the lesions. Other alternatives include dapsone, doxycycline, clofazimine, and cyclosporine. All these drugs influence the migration and other functions of neutrophils.

Course: This is unpredictable without treatment. Spontaneous resolution may occur after weeks to months. The cutaneous lesions of SS usually heal without scarring. Relapse is a possibility following tapering or discontinuation of treatment, especially in patients with malignancy-associated disease.

PYODERMA GANGRENOSUM

Definition: Pyoderma gangrenosum (PG) is a moderately uncommon chronic noninfectious neutrophilic dermatosis, which presents as erythematous papules and pustules, progressing into an inflammatory and ulcerative disorder of the skin. The name is generally a misnomer.

Overview: PG is characterized by neutrophil-predominant infiltrates in the skin. The posited pathogeneses include abnormalities in neutrophil function, genetic variations, and dysregulation of the innate immune system.

Clinical presentation: PG may present as an Inflammatory papule or pustule that progresses to a painful ulcer with a violaceous border and a purulent base (Figure 18.9). Lesions may also be bullous, vegetative, peristomal, and extracutaneous. A common location is the leg, but PG can appear anywhere on the body. Prognosis is influenced by the subtypes and the associated diseases as follows.

Ulcerative (classic) PG: This is the most common subtype. It presents in the lower extremities or trunk on a normal-appearing skin or at a site of trauma as an inflamed papule, pustule, or vesicle, that progresses into an ulcer formation. The ulcer often extends into the subcutaneous tissue or the fascia. Lesions could be single or multiple demonstrating various stages of development. The prognosis is good, and the lesions typically resolve forming atrophic, cribriform scars.

Bullous (atypical) PG: This subtype is less common, superficial, and related to hematologic disease. Commonly affects the arms and face as a rapidly progressing blue-gray, inflammatory bullae, which then erodes forming superficial ulcers. Due to the strong association between bullous PG and hematologic disease, close follow up is recommended to monitor the development of a hematologic disorder.

Pustular PG: This subtype is associated with inflammatory bowel disease (IBD) and tends to present during the IBD flare-up periods. Clinically, it presents as rapidly progressing painful erythematous pustules with concomitant fever and arthralgias.

Vegetative PG: This subtype is known as superficial granulomatous pyoderma and most commonly affects the head and neck. It usually presents as a localized, superficial, indolent, mildly painful nodule, plaque, or ulcer. The borders of the lesions are undermined without purulent bases in the ulcerative form. The prognosis is usually good.

Laboratory studies: Histopathologic examination of a biopsy taken from the earliest lesions of PG will demonstrate perifollicular inflammation and intradermal abscess formation. With more progression, there may be ulceration, epidermal and superficial dermal necrosis with an underlying mixed inflammatory cell infiltrate, and abscess formation as the classic findings (Figure 18.10). There may be pseudoepitheliomatous hyperplasia primarily affecting the epidermis, sinus tracts, and palisading granulomas.

Direct immunofluorescence studies demonstrate deposition of IgM, C3, and fibrin in vessel walls, which are not specific findings.

Differential diagnosis: An underlying hematologic disorder may be ruled out with a complete blood count, antinuclear antibody titer for systemic lupus erythematosus or collagen vascular disorders, antineutrophilic cytoplasmic antibodies for granulomatous vasculitis, hypercoagulability studies for antiphospholipid syndrome, hepatitis panel for hepatitis B or C, rheumatoid factor for cryoglobulinemia and rheumatoid arthritis, and colonoscopy for inflammatory bowel disease.

Management: The guidelines to manage patients with PG are not definitive; however, appropriate wound care is required to enhance the healing. There should be avoidance of surgical

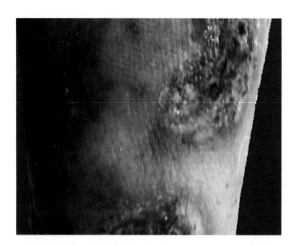

Figure 18.9 Pyoderma gangrenosum, a purulent necrotic ulcer with ragged edges and violaceous border.

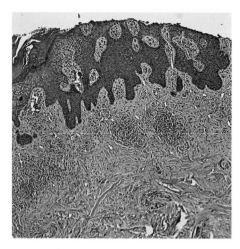

Figure 18.10 Pyoderma gangrenosum. Infundibular hyperplasia, chronic inflammation with extensive fibrosis and changes of suppurative folliculitis and perifolliculitis (hematoxylin and eosin ×60).

debridement and trauma, as this can trigger more destruction. Surgical interventions may be needed in selective with necrotic lesions with high risk of infection to save the movement function. Chemical debridement and occlusive dressings are the mainstay to provide hydration to the wounds. Systemic immunomodulatory agents may be needed.

Wound Management

Sterile saline or a mild antiseptic prior to dressing changes are recommended to promote a moist environment to help healing.

Trauma to the wound and the use of caustic substances (e.g., silver nitrate) should be avoided.

Wound infection signs (e.g., fever, warmth, swelling) should be treated appropriately with antibiotics

Surgery: Surgical procedures are considered only in select cases to remove the necrotic tissue and rescue the neighboring viable tissue.

Local corticosteroids: High potency corticosteroids, such as clobetasol propionate, are usually used once or twice daily. Triamcinolone (6–40 mg/mL) have been reported to help. Corticosteroid injection circumferentially into the ulcer periphery is recommended.

Local calcineurin inhibitors: Topical tacrolimus (0.03–0.3%) has been reported to demonstrate efficacy for PG. The recommended dose is 0.1% ointment once to twice daily.

Systemic glucocorticoids and cyclosporine: prednisolone (initial dose 0.75 mg/kg per day) and patients assigned to cyclosporine (initial dose 4 mg/kg per day) have been reported to induce rapid healing.

Other biologic TNFa inhibitors: Adalimumab (40 mg weekly, 40 mg twice monthly) and etanercept (25–50 mg twice weekly) has been reported to heal ulcers.

Intravenous immune globulin is recommended in divided doses over the course of two to five days, repeated monthly.

Course: More than half of patients with PG have an associated systemic disease, including one or more of inflammatory bowel disease, hematologic disorders, and arthritis, which require attention.

Final comment: PG development is not well understood, but aberrant neutrophil function, genetic susceptibility, and dysregulation of the immune system have been proposed as theories. PG is a diagnosis of exclusion and should include a patient history, physical examination, appropriate laboratory studies, and biopsy to rule out other diseases.

Pyoderma Gangrenosum–Related Levamisole Reaction

Overview: Levamisole is a drug formerly approved for human use by the Food and Drug Administration and now withdrawn. It continues to be approved for veterinary use. Because it is widely used as a filler with illegal heroin and cocaine, such users are at risk for developing this reaction.

Clinical manifestations: Lesions may arise with stunning rapidity, primarily on the lower extremity, and consist of necrotic sites that rapidly expand (Figure 18.9). Somewhat smaller lesions may also arise elsewhere. Lesions characteristically consist of sharply defined areas of black skin that are painless and that subsequently ulcerate.

Laboratory findings: Serum levamisole levels will confirm the diagnosis. Histopathologic examination shows perifollicular inflammation and intradermal abscess formation (Figure 18.10). Ulceration, epidermal and superficial dermal necrosis with an underlying mixed inflammatory cell infiltrate, and abscess formation as the classic findings. There may be pseudoepitheliomatous hyperplasia primarily affecting the epidermis, sinus tracts, and palisading granulomas.

Management: Supportive care with prednisone and local care are indicated.

Final comment: This entity should be considered in patients who abuse heroin and cocaine. They may show refractory ulcers PG in the legs.

MASTOCYTOSIS

Systemic and Cutaneous Mastocytosis

Definition: These are a group of disorders with excessive numbers of mast cells, forming a single tumor or a number of such lesions. The mast cells are usually benign but are hormonally active and can produce flushing reactions when activated. There can even be dangerous drops in blood pressure when severe reactions occur.

Overview: The active vasoactive product released by these cells, predominately serotonin, is responsible for its systemic effects. A widely disseminated cutaneous form, maculopapular cutaneous mastocytosis (MPCM; see the following discussion), arises in adults. Cutaneous masto-cytosis (CM) may be subdivided into subtypes:

Urticaria pigmentosa (UP), also called MPCM,

- Monomorphic affects adult patients

- Polymorphic MPCM affects infants and young children

- Plaque form

Nodular Form

Mastocytoma(s) of the skin affects infants and young children. It resolves spontaneously by the teenage years. Their tendency to suddenly undergo release of vasoactive secretions, predominately serotonin, can produce flushing reactions and dangerous drops in blood pressure.

Clinical presentation: Mastocytomas can additionally arise in the digestive tract, most commonly in the appendix. This tissue is served by the portal circulation, which passes through the liver, where serotonin is inactivated on its way to the systemic circulation. For this reason, clinical manifestations tend to be limited to the abdomen. The differentiation between pediatric and adult types depends on the clinical context, as the pediatric disease is often limited to the skin, while the adult disease can be systemic.

Mastocytomas may arise elsewhere, particularly in the lungs. Such lesions may produce systemic signs and symptoms from the outset. In very rare instances in which a lesion gives rise to a metastasis, systemic signs and symptoms may result from metastasis to the liver. When cutaneous disease is present, the skin may be involved at any site.

Diagnosis of cutaneous mastocytosis may be rendered by skin biopsy. Alternatively, skin involvement may sometimes be suggested by eliciting the Darier sign, in which a lesion is stroked and then urticates to become pruritic, edematous, and erythematous.

Laboratory studies: All tumor sites should be identified using such measures as ultrasound, x-rays, magnetic resonance, and computer-assisted tomography (CAT).

Additional studies include complete blood count with differential (to evaluate for cytopenias and abnormal myeloid and lymphoid lineages), liver function tests, serum total tryptase (tryptase >20 ng/mL is one of the World Health Organization minor criteria for the diagnosis of systemic mastocytosis), bone densitometry (to assess for osteopenia and osteoporosis), *KIT* D816V mutational analysis of peripheral blood by PCR.

Histopathologic study will reveal masses of mast cells (Figure 18.11), which stain with several special stains (e.g., toluidine blue, Giemsa) but more reliably stain with the immunohistochemical marker cKit (CD117).

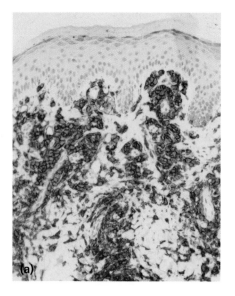 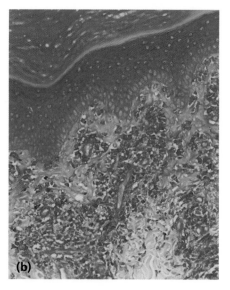

Figure 18.11 Mastocytosis. Cutaneous lesion showing masses of mast cells in the dermis: (a) Giemsa ×360; (b) Immunohistochemical stain cKit (CD117; for mast cells) ×360.

Management: Patients should be referred to an endocrinologist for diagnosis and treatment. Overall, the main recommended management is symptomatic with avoidance of any triggers of mast cell degranulation. H1 antihistamines or antileukotriene agent products can help with pruritis (itching) or flushing. H2 antihistamines can help with gastrointestinal symptoms, such as abdominal pain, heartburn, cramping, and/or diarrhea. As long as tumor masses are present, the possibility exists that one or more may become activated, inducing a potentially disastrous vascular response.

Course: Childhood mastocytosis is almost always a benign disease and usually resolves spontaneously by late childhood or puberty.

Final comment: Mastocytosis is a group of disorders in which excessive numbers of mast cells are present, forming a single tumor or a number of lesions. The mast cells are usually benign but are hormonally active, which can produce flushing reactions when activated.

MACULOPAPULAR CUTANEOUS MASTOCYTOSIS

Synonyms: Telangiectasia macularis eruptiva perstans (TMEP); diffuse cutaneous mastocytosis.

Definition: MPCM is an eruption of pigmented macules (<0.5 cm) with a slightly reddish-brown tinge. It is usually pruritic, but otherwise asymptomatic and persistent. The pathophysiology involves an excessive numbers of mast cells in the skin. To diagnose patients with MPCM, there should generally be no evidence of internal organ involvement.

Clinical presentation: MPCM occurs mainly in adults and is characterized by an eruption of tan to brown macules with telangiectasias (Figure 18.12). Sometimes, the clinical presentation is quite subtle, but unexplained pruritis is usually present. There is an increase in the numbers of mast cells around capillaries and venules of the superficial vascular plexus (Figure 18.13). Severe pruritus and blistering do not usually occur with MPCM. Rarely, it is associated with systemic involvement.

The chief complaint is pruritus which can be triggered by irritation or heat. Flushing or blister formation rarely occur.

Laboratory studies: The diagnosis is based upon characteristic skin findings without systemic disease, which is supported by findings on skin biopsy. Histologically, more than eight mast cells

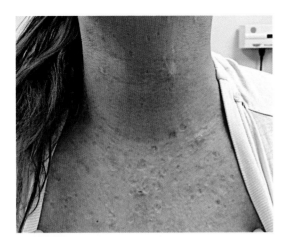

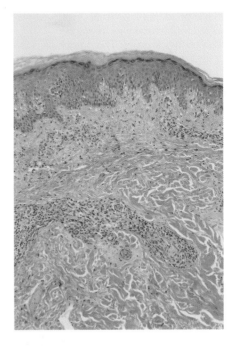

Figure 18.12 Maculopapular cutaneous mastocytosis. Eruption of pigmented macules with a slightly reddish-brown tinge is typical but may be absent.

Figure 18.13 Maculopapular cutaneous mastocytosis. Collections of mast cells are seen surrounding cutaneous blood vessels (hematoxylin and eosin ×340).

surrounding the majority of capillaries is considered diagnostic. Additional laboratory studies are often not needed to diagnose MPCM.

Differential diagnosis: Generalized urticaria and/or angioedema should point toward other allergic disorders. Darier sign is observed in MPCM due to the localized release of mast cell mediators.

Management: This consists of avoiding triggers, such as touching or rubbing the lesion, which can cause mast cell degranulation. Pharmacotherapy for symptomatic relief includes using H1 antihistamines, such as cetirizine, 10 mg daily, fexofenadine 180 mg daily, or loratadine 10 mg daily, and alternatively H2 antihistamines, including famotidine 20 mg twice daily or cimetidine 400 mg twice daily.

Course: The prognosis for young children is excellent, as spontaneous recovery occurs before puberty; however, follow-up is recommended to assure resolution of clinical manifestations. Should the condition last for more than 2 years, systemic mastocytosis should be considered.

Final comment: The prognosis is excellent, and most cases resolve spontaneously. Rarely, some patients may develop systemic mastocytosis.

HISTIOCYTOSIS

Definition: Cutaneous and mucocutaneous Langerhans cell histiocytosis include a wide range of entities localized to the skin and/or mucosa. All are associated with abnormal infiltrates or collections of histiocytes.

Histiocytosis X (Langerhans Cell Histiocytosis)

Overview: Histiocytosis X is a rare disease of infants and small children, which can resemble seborrheic dermatitis. The diagnosis is made by identifying histiocytes in the epidermis on skin biopsy.

Clinical presentation: These are divided into nonspecific inflammatory response with fever, lethargy, and weight loss and organ-related specific manifestations, including cutaneous and noncutaneous signs.

This includes dermatitis, especially in the intertriginous areas and scalp, ranging from scaly erythematous lesions to red papules. Bone can also be affected with pathologic fractures and bone marrow abnormalities, which results in pancytopenia. There may be hepatomegaly, splenomegaly, and lymphadenopathy in up to 50% of cases. Other less frequent findings involve the hypothalamus leading to diabetes insipidus.

Laboratory studies: The diagnosis is made by identifying histiocytes in the epidermis on histology and pancytopenia and confirmed by immunohistochemistry to identify the cell type of the abnormal cells (Figure 18.14).

Differential diagnosis: It should be distinguished from melanoma, mycosis fungoides, Paget disease, and Bowen disease.

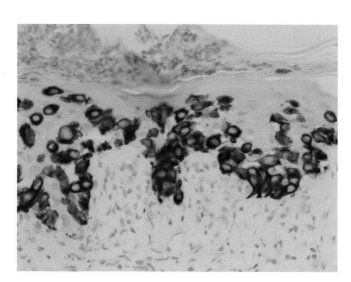

Figure 18.14 Histiocytosis X (Langerhans cell histiocytosis): CD68 immunohistochemical stain (for histiocytes) ×780.

Management: Cutaneous histiocytosis X usually clears spontaneously as the child grows. The limited disease is often managed by local excision, but it may resolve spontaneously. Systemic involvement requires chemotherapy. The prognosis is excellent in the more common limited form of the disease. A comprehensive assessment to identify other sites of disease is very important to address and manage. As spontaneous resolution may occur, a close monitoring is required to rule out multisystem involvement.

Oral methotrexate 20 mg/m^2 weekly is recommended for cutaneous-only disease. 6-mercaptopurine 50 mg/m^2 daily is added, when needed, with dose adjustments made to avoid severe myelosuppression. Hydroxyurea with or without oral methotrexate may also be effective for treating skin involvement in LCH.

Final comment: Histiocytosis X is a rare disease that is diagnosed based on the presence of histiocytes in the tissue. The diffuse disease develops into a chronic form in 60%, achieve remission in 30%, or result in death in up to 10%.

ROSAI-DORFMAN DISEASE

Overview: Rosai-Dorfman disease (R-DD) is a rare, benign disorder with a good prognosis, when the disease is limited to the skin. The etiology of systemic and cutaneous Rosai-Dorfman disease is unknown, but it may be an immune dysfunction reacting to an antigen or infectious organism.

Clinical presentation: Purely cutaneous Rosai-Dorfman disease is rare, and diagnosis is difficult without lymphadenopathy or any distinguishing features of the skin lesion. The lymphadenopathy (Figure 18.15) is usually cervical, painless, and accompanied by fever, neutrophilia, polyclonal hypergammaglobulinemia, hemolytic anemia, and elevated erythrocyte sedimentation rate. The cutaneous disease manifests with nonspecific macules, papules, plaques, or nodules of variable color. Other organ involvement can include the nasal cavity, bone (lytic lesions), orbital tissue, and central nervous system (R-DD may mimic meningioma clinically).

Laboratory studies: A complete blood count is essential. Biopsy of a skin lesion is a crucial part of the diagnosis, and it shows masses of lymphocytes in which collections of histiocytes are noted. The hallmark of the disease is emperipolesis or histiocytes with lymphocytes within their cytoplasm. The histiocytes stain positive for S-100 and CD68 and negative for CD1a and langerin.

Although serologic tests are not conclusive for an etiologic role, many cases of cutaneous Rosai-Dorfman disease have been associated with *Herpes simplex* infection, Epstein-Barr infection, HIV positivity, varicella, or herpes zoster, suggesting that it may be an exaggerated immune response to an infective agent. It is currently recommended that all cases be evaluated for IgG4-positive plasma cells and interpret the level of increase in correlation with an appropriate clinical, serologic, and radiologic context.

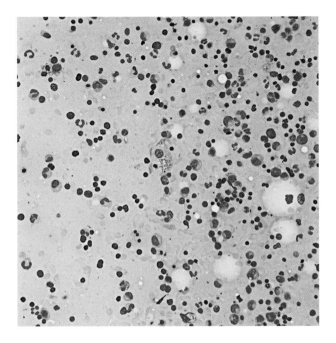

Figure 18.15 Rosai-Dorfman disease. Biopsy showing the accumulation of histiocytes within a broad area of lymphocytes: Trypan blue ×860.

Differential Diagnosis: Cutaneous R-DD should be distinguished from xanthogranuloma. R-DD cases have shown mutations involving genes *MAP2K1, KRAS, NRAS, ARAF,* or *CSF1R*.

Management: Spontaneous regression and recovery often occur over months to years and most cutaneous lesions do not require treatment unless cosmetically unacceptable to the patient. Mortality occurs in up to 10% due to direct complications, infections, and amyloidosis. Patients with asymptomatic and uncomplicated disease may be followed with observation, but surgical excision is recommended in limited or symptomatic lesions. Diffuse irresectable disease requires systemic therapies, including corticosteroids, sirolimus, chemoradiation, and immunomodulatory agents. Targeted therapy for Mitogen-Activated Protein Kinase (MAPK) mutations can be used in severe or refractory disease if driver mutations are identified.

Final Comment: R-DD is a rare histiocytic disorder. It may be sporadic or familial, and the cutaneous disease is considered distinct with unique epidemiologic and clinical features.

XANTHOGRANULOMA

Synonym: Juvenile xanthogranuloma (JXG)

Overview: Xanthogranuloma (XG) is a moderately uncommon, benign, proliferative histiocytic disorder, which originates from dermal factor XIIIa positive dendrocytes. It is the most common of the non-Langerhans cell histiocytosis, occurring predominantly in young children.

Clinical presentation: Typical skin lesions appear as reddish to yellow papules, plaques, or nodules, most often on the head, neck, and upper areas of the trunk (Figure 18.16). Extracutaneous or systemic XG is rare, occurring in up to 4% of all cases, and may involve every organ or system, including the eye.

Laboratory studies: Dermatoscopy shows a yellow-orange central area surrounded by telangiectasias (the "setting sun sign"). In difficult cases, histology and immunohistochemistry are diagnostic; the histopathologic examination shows loss of the rete ridges and sometimes ulceration with a dense infiltrate of foamy histiocytes in the dermis and sometimes in the subcutis. The presence of giant cells and of islands of lymphocytes in the lesion is considered diagnostic (Figure 18.17), although in rare cases one or the other may be absent. A heterogeneous population of inflammatory cells (lymphocytes, plasma cells, eosinophils, and some neutrophils) can be observed.

Differential diagnosis: This may include Langerhans cell histiocytosis (LCH), other xanthomatous lesions, including papular xanthoma, tuberous xanthoma, xanthoma disseminatum, and eruptive xanthoma), Spitz nevusmastocytoma, dermatofibroma, and acrochordon (skin tag).

Management: Cutaneous XG generally regresses spontaneously. Reassurance about the benign course is typically all that is necessary. Surgical removal can be performed.

Final comment: XG is a benign histiocytic disorder with a spontaneous resolution that generally affects predominantly young children. Lesions are commonly found on the head and neck region.

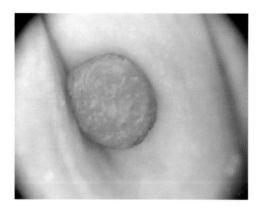

Figure 18.16 Xanthogranuloma. Whitish streak and coalition into small patches.

Source: From Xu J, Ma L. Dermatoscopic Patterns in Juvenile Xanthogranuloma Based on the Histological Classification. Front Med (Lausanne). 2021 Jan 13;7:618946; used under Creative Commons license.

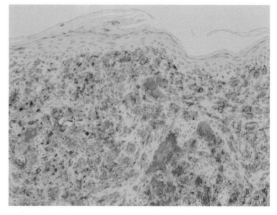

Figure 18.17 Xanthogranuloma of the skin. Note giant cells and collections of lymphocytes in a sea of histiocytes: Immunostain CD68 (histiocyte stain) ×180.

PORPHYRIA

There are a number of different types of porphyria; all are rare except for porphyria cutanea tarda, which is discussed here.

Synonyms: Porphyria cutanea tarda (PCT), symptomatic porphyria, chemical porphyria, toxic porphyria.

Definition: In 1937, Jan Waldenström (1906–1996) named PCT to emphasize the predominant cutaneous manifestations and relatively late onset of disease. PCT is the most common form of porphyria, which is a disease that manifests by an increase in one or more of the porphyrins (heme biochemical products), which causes damage to the skin by a phototoxic process and nervous tissues. There are a number of other types of porphyria, some of which may also produce cutaneous disease; however, all of them are rare.

Overview: PCT is a moderately uncommon disease that occurs due to decreased activity of uroporphyrinogen decarboxylase (UROD), an enzyme responsible for heme biosynthesis. The condition may be inherited (20%) or sporadic (80%), being determined by the presence or absence of heterozygous *UROD* mutations.

Clinical presentation: Risk factors include such activities as alcohol use, smoking, estrogen use (e.g., oral contraceptives), and hepatitis C virus (HCV) infection, as well as hemochromatosis (*HFE*) mutations, which make the individual susceptible for both familial and sporadic disease. Strong occupational hazards include working in machine or automobile body shops or in agriculture, where powerful insecticides are widely used.

Clinically, PCT manifests as chronic blistering photosensitivity, especially on the dorsal hands and other sun-exposed areas (Figure 18.18). This can lead to infection, scarring, and hyper- or hypopigmentation. Particularly prone areas are sites where the underlying tissue undergoes frequent movement as well as sun exposure, such as the dorsal hands and pre-clavicular areas. Early signs may be extremely subtle and may consist entirely of small vesicles on the fingers.

Laboratory studies: Many patients have increased serum transaminases. Plasma and urine total porphyrins are elevated. The measurement of plasma or urinary total porphyrins, if found normal, will exclude PCT and all other blistering cutaneous porphyrias. If total plasma or urine porphyrins are elevated with a predominance of highly carboxylated porphyrins, then plasma peak fluorescence at 620 nm should be tested. Total fecal porphyrins (isocoproporphyrins) in PCT may be either normal or elevated.

A skin biopsy will reveal characteristic histologic features, including subepidermal blisters and deposition of periodic acid Schiff–positive amorphous hyaline material containing immunoglobulin around vessel walls with little inflammation (Figure 18.19). The dermal papillae are frozen in vertical waves, a phenomenon known as "festooning." Such a biopsy is not necessary to diagnose PCT, because the histopathology is not absolutely specific, and documenting the biochemical abnormalities is sufficient to make the diagnosis. Many patients with PCT also have increased hepatic transaminases.

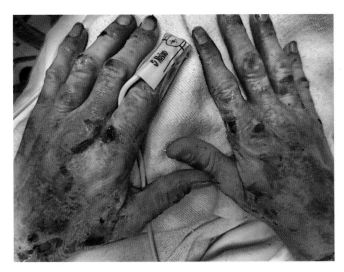

Figure 18.18 Porphyria cutanea tarda. Chronic blistering photosensitivity on the dorsal hands with scarring and hyperpigmentation.

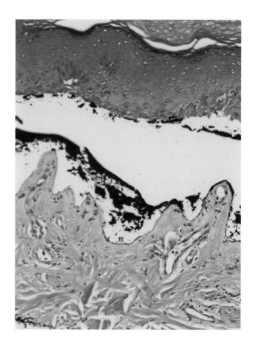

Figure 18.19 Porphyria cutanea tarda. Subepidermal blisters and deposition of periodic acid Schiff–positive amorphous hyaline material containing immunoglobulin around vessel walls with little or no inflammation. The black pigment within the bulla is dye added during processing to identify margins. Periodic acid Schiff stain, ×140.

Management: Phlebotomy and low-dose hydroxychloroquine, 100 mg orally, twice weekly, until at least 1 month after normal plasma levels of porphyrin are achieved. Patients may become anemic, and there may be patient or family resistance to phlebotomy, but it is necessary for proper patient care.

Prognosis: A PCT patient has a normal life expectancy with an excellent prognosis if readily treated. Relapse following successful treatment may occur, especially in patients who resume excessive alcohol intake or occupational hazard. Untreated PCT may predispose to hepatocellular carcinoma or eventually, liver failure.

Final comment: PCT is by far the most common form of porphyria. Clinically, PCT manifests as chronic blistering photosensitivity.

PURPURA

Definition: The word comes from the Latin for *purple*. It represents a subcutaneous or submucosal hemorrhage, which may be related to benign trauma or to a number of life-threatening diseases.

Overview: Purpuric eruptions are subdivided into two types: non-thrombocytopenic (normal platelet) and thrombocytopenic (low platelet). Purpura may result from compromising the vessel walls (trauma, infection, vasculitis, collagen disorders) or due to hemostatic pathology (thrombocytopenia, abnormal platelet function, clotting factor deficiency, or abnormal clotting factor function). Other conditions may be associated with petechiae, including septicemia, immune thrombocytopenia (ITP), hemolytic uremic syndrome, leukemia, and coagulopathies (e.g., hemophilia). Non-thrombocytopenic purpura may result from coagulation disorders, connective tissue disorders, scurvy, or vasculitis. Thrombocytopenic purpura may be due to medications, immune disorders, septicemia, Rocky Mountain spotted fever, or systemic lupus erythematous.

Clinical presentation: Based on size, purpura may be called petechiae (pinpoint hemorrhage less than 2 mm) or ecchymoses (larger confluent lesions). Ecchymoses may be tender or raised. Clinically, lesions of purpura do not blanch, when pressure is applied to the skin, unlike other erythematous or vascular skin lesions.

Patients with COVID-19-related purpura may present with fixed livedo racemose, retiform purpura, or necrotic vascular lesions, which are due to the ability of the virus to induce intravascular coagulopathy of small vessels (Figures 18.20–18.22).

Purpura is common in the elderly (Figure 18.23), due to fracture of vessel walls or to anticoagulant medications. In younger patients, purpura is uncommon and may indicate an underlying disease, which may require immediate attention despite the patient's deceptively normal appearance. In any patient, rapid onset of purpura requires immediate medical evaluation.

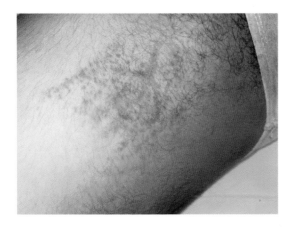

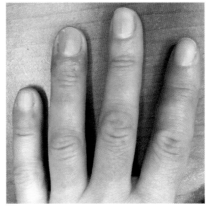

Figure 18.20 COVID-19 patient with a purpuric eruption on the thigh.

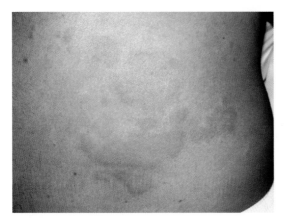

Figure 18.21 Urticaria and dusky erythema (chilblains-like lesions) in a COVID-19 patient. Lesions related to COVID-19 may also appear similar to dermatoses unrelated to COVID-19.

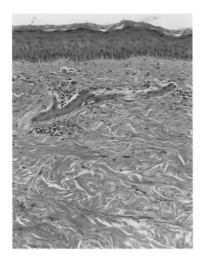

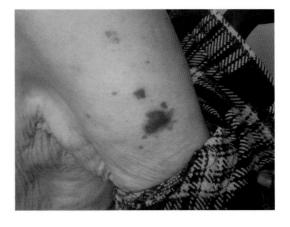

Figure 18.22 Cutaneous intravascular coagulation in COVID-19 related lesions. This finding is often observed even in lesions that appear similar to entities unrelated to COVID-19 (hematoxylin and eosin ×480).

Figure 18.23 Senile purpura.

Palpable purpura may require immediate treatment, possibly with an antimicrobial is the cause is often bacterial. Rocky Mountain spotted fever is a common cause of palpable purpura on the east coast of the United States. Nonpalpable purpura may present as nonpalpable petechiae, such as in cases of fat embolism, and may indicate rapid consumption of platelets. Purpura fulminans is vasculitis that produces palpable ecchymoses, and it is usually progressive and requires immediate attention.

Pigmented purpuric dermatoses (PPDs): It is known as capillaritis, purpura simplex, and inflammatory purpura without vasculitis, are a group of chronic, benign, cutaneous eruptions characterized by the presence of petechiae, purpura, and increased skin pigmentation. PPDs most commonly occur on the lower extremities and may be asymptomatic or pruritic.

Schamberg's disease (Schamberg's purpura; progressive pigmentary purpura) was first described by Jay Frank Schamberg (1870–1934) in 1901. Schamberg's disease presents with discrete, nonblanchable red-brown purpuric patches (Figure 18.24). It is moderately common among middle-aged or elderly individuals and most frequently affects the legs. It is usually asymptomatic, but patients may experience mild pruritus. It takes a chronic course, with numerous exacerbations and remissions. Spontaneous resolution also may occur.

Laboratory studies: Complete blood count (CBC) with a peripheral smear, prothrombin time (PT) with an international normalized ratio (INR), and activated partial thromboplastin time (aPTT) can help establish the diagnosis of any underlying conditions. The CBC identifies abnormalities in different hematologic cell components, including platelet number and presence of anemia or leukopenia, and provides evidence for intravascular hemolysis. The PT evaluates the extrinsic clotting pathway (factors VII, IX, II, X, V, and fibrinogen), and aPTT assesses the intrinsic pathway (factors HWMK, kallikrein, XII, XI, IX, VIII, II, X, V, and fibrinogen).

Management: Patients with purpura who appear ill or are febrile require rapid evaluation and treatment for serious hemorrhage, disseminated intravascular coagulopathy, or infection when present. Patients with abnormal vital signs warrant emergent attention and stabilization. A directed history, physical examination, and pertinent laboratory studies should target likely underlying etiologies, including serious trauma and bacterial sepsis (especially meningococcemia). Empiric antimicrobial treatment is sometimes warranted.

Depending on the cause, other useful treatments may include corticosteroids, intravenous immunoglobulin, and other drug therapies to achieve platelet count ≥50,000/mm³: romiplostim (1 mcg/kg subcutaneous injection once weekly), eltrombopag (50 mg orally once daily) or

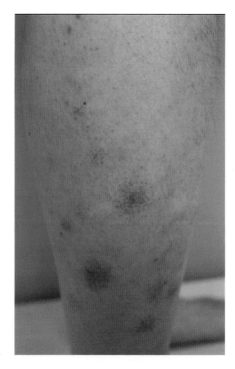

Figure 18.24 Schamberg disease. Characteristic "cayenne pepper" pigmentation on the lower leg.

Source: From: Kim DH, Seo SH, Ahn HH, et al. Characteristics and Clinical Manifestations of Pigmented Purpuric Dermatosis. Ann Dermatol. 2015;27:404–410; used under Creative Commons license.

rituximab (IV infusion: 375 mg/m^2 once weekly for 4 doses). Splenectomy is reserved in some particular cases and causes if medications are not effective. In emergencies, when purpura causes extreme bleeding, transfusions of platelet concentrates, corticosteroids, and immunoglobulin may be used.

FINAL THOUGHT

This group of diseases may represent a disparate number of cutaneous maladies, some of which resolve on their own and others that require significant attention.

ADDITIONAL READINGS

Abla O, Jacobsen E, Picarsic J, et al. Consensus recommendations for the diagnosis and clinical management of Rosai-Dorfman-Destombes disease. Blood. 2018;131:2877–2890.

Atmatzidis DH, Hoegler K, Weiss A, et al. Unsafe deposits: overlapping cutaneous manifestations of porphyria cutanea tarda, ochronosis, hemochromatosis, and argyria. Skinmed. 2019;17:161–170.

Bankova LG, Walter JE, Iyengar SR, et al. Generalized bullous eruption after routine vaccination in a child with diffuse cutaneous mastocytosis. J Allergy Clin Immunol Pract. 2013;1:94–96.

Buck T, González LM, Schwartz RA, et al. Acute neutrophilic dermatosis (Sweet's syndrome) with hematologic disorders: a review and reappraisal. Int J Dermatol. 2008;47:775–782.

Hartmann K, Escribano L, Grattan C, et al. Cutaneous manifestations in patients with mastocytosis: consensus report of the European Competence Network on Mastocytosis; the American Academy of Allergy, Asthma & Immunology; and the European Academy of Allergology and Clinical Immunology. J Allergy Clin Immunol. 2016 Jan;137:35–45.

Lima AL, Illing T, Schliemann S, et al. Cutaneous manifestations of diabetes mellitus: a review. Am J Clin Dermatol. 2017;18:541–553.

Méni C, Bruneau J, Georgin-Lavialle S, et al. Paediatric mastocytosis: a systematic review of 1747 cases. Br J Dermatol. 2015;172:642–651.

Newman B, Hu W, Nigro K, et al. Aggressive histiocytic disorders that can involve the skin. J Am Acad Dermatol. 2007;56:302–316.

Piette EW, Rosenbach M. Granuloma annulare: pathogenesis, disease associations and triggers, and therapeutic options. J Am Acad Dermatol. 2016;75:467–479.

Rochet NM, Chavan RN, Cappel MA, et al. Sweet syndrome: clinical presentation, associations, and response to treatment in 77 patients. J Am Acad Dermatol. 2013;69:557–564.

Schwartz RA, Lambert WC. COVID-19 Specific skin changes related to SARS-CoV-2: visualizing a monumental public health challenge. Clin Dermatol (in press).

19 Benign Neoplasms

Abdullah Demirbaş, Ömer Faruk Elmas, and Necmettin Akdeniz

CONTENTS

Overview: Most benign cutaneous neoplasms can be diagnosed clinically. If the diagnosis is uncertain clinically, especially when there have been unexpected changes in the appearance of the lesion, a biopsy is indicated.

LENTIGO SIMPLEX

Synonyms: Simple lentigo

    Definition: This is a small melanocytic lesion characterized by proliferation of benign melanocytes on the basal layer without nesting.

    Overview: Lentigo simplex is a common, benign, hyperpigmented macule located anywhere on the body. These lentigines typically occur early in life and are not associated with exposure to sunlight. This is due to a slight increase in the number of normal epidermal melanocytes that produce increased amounts of melanin.

    Clinical presentation: Lesions are small hyperpigmented macules with a diameter generally not exceeding 5 mm. They are located anywhere on the trunk, extremities, genitals, and mucous membranes. (Figure 19.1) The number of lesions may range from few to many. Lentigines may also be seen in patients with xeroderma pigmentosum, Peutz-Jegher disease, Addison disease, Carney complex, LEOPARD (lentigines, ECG changes, ocular hypertelorism, pulmonary stenosis, abnormal genitalia, growth retardation, and deafness), Laugier Hunziker, and Bannayan-Riley-Ruvalcaba.

    Xeroderma pigmentosum is a rare autosomal recessive disorder characterized by photosensitivity, pigment changes, premature aging of the skin, and the development of malignant tumors. These symptoms are caused by a cellular hypersensitivity to ultraviolet (UV) radiation as a result of a DNA repair defect.

DOI: 10.1201/9781003105268-19

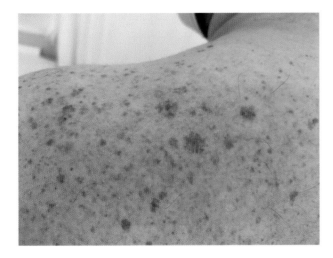

Figure 19.1 Numerous lentigo simplexes due to sun damage are seen on the back of the patient.

Source: Courtesy of Istanbul Medeniyet University Dermatology Clinic.

Peutz-Jeghers syndrome (PJS) is an autosomal dominant hereditary disorder characterized by intestinal hamartomatous polyps associated with a distinct pattern of cutaneous and mucosal melanin deposition.

Addison's disease is delineated by mucocutaneous pigmentation, usually with autoimmune destruction of adrenal cortex cells.

Carney complex is an autosomal dominant condition with spotty skin pigmentation, endocrinopathy, and endocrine and non-endocrine tumors.

Laugier-Hunziker syndrome (LHS) is an idiopathic macular hyperpigmentation characterized by mucosal brownish-black patches and longitudinal melanonychia.

Bannayan-Riley-Ruvalcaba syndrome is characterized by macrocephaly, pigmented macules on the glans penis and benign mesodermal hamartomas.

Laboratory studies: Dermatoscopy may show a reticular pattern, while histologic examination will reveal melanocytic proliferation and epidermal hyperplasia.

Differential diagnosis: There may be confusion with *in situ* lentiginous melanoma, lentiginous junctional nevus, dysplastic nevus, and solar lentigo, especially the Spitzoid lentigo variant.

Management: Surgical removal is indicated only when there is a question in the differential diagnosis. Chemical peels, cryosurgery, and laser treatments can lighten or remove lesions.

MELANOTIC MACULE

Definition: This represents a well-defined pigmented lesion due to basal cell pigmentation.

Overview: The melanotic macule is a benign hyperpigmentation of mucous membranes found in about 3% of the general population. There is an increase in focal melanin accumulation without an increase in melanocytes. Lesions are most often located on the vermillion border of the lip, more often on the upper lip.

Clinical presentation: This well-circumscribed lesion has a diameter less than 1 cm, typically due to trauma to the lip. It can also be found on the buccal or genital mucosa, nail bed, and nail matrix. There be an association with LHS and Peutz-Jeghers syndrome. Long-term psoralen plus UVA (PUVA) therapy may also create such a melanocytic macule.

LHS is a rare, benign macular hyperpigmentation of mucocutaneous surfaces and the nails. Although there have been a small number of familial cases reported, no putative genetic abnormalities have been confirmed, and this is usually believed to be an acquired disorder. PJS is a rare autosomal dominant syndrome associated with both mucocutaneous pigmentation and multiple hamartomatous intestinal polyps.

Laboratory studies: Histologic study will reveal significant epidermal pigmentation without an increase in melanocytes and pigment-laden macrophages in the papillary dermis.

Differential diagnosis: Melanoma and melanoacanthoma should be considered; however, primary and metastatic melanoma are rarely seen intraorally. Melanoacanthoma is an uncommon condition that is most often found on the buccal mucosa in young African American women. The lesion is typically much larger (>1 cm or) than a melanotic macule and usually follows a characteristic spontaneous cycle of evolution within days to weeks.

Management: This is optional with cryosurgery If treatment is required, macules can be treated with cryotherapy or laser surgery

SOLAR LENTIGO

Synonyms: Actinic lentigo, lentigo senilis

Definition: These are brown macules occurring on sun-exposed areas.

Overview: This represents a benign patch of darkened skin. It results from exposure to UV light, which induces local melanocyte proliferation and melanin aggregation in the keratinocytes. Solar lentigines are very common, especially in people older than 40 years of age.

Clinical presentation: Lesions are characterized by milky dark brown macules with irregular borders following chronic ultraviolet exposure. Lesions are more predominant in older patients with lighter skin phenotypes. Dermatoscopy of a solar lentigo may show a faint pigment network, fingerprint structures, or uniform pigmentation. A "moth-eaten border," or a sharply demarcated indentation, can be seen.

Laboratory studies: Histologic examination shows a significant increase in pigmentation in the basal layer together with solar elastosis and pigment-laden macrophages in the dermis.

Differential diagnosis: This lesion may resemble a seborrheic keratosis or simple lentigo.

Management: Treatment with keratolytics, cryosurgery, laser surgery, or curettage and electro-desiccation is optional.

MELANOCYTIC NEVUS

Synonym: Mole

Definition: Melanocytic nevus is a common hamartomatous lesions that can first occur in childhood.

Overview: This represents a pigmented or nonpigmented lesion, which typically appears within the first 6 months of life, reaches maximum size and number in young adulthood, and then disappears with advancing age. Common acquired nevi are made up of nevomelanocytic nests and are classified according to the nests' histologic location (e.g., junctional, compound, or intradermal).

Clinical presentation:

- Junctional nevus is a brown-black well-circumscribed macule with a diameter smaller than 0.5 cm. (Figure 19.2)

- Compound nevus are brown nodules or papules arising from the surface. (Figure 19.3)

- Intradermal nevus (dermal) is a skin-colored or light-brown polypoid lesions, often without pigment. (Figure 19.4)

- Variants include balloon cell nevus, inverted type A nevus, eccrine-centric nevus, and Cockade nevus.

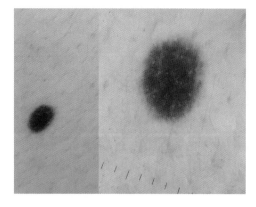

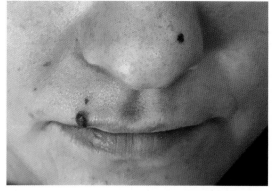

Figure 19.2 (a) Junctional nevus and (b) dermoscopic view on the skin of the back.

Source: Courtesy of Istanbul Medeniyet University Dermatology Clinic.

Figure 19.3 A compound nevus on the upper lip vermilion and a junctional nevus on the nose.

Source: Courtesy of Istanbul Medeniyet University Dermatology Clinic.

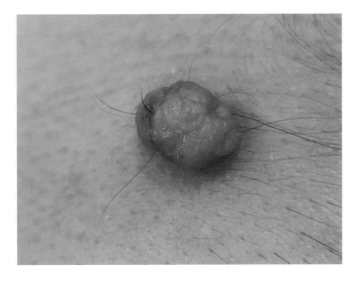

Figure 19.4 Dermal nevus is seen the skin above the eyebrow.

Source: Courtesy of Istanbul Medeniyet University Dermatology Clinic.

Laboratory studies: This consists of intraepidermal and dermal collection of nevus cells. The cells have round, ovoid, or fusiform shapes within the junctional nests and are arranged in cohesive nests. The cells generally have epithelioid cell features in the superficial part of the dermis and contain amphophilic cytoplasm and, frequently, granular melanin. The nucleus has uniform chromatin with a slightly clumped texture. Deeper in the dermis, there is reduced cytoplasm content. Acquired nevi are classified as junctional, compound, or intradermal according to their histologic features. Melanocytes in junctional and compound nevus are positive for HMB-45, Melan A, and NKI/C3, while loss of HMB-45 expression can be observed in melanocytes in intradermal nevus.

Differential diagnosis: The most important differential diagnosis of acquired melanocytic lesions is melanoma. Histologically, lesions differ from melanoma by having small nucleolus of the melanocytes, absence of atypical mitoses, uniformity of cells, normal maturation, and nesting.

Management: Total surgical excision may be performed when there is concern for a melanoma. Because a nevus generally about 30s, removal is generally optional.

CONGENITAL NEVUS

Synonym: Birth mark

Definition: Congenital nevi appear at birth and are caused by benign melanocyte proliferation in the dermis, epidermis, or both. Occasionally, nevi that are not present at birth but are histologically similar to congenital nevi may develop within the first 2 years of life. Tardive congenital nevus is the term for this condition.

Overview: It results from a proliferation in the dermis, epidermis, or both of benign melanocytes. Nevi that are not present at birth but are histologically identical to congenital nevi, may develop during the first 2 years of life. The estimated incidence is approximately 1% and are classified separately due to their frequently unique clinical and pathologic characteristics, which make it possible to distinguish between commonly acquired nevi.

Clinical presentation: It is most common on the trunk or extremities. They are defined as small (<1.5 cm in diameter), medium (1.5–19 cm), and giant congenital nevi (>20 cm) according to their size (Figure 19.5). Small and medium-sized congenital nevi are often ovoid and sharply circumscribed. These lesions may be skin-colored or light brown. In addition, hypertrichosis and perifollicular hyperpigmentation may be observed. Giant congenital nevi are often asymmetric with irregular borders and dark brown with hairs within. Over time, a nodular or verrucous lesion may occur within. Satellite lesions can be observed around medium and giant congenital nevi. Variants include the desmoplastic congenital nevus and kissing nevus.

Laboratory studies: Histologically, congenital nevi can resemble junctional, compound, and intradermal melanocytic lesions; however, unlike the acquired nevus, melanocytes show a diffuse distribution by spreading between the reticular dermis, collagen fibers in subcutaneous adipose tissue, and fat cells. They can also be seen in the surrounding eccrine glands, sebaceous glands,

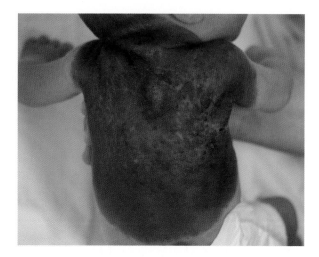

Figure 19.5 Giant congenital nevus is seen, which covers a large part of the body of the baby.

Source: Courtesy of Istanbul Medeniyet University Dermatology Clinic.

and hair follicles. This is called adnexal colonization. In addition, melanocytes may also show intraepidermal spread.

Differential diagnosis: Dysplastic nevus and congenital melanoma should be considered in the differential.

Prognosis: The risk of melanoma in giant congenital nevi is much higher than in the normal population. About 70% of childhood melanomas may be caused by giant congenital nevi. In contrast, the rate of melanoma development is low in small and medium-sized congenital nevi.

Management: Two factors are primarily associated with the treatment of congenital melanocytic nevi: their increased risk of progression to melanoma and their cosmetically disfiguring appearance. The decision to remove a congenital nevus is individually tailored and based on melanoma risk, age, anatomy, location, nevus quality, cosmetic outcome, and complication rates. Routine excision of small and medium-sized congenital nevi is not performed due to low risk for melanoma. Baseline photography and annual observation is an acceptable alternative. Giant congenital nevi can be observed closely, or removal can be considered. Apart from surgery, laser treatments can be used as an alternative.

HALO NEVUS

Synonym: Halo nevus of Sutton

Definition: This is a well-circumscribed nevus with a slightly raised, pigmented area and a surrounding depigmented halo, first described by Richard L. Sutton, Sr. (1879–1952).

Overview: This is a unique lesion where a centrally placed, generally pigmented nevus is surrounded by a hypo- or depigmentation halo of about 1–5 mm. It typically occurs in younger patients. The cause of spontaneous pigmentation loss is unknown, but melanocytes and nevus cells appear to be linked to immunologic destruction.

Clinical presentation: It is characterized as a 0.5-cm lesions with a dark brown to black area in the center with a depigmented halo. (Figure 19.6) This nevus, which is often solitary, is typically located on the trunk. Observations have shown that the halo nevi lasts for 10 years or longer, but a wide subgroup goes through different phases, eventually regressing entirely. The process takes an average of 8 years.

Laboratory studies: Histologically, it is characterized by a dense lymphocyte and histiocyte dermal infiltration intersperse between melanocytes.

Differential diagnosis: In patients who present with a halo nevus at an older age, melanoma of any location should be suspected. As compared with the symmetry found in the halo nevus, an asymmetric, irregular halo may be seen with melanoma, but asymmetry does not equate with malignancy. Melanoma is typified by other attributes such as generally >1 cm in size, irregular or notched borders, and marked color irregularity. Multiple halo nevi may be a sign of ocular or cutaneous melanoma elsewhere, particularly in older adults.

Management: A patient with a halo nevus should be given a total body scan and about a personal or family history of cutaneous melanoma, atypical nevi, and vitiligo. If the lesion is atypical, it should be removed.

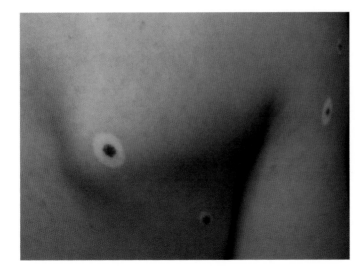

Figure 19.6 Halo Nevi: Depigmented areas are seen around the multiply pigmented nevi on the back of the body.

Source: Courtesy of Istanbul Medeniyet University Dermatology Clinic.

SPITZ NEVUS

Synonym: Spindle and epithelioid nevus, juvenile melanoma

Definition: Spitz nevi are This is a benign melanocytic lesion commonly found in childhood and first described by Sophie Spitz (1910–1956).

Overview: It is a rare type of melanocytic nevus that typically presents as a solitary, small pink to reddish-brown papule primarily on faces and extremities of children.

Clinical presentation: It is a pink to red well-circumscribed papule that may occur more often in childhood and adolescence than in adults. It is frequently located on the face, head, neck, arms, and legs and is typically less than 0.5 cm in diameter. Variants include the desmoplastic, plexiform, angiomatoid, pigmented spindle cell, and pagetoid type.

Laboratory studies: Histologic examination demonstrates acanthosis and hyperkeratosis in the epidermis, edema in the papillary dermis, and telangiectatic vessels. At the dermo-epidermal junction, there are vertically located melanocytes forming large nest structures. In addition, eosinophilic structures, known as Kamino bodies, consisting of collagen fibers can be seen in the subepidermal area.

Differential diagnosis: A spitzoid malignant melanoma differs from a Spitz nevus, which is symmetric, well circumscribed, and without atypical mitoses.

Management: Lesions can be removed for histologic assessment due to the diagnostic difficulties encountered in the classification of Spitz nevi; however, follow-up of lesions that are not clinically atypical is recommended. In addition, it is recommended that patients with atypical lesions have periodic evaluations.

BLUE NEVUS OF JADASSOHN

Definition: This is a benign nevus composed of melanocytes with pigmented dendritic cells in the dermis, first described by Josef Jadassohn (1863–1936).

Overview: It is a smooth macule, papule, or plaque that is gray-blue to bluish-black in color. Lesions are usually solitary and found on the head and neck, sacral region, and dorsal aspects of the hands and feet.

Clinical presentation: A lesion is typically a blue to gray-black papule, no more than to 1 cm in diameter. It occurs more often in women, with no age preference, on the dorsal surface of the hand or foot and sometimes on the face, scalp, or thigh (Figure 19.7).

Laboratory studies: Histologically, the dermis contains darkly pigmented bipolar dendritic cells and melanophages extending parallel to the epidermis. Melanocytes will stain positive with HMB-45, Melan A, MITF-1, and S-100. The common blue nevus is associated with nests and fascicles of spindle-shaped cells with abundant pale cytoplasm containing little or no melanin.

Differential diagnosis: This may be confused with a desmoplastic Spitz nevus, dermatofibroma, tattoo, graphite tattoo, or melanoma.

Prognosis: Malignant transformation is rare.

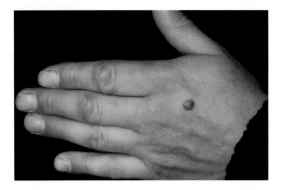

Figure 19.7   Blue nevus on hand.

Source: Courtesy of Istanbul Medeniyet University Dermatology Clinic.

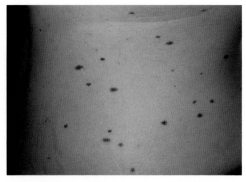

Figure 19.8   Multiple dysplastic nevi are seen on the trunk of the patient with dysplastic nevus syndrome.

Source: Courtesy of Istanbul Medeniyet University Dermatology Clinic.

Management: There is no need to remove a single blue nevus, unless there are atypical features or the development of multinodular or plaque-like lesions or changing lesions.

NEVUS OF ITO/OTA

Synonym: Oculodermal melanocytosis, nevus fuscoceruleus opthalmomaxillaris, nevus fuscoceruleus acromiodeltoideus

Definition: Lesions are gray-bluish nevi composed of bipolar dendritic melanocytes in the dermis.

Overview: The nevus of Ota is a blue-gray or brown patch found on the face in the distribution of the first and second branches of the trigeminal nerve (i.e., the forehead, periorbital, temple, and cheek regions), while the nevus of Ito w is restricted to the neck, shoulder, and adjacent areas of the arm. Both nevus of Ota and Ito persist into adulthood and sometimes darken in appearance. They may accompany vascular malformations, including Sturge-Weber or Klippel-Trenaunay syndromes.

Clinical presentation: Nevus of Ota occurs at birth and is seen in areas innervated by the ophthalmic and maxillary branches of the trigeminal nerve, where there may be periocular pigmentation, often including the sclera and conjunctiva. In the nevus of Ito, which is found on the shoulder or scapula, the pigmented areas that are innervated by the localized nerves.

Laboratory studies: In both nevus of Ota and Ito, histology is characterized by increased epidermal basal pigmentation and bipolar dendritic melanocytes in the dermis.

Differential diagnosis: Similar lesions include the sun nevus (acquired nevus of Ota) and Hori nevus. Acquired bilateral nevus of Ota-like macules, also known as Hori nevus, is one of the most frequently acquired dermal facial melanocytosis in dark-skinned people, particularly in Asian women. Other presentations that could be considered are blue nevus of Jadassohn, congenital dermal melanocytosis, cutaneous melanoma, drug-induced pigmentation, hairy nevus, lentigo, melasma, ochronosis, and phytophotodermatitis.

Prognosis: Rarely nevus of Ito may progress to cutaneous melanoma.

Management: Laser treatment is optional.

CONGENITAL DERMAL MELANOCYTOSIS

Synonyms: Mongolian blue spot, slate gray nevus, lumbosacral dermal melanocytosis

Definition: This lesion represents gray-blue dermal melanosis on the lumbosacral area.

Overview: Congenital dermal melanocytosis is a type of birthmark. They are flat blue or bluegrey patches with an irregular border that usually occur at birth or soon after. The most common locations of congenital dermal melanocytosis are the base of the spine, buttocks, back, and shoulders. It is frequently observed in those of Asian and African ancestry.

Clinical presentation: The typical lesion is a congenital blue-gray patch on the lower part of the back or the buttocks and can spread to cover large areas. It may also be seen in other areas, such as the legs, abdomen, and arms, including the shoulder. Congenital dermal melanocytosis may accompany cleft palate and Hurler syndrome. Usually, the lesion regresses by adolescence.

Laboratory studies: Histologic study reveals melanocytes in the reticular dermis that extend parallel to the epidermis, which can also spread to the subcutaneous adipose tissue.

Differential diagnosis: Nevus of Ota, nevus of Ito, Hori nevus, and ecchymosis should be considered in the differential.

Management: The lesion may be removed for cosmetic reasons or to allay concern over malignancy. This may be accomplished by surgical excision or by laser surgery.

DYSPLASTIC NEVUS

Synonyms: Atypical nevus, Clark's nevus (see Chapter 20).

Recurrent Nevus

Synonym: Persistent nevus

Definition: This represents the reappearance of a melanocytic nevus in scar tissue following incomplete removal, first recognized by Wallace Clark (1924–1997).

Overview: This results from an incomplete excision by superficial shaving techniques, which is a typical practice for the management of benign pigmented lesions and biopsies.

Clinical presentation: Lesions represent the irregular reproliferation of melanocytes in the prior procedural area. These nevi often mimic melanoma and have even been called pseudomelanoma. Recurrent nevi can develop months to years after the procedure.

Laboratory Studies: Histologic examination may reveal asymmetric lentiginous proliferation and irregular nest structures in the scar tissue. In a recurrent nevus, melanocytic proliferation generally does not exceed the borders of scar tissue.

Differential diagnosis: Melanoma should be considered, as the tumor could have regressed. Other lesions to consider include a benign nevus, dysplastic nevus, halo nevus of Sutton, acquired nevus of Ota (sun nevus), or Hori nevus.

Management: No treatment is generally required for a recurrent nevus due to the supportive clinical history and the benign nature of the previously removed nevus. If the patient cannot provide the history of the previous removal, the current lesion should be excised.

Ephelis

Synonym: Freckle

Definition: These are small, well-circumscribed pigmented macules seen in sun-exposed areas.

Overview: This is a small, well-demarcated, hyperpigmented macule present often in large numbers on sun-exposed skin. Most ephelides develop during childhood in susceptible light-skinned individuals. Lesions are usually darkened with prolonged sun-exposure.

Clinical presentation: Ephelides are seen as light tan to dark brown pigmented macules with a diameter of 1–3 mm in sun-exposed areas, such as the face, dorsal surfaces of the arms and legs, chest, and upper portion of the back (Figure 19.9). Lesions are more prominent in fair-skinned individuals, particularly of Celtic ethnicity. Lesions may increase in numbers as the patient grows older and probably has had additional sun exposure.

Laboratory studies: Histologically, the number of melanocytes remains the same, while the number of melanosomes increases. This is due to a rise in melanin pigment transfer from increased melanogenesis.

Differential diagnosis: Lentigo simplex, solar lentigo, cafe au lait macules, and junctional nevi should be considered in the differential.

Management: Because ephelides occur and darken with increased UV radiation, it is helpful to decrease sun exposure. Use of sunscreen year-round can be helpful. Topical treatments, such as hydroquinone and retinoids, can help lighten lesions, and laser treatments can be effective as well.

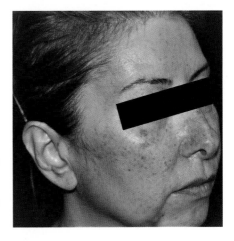

Figure 19.9 A large number of ephelids are seen on the face.

Source: Courtesy of Istanbul Medeniyet University Dermatology Clinic.

237

BECKER'S NEVUS

Synonyms: Becker melanosis, Becker's pigmentary hamartoma, nevoid melanosis, pigmented hairy epidermal nevus

Definition: A Becker's nevus is a unilateral, hyperpigmented, and hypertrichotic patch that is often seen in men.

Overview: Becker nevus is a late-onset epidermal nevus or birthmark found predominantly in men. It is caused by overgrowth of the epidermis, melanocytes, and hair follicles. It occurs on the shoulders or upper part of the trunk during childhood or adolescence, but rarely elsewhere. Circulating androgens have been implicated, which is why it can occur in men during puberty. It was first described by Samuel Becker, Jr. (1924–2007).

Clinical presentation: Becker's nevi are seen in young adulthood and may occur after intense UV exposure. Lesions generally have a unilateral distribution. Although lesions often involve the shoulder area, they can also be seen on the face, neck, arms, legs, and gluteal regions. Lesions are light to dark brown in color and range in size from a few centimeters to 15 cm. Hypertrichosis may develop in lesions (Figure 19.10).

Laboratory studies: Histologic study will show papillomatosis, acanthosis, and hyperkeratosis. In addition, melanin transfer from melanocytes to keratinocytes increases, and the number of melanocytes can be observed as normal or slightly increased without causing a nest.

Differential diagnosis: Lesions may be confused with cafe au lait macules, congenital melanocytic nevus, neurofibroma, and congenital smooth muscle hamartoma.

Prognosis: Patients with Becker nevus can be investigated for soft tissue and boney anomalies.

Management: Laser treatments can reduce hyperpigmentation and hypertrichosis.

CAFE AU LAIT MACULES

Definition: Cafe au lait macules (CALMs) are well-circumscribed, uniform, light to dark brown macules or patches that are typically between 2–5 cm.

Overview: CALMs are hyperpigmented lesions that can differ in color from light to dark brown. They are caused by the aggregation of pigment-producing melanocytes in the epidermis. These spots are usually permanent and can grow or increase in number over time. CALMs are mostly harmless, but syndromes, such as neurofibromatosis type 1 and McCune Albright syndrome, can be associated.

Clinical presentation: CALMs are homogeneous light to dark brown macules or patches with sharp borders. They can be observed anywhere on the body, except for the mucosa. Lesions typically occur in infancy and early childhood. They can be seen in 10% of the normal population without any underlying disease (Figure 19.11).

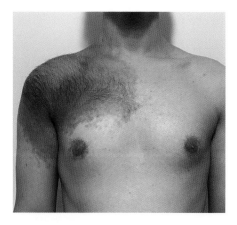

Figure 19.10 Becker nevus covering the acromiodeltoid region.

Source: Courtesy of Istanbul Medeniyet University Dermatology Clinic.

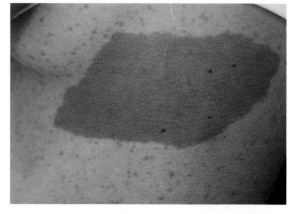

Figure 19.11 Giant cafe au lait macules lait in a patient with neurofibromatosis.

Source: Courtesy of Istanbul Medeniyet University Dermatology Clinic.

Laboratory studies: Histologic study will reveal a normal epidermis but with an increase of melanin in the basal layer keratinocytes.

Differential diagnosis: Other similar lesions include Becker's nevus, linear nevoid hyperpigmentation, nevus spilus, and mastocytoma.

Management: Laser treatment can be helpful in lightening lesions. Greater response has been described in lesions with jagged borders in contrast to those with smooth borders.

CHERRY ANGIOMA

Synonyms: Cherry hemangioma, Senile angioma, Campbell de Morgan spot

Definition: This is the most common adult type of cutaneous vascular lesions, and its frequency increases with age. It was first described by Campbell de Morgan (1811–1876).

Overview: Although its pathogenesis is unclear, the increase in number and size during pregnancy and its disappearance in the postpartum period indicates that hormonal factors may play a role. In addition, a cherry angioma has been reported in women with high serum prolactin levels. Lesions can be seen in both sexes. Some lesions occur in young adulthood, but the incidence gradually increases over the age of 30 years. Originally thought to be paraneoplastic, cherry angiomas are benign.

Clinical presentation: It is a few millimeters in size and is polypoid, bright to deep red, slightly raised papule (Figure 19.12). They are most common on the trunk and proximal aspects of the arms and legs. It often remains unchanged but can bleed when traumatized.

Laboratory studies: Histologic presentation include congestion and ectatic vascular proliferation in the papillary dermis.

Differential diagnosis: Glomeruloid hemangiomas seen in polyneuropathy, organomegaly, endocrinopathy, monoclonal gammopathy, and skin lesions (POEMS) syndrome, angiokeratoma, pyogenic granuloma, and angiosarcoma can be considered. POEMS syndrome is a rare multisystemic condition that occurs in the setting of plasma cell dyscrasia.

Management: Surgical removal, electrocauterization, or laser treatment can be performed for cosmetic reasons.

CYSTS

Definition: Cutaneous cysts are sac-like lesions containing liquid or semisolid material. Although genetic and environmental factors can impact the occurrence of cysts, the etiologic reasons are unclear. There are many types of cysts that differ in their histologic features.

Infundibular Cyst

Synonyms: Epidermoid cyst, keratinous cyst, epidermal inclusion cyst, wen

Overview: This is a benign lesion characterized by an epithelial wall containing all layers of the epidermis. It is located in the dermis and subcutis. It constitutes 80–90% of all cysts and can originate from epithelial cells in the follicular infundibulum region for no apparent reason or develop either as result of trauma or surgical implantation of follicular or epithelial cells.

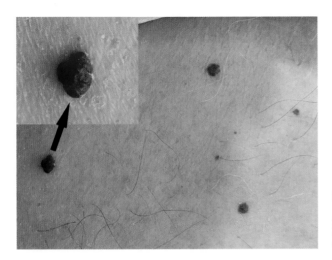

Figure 19.12   Cherry angiomas.

Source: Courtesy of Istanbul Medeniyet University Dermatology Clinic.

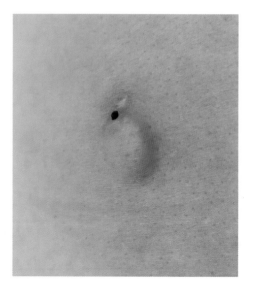

Figure 19.13 Epidermal inclusion cyst: Contains cyst and a black punctum.

Source: Courtesy of Istanbul Medeniyet University Dermatology Clinic.

Clinical presentation: It can create an irregular nodule on the skin surface. This is dependent on its proximity to the epidermis and size of the cyst. Although an epidermoid cyst can appear anywhere on the body, the most commonly location includes the head, neck, chest, and back (Figure 19.13). It is usually asymptomatic and only of cosmetic concern, but when infected, inflamed, or traumatized, there can be erythema, sensitivity, warmth, tenderness, and pain.

Laboratory studies: Histologic study will show a lining mimicking the epidermis with the granular cell layer present.

Differential diagnosis: A tumor, skin metastasis, calcinosis cutis, and foreign body granuloma can be considered. If multiple infundibular cysts are present, the possibility of relevant syndromes should be investigated in the right clinical context, including Gardner's syndrome, Gorlin's syndrome, and pachyonychia congenita type 2.

Management: Treatment includes intralesional steroid injection, incision and drainage, surgical removal, or cryosurgery. Antimicrobials may be used if infected or for anti-inflammatory properties. Even with intervention, a cyst may recur.

Milium

Overview: Milia can be congenital or acquired and are common in all age groups. The congenital type can be seen as many small papules around the nose, which can regress spontaneously in 3–4 weeks. Diseases, such as Maria-Unna hypotrichosis and oral-facial-digital syndrome, should be considered for congenital types that are more generalized and do not disappear spontaneously. Acquired milia can also occur secondary to diseases that cause subepidermal bulla formation, such as epidermolysis bullosa, porphyria cutanea tarda, and bullous pemphigoid.

Clinical presentation: A milium is a small, superficial type of cyst with a diameter of 1–2 mm and white-yellow color.

Laboratory studies: Its histology is similar to a very small epidermoid cyst.

Differential diagnosis: The differential diagnosis of milium involves sebaceous hyperplasia, syringoma, molluscum contagiosum, lichen nitidus, closed comedones, cutaneous myxoma, and calcinosis cutis.

Management: Treatment can be performed through incision of the epidermis overlying the lesion with a lancet or needle tip and extraction of the lesion. Electrodestruction is an alternative.

Dermoid Cyst

Overview: The tumor is surrounded by a thick dermis-like wall that includes multiple sebaceous glands and nearly all skin adnexa. Hairs and vast quantities of fatty masses can surround complexes originating from the ectoderm. Dermoid cysts can include substances such as nails and dental, cartilage-like, and bone-like structures, depending on the lesion site.

Clinical presentation: Cutaneous dermoid cysts are typically observed as subcutaneous nodules with a 1–4 cm diameter, located on the embryonic fusion lines in infants. The most common location is around the eyes. Very often, these are found near or underneath the outer part of the eyebrows.

Laboratory studies: On histology, there is a lining with stratified squamous epithelium, as well as associated hair follicles and sebaceous glands. Eccrine and apocrine glands can be present, and the lesions can be filled with semisolid material and hair.

Differential diagnosis: Other cysts can also be considered. Heterotopic neural tissue can be in the differential, so radiologic imaging should be performed in the right context to exclude a neurologic connection.

Management: Treatment is excision.

Pilonidal Cyst

Overview: It is a component of the follicular occlusion tetrad that includes acne conglobata, hidradenitis suppurativa, and dissecting cellulitis of the scalp. It often has a chronic course and may have a genetic component.

Clinical presentation: It presents as an inflamed, painful, nodule in areas such as sacrococcygeal, axillary, umbilical, and anogenital regions. It can occur due to a foreign body reaction to hair accumulation, which is associated with occlusion and inflammation.

Laboratory studies: Histologic findings include a mixed type of inflammation with hair and keratin material at its center.

Management: While intralesional steroids may flatten the lesion, but removal may be required.

Isthmic Cyst

Synonyms: Pilar cyst, trichilemmal cyst, follicular isthmus cyst

Clinical presentation: It develops from the isthmic part of the hair follicle and is filled with hair keratin material. About 90% of lesions are localized to the scalp. It is the most common type of cyst after the infundibular cyst. There is often an autosomal dominant genetic pattern, where such cysts may be found as solitary or multiple.

Laboratory studies: Histologic study demonstrates a cystic structure that is covered with homogeneous eosinophilic keratin from its lumen and a stratified squamous epithelium that does not contain a surrounding granular cell layer.

Differential diagnosis: Cylindroma, eccrine poroma, and skin metastases should be considered in the differential as well as other types of cysts.

Management: Surgical excision is recommended.

Mucocele

Synonym: Mucous cyst

Overview: This is a persistent epithelial cyst which occur in the presence of an obstructed sinus ostium or minor salivary gland duct in the sinuses. They have the ability for substantial concentric expansion beyond the sinus, which can lead to bony erosion and extension.

Clinical presentation: It presents as a clear to white lesion filled with mucin, commonly localized to the mucosa of the lower lip. (Figure 19.14) The lesion surface is covered with

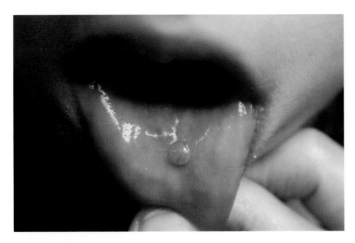

Figure 19.14 Mucocele: A benign artificial lesion of accessory salivary gland.

Source: Courtesy of Istanbul Medeniyet University Dermatology Clinic.

normal-appearing mucosa and may appear red to purple due to bleeding or white due to keratinization.

Laboratory studies: Histologically, it is not a true cyst but a pseudocyst due to the lack of lining.

Differential diagnosis: A venous lake, fibroma due to a bite, or a pyogenic granuloma can be considered.

Management: Treatment includes destructive modalities, such as surgical excision, incision and drainage, curettage, electrosurgery, cryotherapy, and laser surgery.

Steatocystoma

Overview: This is a solitary or multiple that may have an autosomal dominant pattern of inheritance and occurs in adolescence and young adulthood.

Clinical presentation: The lesion or lesions appear as multiple skin- to yellow-colored dermal cysts varying in size from 3 mm to 3 cm. Single cysts range from elastic to solid and can also move freely. Lesions do not have a central punctum and contain an odorless substance or sticky jelly. Individual steatocystoma multiplex lesions can become suppurative, increase in size, and become vulnerable to rupture. In such cases, secondary bacterial colonization often results in a malodorous discharge. Lesions are most commonly located on the face, neck, chest, and axilla.

Laboratory studies: Histologic examination shows a wavy cyst wall lined by squamous epithelium and a corrugated eosinophilic cuticle surface. Typically no granular layer is seen. Flattened lobules of sebaceous glands in different sizes are found inside or adjacent to the cyst wall. Cystic space may contain keratin, vellous hair, sebum, and so on.

Differential diagnosis: Idiopathic scrotal calcification, epidermoid cyst, and cystic lesions of acne vulgaris should be considered in the differential diagnosis. In addition, pachyonychia congenita type 2 should be investigated in patients with multiple steatocystomas.

Management: Treatment includes destructive modalities, such as surgical excision, incision and drainage, curettage, cryotherapy, electrosurgery, and laser surgery.

Dermatofibroma

Synonym: Histiocytoma

Definition: This is a commonly acquired fibrohistiocytic tumor of the skin.

Overview: Although its etiology is unknown, it is thought to occur from the activation of fibroblasts, histiocytes, and endothelial cells due to the stimulating effect of physical trauma, especially an arthropod bite.

Clinical presentation: A dermatofibroma is a solid papule that is slightly raised with a smooth surface and diameter of about 0.5–1 cm. (Figure 19.15) Although a lesion is primarily located on the lower extremities, they can occur on any part of the body. It can appear pink to brown and can

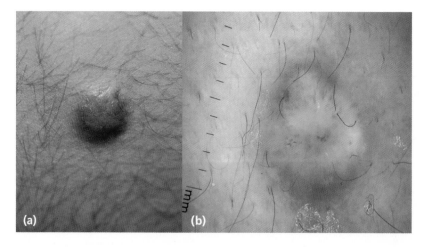

Figure 19.15 (a) Dermatofibromas are multiple 0.5–1cm nodular lesions at the skin level or slightly raised from the skin; (b) Dermatoscopic view.

Source: Courtesy of Istanbul Medeniyet University Dermatology Clinic.

be darker than the surrounding skin. When the lesion is slightly compressed, the shrinkage and downward displacement of the lesion creates a dimple.

The lesion is generally single or sometimes multiple; however, the sudden appearance of multiple lesions may suggest an autoimmune disease, such as systemic lupus erythematosus, Sjögren's syndrome, pemphigus vulgaris, and myasthenia gravis as well as immunosuppressive patients, such as with HIV infection.

Laboratory studies: The histology is characterized by a poorly defined proliferation of fibrohistiocytic cells with an overlying grenz zone within the dermis. Collagen is trapped on the periphery of the lesion. With enhanced pigmentation of the basal layer, the overlying epidermis can be acanthotic. Smooth muscle actin, factor XIIIA, CD68, CD163 are positive, and CD34 is negative in dermatofibromas.

Differential diagnosis: Dermatofibrosarcoma protuberans (DFSP), blue nevus, Spitz nevus, pilomatrixoma, desmoplastic melanoma, keloid, and skin metastases can be considered, depending on the clinical context and history. DFSP is CD34 (+) and factor XIIIA (–), which is in contrast to dermatofibroma, which is CD34 (–) and factor XIIIA (+).

Management: Treatment is done for cosmetic reasons, and surgical excision or lasers can be used. Recurrence can occur.

Infantile Hemangioma

Synonyms: Juvenile hemangioma

Definition: Infantile hemangiomas are benign vascular neoplasms with a distinct clinical pattern characterized by early proliferation and spontaneous involution.

Overview: This lesion is usually sporadic, but there may be an autosomal dominant component. It is thought to be due to the proliferation of endothelial progenitor cells secondary to hypoxia resulting in ischemia to the placenta. In addition, GLUT1, which is A placental protein, is positive in infantile hemangiomas but not in other hemangioma types. Contrary to folklore, it is not due to the stork holding nape.

Clinical presentation: Infantile hemangioma is the most common tumor of infancy, with a rate of 2–10% in newborns. This tumor, which is more common in girls, typically occurs within the first weeks of life. It located in the skin and soft tissues as a solitary lesion on the head or neck (Figure 19.16). It can also occur on the trunk, arms, legs, and visceral organs.

Internal organ involvement is more common if there are multiple lesions. Hemangiomas with segmental involvement can be associated with some syndromes, including PHACE (posterior fossa abnormalities hemangiomas, arterial anomalies, cardiac anomalies, eye abnormalities), PELVIS (perineal hemangioma, external genital malformations, lipomyelomeningocele, vesicorenal abnormalities, imperforate anus, skin tag), and SACRAL (spinal dysraphism with anogenital, cutaneous, renal, and urologic anomalies, associated with an angioma of lumbosacral localization).

The lesion appears as telangiectatic red papules and plaques, while those that are deep-seated can be blue to purple nodules. The early months in which the lesion grows rapidly after birth is

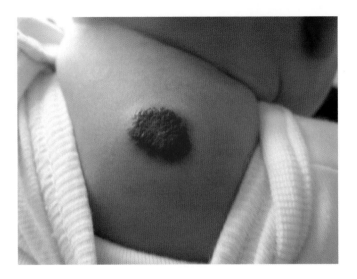

Figure 19.16 An infantile hemangoma of the shoulder.

Source: Courtesy of Istanbul Medeniyet University Dermatology Clinic.

called the *proliferative phase*. Lesions generally continue to develop until the age of 1, and most lesions show spontaneous regression by the age of 5–7 years. Complications, such as ulceration, infection, and hemorrhage, can occur, especially during periods of rapid growth.

Laboratory studies: The histology can vary according to the phase of growth. In the proliferative phase, it consists of large lobules of capillary vessels lined with large endothelial cells and pericytes, plus increased mitoses. In the maturation phase, capillary vessels show enlargement of the vascular spaces and flattening of the endothelial cells. In the involution phase, the lobules diverge due to interstitial fibrosis and prominence in adipose tissue. Hemangiomas slowly regress, leaving behind fat and fibrous tissue.

Differential diagnosis: Pyogenic granuloma, tufted hemangioma, vascular malformations, and kaposiform hemangioendothelioma can be considered. While these lesions are GLUT1 (–), infantile hemangioma is GLUT1 (+).

Management: Intervention is not always required, as small lesions may regress spontaneously. Systemic and intralesional steroids, topical and systemic beta blockers, imiquimod, interferon-a, and laser treatments can be used in larger lesions or those on cosmetically sensitive areas, such as the face. Pulsed dye lasers have had tremendous efficacy. Giving regimen for beta-blockers.

SEBORRHEIC KERATOSIS

Synonyms: Seborrheic verruca, senile wart, basal cell papilloma, old age spot

Definition: This represents the most common benign tumor, originating from epidermal keratinocytes usually in older patients.

Overview: No specific etiologic factor has been identified; however, the papilloma virus has periodically been implicated. The pathophysiology is believed to involve the clonal expansion of mutated epidermal keratinocytes and due to gene encoding *FGFR3*, *PIK3A*, *RAS*, and *AKT1* with changes in the distribution of the epidermal growth factor (EGF) receptors contributing. Chronic ultraviolet damage has also been questioned.

Clinical presentation: A lesion may develop anywhere on the body, except the palms, soles, and mucous membranes, usually after the third or fourth decade of life. It begins as a sharply circumscribed, tan to brown, macule or papule. It can then have a verrucous or velvety appearance, with light surface crusting. A single lesion is usually about 1 cm in diameter (Figure 19.17). It may be traumatized by rubbing against clothing or scratching.

The Leser-Trélat Sign is the simultaneous occurrence of multiple seborrheic keratoses on the body, which is associated with internal malignancy, most commonly a gastrointestinal adenocarcinoma. This is a questionable association. Additionally, eruptive seborrheic keratosis may also develop after an inflammatory dermatosis. It is thought to be associated with excessive secretion of growth factors.

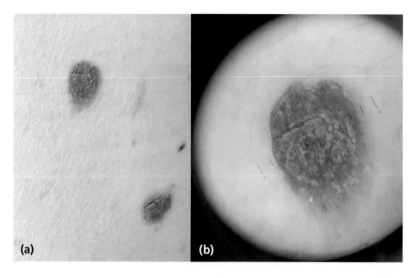

Figure 19.17 (a) Seborrheic keratosis; (b) dermatoscopic view.

Source: Courtesy of Istanbul Medeniyet University Dermatology Clinic.

Examples of clinical variants include the following:

- *Dermatosis papulosa nigra:* This is a clinically different entity but is considered a variant of seborrheic keratosis. The lesion is seen in a darker-skinned patient, more common in women. It is characterized by numerous pigmented papules on the face, neck, and trunk.

- *Stucco keratosis:* This represent a smaller variant of seborrheic keratoses and has a light tan to gray color with multiple lesions and symmetric distribution, especially on the calves and may be somewhat flat.

- *Inverted follicular keratosis:* The lesion often appears as solitary nonpigmented verrucous papule on the face. This is considered by some to be an endophytic variant of inflamed seborrheic keratosis, which originates from the follicular infundibulum. Histology is generally needed for diagnosis and confirmation.

Laboratory studies: Various histologic types of seborrheic keratoses have been described. Oftentimes, more than one can be present in the same lesion. Low molecular weight cytokeratin, filaggrin, and BCL-2 expression can be seen, which may vary based on histologic subtype; however, a common finding is Borst-Jadassohn phenomenon.

Examples of histologic variants include the following:

- *Acanthotic type:* This is the most common histologic pattern. Characteristically, there can be hyperkeratosis, papillomatosis, pseudo-horn cysts, and hyperpigmentation.

- *Hyperkeratotic type:* This has prominent papillomatosis, orthohyperkeratosis, mild acanthosis, and cyst-like structures. There is no hyperpigmentation.

- *Clonal type:* This is characterized by the localized proliferation and clonal expansion of basaloid cells.

- *Adenoid type:* This demonstrates anastomoses from basaloid epidermal cells to the epidermis. Horn and pseudo-horn cysts are not seen; however, hyperpigmentation is common.

- *Irritated/inflamed type:* Lichenoid inflammation is observed. It can be confused with squamous cell carcinoma in some cases. Acantholysis, dyskeratosis, and spongiosis can be seen.

Differential diagnosis: A seborrheic keratosis may mimic an epidermal nevus, actinic keratosis, squamous cell carcinoma in situ, verruca vulgaris, and melanocytic lesions.

Prognosis: Although lesions are benign tumors, secondary tumors, such as Bowen disease, BCC, SCC, keratoacanthoma, or malignant melanoma may infrequently occur within or adjacent to the lesion. This is called the "collision theory," and it is seen when two different neoplasia occur in the same area, separate from each other.

Management: Destructive methods, such as cryotherapy, curettage, laser, shave excision, electrocautery, and chemical peels, can be performed for aesthetic purposes.

FINAL THOUGHT

Moles are a common finding that require intervention only when there is concern for a malignancy or when they are cosmetically unacceptable.

ADDITIONAL READINGS

Bsirini C, Smoller BR. Histologic mimics of malignant melanoma. Singapore Med J. 2018 Nov;59:602–607.

Buslach N, Foulad DP, Saedi N, et al. Treatment modalities for Cherry Angiomas: a systematic review. Dermatol Surg. 2020;46:1691–1697.

Damsky WE, Bosenberg M. Melanocytic nevi and melanoma: unraveling a complex relationship. Oncogene. 2017;36:5771–5792.

Dika E, Ravaioli GM, Fanti PA, et al. Spitz Nevi and other spitzoid neoplasms in children: overview of incidence data and diagnostic criteria. Pediatr Dermatol. 2017;34:25–32.

Iacobelli J, Harvey N, Waldman RA, et al. Skin diseases of the breast and nipple: benign and malignant tumors. J Am Acad Dermatol. 2019;80:1467–1481.

Iacobelli J, Harvey NT, Wood BA. Sebaceous lesions of the skin. Pathology. 2017;49:688–697.

Karadag AS, Parish LC. The status of the seborrheic keratosis. Clin Dermatol. 2018;36:275–277.

Mavrogenis AF, Panagopoulos GN, Angelini A, et al. Tumors of the hand. Eur J Orthop Surg Traumatol. 2017;27:747–762.

Stanoszek LM, Wang GY, Harms PW. Histologic mimics of basal cell carcinoma. Arch Pathol Lab Med. 2017;141:1490–1502.

Zalaudek I, Cota C, Ferrara G, et al. Flat pigmented macules on sun-damaged skin of the head/neck: junctional nevus, atypical lentiginous nevus, or melanoma in situ? Clin Dermatol. 2014;32:88–93.

20 Premalignant Neoplasms

Alex Sherban and Matthew Keller

CONTENTS

Overview: Premalignant neoplasms comprise a group of lesions with a specific risk for malignant transformation (Table 20.1).

ACTINIC KERATOSIS

Definition: Actinic keratoses (AKs) are composed of epidermal keratinocytes with varying degrees of dysplasia that result from ultraviolet (UV) radiation. Opinions differ as to whether they are premalignant neoplasms, *in situ* malignancies, or epiphenomena reflecting chronic UV exposure.

Overview: AKs are the result of chronic sun exposure. Generation of arachidonic acid metabolites promotes inflammation, while UVA radiation-induced reactive oxygen species damage nucleic acids and cell membranes. UVB exposure classically converts cytosine to thymine and inactivates tumor suppressor p53, which further promotes carcinogenesis.

Clinical Presentation: AKs most commonly present on sun-exposed skin as erythematous and scaly macules, papules, or plaques with poorly defined borders (Figure 20.1). They are often better felt than seen due to their rough texture. Colors may vary from skin-colored to erythematous, pink, or brown. Although lesions are often asymptomatic, they can be tender or pruritic. Several clinical variants exist, including hyperkeratotic, atrophic, and pigmented (Figure 20.2).

While UV radiation is responsible for their generation, other risk factors include Fitzpatrick skin types I and II, red hair, older age, male sex, residence near the equator, personal and family history of skin cancer, smoking, and immunosuppression. Organ transplant patients are at particularly high risk, being 250 times more likely to develop an AK. The influence of the human papillomavirus (HPV) on risk remains controversial.

Laboratory studies: Most AKs are diagnosed clinically, but histopathologic examination may be needed. Their morphologic variation and lack of standardized definition may lead to

Table 20.1 Overview of Premalignant Lesions

	Prevalence	Rate of Malignant Transformation of a Single Lesion (unit time)
Actinic Keratosis	11–25% of Caucasians	0.6% (per year)
Dysplastic Nevus	10–50% of Caucasians	1/3,000 to 1/200,000 (lifetime risk)
Actinic Cheilitis	0.9–43.24%	10–30% (lifetime risk)
Porokeratosis	*Unknown*	*Disseminated superficial actinic porokeratosis (DSAP)**
		3.4% (30-year risk)
		LP: 19% (30-year risk)
Leukoplakia	1.49–4.9%	*Homogeneous*: 0.6–5% (lifetime risk)
		Nonhomogeneous: 20–25% (lifetime risk)
		PVL: 70–100% (lifetime risk)

Note:*Malignant transformation rates of DSAP may be inflated due to the inclusion of suspected *de novo* malignancies arising in fields of cancerization concurrently occupied by DSAP.

DOI: 10.1201/9781003105268-20

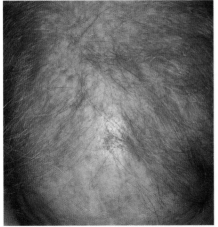

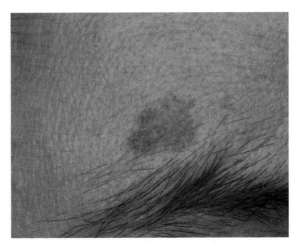

Figure 20.1 Actinic keratosis.

Figure 20.2 Pigmented actinic keratosis.

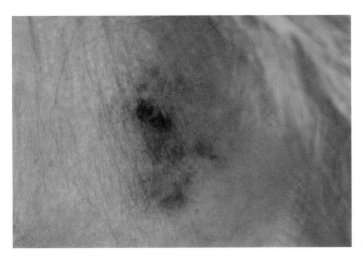

Figure 20.3 Lentigo maligna.

misdiagnosis. Dermatoscopy can be helpful in clinically suspect cases. Facial AKs can have a characteristic strawberry pattern due to the formation of a vascular pseudo network around hair follicles, while nonfacial AKs can display erythema and superficial scale.

Differential diagnosis: The most common considerations are squamous cell carcinoma (SCC) and Bowen's disease. Less common diagnoses include lichen planus, lichen keratosis, and seborrheic keratoses. Pigmented AKs may mimic lentigo maligna (Figure 20.3).

Management: AKs may be managed medically with topical or destructive approaches. Topical therapies include 5-fluorouracil (5-FU), imiquimod, ingenol mebutate, and photodynamic therapy. Destructive therapies include cryotherapy, curettage, and ablative laser resurfacing. Transplant patients given low-dose acitretin or isotretinoin can have significant reductions in the number of lesions. Oral nicotinamide may be effective for prevention in high-risk groups.

Prognosis: AKs ultimately have three fates: remission with risk of recurrence, persistence without progression, or malignant transformation. About 50–70% regress spontaneously, and the rate of progression to SCC within one year is around 0.6%, with studies ranging from 0–20%. Up to 16% of AKs may progress to SCC within 10 years if left untreated.

Final comment: AKs are premalignant neoplasms due to UV-induced dysplasia. They affect up to 25% of Caucasians worldwide, most commonly in areas with increased sun exposure. Diagnosis can often be made from clinical examination. A variety of treatment modalities exist, and field treatment can be helpful for generalized areas of involvement.

247

ACTINIC CHEILITIS

Definition: Actinic cheilitis (AC) is a UV-radiation induced premalignant lesion of the vermillion border of the lip. Clinically similar to AKs, AC is characterized by atrophy, dryness, and an obscured indistinct border.

Overview: AC is due to UV radiation-induced disruptions in cellular proliferation, tumor suppression, and intracellular signaling. Alterations in the tumor suppressor p53 and antiapoptotic proteins have been implicated.

Clinical presentation: AC most commonly appears as white, dry, atrophied plaques of varying thickness with scale, focal erosions, indistinct borders, and surrounding erythema on the vermillion border of the lip (Figure 20.4). Their color may range from white to gray or brown, and more than 90% develop on the lower lip. Like AKs, AC has a rough sandpaper-like texture that may be better felt than seen. Men older than 40 years with a history of chronic UV exposure appear to be the most affected. Although chronic UV exposure is the most significant risk factor, Fitzpatrick skin types I and II, geographic latitude, older age, male sex, and at-risk occupations have also been implicated. Immunosuppression, tobacco, and alcohol may increase the risk of AC, but the evidence is limited.

Laboratory studies: A definitive diagnosis often requires histologic examination, which reveals hyperkeratosis with various degrees of atypia. Perivascular inflammation, solar elastosis, and vasodilation are the most commonly observed features. Epithelial dysplasia may be evident. Dermatoscopy can aid in the diagnosis, which reveals poorly defined borders, vascular telangiectasias, and white projections surrounding ulcerated areas.

Differential diagnosis: Clinically, AC may be confused with SCC *in situ*.

Management: Limited data exist on the management of AC. There is no accepted standard of treatment. Treatment options include curettage and electrodesiccation, excision, cryosurgery, ablative laser therapy, and topical 5-FU and imiquimod.

Prognosis: AC is 2.5 times more likely to progress to SCC than AKs. Although rates of malignant transformation vary widely from 10–30%, about 95% of SCC on the lip have been thought to arise from preceding AC. Years of chronic UV exposure are likely necessary for progression to SCC. SCC that arises from AC is 3–5 times less likely to metastasize when compared to *de novo* SCC. Although patients younger than 40 rarely develop SCC (less than 7% of all SCC on the lip), these cancers have relatively higher rates of cervical node metastasis.

Final comment: AC represents a premalignant entity similar to AKs, which present as atrophied, scaly, rough areas on the vermillion border of the lip. A biopsy is typically needed for definitive diagnosis, and more aggressive surgical treatments may be required for complete clearance.

POROKERATOSIS

Definition: Porokeratosis (PK) is a rare acquired or hereditary disorder of keratinization capable of undergoing malignant transformation. Several clinical variants exist, including porokeratosis of Mibelli (PM), disseminated porokeratosis (DSP), disseminated superficial actinic porokeratosis (DSAP), and linear porokeratosis (LP). Of these variants, DSAP is the most common and least likely to progress to carcinoma, while LP is the most likely to undergo malignant transformation.

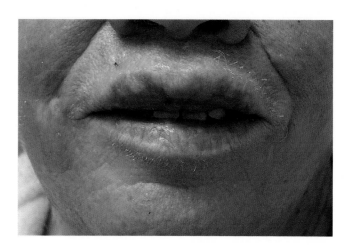

Figure 20.4 Actinic cheilitis.

Source: Courtesy of Dr. Robert Schwartz and the *Journal of the American Academy of Dermatology.*

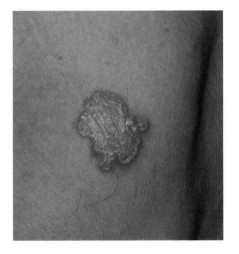

Figure 20.5   Porokeratosis of Mibelli.

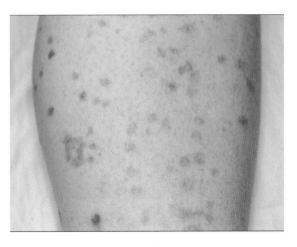

Figure 20.6   Disseminated superficial actinic porokeratosis.

Overview: Although confirmed pathogenesis of PK remains unknown, it is thought to be due to a dysregulation of terminal differentiation and proliferation of abnormal epidermal keratinocytes beneath the coronoid lamella. Familial inheritance has been observed, and several attributable genetic loci have been identified. HIV, leukemia, lymphoma, autoimmune disease, and immunosuppressive agents have been associated with PK. Certain medications, such as diuretics, antibiotics, and TNFα inhibitors, have been implicated as having a causal or exacerbating role with the DSP variant. UV radiation has been associated with the DSAP variant.

Clinical presentation: Lesions typically present as a slowly enlarging, brown papule that extends from its center until it develops into a 1–10 mm, well-circumscribed plaque with hyperkeratotic rim and atrophic center. Although lesions are primarily located on the extremities, they can appear on the lips, genitals, or mucosa. Overall, PK has a slight male predominance, but DSAP and LP variants have a slight female predominance. Given the rarity of the disease, the exact incidence is unknown. Caucasians tend to be at the highest risk of PK. Organ transplant patients have a reported incidence of 0.34–10.68%, with the highest rates associated with renal transplant.

PM, DSAP, and DSP are the most common variants. PM typically presents as one or a few papules that develop into an atrophic center with a hyperkeratotic rim (Figure 20.5). Onset usually occurs during childhood. Lesions may involve any area of the body, but most commonly occur on an extremity. DSAP is the most common clinical variant, presenting in the third and fourth decades. Like PM, DSAP begins as keratotic papules that progress to hyperkeratotic rings with an atrophic center (Figure 20.6). They are predominantly located bilaterally on the extremities. One-third of patients report pruritus, and nearly half experience exacerbations during the summer due to UV radiation. The DSP variant presents similarly to DSAP; however, DSP is not exacerbated by sun exposure and presents much earlier (5–10 years of age). LP is a rare variant that presents in younger patients, often near birth. It presents as linearly distributed hyperkeratotic plaques that follow Blaschko's lines (Figure 20.7).

Laboratory studies: Clinical examination is often all that is necessary for diagnosis. Biopsy of the hyperkeratotic rim will reveal the characteristic coronoid lamella (Figure 20.8), which is a stack of parakeratotic cells extending through the stratum corneum. Dermatoscopy can be helpful, which shows a skin-colored coronoid lamella with centrally located vessels.

Differential diagnosis: The most common considerations include AKs and Bowen's disease. DSAP may mimic guttate psoriasis. Other less common diagnoses include seborrheic keratoses, stucco keratoses, elastosis perforans serpiginosa, and lichen planus. Epidermal nevus, linear psoriasis, and lichen striatus are included in the differential for LP.

Management: Most therapies do not provide definitive clearance without recurrence. Management involves prevention with sunscreen, as well as regular skin examinations for malignancy surveillance. Treatment options include phototherapy, cryotherapy, ablative laser treatment, and a variety of topical therapies. PM has reported positive outcomes with topical imiquimod. DSAP has effectively been treated with long-term use of vitamin D analogs. Refractory DSAP may

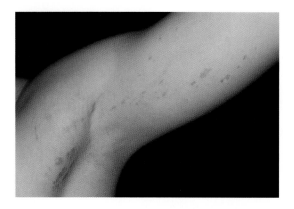

Figure 20.7 Linear porokeratosis.

Source: Used with permission from Eicher L, Flaig MJ, Senner S, Betke M, Lineare Porokeratose, *Der Hautarzt*; 2020: 71;54–56.

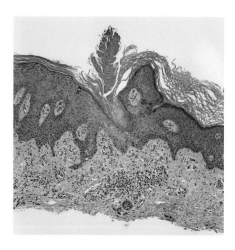

Figure 20.8 Cornoid lamella of porokeratosis on histology.

respond well to photodynamic therapy. Oral or topical retinoids have been effective against LP. Surgical excision may be helpful in areas where topicals are contraindicated or if few lesions are present. Anti-inflammatories, such as topical corticosteroids, can provide relief of pruritus; however, they are not effective in lesion clearance.

Prognosis: Although some lesions may spontaneously regress, they typically progress in size and number. Despite ablative and topical treatment options, recurrence is common. When PK is associated with immunodeficiency, the severity of the disease may fluctuate with the degree of immunosuppression. The rate of malignant transformation is between 3.4–19%. While the PM variant, persistent lesions, and those in immunocompromised patients are at increased risk, the LP variant has the greatest risk of progression to carcinoma with a rate of 19%. The most common form of PK, the DSAP variant, is the least likely to undergo malignant transformation, with rates reported as low as 3.4%. It is important to note that data are limited and from small studies.

Final comment: PK is a rare disorder of keratinization that has a slight male predominance with several clinical variants. Initially presenting as a brown papule, PK typically progresses to hyperkeratotic, annular plaques with atrophic centers that have characteristic coronoid lamella. Clinical presentation, epidemiology, and effective management strategies are unique to each variant.

LEUKOPLAKIA

Definition: Leukoplakia represents an oral white plaque or patch with varying risk of progression to SCC. It remains a diagnosis of exclusion.

Overview: The evolution of dysplasia progressing to invasive malignancy is believed to occur through stepwise progression, which is believed to involve genetic and epigenetic mutations. DNA aneuploidy, loss of heterozygosity, and telomerase dysfunction have been implicated, as well as mutations in tumor suppressors p53 and p16.

Clinical presentation: There are white patches or plaques with well-defined margins on the floor of the mouth, tongue, or soft palate (Figure 20.9). It is divided into two types based on appearance and risk of malignant transformation: homogeneous or nonhomogeneous. The homogeneous type presents with uniformly white, thin, flat lesions that are typically localized, affect men, and are associated with tobacco use. The nonhomogeneous subtype carries higher rates of malignant transformation and can further be divided into three variants: nodular, verrucous, and erythroplakia, the last having a speckled or erythematous appearance.

Of the nonhomogeneous variants, the proliferative verrucous leukoplakia (PVL) is the most concerning. PVL is an aggressive, progressive, and persistent lesion that can involve both keratosis and carcinoma most commonly affects women and is only weakly associated with tobacco use. The most characteristic features include its multifocality and requisite involvement of the gingiva. It tends to involve the buccal mucosa or alveolar ridge and typically spares the tongue. PVL is initially uniform in color and texture before becoming exophytic, verrucous, and erythematous.

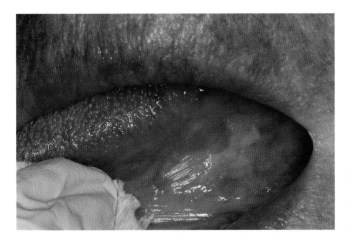

Figure 20.9 Leukoplakia.

Source: Courtesy of Dr. Alessandro Villa and the *Journal of Oral Maxillofacial Surgery.*

The prevalence of leukoplakia is estimated to be 1.49–4.9%. Unfortunately, most epidemiologic data are outdated and retrospective. Risk factors include tobacco use, alcohol use, areca nut use, UV exposure, age, family history of cancer, and immunosuppression. HPV has been implicated in epithelial dysplasia.

Laboratory studies: It is based on historical, clinical, and histologic factors after other conditions without the risk of cancer have been ruled out. The histologic examination may be required to confirm the diagnosis in clinically suspect lesions, but there are no pathognomonic features. Biopsy typically shows either hyperkeratosis or parakeratosis with varying levels of dysplasia that may include *in situ* or invasive malignancy. A variety of methods have been used as screening tools for suspicious lesions: brush biopsies, stains, fluorescent examination, and examination of serologic, salivary, and cellular biomarkers. Unfortunately, these methods have poor specificity and incur a high rate of false positives.

Differential diagnosis: The most common diseases to be considered include alveolar ridge keratosis, candidiasis, frictional keratosis, smoker's lesions, and hairy leukoplakia.

Management: Its management can be challenging due to its location. Treatment options may involve observation, lesion-directed therapies, topical medications, systemic medications, or a combination. Definitive treatment is preferred in younger patients, whereas it may be more appropriate to observe lesions in those who are older.

Ablative laser therapies are effective, but the risk of recurrence or malignancy ranges between 0–15%. Photodynamic therapy has been used with mixed results. There have been reports that mild epithelial dysplasia has spontaneously regressed without intervention, which makes observation a reasonable initial approach in certain cases; however, these reports may reflect trauma-induced reactive changes that are distinct from the characteristic dysplastic lesions that carry the risk of progression to carcinoma.

Biopsy-confirmed carcinoma or dysplasia should be surgically excised. A histopathologic diagnosis of SCC should prompt referral for evaluation by a head and neck oncologist because surgery, radiation, or chemotherapy may be necessary. The aggressive PVL variant is notorious for its high recurrence rates despite multiple treatment modalities having been studied.

Prognosis: The rate of malignant transformation for non-PVL leukoplakia ranges between 0.13–34% with older patients and women being at the greatest risk. It may be more useful to approach rates of malignant transformation based on the extent of oral involvement or subtype. The homogeneous subtype is the most benign with rates of progression ranging between 0.6–5%. Localized, singular lesions of either subtype carry a slightly higher lifetime risk, which ranges between 3–15% with 1–3% transforming within one year. Overall, the nonhomogeneous subtype has a rate of progression of 20–25%. PVL has the highest rate of malignant transformation, where 70–100% can progress to carcinoma. The location of the lesion may give insight into the risk of progression; the floor of the mouth, anterior tongue, and the soft, non-keratinized palate carries the greatest risk. Other risk factors for malignant progression include lesion size (>200 mm^2) and female gender (15.2% vs 1.7% in men).

Final comment: It represents a challenging clinical entity, often requiring historical, clinical, and histopathologic investigation to confirm the diagnosis. Although it typically presents as white plaques or patches in the mouth, there are no defining characteristics, and it remains a diagnosis of exclusion. The risk of progression to carcinoma varies widely.

DYSPLASTIC NEVI

Definition: Dysplastic nevi have a complex history and were originally thought of as premalignant neoplasms in melanoma-prone families. Although various familial syndromes with different nevi counts and risks of melanoma were discovered, "dysplastic nevus" entered the dermatologic lexicon and was often erroneously grouped with these distinct syndromes that were associated with increased risk of melanoma.

Overview: Current recommendations are for the adoption of the term "nevus with architectural disorder," because the term *dysplastic* implies the risk of malignant transformation that was not fully understood. Dysplastic nevi were originally described as dysplastic due to their histologic atypia and architectural distortion. Despite this recommendation, the term *dysplastic nevus* is still commonly used, and their diagnostic criteria and premalignant status remain controversial.

Dysplastic nevi are often described as irregular and asymmetrical lesions that have color variation, are greater than 5 mm in diameter and may be observed in up to 50% of Caucasians. There is no standardized clinical or histologic definition accepted by dermatologists, but it is understood that at least a subset of dysplastic nevi exists on a spectrum between benign melanocytic nevus and malignant melanoma.

The etiology of dysplastic nevi involves multiple genetic and environmental factors. Although many different genetic mutations have been observed, they occur less frequently than in melanoma. From the subset of dysplastic nevi capable of progressing to melanoma, mutations were found in *CDKN2a*, non-V600E *BRAF*, *NRAS*, and *TERT* genes, as well as the MAPK genes *HRAS*, *NF1*, *MAP2Kt*, and *GNA11*. Of note, *CDKN2a* mutations are found in only 20–30% of melanoma-prone families, which suggests that malignant transformation may be complex and multifactorial.

UV radiation has been implicated because dysplastic nevi have been found in greater numbers on chronically and intermittently sun-exposed areas. People living in climates with increased sun exposure and those receiving UVB phototherapy can also have more dysplastic nevi. There is evidence that patients with dysplastic nevi may be more sensitive to UV radiation. Other immunologic factors are known to contribute to the diagnosis, including greater numbers of T cells, antigen-presenting cells, and reactive oxygen species.

Clinical presentation: The clinical characteristics of dysplastic nevi have been refined to include lesions ≥5 mm in diameter with a macular component, variable pigmentation, asymmetry, and irregular, indistinct borders (Figure 20.10), as outlined by the 1990 International Agency for Research on Cancer. There is significant overlap with the ABCDE (asymmetry, border, color, diameter, evolution) criteria of melanoma, which contributes to the diagnostic gray area. Their color is usually tan to brown, and they are often no greater than 10 mm in diameter. The incidence is unknown because most dysplastic nevi are clinically examined without histologic confirmation of dysplasia, but studies have estimated the prevalence to be 10–50% in Caucasians. They are often observed in young adults with lesions presenting during childhood.

Laboratory studies: Although there have been efforts to find a consensus on the clinical appearance of dysplastic nevi, definitive diagnosis requires histologic examination for evidence of dysplasia. Dysplastic nevi were originally described histologically as having atypical melanocytic hyperplasia, cytologic atypia, fibroplasia of the papillary dermis, and lymphocytic infiltrate.

Other organizations, including the World Health Organization (WHO), have put forth additional histologic criteria. Major criteria include atypical melanocytic proliferation or nesting in the basal layer, which creates bridges of melanocytes between at least 3 adjacent rete ridges. Minor criteria include lamellar or concentric eosinophilic fibrosis, neovascularization, inflammation, and fusion of rete ridges. According to the WHO, a diagnosis requires both major criteria and at least 2 minor criteria. The WHO further divides dysplastic nevi into either high-grade (previously severe) or low grade (previously moderate). The abandoned "mild" category has been reclassified as a lentiginous nevus.

Differential diagnosis: The most common considerations in diagnoses for atypical nevi include the common melanocytic nevus, melanoma *in situ*, malignant melanoma (Figure 20.11), and lentigo maligna (Figure 20.4).

Management: Prophylactic excision of all dysplastic nevi is not recommended, because this does not reduce the overall risk for melanoma. Most melanomas arise *de novo*, and most dysplastic nevi do not undergo malignant transformation. It is recommended that patients with dysplastic nevi undergo routine skin surveillance and avoid excessive UV exposure. Patients with high nevus counts (>100) or large nevi (>4.4 mm) should undergo routine surveillance for malignancy.

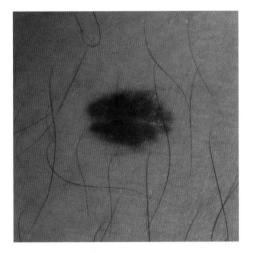

Figure 20.10 Dysplastic nevus.

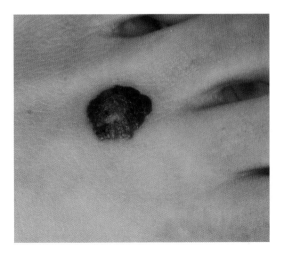

Figure 20.11 Malignant melanoma.

Photography can be used to monitor nevi over time for suspicious changes. Nevi in sun-exposed areas, nevi that change in appearance, and nevi of patients with a personal or family history of melanoma should be carefully scrutinized. Suspicion for melanoma should prompt excision, but little evidence justifies aggressive treatment and excision of dysplastic nevi.

Prognosis: Due to the lack of established diagnostic criteria and the common practice for dysplastic nevi to be evaluated only clinically, there remains conflicting evidence on their rate of progression to melanoma. It is currently believed by some that a subset of lesions exists as an intermediate form between common nevi and melanoma, which possess the ability to undergo malignant transformation. Several studies have demonstrated an increased risk of melanoma among those with dysplastic nevi, ranging 5–15-fold; however, dysplastic nevi are generally considered to be more of a marker for overall melanoma risk than a premalignant lesion. Terminology and grading of dysplasia have erroneously implied that dysplastic nevi invariably progress to melanoma, which is not the case.

FINAL THOUGHT

Classification of dysplastic nevi is controversial. The current consensus is that only a subset of nevi represents a continuum between a common melanocytic nevus and malignant melanoma. Although definitive diagnosis requires histologic examination, dysplastic nevi are often identified clinically. Dysplastic nevi may be a marker for patients with increased risk, and routine skin surveillance should be recommended.

ADDITIONAL READINGS

Duffy K, Grossman D. The dysplastic nevus: from historical perspective to management in the modern era. J Am Acad Dermatol. 2012;67:1.e1–16.

Fernandez Figueras MT. From actinic keratosis to squamous cell carcinoma: pathophysiology revisited. J Eur Acad Dermatol Venereol. 2017;31 Suppl 2:5–7.

Jadotte YT, Schwartz RA. Solar cheilosis: an ominous precursor. J Am Acad Dermatol. 2012;66:173–184.

Kanitakis J. Porokeratoses: an update of clinical, etiopathogenic and therapeutic features. Eur J Dermatol. 2014;24:533–544.

Lai M, Pampena R, Cornacchia L, et al. Treatments of actinic cheilitis: a systematic review of the literature. J Am Acad Dermatol. 2020;83:876–887.

Rosendahl CO, Grant-Kels JM, Que SK. Dysplastic nevus: fact and fiction. J Am Acad Dermatol. 2015;73:507–512.

Sertznig P, Felbert VV, Megahed M. Porokeratosis: present concepts. J Eur Acad Dermatol. Venereol. 2011;26:404–412.

Siegel J, Korgavkar K, Weinstock M. Current perspective on actinic keratosis: a review. Br J Dermatol. 2016;177:350–358.

Villa A, Woo SB. Leukoplakia—a diagnostic and management algorithm. J Oral Maxillofac Surg. 2017;75:723–734.

Warnakulasuriya S, Ariyawardana A. Malignant transformation of oral leukoplakia: a systematic review of observational studies. J Oral Pathol Med. 2015;45:155–166.

21 Malignant Neoplasms

Mark Biro and Vesna Petronic-Rosic

CONTENTS

Overview: Cutaneous neoplasms are the most common form of human malignancies. This chapter outlines the clinical presentation, pathologic findings, and subsequent treatment of various cutaneous neoplasms.

BASAL CELL CARCINOMA

Synonyms: Basal cell epithelioma, rodent ulcer

Definition: Basal cell carcinoma (BCC), previously known as basal cell epithelioma, is a locally invasive, destructive tumor of basal keratinocytes.

Overview: BCC is the most common human cancer. The average age of patients diagnosed with BCC is 60 years old, with a higher incidence in men. Additional risk factors include ultraviolet light exposure, immunosuppression, solid organ transplant, fair skin complexion, xeroderma pigmentosum, albinism, and basal cell nevus syndrome. Tumorigenesis involves mutations that activate the sonic hedgehog protein (SHH) and promote the binding of SHH to the PTCH1 receptor. The binding of SHH to PTCH1 prevents PTCH1 inhibition of both SMO and cyclin proteins. Without inhibition from PTCH1, SMO promotes continuous activation of the SHH pathway. Cyclin proteins enter the cell nucleus and bind to genes to promote constitutive cell growth. The understanding of this pathway has allowed for the development of targeted therapy.

Clinical presentation: BCC is found in areas of sun exposure, such as the head and neck region, chest, back, and forearms (Figure 21.1, Table 21.1). Typically, patients will describe a slow growing, pimple that will not pop or a wound not healing with time.

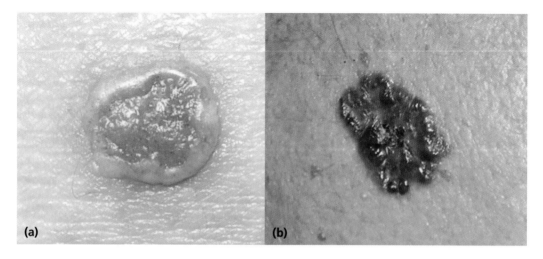

Figure 21.1 Pearly (a) pink and (b) brown nodule with central ulceration, rolled border, and telangiectasias.

DOI: 10.1201/9781003105268-21

Table 21.1 Three Important Clinical Variants of BCC

BCC Subtype	Epidemiology	Common Location	Clinical Presentation
Nodular BCC	~50% of BCC	Head & neck	A shiny, pearly, papule with rolled borders and arborizing telangiectasias that may ulcerate. This was previously described as the "rodent ulcer."
Superficial BCC	~10–30% of BCC	Trunk & extremities	An erythematous, plaque, with a thin rolled border and telangiectasias. Often there is central clearing, scaling, and an overlying crust.
Morpheaform BCC	< 10% of BCC	Head & neck	An infiltrated, white, scar-like plaque with poorly defined borders. This subtype has the greatest potential for extensive local invasion.

Table 21.2 Histologic Variants of Basal Cell Carcinoma

Histologic Variant	Pathologic Findings
Nodular	Intradermal nodules of basaloid cells demonstrating a peripheral palisading pattern and stromal cleft formation
Superficial	Superficial foci of peripherally palisaded basaloid cells invading downward from the epidermis and stromal cleft formation
Morpheaform	Interspersed cords of basaloid cells within sclerotic collagenous stroma, which often lacks a peripheral palisading pattern and stromal cleft formation
Micronodular	Small islands of interconnected tumor foci with peripheral palisading and stromal cleft formation
Basosquamous	Features of the nodular or superficial basal cell carcinoma with a deeper component demonstrating overlapping features with squamous cell carcinoma

Laboratory studies: Approximately 26 different subtypes of BCC have been described. Histopathologic examination demonstrates basophilic epidermal cells with dermal invasion into the dermis in a peripheral palisading pattern accompanied by retraction artifact, that may be related to poor intercellular adherence (Table 22.2).

Differential diagnosis: A BCC may be confused clinically with sebaceous gland hyperplasia, squamous cell carcinoma (SCC), facial angiofibroma, trichoepithelioma, morphea, melanoma, or even a scar. The clinical picture, with histopathologic confirmation, makes the diagnosis.

Management: BCC is commonly treated surgically with electrodessication and curettage, surgical excision, or Mohs micrographic surgery. For low-risk cancers, surgical excision and electrodessication and curettage are the standard of care. Current guidelines recommend 4-mm margins to be used during surgical excision. One limitation of electrodessication and curettage is that it cannot be completed on hair bearing areas. For cancers that pose a high risk of recurrence and morbidity, Mohs micrographic surgery has the highest cure rate and appropriate use criteria have been developed for its use in BCC. Guidelines do not recommend topically based therapies or cryotherapy destruction for their treatment.

Rarely, BCC will demonstrate evidence of metastatic disease and recently targeted agents including Vismodegib, which inhibits smoothened (SMO) within the SHH pathway, has been approved for the treatment of metastatic BCC.

Prognosis: In general, studies have demonstrated 5-year cure rates more than 90% for Mohs micrographic surgery, excision, and electrodessication and curettage. When appropriate, Mohs micrographic surgery has the highest cure rate. Following the diagnosis of BCC, patients should undergo a total body skin examination at least annually, because they have a higher risk for developing additional keratinocyte carcinomas and melanoma.

Final comment: BCC is a malignant proliferation of basal keratinocytes that often presents as a shiny, pearly papule, with rolled borders and arborizing telangiectasias on sun-exposed areas.

Pathology demonstrates basophilic islands of tumor cells in a palisaded pattern, and surgical treatments have a high cure rate. Patients diagnosed with BCC have a higher incidence of future skin cancers and should be closely monitored by a dermatologist.

BOWEN DISEASE

Synonym: Squamous cell carcinoma *in situ*

Definition: Bowen disease (BD) or SCC *in situ*, represents full thickness atypia of keratinocytes limited to the epidermis.

Overview: BD is usually seen in patients older than 60 years, and common risk factors include ultraviolet light exposure, previous BCC or SCC, HPV infection, arsenic exposure, and immunosuppression. The etiology of BD is akin to SCC (see the following discussion).

Clinical presentation: BD presents as a well-demarcated, erythematous, scaly plaque with irregular borders found in sun-exposed areas (Figure 21.2). BD is generally asymptomatic, but larger lesions may be pruritic. Different regional variants include erythroplasia of Queyrat, which presents as a red, velvety patch on the glans penis and Bowenoid papulosis, which present as multiple red brown, papules often found on the penile shaft and associated with HPV-16 infection. Approximately 3–10% of all BD progresses to invasive SCC.

Laboratory studies: Histopathologic examination demonstrates full thickness atypia of keratinocytes, buckshot scattered atypical keratinocytes within the epidermis, involvement of the hair follicles, and parakeratosis. BD does not invade through the basement membrane, unlike invasive SCC.

Differential diagnosis: BD may resemble actinic keratosis (AK), keratoanthoma (KA), invasive SCC, BCC verruca vulgaris, or prurigo nodularis, but the diagnosis is made histopathologically.

Management: Electrodessication and curettage, excision, Mohs micrographic surgery, chemotherapeutic agents, topical immunomodulators, and photodynamic therapy all may be used in the treatment of BD.

Prognosis: Patients with BD have an excellent prognosis. Tumors more than 1.4 cm in width have greater than two times higher odds of recurrence than smaller lesions and are commonly associated with invasive SCC.

Final comment: BD refers to full thickness keratinocyte atypia confined to the epidermis that can be clinically managed with multiple modalities and overall has an excellent prognosis.

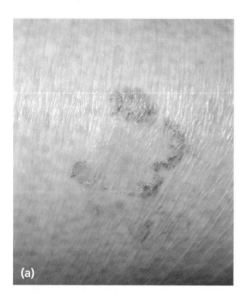
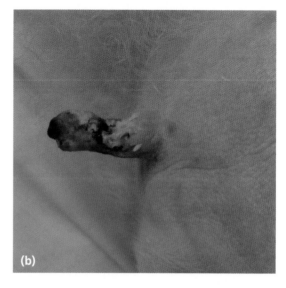

Figure 21.2 (a) Well-demarcated, erythematous, scaly plaque with irregular borders on sun damaged skin; (b) cutaneous horn in an albino skin of color patient.

SQUAMOUS CELL CARCINOMA

Definition: Invasive SCC is a malignant proliferation of keratinocytes with metastatic potential.

Overview: The mean age at the time of diagnosis for invasive SCC is age older than 60 years old and occurs more frequently in men and Caucasians. Previously, SCC occurred less frequently than BCC, but recently both have developed a similar incidence. SCC is most often the result of excessive sun exposure, but other contributing factors include immunosuppression, solid organ transplantation, chronic wounds and inflammation, xeroderma pigmentosum, albinism, and arsenic exposure. Tumor protein 53, a tumor suppressor gene, mutation is the most commonly associated mutation involved in tumorigenesis of SCC. With continued UV damage or inflammation, additional mutations accumulate, leading to unregulated cell growth and progression to SCC.

Clinical presentation: SCC can develop on any skin surface but is most commonly found on the sun-exposed areas of the head and neck. It can vary in size, with growth occurring over months and even years, while presenting as a firm pink to red hyperkeratotic scaly papule or plaque. There may be ulceration, hemorrhagic crusting, and pain. SCC may vary in size from less than 1 cm to several centimeters in diameter, and it can metastasize unlike a BCC, which rarely does.

Laboratory studies: Histopathologic study will reveal full thickness keratinocyte atypia invading into the dermis, horny pearls, acantholysis, and desmoplasia. An SCC may be graded from well differentiated to poorly differentiated based on its appearance and approximate percentage of cells that resemble native keratinocytes.

When there is palpable lymphadenopathy, an ultrasound guided fine needle aspirate may be completed to assess for lymphatic metastasis. If there are no palpable lymph nodes but the cancer is stratified as high risk, computed tomography (CT) or other advanced imaging, including magnetic resonance imaging (MRI) or positron emission tomography, should be considered. When there is concern for local metastasis, a sentinel lymph node biopsy will rule out metastatic disease.

Differential diagnosis: SCC may resemble BD, KA, hypertrophic actinic keratosis, BCC, verruca vulgaris, and prurigo nodularis.

Management: Standard excision, Mohs micrographic surgery, or electrodessication and curettage are frequently used in the treatment of SCC. For standard excision, 4–6-mm margins are recommended and for tumors with high-risk features or cosmetically sensitive locations Mohs micrographic surgery is completed. For patients with low-risk tumors in areas without terminal hair growth, electrodessication and curettage may be used for SCC. If surgical therapy is not feasible, radiation therapy or cryosurgery may be considered.

Prognosis: Locally invasive SCC has an excellent prognosis as standard excision and Mohs micrographic surgery have cure rates over 90%. Risk of distant metastasis is approximately 3–4%, but it is up to 2–3 times higher in solid organ transplant recipients. Risk factors for nodal metastasis and local recurrence include poorly differentiated tumors, depth greater than 2 mm, and perineural involvement. The largest risk factor for tumor related death is a tumor >2 cm in size in a solid organ transplant patient. The lip and ear are the clinical sites with the highest risk of recurrence and distant metastasis.

Patients diagnosed with one SCC have a 40.7% risk of developing another SCC or BCC within 5 years. This risk increases to 82% in patients previously diagnosed with more than one SCC.

Final comment: Cutaneous SCC characteristically presents as a red or brown, scaly, often crusted, papule or plaque in sun exposed areas (Figure 21.3). Cutaneous SCC is commonly treated surgically, and patients require close follow up with dermatology for total body skin examinations following diagnosis, as they are at a higher risk for developing additional skin cancers.

Table 21.3 Brigham and Women's Hospital Tumor Classification

Risk Factors	Number of Risk Factors	Stage
Tumor diameter >2 cm	0	T1
Poor cell differentiation	1	T2a
Perineural invasion	2–3	T2b
Tumor invasion beyond the subcutis	4	T3

Source: From Kim JYS, Kozlow JH, Mittal B, Moyer J, Olenecki T, Rodgers P. Guidelines of care for the management of cutaneous squamous cell carcinoma. J Am Acad Dermatol. 2018; 78:560–578, used with permission; adapted from Jambusaria-Pahlajani A, Kanetsky PA, Karia PS, et al. Evaluation of AJCC tumor staging for cutaneous squamous cell carcinoma and a proposed alternative tumor staging system. JAMA Dermatol. 2013;149:402–410.

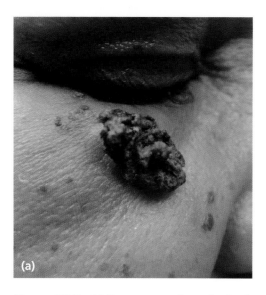
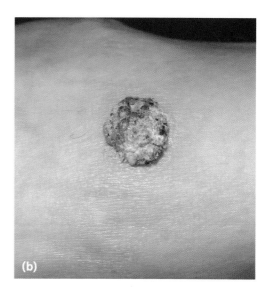

Figure 21.3 (a) Brown crusted exophytic plaque and (b) red keratotic papule, both on sun exposed skin.

KERATOACANTHOMA

Definition: A KA is a solitary keratin-filled, crater-like papulonodular tumor produced by squamous epithelium that rapidly grows, matures, and involutes over a period of months.

Overview: The mean age at diagnosis for KA is 50 years of age, and it most commonly effects Caucasian patients. Risk factors for development are similar to SCC and include ultraviolet light exposure, immunosuppressive drugs, trauma, chemotherapeutic agents including BRAF inhibitors, vemurafenib, and dabrafenib, and sonic hedgehog pathway inhibitors, vismodegib. Development of multiple KAs is associated with several rare genetic syndromes including Ferguson-Smith syndrome, Grzybowski syndrome and Muir-Torre syndrome discussed in Table 21.4.

Clinical presentation: A KA will most frequently develop in sun exposed areas. The typical clinical presentation is of a rapidly evolving, crater-like papule or nodule that may be a few millimeters to several centimeters in diameter (Figure 21.4). These tumors will undergo an initial growth phase, a proliferative phase, and a regressive phase within a timeframe of several months.

Laboratory studies: Histopathologic examination of KA will demonstrate a keratin-filled crater surrounded by variable squamous epidermal hyperplasia, neutrophilic abscesses, dermal fibrosis, and inflammation. Generally, KA lack atypical mitosis often seen in conventional cutaneous SCC. In contrast to SCC, KA is assumed to originate from the hair follicle.

Differential diagnosis: KA may resemble a conventional SCC, verruca vulgaris, prurigo nodularis, and milker's nodule.

Management: There are currently no formal guidelines regarding management of KA, although it is generally treated similar to SCC. One explanation is that only a fraction of the biopsied tissue

Table 21.4 **Keratoacanthoma Syndromes**

Keratoacanthoma Syndrome	Comments
Ferguson-Smith syndrome	• Autosomal dominant mutation of *TGFBR1*
	• Multiple KA's in patient's early adulthood
Grzybowski syndrome	• Thousands of milia-like KA's developing rapidly with self-resolution, leading to scarring
Muir-Torre syndrome	• Autosomal dominant condition associated with DNA mismatch repair genes
	• Associated with colon cancer, genitourinary cancer and multiple KAs

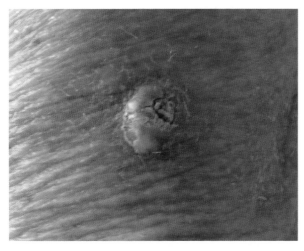

Figure 21.4 Crateriform papule with keratotic center.

specimen is examined by traditional histopathologic bread-loafing, and therefore, it is impossible to rule out foci with severe atypia within a KA specimen. For excision-based therapy, most clinicians extrapolate similar surgical margins recommended for SCC as guidance. In cases of giant KA or in cosmetically sensitive areas, Mohs micrographic surgery may be employed.

Prognosis: KA has an excellent prognosis; however, if the KA is refractory to treatment, SCC should be considered as an alternate diagnosis. There are no known confirmed cases of fatal KA.

Final comment: KA is a keratin-filled crater-like papulonodular tumor most commonly found in sun exposed areas and is thought to be related to or a subtype of SCC. KA's are usually treated with surgical excision and overall have an excellent prognosis.

MELANOMA

Definition: This represents a malignant proliferation of melanocytes. It accounts for the majority of skin cancer–related deaths.

Overview: In 2017, there were an estimated 87,110 new cases of melanoma and 9,730 melanoma-related deaths in the United States. The mean age at the time of melanoma diagnosis is 55 years old, and men are more frequently diagnosed with melanoma in the United States. The strongest risk factors for the development of melanoma include ultraviolet light exposure, fair skin complexion, having over 100 nevi, and a family history of melanoma. Multiple genes, including *CDKN2A*, which serves as a tumor suppressor gene, have been associated with the development of familial melanoma. Multiple gene mutations have been implicated in cutaneous melanoma. The *BRAF* gene and pathway, which regulates cell differentiation, growth, and proliferation, is commonly mutated in melanoma and is the target of new therapeutic agents.

Clinical presentation: Melanoma can develop either from preexisting nevi or *de novo*. Clinical features suggestive of melanoma include asymmetric shape, notched or irregular borders, color variation, diameter over 6 mm, and evolution of a pigmented lesion. These commonly employed criteria, referred to as the ABCDE's of melanoma, are used in the clinical setting to evaluate melanocytic growths. Additionally, the *ugly duckling sign*, a nevus that is not consistent with a patient's individual nevus pattern, can help making the diagnosis of melanoma. Important clinical variants of melanoma are covered in Table 21.5.

Laboratory studies: When there is concern for melanoma, an excisional biopsy is indicated with 1–3-mm margins around the lesion of interest. Histopathologic examination demonstrates asymmetric proliferation of atypical melanocytes and may have features characteristic of a radial and/or vertical growth phase.

Additional factors used in the histopathologic evaluation of melanoma include the mitotic rate, presence of lympho-vascular or perineural invasion, and regression of the tumor. Immunohistochemical staining for melanocytic makers can aide in the assessment of cutaneous melanoma; however, the diagnosis is traditionally made based on hematoxylin and eosin staining.

Melanoma staging is determined according to the American Joint Committee on Cancer (AJCC) staging system. The AJCC staging system uses the TNM scale, where T corresponds to tumor thickness, also known as Breslow's depth, N corresponds to nodal involvement, and M corresponds to sites of metastatic disease (Tables 21.7 and 21.8). Breslow's depth is the most important

Table 21.5 Clinical Subtypes of Melanoma

Clinical Variant	Epidemiology	Common Location	Clinical Presentation
Superficial spreading melanoma	Most common form of melanoma	Trunk & extremifies	Can develop from an existing nevus or *de novo* in sun exposed areas. This subtype has a slow radial growth phase, prior to invasion.
Nodular melanoma	Second most common form of melanoma	Head, neck & trunk	Thick, blue to black or pink-colored nodule with a rapid vertical growth phase. This variant is often diagnosed at advanced stages.
Lentigo maligna melanoma Synonym: Hutchinson's freckle	Common in elderly patients	Head & neck	Slow-growing, asymmetric, irregular brown patch with a long radial growth phase
Acral lentiginous melanoma	Similar incidence across all ethnic and racial groups	Palms, soles, or within the nail unit	An asymmetric brown to black macule with irregular borders

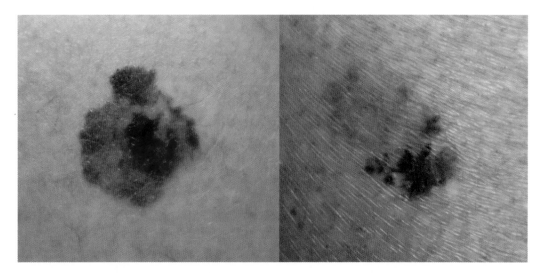

Figure 21.5 Superficial spreading melanoma: Asymmetrical plaque with scalloped borders and various shades of brown color and focal crust.

Table 21.6 Histopathologic Observations

Growth Phase	Pathology Findings
Radial growth phase	Confluent atypical melanocytes along the dermal-epidermal junction in addition to a "pagetoid" pattern of spread where melanocytes extend upward through the epidermis resembling Paget's disease of the breast. Additionally, this may include intra-epidermal nests of atypical melanocytes.
Vertical growth phase	Vertical, asymmetric growth of atypical melanocytes within or below the epidermis forming a tumor. This phase is characterized by the presence of dermal nests of atypical melanocytes that fail to mature and are larger or cytologically different than those in the overlying epidermis.

Table 21.7 Adapted American Joint Committee on Cancer TNM Definitions for Cutaneous Melanoma

Tumor Depth, Breslow Depth	
T1 <1.0 mm	a. <0.8 mm without ulceration
	b. <0.8 mm with ulceration or 0.8–1.0 mm with or without ulceration
T2 >1.0 to 2.0 mm	a. Without ulceration
	b. With ulceration
T3 >2.0 to 4.0 mm	a. Without ulceration
	b. With ulceration
T4 > 4.0mm	a. Without ulceration
	b. With ulceration
Lymph Node Involvement	
N1: 1 node or in-transit, satellite, and/or microsatellite metastases with no tumor-involved nodes	a. Clinically occult*
	b. Clinically detected**
	c. Intralymphatic metastases without regional lymph node disease***
N2: 2–3 nodes or in-transit, satellite, and/or microsatellite metastases with 1 tumor-involved node	a. Clinically occult*
	b. Clinically detected** ≥1 lymph node
	c. Intralymphatic metastases*** with 1 occult or clinically detected regional lymph node
N3: ≥4 tumor-involved nodes or in-transit, satellite, and/ or microsatellite metastases with ≥2 tumor-involved nodes, or any number of matted nodes without or with in-transit, satellite, and/ or microsatellite metastases	a. >4 metastatic clinically occult nodes* with no intralymphatic metastases
	b. >4 metastatic nodes** (≥1 clinically detected), or matted nodes (any number) with no intralymphatic metastases
	c. >2 clinically occult or clinically detected nodes and/or presence of matted nodes (any number) with intralymphatic*** metastases
Metastasis	
M1a: Distant skin, soft tissue (including muscle), and/or nonregional lymph nodes	With or without elevated LDH level
M1b: Lung metastasis with or without M1a	With or without elevated LDH level
M1c: Distant non-CNS visceral with or without M1a or M1b	With or without elevated LDH level
M1d: Distant metastasis to CNS with or without M1a, M1b, or M1c	With or without elevated LDH level

Source: From Swetter SM, Tsao H, Bichakjian CKet al. Guidelines of care for the management of primary cutaneous melanoma. J Am Acad Dermatol. 2019; 80: 208–250; adapted from Gershenwald JE, Scolyer RA, Hess KR, et al. Melanoma of the skin. In: Amin MB, Edge SB, Greene FL, et al. eds. AJCC Cancer Staging Manual. 8th ed. New York, NY: Springer International Publishing; 2017, used with permission.

Abbreviations: LDH, lactic dehydrogenase; CNS, central nervous system.

Notes: *Clinically occult tumor-involved regional lymph nodes are microscopically diagnosed after sentinel lymph node biopsy; **Clinically detected tumor-involved regional lymph nodes are defined as clinically evident nodal metastases confirmed by fine-needle, aspiration, biopsy and/or therapeutic lymphadenectomy; ***Intralymphatic metastases are defined by the presence of clinically apparent in-transit/satellite metastasis and/or histologically evident microsatellite metastases in the primary tumor specimen.

Table 21.8 Adapted AJCC Staging for Cutaneous Melanoma

T	N	M	Pathologic Stage
In situ	N 0	M0	0
T1a	N 0	M0	1a
T1b	N 0	M0	1a
T2a	N 0	M0	1b
T2b	N 0	M0	2a
T3a	N 0	M0	2a
T4a	N 0	M0	2b
T4b	N 0	M0	2c
T0, no identified primary melanoma	N1b–N1c	M0	3b
T0, no identified primary melanoma	N2b–N2c or N3b–N3c	M0	3c
T1a–T2a	N1a or N2a	M0	3a
T1a–T2a	N1b–N1c or N2b	M0	3b
T2b–T3a	N1a–N2b	M0	3b
T1a–T3a	N2c–N3c	M0	3c
T3b–T4a	N1a–N3c	M0	3c
T4b	N1a–N2c	M0	3c
T4b	N3a–N3c	M0	3d
Any T grade	Any N grade	M1a–M1d	4

Source: From Swetter SM, Tsao H, Bichakjian CK, et al. Guidelines of care for the management of primary cutaneous melanoma. J Am Acad Dermatol. 2019; 80: 208–250, used with permission, adapted from Gershenwald JE, Scolyer RA, Hess KR, et al. Melanoma of the skin. In: Amin MB, Edge SB, Greene FL, et al. eds. AJCC Cancer Staging Manual. 8th ed. New York, NY: Springer International Publishing; 2017.

staging characteristic and is measured from the granular layer to the deepest part of the melanoma. Presence of tumor ulceration increases the grade of the tumor. Depending on the stage of melanoma at the time of diagnosis, patients may require sentinel lymph node biopsy. If further metastatic evaluation is warranted, computer-assisted tomography (CAT) scan with contrast of the chest, abdomen, and pelvis or total body positron emission tomography may be completed. If there are findings suggestive of brain involvement, a brain MRI is recommended.

Differential diagnosis: This includes an atypical nevus, Spitz nevus, blue nevus of Jadassohn, pigmented BCC, solar lentigo, seborrheic keratosis, and black heel.

Management: The treatment of melanoma is based on tumor stage. Early diagnosis combined with appropriate surgical therapy is currently the only curative treatment for melanoma. Surgical modalities used for the treatment of melanoma include wide local excision, with or without sentinel lymph node biopsy, and Mohs micrographic surgery. For wide local excision, surgical margins are based on the depth of tumor invasion. If a sentinel lymph node biopsy is recommended, the procedure is completed simultaneously with wide local excision.

For patients with melanoma *in situ* or lentigo maligna, modified Mohs micrographic surgery may be completed. For metastatic melanoma new targeted therapies are available including BRAF inhibitors, MEK inhibitors, CTLA-4 inhibitors and PDL-1 inhibitors. Both BRAF and MEK inhibitors target tumor growth pathways and are used as combination therapy, whereas CTLA-4 inhibitors and PDL-1 inhibitors potentiate T-cell mediated inflammation of destruction of tumor cells in melanoma.

Prognosis: Recent data suggest 5-year and 10-year survival of >95% in patients diagnosed with Stage I melanoma, whereas this number substantially drops with more advanced stage at the time

Table 21.9 Recommended Follow-up Intervals

Melanoma Stage	Recommended Follow-Up Interval
Melanoma in-situ	Every 6–12 months for 1–2 years then annually
Stage IA–IIA	Every 6–12 months for 2–5 years then annually
Stage IIB–IVC	Every 6 months for 3–5 years and then annually

of diagnosis and is worst in patients with metastatic disease. New studies suggest that BRAF and MEK inhibitors, in addition to PD1 inhibitors, are similarly effective in the treatment of metastatic disease and provides for optimism related to the treatment of metastatic disease. Recommended follow-up total body skin examinations are listed in Table 21.9.

Final comment: Melanoma is an invasive, potentially fatal malignant neoplasm of melanocytes. Clinical evaluation of melanocytic growths with the ABCDE criteria and the ugly duckling sign allow for increased clinical sensitivity in diagnosing melanoma. It is characterized by asymmetric growth of atypical melanocytes in the radial or vertical growth phase. Primary treatment is surgical excision, with or without lymph node biopsy and new therapeutics targeting the BRAF pathway or that enhance immune cell activation have provided new optimism for the treatment of patients diagnosed with metastatic melanoma.

MERKEL CELL CARCINOMA

Definition: Merkel cell carcinoma (MCC) is an aggressive malignant proliferation of neuroendocrine cells, presenting with locally invasive and metastatic behavior.

Overview: The mean age at diagnosis for MCC is 75 years old, and it is more commonly found in Caucasian patients. MCC is associated with integration of Merkel cell polyomavirus DNA into host cells, eventually leading to loss of cell cycle regulation in Merkel cells. Although approximately 60–80% of the general population have been infected by the Merkel cell polyomavirus, other host factors associated include ultraviolet radiation, immunosuppression, organ transplantation, and HIV infection.

Clinical presentation: MCC is most often diagnosed in sun exposed areas and presents as a solitary pink to purple smooth indurated plaque or nodule, most often on the head neck. The lesion may be ulcerated, sometimes, tender, and associated with palpable regional lymphadenopathy.

Laboratory studies: Histopathologic examination of MCC demonstrates intradermal sheets, nests, or trabeculae of uniform, small, round blue cells with scant cytoplasm, frequent mitoses, and necrotic cells. Immunostaining for MCC is positive for cytokeratin 20, chromogranin, CD56 and neuron specific enolase. Additional immunohistochemistry stains including S100 or SOX10, are used to rule out melanoma, and CD43 to rule out lymphoma.

When there is concern for metastatic disease, a CAT scan with contrast of the chest, abdomen, and pelvis is indicated.

Differential diagnosis: Clinically, BCC, SCC, and amelanotic melanoma may resemble MCC, and histologically melanoma metastatic neuroendocrine carcinoma, and lymphoma may resemble MCC.

Management: The AJCC eighth edition guidelines recommend excision with 1–2-cm margins and sentinel lymph node biopsy as initial treatment for MCC. For small tumors, Mohs micrographic surgery may be used as well. In addition to surgical removal, patients who undergo local radiation following excision have improved outcomes. For tumors that are not amenable to surgery, radiation therapy may be used. Finally, studies have anti-PDL1 immunotherapy, including pembrolizumab, can be used for MCC. Patients diagnosed with MCC should undergo total body skin examination and lymph node examination every 3–6 months for the first 3 years following diagnosis and every 6–12 months thereafter.

Prognosis: MCC patients have a 5-year survival rate of 51% in patients with local disease, 35% of patients with nodal disease, and 14% with metastatic disease. In patients with local disease, life expectancy is similar to their age matched peers, which may be related to the association with development of MCC late in life.

Final Comment: MCC is a malignant proliferation of Merkel cells that presents as a solitary pink to purple plaque or nodule commonly located in the head and neck region of older adults. This tumor demonstrates aggressive behavior, and many patients have invasive disease at the time of diagnosis. Current guidelines recommend surgical excision with lymph node biopsy for initial management. Overall, patients with limited disease and those who are amenable to curative surgical therapy have a similar life span to their peers, whereas patients with advanced disease have a grim prognosis.

DERMATOFIBROSARCOMA PROTUBERANS

Definition: Dermatofibrosarcoma protuberans (DFSP) is a locally invasive cutaneous sarcoma of spindled cells with metastatic potential.

Overview: The mean age at diagnosis for DFSP is 43 years old, with a slightly higher incidence in women than men. Multiple DFSP tumors have been observed in children with adenosine deaminase deficient severe combined immunodeficiency. The pathogenesis involves a translocation between chromosomes 17 and 22, creating a tyrosine kinase fusion gene involving collagen type 1 alpha 1 and the platelet-derived growth factor subunit b. This new oncogene enables constitutive expression of platelet-derived growth factor subunit b and unregulated proliferation of the tumor.

Clinical presentation: DFSP initially presents as an asymptomatic, slow-growing skin-colored to purple-brown plaque that becomes more indurated and nodular over time (Figure 21.6). The tumor is found on the trunk in the majority of patients, often favoring the shoulder and pelvic girdle.

Laboratory studies: If there is concern DFSP, a deep incisional biopsy is required to determine the extent of local invasion; otherwise, this tumor may be mistaken for dermatofibroma, as they can resemble one another both clinically and histologically. The classic histopathologic findings of DFSP include proliferation of dermal spindle cells arranged in a storiform pattern. Immunostaining aids in diagnosis, and most histologic variants stain positive for CD34 and negative for factor XIIIa. In contrast, a dermatofibroma stains positive for factor XIIIa but not CD34.

Differential diagnosis: DFSP may resemble dermatofibroma, morpheaform BCC, neurofibroma, lipoma, sebaceous cyst, hypertrophic scar, and cutaneous metastasis.

Management: Definitive management of localized DFSP includes surgical excision or Mohs micrographic surgery (MMS). DFSP tumors excised with positive histopathologic margins have >50% likelihood of recurrence. For this reason, MMS is recommended for cosmetically sensitive area's including the head and neck, whereas conventional excision is utilized for involvement of the trunk and extremities. If there is concern for local involvement of deeper or vital structures, a CAT scan or an MRI may be used to determine the extent of tumor invasion prior to definitive treatment. If there are concerns for distant spread, CAT imaging with contrast dye can evaluate for sites of distant metastasis. For metastatic DFSP or tumors nonamenable to surgery, tyrosine kinase inhibitors, such as imatinib, as well as radiation therapy can be used as adjuvant therapy.

Prognosis: The most common complication is local recurrence. In DFSP treated with MMS, the risk of recurrence is decreased, because the surgical margins are analyzed intraoperatively. Metastatic disease occurs in less than 5% of cases, and the lungs are the most common sites for metastasis. Metastatic disease is more common in recurrent tumors that were not completely excised at the time of initial diagnosis. A poor prognosis is related to older age, male gender, and tumor size at the time of diagnosis.

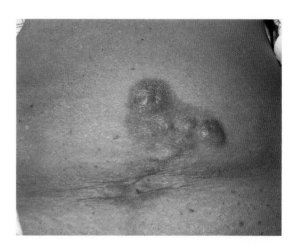

Figure 21.6 Brown multinodular plaque.

FINAL THOUGHT

DFSP is a cutaneous sarcoma that presents as a slow-growing, skin-colored to purple or brown indurated asymptomatic plaque. Histology demonstrates spindle cells in a storiform pattern, and excision-based therapies are recommended for treatment. Overall prognosis for DFSP patients is good; however, the risk of local recurrence is high for incompletely excised tumors.

ADDITIONAL READINGS

Coggshall K, Tello TL, North JP, et al. Merkel cell carcinoma: an update and review: pathogenesis, diagnosis, and staging. J Am Acad Dermatol. 2018;78:433–442.

Criscito MC, Martires KJ, Stein JA. Prognostic factors, treatment, and survival in dermatofibrosarcoma protuberans. JAMA Dermatol. 2016;152:1365–1371.

Ferrándiz C, Malvehy J, Guillén C, et al. Precancerous skin lesions. Actas Dermosifiliogr. 2017;108:31–41.

Kim DP, Kus KJB, Ruiz E. Basal cell carcinoma review. Hematol Oncol Clin North Am. 2019;33:13–24.

Kim JYS, Kozlow JH, Mittal B, et al. Guidelines of care for the management of basal cell carcinoma. J Am Acad Dermatol. 2018;78:540–559.

Kim JYS, Kozlow JH, Mittal B, et al. Guidelines of care for the management of cutaneous squamous cell carcinoma. J Am Acad Dermatol. 2018;78:560–578.

Rogers HW, Weinstock MA, Feldman SR, et al. Incidence estimate of nonmelanoma skin cancer (Keratinocyte Carcinomas) in the US Population, 2012. JAMA Dermatol. 2015;151:1081–1086.

Siegel R, Miller K, Fedewa S, et al. Cancer statistics, CA. Cancer J Clin. 2017;67:7–30.

Swetter SM, Tsao H, Bichakjian CK, et al. Guidelines of care for the management of primary cutaneous melanoma. J Am Acad Dermatol. 2019;80:208–250.

Ugurel S, Röhmel J, Ascierto PA, et al. Survival of patients with advanced metastatic melanoma: the impact of novel therapies. Eur J Cancer. 2016;53:125–134.

22 Cutaneous Lymphomas

Emily Correia, Shalini Krishnasamy, and Neda Nikbakht

CONTENTS

Overview: Primary cutaneous lymphomas are defined as a heterogenous group of non-Hodgkin lymphomas with varying clinical presentations and disease courses that initially present in the skin but may progress to having extracutaneous involvement. Primary cutaneous lymphomas are broadly classified as cutaneous T-cell lymphomas and cutaneous B-cell lymphomas. These classifications include several distinct entities, as outlined by the most recent 2018 update of the World Health Organization/European Organisation for Research and Treatment of Cancer (WHO/EORTC) classification (Table 22.1).

CUTANEOUS T-CELL LYMPHOMAS

Definition: Cutaneous T-cell lymphomas compose approximately 75% of all primary cutaneous lymphomas. Included in this classification are mycosis fungoides and its leukemic variant, Sézary syndrome, CD30+ lymphoproliferative disorders, and other entities including subcutaneous panniculitis-like T-cell lymphoma, extranodal natural killer (NK)/T-cell lymphoma nasal type, primary cutaneous peripheral T-cell lymphoma not otherwise specified, and adult T-cell leukemia/lymphoma. See Table 22.2.

MYCOSIS FUNGOIDES

Definition: Mycosis fungoides (MF) is the most common type of cutaneous T-cell lymphoma and accounts for almost 50% of all primary cutaneous lymphomas. MF is an indolent, mature T-cell lymphoma characterized by aberrant and excessive proliferation of CD4 T-cells in the skin, with possible progression to involve lymph nodes, blood, and viscera.

The etiology of MF is largely unknown. Many infectious agents have been investigated for putative roles in development of MF; however, the data are limited, and studies have yielded contradictory results to reliably implicate any single infectious agent, including HTLV-1. It has also been hypothesized that MF may arise from malignant transformation of activated T-cells in the setting of persistent antigen stimulation or chronic inflammation.

DOI: 10.1201/9781003105268-22

Table 22.1 WHO-EORTC Classification of Cutaneous Lymphomas

Cutaneous T-Cell and Natural Killer (NK)-Cell Lymphomas

Mycosis fungoides

Folliculotropic MF

Pagetoid reticulosis

Granulomatous slack skin

Sezary syndrome

Adult T-cell leukemia/lymphoma

Primary cutaneous CD30+ lymphoproliferative disorders

Lymphomatoid papulosis

Primary cutaneous anaplastic large cell lymphoma

Subcutaneous panniculitis-like T-cell lymphoma

Primary cutaneous peripheral T-cell lymphoma, rare subtypes

Cutaneous γ/δ T-cell lymphoma (provisional)

Primary cutaneous aggressive epidermotropic CD8+ T-cell lymphoma (provisional)

Primary cutaneous CD4-positive small/medium pleomorphic T-cell lymphoproliferative disorder

Primary cutaneous acral CD8+ T-cell lymphoma (provisional)

Primary cutaneous peripheral T-cell lymphoma, NOS

Extranodal NK/T-cell lymphoma, nasal type

Cutaneous B-Cell Lymphomas

Primary cutaneous marginal zone B-cell lymphoma

Primary cutaneous follicle center lymphoma

Primary cutaneous diffuse large B-cell lymphoma

Source: Adapted from WHO/EORTC 2018 classification for cutaneous lymphomas.

Currently, there is little information on the founder and driver mutations responsible for early transformation of T cells in MF; however, some studies identified mutational hotspots at genes involved in important signaling pathways for T-cell activation (e.g., T-cell receptor, JAK/STAT, CD28, phospholipase C gamma) as well as canonical cancer-associated genes, such as MAPK and chromatin modifying genes.

Clinical presentation: The overall incidence of MF is approximately 5.6 per million persons per year. Men are more commonly affected (incidence rate ratio IRR = 1.6–2:1), and blacks have a higher incidence than whites (IRR:1.57). MF primarily affects middle-aged to older adults (median age at diagnosis: 55–60) but may occur in children and adolescents. Notably, black patients are diagnosed younger (mean age of diagnosis of 53 years, compared to 63 years for whites) and have worse survival compared to whites regardless of age and stage.

MF is characterized by various cutaneous manifestations, including patches, plaques, or tumors (Figures 22.1–22.3), most commonly involving sun-protected areas, although any area may be affected. Patients may also present with generalized erythroderma, and in this case, the possibility of leukemic disease should be investigated. Patients can have different types of lesions simultaneously.

Early patch-stage MF is characterized by the presence of erythematous lesions of variable size with fine scale, frequently occurring on covered areas of the trunk and limb, particularly the buttocks, lower part of the abdomen, and thighs. The lesions may have an atrophic surface or may present as poikiloderma with mottled dyspigmentation or telangiectasia. In general, patch-stage lesions often resemble dermatitis, being round or ovoid, although arciform, polycyclic, and annular configurations can occur.

With progression, thicker, more infiltrated reddish-brown scaling plaques can develop in a more generalized distribution and may resemble psoriasis. The palms and soles may be involved with hyperkeratotic, psoriasiform, and fissuring plaques. Over time, involvement can become widespread through coalescence of plaques, but there are usually patches of normal skin interspersed.

Table 22.2 Summary of Cutaneous T-Cell Lymphomas

Name	Clinical Presentation	Histology	Immunophenotype	5- Year Survival
Mycosis Fungoides	• Patches, plaques, or tumors that may be pruritic and ulcerate • Lymph nodes and visceral organs my become involved • Variants include folliculotropic, pagetoid reticulosis, and granulomatous slack skin	T lymphocytes with cerebriform nuclei confined to the epidermis	Aberrant CD2, CD3, CD5 Loss of CD7	88%
Sezary Syndrome	• Triad of erythroderma, peripheral lymphadenopathy, and atypical cellular infiltrates • Alopecia, onychodystrophy, palmoplantar hyperkeratosis	Cellular infiltrates in epidermis	CD3+, CD4+ Loss of CD7 and CD26	24%
Primary Cutaneous CD30+ Lymphomatoid papulosis	• Recurrent papular, papulonecrotic, or nodular lesions that regress spontaneously in 3–8 weeks	• CD30+ cells with inflammatory cells in dermis that may resemble non-Hodgkin's lymphoma	CD3+, CD4+, CD8-	100%
Cutaneous Anaplastic Large Cell Lymphoma	• Solitary or localized papules, nodules, and tumors that may ulcerate and occasionally regress	• Nonepidermotropic CD30+ cells with irregularly shaped nuclei	Loss of CD2, CD5, CD3	95%
Adult T-Cell Lymphoma	• Leukemia, lymphadenopathy, organomegaly, hypercalcemia • Generalized papules or plaques, nodules, or tumors	Superficial or diffuse infiltrate of various T-cell sizes with pleomorphic nuclei Epidermotropism	CD3+, CD4+, CD25+ CD8-	N/a
Subcutaneous Panniculitis-like T-Cell Lymphoma	• Solitary or multiple nodules and plaques, commonly on legs • Commonly accompanies by fever, fatigue, weight loss	Panniculitis-like subcutaneous infiltrates with pleomorphic T-cells containing hyperchromatic nuclei and macrophages	CD3+, CD8+, βF1+ CD4-, CD56-	82%
Extranodal NK/T Cell Lymphoma, Nasal Type	• Multiple plaques or tumors on trunk and extremities, or destructive midfacial tumor • Fever, malaise, weight loss, hemophagocytic syndrome	Dense infiltrates in dermis and subcutis with angiocentricity, angiodestruction, and necrosis	CD2+, CD3+ (cytoplasmic), TIA-1+, EBER-1+, CD56+, granzyme B+, perforin+ CD4-	N/a
Primary Cutaneous Peripheral T-Cell Lymphoma Primary Cutaneous Aggressive	• Localized or disseminated eruptive papules, nodules and tumors that may ulcerate and necrose	Atrophic epidermis, necrotic keratinocytes, ulceration, and spongiosis; epidermotropism	βF1+, CD3+, CD8+, granzyme B+, perforin+, TIA-1+, CD45RA+ CD45RO-, CD2-, CD4-, CD5-	18%

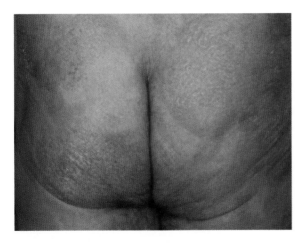

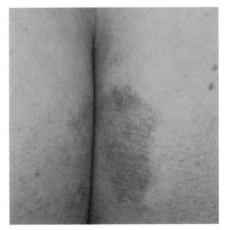

Figure 22.1 Erythematous patches in a bathing suit distribution. There may be varying amounts of scale.

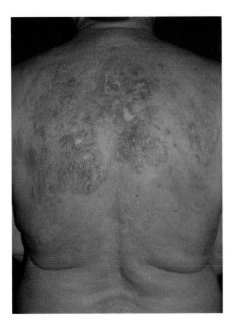

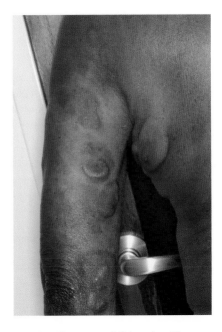

Figure 22.2 Well-defined erythematous plaques with some crusting and hyperpigmentation.

Figure 22.3 Tumors exhibit a significant vertical growth phase and must measure at least 1 cm in diameter and may or may not ulcerate.

The lesions can progress to the tumor stage, characterized by nodules of varying size on infiltrated plaques as well as on normal appearing skin. Tumors have a propensity to form on the trunk, although they can occur anywhere on the skin.

In 30% of cases, patches or plaques are limited to less than 10% of the skin surface, and more generalized patch/plaque involvement is observed in approximately 35% of cases. Tumors and erythroderma are seen in approximately 20% and 15% of cases, respectively.

Besides the conventional presentation of classic MF as detailed above, several variants of MF exist including folliculotropic (pilotropic) MF, localized pagetoid reticulosis (Woringer-Kolopp), and granulomatous slack skin. MF with large cell transformation is defined by the presence of large cells (>4 times the size of a small lymphocyte) comprising greater than 25% of the lesion infiltrate or the presence of microscopic nodules of large cells.

See Tables 22.3a, 22.3b, and 22.3c for clinical features, histology, and staging.

269

Table 22.3a Clinical Features and Histopathology of Mycosis Fungoides (MF)

MF Variant	Clinical Features	Histopathology
Folliculotropic	• Grouped follicular papules, acneiform lesions, indurates plaques, and sometimes tumors that preferentially involve the head and neck • Associated with alopecia and mucinorrhea	Perivascular and periadnexal localization of dermal infiltrates with variable infiltrations of the follicular epithelium
Pagetoid reticulosis	• Solitary patch or plaque, usually localized on the extremities • Slowly progressive	Hyperplastic epidermis with marked infiltration by atypical pagetoid cells, either singly or in clusters
Granulomatous Slack Skin	• Circumscribed areas of pendulous lax skin with predilection for axillae and groin	Dense granulomatous dermal infiltrates containing atypical T cell, macrophages and destruction of elastic tissue

Table 22.3b TNMB Staging of Mycosis Fungoides and Sezary Syndrome

	T	N	M	B
0	–	No enlargement	No involvement	No involvement
1	Patches, papules, plaques <10%*	Enlarged lymph nodes+	Involvement no histological involvement	Low number of circulating atypical cells**
2	Patches ≥10%* (2A) Patches and/or plaques ≥10%* (2B)	Enlarged lymph nodes+ histological involvement (nodal architecture not effaced)	–	High number of circulating atypical cells***
3	≥1 tumor ≥1cm diameter	Enlarged lymph nodes+ histological involvement (nodal architecture partially effaced)-	– –	– –
4	Confluent erythema >80%*	–	–	–
X	–	Abnormal involvement No histology acquired	Abnormal involvement+ No histology acquired	–

Source: Adapted from NCCN *Primary Cutaneous Lymphomas* 2020 guidelines.

Abbreviations: T, skin involvement; N, lymph node involvement; M, visceral metastasis; B, blood involvement.

*of body surface area

**>5% Sezary cells OR >15% CD4+CD26−/CD4+CD7− cells of total lymphocytes

***≥1000 Sezary cells/microliter OR ≥30% CD4+CD26− cells OR ≥40% CD4+CD7− cells

Laboratory studies: Patients with suspected MF should have a full clinical examination and biopsies taken from patches, plaques, and tumors. Typically, broad shave biopsies are used for patch or plaque lesions, while nodular and tumoral lesions require punch or incisional biopsies. Subsequently, histology of the biopsy is viewed and immunophenotypic and molecular studies are conducted. Polymerase chain reaction for T-cell receptor rearrangement to identify mono-clonality or next generation high-throughput sequencing to identify dominant malignant T-cell clones should be done. Blood work, including a routine complete blood count, biochemistry, serum lactate dehydrogenase, HTLV-1 serology, blood smear review to identify Sezary cells, and flow cytometry to identify lymphocyte subsets (CD4, CD8, CD26, CD7 included) is also required. These studies are important to determine which patients have peripheral blood T-cell clones along with the skin malignancy, which would correlate to a worse prognosis.

Table 22.3c Clinical staging of Mycosis Fungoides and Sezary Syndrome

I	A	T_1	N_0	M_0	B_{0-1}
	AB	T_2	N_0	M_0	B_{0-1}
II	A	T_{1-2}	N_{1-2}	M_0	B_{0-1}
	B	T_3	N_{0-1}	M_0	B_{0-1}
III	A	T_4	N_{0-2}	M_0	B_{0-1}
	B	T_4	N_{0-2}	M_0	B_1
IV	A_1	T_{1-4}	N_{0-2}	M_0	B_2
	A_2	T_{1-4}	N_3	M_0	B_{0-2}
	B	T_{1-4}	N_{0-3}	M_1	B_{0-2}

Source: From Bolognia J, et al., Dermatology Essentials, Elsevier 2014, with permission

Imaging (CT scan or PET-CT) of the neck, chest, abdomen, and pelvis can be performed and should be part of the workup for patients with significant skin involvement or any extracutaneous disease. The use of PET scans in cutaneous lymphomas is still being investigated; however, it may increase the detection rate of systemic disease. Lymph node excision or core biopsies should be done on patients with palpable lymph nodes, or nodes that are greater than 1.5 cm.

Histopathologically, MF is characterized by an epidermotrophic proliferation of small to medium-sized pleiomorphic lymphocytes with cerebriform nuclei surrounded by a clear cytoplasm (haloed cells) which can form intraepidermal collections known as Pautrier's microabscesses (Figure 22.4). It should be noted that marked epidermotropism and Pautrier's microabscesses, the two histopathologic hallmarks of the disease most valuable for diagnosis, are absent in a majority of early MF specimens. Additional useful clues include presence of papillary dermal fibrosis and lymphocytic apposition to basal keratinocytes. Although histopathologic criteria for the diagnosis of early MF are available, many of them are similar to those seen in inflammatory dermatoses. In many cases, a definitive diagnosis is only possible with careful clinicopathologic correlation.

Immunohistochemical studies are often used to aid in diagnosis of MF and can be helpful in differentiating MF from inflammatory dermatoses. In classic MF, the atypical lymphocytes are CD3+, CD4+, CD8−, and CD56−. Generally, the overall infiltrate should have a skewed CD4 > CD8 ratio (find normal ratio), although it should be noted that this finding can also be seen in some benign inflammatory dermatoses. Loss of T-cell antigens, such as CD2 and CD5, may further support a neoplastic process, but loss of CD7 should be interpreted with caution because it can be lost in a variety of benign dermatoses. Finally, it is important to note aberrant phenotypes observed in MF, including CD56 positive MF, double negative MF (CD4−CD8−) and CD8-positive

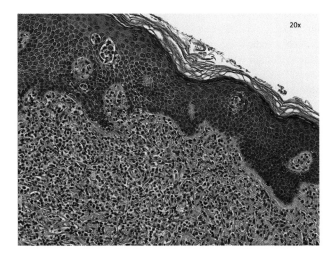

20x

Figure 22.4 Mycosis fungoides: Dense lymphocytic infiltrates in the dermis. Epidermis features Pautrier's microabscesses containing Langerhans cells and lymphocytes.

MF (CD4−CD8+). In these cases, histopathology and clinical correlation is crucial, particularly in cases with cytotoxic phenotype in order to exclude other cytotoxic lymphomas, such as cutaneous aggressive epidermotropic CD8+ cytotoxic T-cell lymphoma, cutaneous γ/δ T cell lymphoma, or cytotoxic lymphopapulosis.

The T-cell receptor (TCR) genes are clonally rearranged in the majority of cases of MF, so evaluation for clonal TCR gene rearrangement in skin should be performed. Assays used to assess T-cell clonality include polymerase chain reaction (PCR) and, most recently, next-generation high-throughput sequencing. High-throughput sequencing of the TCR gene, which permits identification of a T-cell clone through the sequence of its CDR3 region with superior sensitivity compared with traditional TCR PCR is the single greatest advancement to aid in diagnosis of MF. MF can present or progress to a large cell transformed histologic variant, which corresponds to poor prognosis and reduced survival. MF with large cell transformation is defined by the presence of large cells (>4 times the size of a small lymphocyte) composing greater than 25% of the lesion infiltrate or the presence of microscopic nodules of large cells.

Differential diagnosis: Due to overlapping clinicopathologic features with many benign and malignant conditions, MF has a broad differential diagnosis. Benign dermatoses that MF can resemble include psoriasis, chronic dermatitis, and lymphomatoid drug eruptions, among others. Pityriasis lichenoides, including pityriasis lichenoides chronica (PLC) and pityriasis lichenoides et varioliformis acuta (PLEVA), can resemble MF clinically and overlap with MF pathologically; particularly, PLC patients should be monitored as they may over time develop MF.

Management: Treatment is guided by degree of body surface area involvement and stage (Table 22.4). Early-stage MF (Stages IA–IIA) is managed with skin-directed therapies including topical corticosteroids and phototherapy. Topical bexarotene, topical nitrogen mustard, imiquimod, local radiation, and psoralen plus ultraviolet A (PUVA) are additional options. Treatment options for more advanced disease include oral bexarotene, extracorporeal photopheresis, interferon therapy (IFNa and IFNg), total skin electron beam therapy (TSEBT), methotrexate, monoclonal antibodies such as brentuximab vedotin and mogalizumab, and epigenetic modulators such as

Table 22.4 MF Treatment Based on Clinical Stage

Stage IA/IIA (T1) with B0	• Skin directed therapy* (limited)
Stage IB/IIA with B0	• Skin directed therapy (generalized)
Stage IA/IB/IIA with B1	• Systemic biologic therapies
Stage IIB with B0	• Local radiation for tumors
	• Systemic biologic therapies
	• Skin-directed therapies any patch/plaque disease
Stage IIB with B0 or IIB with B1	• Total skin electron beam therapy with or without adjuvant systemic biologic therapy
	• Combination therapies
	• Systemic chemotherapies**
	• Skin-directed therapy for path/plaque disease
Stage III with B0	• Skin-directed therapy (generalized)
	• Systemic biologic therapies
Stage III with B1	• Systemic biologic therapies with or without skin-directed therapy
Stage IV: Sezary syndrome and/or lymph node involvement	• Systemic biologic therapies
	• Combination therapies
Stage IV: Visceral disease or lymph node disease (not SS)	• Systemic chemotherapies
	• Possible radiation therapy

Source: Adapted from Bolognia J, et al., Dermatology Essentials, Elsevier 2014.

* Skin-directed therapies include topical corticosteroids, topical retinoids (tazarotene, bexarotene), topical imiquimod, topical chemotherapy (nitrogen mustard, carmustine), local radiation, phototherapy (narrowbeam UVB and PUVA), total skin electron beam radiation therapy; ϙ systemic biologic therapies include interferon α and β, methotrexate, oral retinoids (bexarotene, isotretinoin, acitretin), extracorporeal photophoresis, brentuximab, vorinostat, and romidepsin.

** Systemic chemotherapies include doxurubicin, gemcitabine, and the like.

histone deacetylase inhibitors, including vorinostat and romidepsin, as well as single and multi-modal chemotherapy.

Course: Prognosis of MF is affected by disease stage at time of diagnosis. Most patients with MF present with early-stage disease and have an indolent course with low risk of disease progression. Individuals with patch/plaque stage MF with limited body surface area involvement have a life expectancy unchanged from age, sex, and race-matched controls. Prognosis worsens in patients with extensive skin involvement, the presence of tumor stage lesions, and extracutaneous involvement. Apart from advanced stage, age greater than 65 years, male gender, African American race, high plasma lactate dehydrogenase (LDH), nodal involvement, and large cell transformation have been associated with worse overall survival. The 5-year survival rate is 88%.

SEZARY SYNDROME

Overview: Sezary syndrome is the classic triad of erythroderma, lymphadenopathy, and atypical clonal T cells (Sezary cells) in the skin, lymph nodes, and peripheral blood. Like other forms of cutaneous T-cell lymphoma (CTCL), the etiology of Sezary syndrome is mostly unknown, but it is linked to the monoclonal proliferation of T cells and the spread of these lymphocytes to the peripheral blood.

Clinical presentation: Sezary syndrome commonly presents in elderly men. Although patients may sometimes have had a previous history of the disease, it is rarely a progression of MF. Typically, patients complain of a long history of dermatitis. Presenting features of Sezary syndrome are exfoliative, edematous, and pruritic erythroderma (Figure 22.5). Patients may have systemic problems, such as high-output cardiac failure, due to blood trafficking through dilated cutaneous vessels. Patients may also have alopecia, palmoplantar hyperkeratosis, fissuring of the nails, and peripheral lymphadenopathy. Lichenification and ectropion is also seen, and bacterial or dermatophyte infections can occur in areas of excoriation.

Laboratory studies: The diagnosis requires the presence of Sezary cells in the peripheral blood; these cells are cerebriform and mononuclear. On complete blood count, a normal white blood cell count can be seen or there can be a moderate leukocytosis. In order to diagnose Sezary syndrome, there must be a Sezary cell count of at least 1000 cells per microliter. The buffy coat may also contain 15–30% Sezary cells.

Similar to MF, the histology may also demonstrate epidermotropism with abnormal cells in the dermis; however, nonspecific findings may be seen on histology. Lymph nodes involved in the disease process typically demonstrate a dense infiltrate of Sezary cells with effacement of lymph node architecture. Immunophenotypically, Sezary cells are CD3+, CD4+, CD7-, CD8-, and CD26-.

The diagnostic criteria for Sezary syndrome require the triad of erythroderma, lymphadenopathy, and Sezary cells in blood (at least 1000 cells per microliter), along with evidence of monoclonality of T cells, typically determined by PCR assay or HTS.

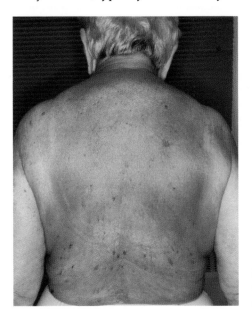

Figure 22.5 Sezary syndrome: Erythroderma is one of the common presenting symptoms of Sezary syndrome.

Differential diagnosis: Similar to that for erythroderma, the differential diagnoses of Sezary syndrome includes psoriasis, atopic dermatitis, chronic lymphocytic leukemia, drug reaction, or pityriasis rubra pilaris. Sezary syndrome must be differentiated from MF based on the degree of peripheral blood involvement. See Tables 22.3B and 22.3C.

Management: Early diagnosis and treatment are essential in improving the response; however, relapses can occur. Treatment should include skin-directed therapy, but systemic treatments need to be initiated to address blood involvement. Systemic therapies include extracorporeal photopheresis with or without other treatment modalities, such as interferon-a, mogamulizumab, and systemic chemotherapy. Skin-directed therapy includes topical corticosteroids, topical nitrogen mustards such as mechlorethamine and carmustine, topical bexarotene, phototherapy, and electron beam therapy.

Course: The 5-year survival for Sezary syndrome is 36%, with a median survival of 2–4 years, emphasizing the importance of early diagnosis and treatment. Lymphadenopathy, degree of peripheral blood involvement, increased age, and male gender are all key prognostic factors. Many patients with Sezary syndrome may die from opportunistic infections.

Final comment: Sezary syndrome is an aggressive form of CTCL characterized by erythroderma and leukemic involvement of clonal T-cells, which requires prompt diagnosis and aggressive treatment.

ADULT T-CELL LYMPHOMA

Definition: Adult T-cell lymphoma (ATCL) is a T-cell malignancy caused by human T-cell leukemia virus-1 (HTLV-1). Malignancy usually presents with disseminated disease with manifestations in skin lesions; however, chronic and smoldering skin-limited variants are also observed.

Overview: The etiology of ATCL is a malignant transformation of T-cells infected with retrovirus HTLV-1. Only 1–5% of patients seropositive for HTLV-1 develop ATCL, typically after more than 2 decades of viral disease. In places with a high prevalence of HTLV-1, such as southwestern Japan, the Caribbean Islands, South America, and parts of Central America, ATCL is endemic. Additionally, ATCL is prevalent in a small Sephardic Jewish population with ancestors from Mashad and Iran. Vertical transmission from virally infected mothers with this retrovirus is common in endemic areas.

Clinical presentation: Patients usually present with acute ATCL, in which there is leukemia, lymphadenopathy, organomegaly, and hypercalcemia. Skin lesions are found in about half of patients and consist of nodules or tumors, generalized papules, or plaques. Two variants of ATCL, chronic and smoldering, commonly present with skin lesions mimicking MF without circulating neoplastic T cells. ATCL has a predilection for adult males.

Laboratory studies: The histopthology shows a superficial or diffuse infiltrate of various sizes of T cells with pleomorphic nuclei and epidermotropism, making it indistinguishable from MF. Immunophenotypically, cells are CD3+, CD4+, CD8–, and CD25+. Cells show T-cell receptor monoclonality. Integrated HTLV-genes and antibody titers help differentiate between chronic or smoldering variants and MF.

Differential diagnosis: Differential diagnosis includes MF and distinguishing between chronic and smoldering variants.

Management: Systemic chemotherapy is required in most cases; however, in chronic and smoldering cases, therapies used for MF are effective treatments.

Course: Prognosis is influenced by clinical subtype, where survival in acute and lymphomatous variants ranges from 2 weeks to more than 1 year. Chronic and smoldering variants of disease may have a protracted course, or progress to a high-grade malignancy.

CD30 LYMPHOPROLIFERATIVE DISORDERS

Primary cutaneous CD30+ lymphoproliferative disorders are the second-most common group of CTCL and account for approximately 25–30% of cases. Included in this classification is primary cutaneous anaplastic large-cell lymphoma and lymphomatoid papulosis.

LYMPHOMATOID PAPULOSIS

Definition: Lymphomatoid papulosis (LyP) is a chronic T-cell lymphoproliferative disease in which eruptions of red-brown papulonodular and papulonecrotic lesions recur and self-resolve within 3–8 weeks, with no systemic or nodal involvement.

Overview: The etiology of LyP is mostly unknown, and there is continued debate about whether the disease is benign or malignant. Although this disease appears as a CD30+ malignant lymphoma on histology, it is clinically considered benign by most practitioners.

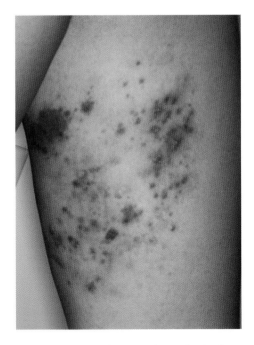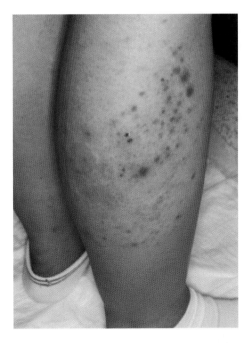

Figure 22.6 Lymphomatoid papulosis: Crusted papules of lymphomatoid papulosis on lower extremities.

Clinical presentation: LyP typically occurs in adults around the age of 45–50 and is more prevalent in men. LyP can also occur in children, in which more women are affected. The characteristic lesions seen in this disease are recurrent dome-like papules that typically erupt on the trunk and extremities. The lesions become necrotic, ulcerated, and crusted over the course of a few days and can be at different stages of development (Figure 22.6). Episodes of these lesions can last from 3–12 weeks and are normally self-resolving; however, superficial scars can remain. These relapsing-remitting episodes may last 20–40 years. Eventually, there is persistent remission in which lesions do not recur. LyP may be associated with other lymphomas.

Laboratory studies: Histologically, LyP shows inflammatory infiltrates with atypical cells in the dermis. There are many histologic subtypes of LyP, including subtypes A to C, which can occur simultaneously in an individual. Type A reveals large atypical CD30+ cells, a wedge-shaped dermal infiltrate, and may resemble Hodgkin's lymphoma with Reed-Sternberg-like, CD30+ cells. Type B is CD30− with a bandlike dermal infiltrate and appears similar to MF under the microscope due to epidermotropism. Type C includes large groups of CD30+ T-cells and resembles anaplastic large-cell lymphoma. Immunohistochemically, LyP types A and C display a similar phenotype to ALCL, while type B is CD3+, CD4+, CD8−, and CD30−. Ultimately, when LyP histopathology overlaps with MF or ALCL, clinical evaluation is necessary for diagnosis.

Differential diagnosis: Historically, duration and reoccurrence are important in the diagnosis of LyP. LyP can commonly be confused with bites from arthropods, scabies, and cutaneous leishmaniasis. This disease may also be mistaken as pityriasis lichenoides et varioliformis acuta (PLEVA), which presents similarly; however, PLEVA has no recurrence. Other diseases on the differential diagnosis include folliculitis, viral infections, and myelodysplastic syndromes. Hodgkin's lymphoma should be ruled out due to CD30+ and similar histologic features.

Management: Typical LyP resolves without any interventions; however, therapy can be used for symptomatic individuals. Low-dose methotrexate is currently the preferred and most effective treatment. Tetracyclines, topical or systemic corticosteroids, and narrow band ultraviolet-B (NBUVB) are alternative options; however, no curative therapy is available.

Course: LyP typically has no impact on overall health and has an excellent prognosis, with 100% overall survival at 5 years; however, in 20% of patients LyP may be associated with other malignancies, such as MF, Hodgkin's lymphoma, and cutaneous anaplastic large-cell lymphoma, which would worsen prognosis.

Final comment: As a lymphoproliferative disorder, LyP may not be malignant, but it is extremely important to monitor due to emotional distress and association with other malignancies.

CUTANEOUS ANAPLASTIC LARGE CELL LYMPHOMA

Definition: Cutaneous anaplastic large cell lymphoma (ALCL) is a primarily cutaneous CD30+ malignancy composed of large cells with anaplastic, pleomorphic immunoblastic cytomorphology.

Clinical presentation: ALCL normally occurs in patients in their 60s with a 2:1 male to female predominance. This disease may present with an erythematous or violaceous nodule, tumor, or plaque that may ulcerate. Most commonly, these lesions are found on the head and extremities, and they can be solitary or multifocal. Unlike LyP, these lesions usually do not regress and represent a malignant process. Cutaneous ALCL should be differentiated from systemic ALCL, which presents with additional lymph node and/or extracutaneous site involvement.

Laboratory studies: ALCL on histology characteristically demonstrates sheets of large, non-epidermotropic, CD30+ atypical cells with anaplastic morphology in the dermis. Cells are round, oval, or have irregularly shaped nuclei, with prominent eosinophilic nucleoli and abundant cytoplasm. Cells may express the CD4+ phenotype and other T-cell markers, such as CD2, CD3, and CD5. Necrosis and ulceration with areas of more inflammatory cells may be seen and reactive lymphocytes are typically present at the periphery. Expression of anaplastic lymphoma kinase (ALK) and epithelial membrane antigen (EMA) on malignant cells should highly raise suspicion of systemic involvement of ALCL.

Differential diagnosis: Cutaneous ALCL should be differentiated from other CD30+ lymphoproliferative or malignant disorders including LyP, LCT-MF, and Hodgkin's lymphoma. In appropriate settings, systemic ALCL should be ruled out.

Management: If systemic involvement is suspected, complete staging workup, including flow cytometry, imaging studies, and bone marrow biopsies, should be conducted. For cutaneous ALCL, radiation therapy and surgical excision are the mainstays of therapy due to low recurrence rates; however, spontaneous resolution of lesions is also seen in some patients, making observation a reasonable option. In systemic cases, chemotherapy including CHOP (cyclophosphamide, doxorubicin, vincristine, prednisone) and methotrexate can be effective.

Course: Cutaneous ALCL has a great prognosis, with a 5-year survival of over 90%.

SUBCUTANEOUS PANNICULITIS-LIKE T-CELL LYMPHOMA

Definition: Subcutaneous panniculitis-like T-cell lymphoma (SPTL) is a CD8+ cytotoxic T-cell lymphoma with predilection for the subcutaneous fat clinically resembling panniculitis.

Clinical presentation: SPTL may present in both children and adults and affects both sexes equally. Typically, patients present with solitary or multiple nodules and plaques that commonly arise on the legs (Figure 22.7). Fever, fatigue, and weight loss may accompany the lesions, while ulceration of lesions and dissemination to extracutaneous sites is uncommon. A life-threatening hemophagocytic lymphohistiocytosis (HLH) may seldom occur and can correspond with a rapidly progressive course. The diagnosis of SPTL may be preceded by a seemingly benign panniculitis.

Laboratory studies: Histopathologic examination may indicate panniculitis. Pleomorphic T cells of different sizes with hyperchromatic nuclei and many macrophages are seen. Commonly, necrosis,

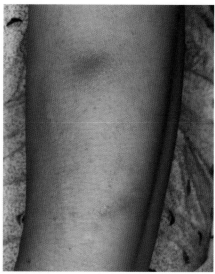

Figure 22.7 Subcutaneous panniculitis-like T-cell lymphoma: Subcutaneous nodules on the arm of a patient with subcutaneous panniculitis-like T-cell lymphoma.

karyorrhexis, and cytophagocytosis in so-called beanbag cells is seen. In the early stages of disease, inflammatory cells may predominate, while neoplastic cells may lack significant atypia. Immunophenotypically, cells demonstrate α/β+ (Beta F1+), CD3+, CD4−, CD56−, and CD8+ markers with expression of cytotoxic proteins (TIA-1+, granzyme B+, and perforin+). The clonality test for TCR gene rearrangement is generally positive.

Differential diagnosis: SPTL should be differentiated from cutaneous γ/δ T-cell lymphoma (CGD-TCL) by confirmation of α/β+ (Beta F1+) T-cell phenotype. Of note, cutaneous γ/δ (CGD)–TCL was previously known as SPTL with a γ/δ phenotype. This distinction is important, since SPTL has an indolent course with high survival while CGD-TCL has a grim prognosis.

Management: Immunosuppressive therapy, such as systemic corticosteroids, cyclosporine, or hydroxychloroquine, is utilized in treatment of SPTL with no accompanying HLH or systemic involvement. More aggressive treatment strategies, including chemotherapy, should be considered for SPTL patients with HLH or systemic involvement.

Course: Generally, patients with SPTL with a CD8+, α/β+ phenotype have an indolent clinical course with recurrent lesions without extracutaneous involvement. 5-year survival is around 82%.

PRIMARY CUTANEOUS PERIPHERAL T-CELL LYMPHOMA, RARE CUTANEOUS Γ/Δ T-CELL LYMPHOMA

Definition: Cutaneous γ/δ T-cell Lymphoma (CGD-TCL) is a clonal proliferation of mature cytotoxic γ/δ T-cells. It was previously known as a SPTL with an γ/δ phenotype.

Clinical presentation: Patients typically present with disseminated plaques, nodules, or tumors that are generally on the extremities. Mucosal and other extranodal sites may also be involved; however, lymph node, spleen, and bone marrow involvement is rare. HLH may accompany.

Laboratory studies: CGD-TCL may present with an epidermotropic, dermal, or subcutaneous histologic pattern. Multiple patterns may be present within a single patient or biopsy specimen. Microscopically, medium to large malignant cells with clumped chromatin expressing CD56 and γ/δ T-cell receptor are seen. Apoptosis and necrosis with angioinvasion are also common, and subcutaneous specimens may show rimming around fat cells, similar to SPTL. Immunophenotypically, cells are γ/δ+, BetaF1−, CD56+, CD3+, CD2+, CD5−, express cytotoxic proteins, and commonly lack CD4 and CD8 expression.

Differential diagnosis: This includes SPTL, as they present similarly with subcutaneous nodules. The distinction between the two must be made with immunohistochemistry to distinguish γ/δ and α/β phenotype, in addition to the other criteria listed in Table 22.5.

Management: Patients are treated with systemic chemotherapies as previously described.

Course: CGD-TCL is often an aggressive disease resistant to multiagent chemotherapy and radiation. Subcutaneous fat involvement is a predictor of a poorer prognosis than epidermal or dermal disease. Median survival is 15 months.

Table 22.5 Comparison of Subcutaneous Panniculitis-Like T-Cell Lymphoma (SPTL) and Primary Cutaneous γ/δ T-Cell Lymphoma

	SPTL	CGD-TCL with Subcutaneous Involvement
Phenotype	α/β T-cell phenotype	γ/δ T-cell phenotype
T-cell receptor	βF1+, TCRδ1−	βF1−, TCRδ1+
T-cell phenotype	CD4−, CD8+, CD56−	CD4−, CD8−, CD56+
Histological features	Rimming of CD8+ neoplastic T cells around adipocytes	May display fat rimming mimicking SPTL
	No epidermotropism and lichenoid interface	Epidermotropism and lichenoid interface
Clinical features	Nodules and plaques	Nodules and plaques
	Rarely ulceration	Ulceration common
Hemophagocytic syndrome	Uncommon	Common
Survival (5-year)	82%	11%

PRIMARY CUTANEOUS AGGRESSIVE EPIDERMOTROPIC CD8+ CYTOTOXIC T-CELL LYMPHOMA

Definition: This lymphoma is a proliferation of CD8+ cytotoxic T-cells in the epidermis with aggressive clinical features.

Clinical presentation: It presents with localized or disseminated eruptive papules, nodules, and tumors that may ulcerate and necrose, or with superficial, hyperkeratotic patches and plaques (Figure 22.8). Spread to visceral sites, such as the lung, testis, central nervous system, and oral mucosa may occur, but lymph node involvement is uncommon.

Laboratory studies: Under the microscope, epidermotropism in a linear or diffuse pattern with pleomorphic CD8+ T cells is present. Necrotic keratinocytes, ulceration, invasion and destruction of adnexal skin, angiocentricity, and angioinvasion are commonly seen (Figure 22.9). Malignant cells are CD8+ T cells expressing cytotoxic proteins (granzyme B+, perforin+, TIA-1+). Immunophenotypically, they are BetaF1+, CD3+, CD2−, CD4−, and CD5−. Furthermore, clonal TCR gene rearrangements are seen.

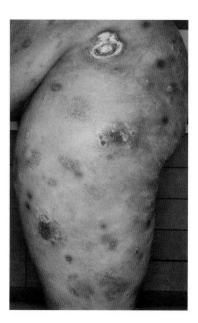
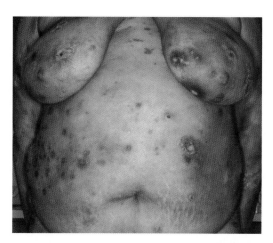

Figure 22.8 Primary cutaneous aggressive epidermotropic CD8+ cytotoxic T-cell lymphoma: Ulcerated disseminated eruptive plaques on a patient with CD8+ cytotoxic T-cell lymphoma.

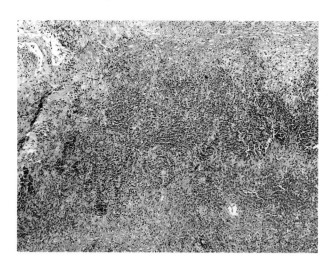

Figure 22.9 Primary cutaneous aggressive epidermotropic CD8+ cytotoxic T-cell lymphoma: This specimen is notable for fragmentation of the epidermis away from the dermis. The epidermis has significant epidermal necrosis, along with scattered epidermotropic hyperchromatic and irregularly contoured lymphocytes.

Management: These lymphomas have an aggressive clinical course and should be treated with multiagent chemotherapy.

Course: The median survival for patients with this aggressive lymphoma is 32 months, and disease specific 5-year survival is 18%.

PRIMARY CUTANEOUS CD4-POSITIVE SMALL/MEDIUM PLEOMORPHIC T-CELL LYMPHOPROLIFERATIVE DISORDER

Definition: This disorder is a newly described entity with a benign clinical course that does not reflect a frank malignancy.

Clinical presentation: Primary cutaneous CD4-positive small/medium pleomorphic T-cell lymphoproliferative disorder presents as a solitary plaque of nodule typically on the head, neck, or upper portion of the trunk. Staging is not recommended due to its excellent prognosis.

Laboratory studies: Histopathologic study may reveal dense dermal and subcutaneous infiltrate of small to medium lymphocytes. Minimal to no epidermotropism is seen. Cells are CD4+, CD8−, CD3+ and CD30− and are histologically indistinguishable from tumor stage MF; however, it lacks preceding MF patches or plaques.

Differential diagnosis: The differential diagnosis includes MF.

Management: Lesions may respond spontaneously after biopsy or may be treated with intralesional corticosteroids, surgical excision, or rarely radiotherapy.

Course: Primary cutaneous CD4-positive small/medium pleomorphic T-cell lymphoproliferative disorder has a 5-year survival rate of 100%.

PRIMARY CUTANEOUS ACRAL CD8+ T-CELL LYMPHOMA

Definition: Primary cutaneous acral CD8+ T-cell lymphoma is a newly described provisional entity in the updated WHO-EORTC classification.

Clinical presentation: It presents as a solitary plaque or nodule on an acral site, such as the ear or nose. It is clinically very indolent.

Laboratory studies: The histopathology consists of dense dermal CD8+ infiltrate of lymphocytes. Cells are CD8+, TIA1, and CD3+ and have a dot-like pattern of CD68; however, they are negative for cytotoxic proteins.

Differential diagnosis: This is similar to that of MF.

Management: Aggressive treatment is unnecessary, and lesions may be treated with topical corticosteroids, surgical excision, radiotherapy, or observation.

Course: Primary cutaneous acral CD8+ T-cell lymphoma has an excellent prognosis with a 5-year survival rate of 100%.

PRIMARY CUTANEOUS PERIPHERAL T-CELL LYMPHOMA, NOT OTHERWISE SPECIFIED

Definition: This is a diagnosis maintained for heterogeneous cutaneous T-cell lymphomas that do not fit into a well-defined subtype. It accounts for 26% of all peripheral T-cell lymphomas.

Clinical presentation: It is a clinically aggressive disease with a predilection for men. Patients are typically adults that may present with solitary, localized, or disseminated plaques, nodules, or tumors with no site predilection. Patients commonly have constitutional symptoms (B symptoms) and pruritus.

Laboratory studies: Other categories of T-cell lymphomas must be excluded before diagnosis of primary cutaneous peripheral T-cell lymphoma, not otherwise specified (PTCL-NOS) can be made. Dermatopathology typically shows nodular or diffuse infiltrates with medium or large size pleomorphic or immunoblastic-like T-cell. Epidermotropism is typically mild or lacking. Generally, cases show an aberrant CD4+ T-cell expression. CD30 is usually mild or negative, while some cases may show CD56 co-expression.

Differential diagnosis: This includes all subtypes of cutaneous T-cell lymphomas, and these must be excluded before this diagnosis can be made.

Management: Patients are treated with multiagent chemotherapies.

Course: PTCL-NOS has a poor prognosis with a 5-year survival of less than 20%.

EXTRANODAL NK/T-CELL LYMPHOMA, NASAL TYPE

Definition: Extranodal NK/T-cell lymphoma, nasal type is typically an Epstein-Barr virus (EBV) associated aggressive lymphoma. After the nasal cavity and nasopharynx, skin is the second-most common site of involvement. Both primary or secondary cutaneous lesions show aggressive behavior.

Clinical presentation: Extranodal NK/T-cell lymphoma, nasal type is commonly seen in Asia, Central America, and South America and predominantly affects adult males. Typical presentation involves multiple plaques or tumors on the trunk and extremities, or a destructive midfacial tumor previously called lethal midline granuloma. Fever, malaise, weight loss, and other systemic symptoms may be seen, along with HLH and ulceration of lesions.

Laboratory studies: Under the microscope, dense infiltrates of cells expressing CD2, CD56, cytotoxic proteins (granzyme B+, perforin+, TIA-1+), and cytoplasmic CD3 (but not surface CD3) involving the dermis and subcutaneous tissue is visualized. Pathology also demonstrates angiocentricity, angiodestruction with necrosis, and a heavy inflammatory infiltrate. EBV-encoded small RNAs (EBER) is expressed in almost all cases and is a diagnostic feature.

Management: Systemic chemotherapy is recommended; however, due to the aggressive nature of disease, results are commonly unsatisfactory.

Course and/or Prognosis: This highly aggressive neoplasm has a median survival of less than 12 months; however, those with solely skin lesions at presentation have a median survival of 27 months.

CUTANEOUS B-CELL LYMPHOMAS

Overview: Cutaneous B-cell lymphomas are a group of B-cell malignancies that arise in the skin and compose about 25% of cutaneous lymphomas. Cutaneous B-cell lymphomas include marginal zone lymphomas, follicle center cell lymphoma, and primary cutaneous diffuse large B-cell lymphoma (Table 22.6).

PRIMARY CUTANEOUS MARGINAL ZONE B-CELL LYMPHOMA

Definition: This is a B-cell lymphoma with an indolent clinical course.

Clinical presentation: Primary cutaneous marginal zone B-cell lymphoma (PCMZL) has a slight male predominance with a median age of 39 years. This typically presents as solitary or multifocal red to violaceous papules, plaques, or nodules commonly on the trunk or extremities (Figure 22.10). Spontaneous resolution of lesions can occur, and recurrence is common. A relationship between *B. burgdorferi* infection and PCMZL is observed, particularly in cases reported in Europe.

Laboratory studies: Histopathologically, PCMZL shows nodular to diffuse infiltrates of atypical marginal zone B-cells (small lymphocytes with irregular nuclei and abundant pale cytoplasm), reactive T-cells, and plasma cells. The infiltrate may be seen in the dermis and subcutis and may be accompanied by surrounding lymphoid follicles and germinal centers. Reactive plasma cells

Table 22.6 Summary of Cutaneous B-Cell Lymphomas

Name	Clinical Presentation	Histology	Immunophenotype	5- Year Survival
Primary cutaneous marginal zone B-cell lymphoma	• Red to violaceous papules, plaques, or nodules typically on trunk and upper extremities	Nodular or diffuse infiltrates of small lymphocytes, centrocyte cells, lymphoplasmacytoid cells and plasma cells that spare epidermis	CD20, CD79a, Bcl-2 Negative for CD5, CD10, Bcl-6	98–100%
Primary cutaneous follicle center cell lymphoma	• Solitary or grouped plaques and tumors, typically on forehead and trunk that may be surrounded by erythematous papules and indurated plaques • May increase in size over years if left untreated	Diffuse infiltrates in the dermis with a zone of normal collagen that separates the lymphocytes called the Grenz zone	CD20, CD79a, Bcl-6 CD5 and CD43 negative MUM1 negative	94–97%
Primary cutaneous diffuse large B-cell lymphoma, leg type	• Rapid growing red or violaceous tumor on leg(s) • Often disseminate extracutaneously	Diffuse infiltrate of large neoplastic cells such as centroblasts and immunoblasts in the dermis, with many mitotic figures	CD20, CD79a, Bcl-2 CD10 negative MUM1 positive	55%

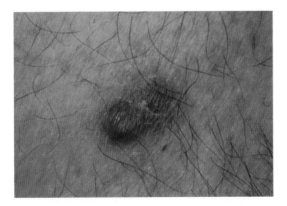

Figure 22.10 Primary cutaneous marginal zone B-cell lymphoma: Solitary red to violaceous papule on a patient with cutaneous marginal zone lymphoma.

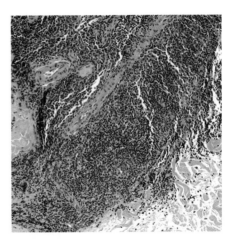

Figure 22.11 Primary cutaneous marginal zone B-cell lymphoma: The specimen shows diffuse and nodular infiltrates of atypical lymphoid cells in dermis and superficial subcutis. Plasma cells and plasmacytoid cells are conspicuous at the periphery of the nodular infiltrates.

can be found at the periphery of the infiltrate (Figure 22.11). If plasma cells predominate, it is classified as a PCMZL plasmacytic variant. Immunophenotypically, marginal zone B cells express positivity for CD20 and Bcl-2. Additionally, they are Bcl-6−, CD10−, CD79a+, MUM1−, and CD5−. The reactive germinal centers are Bcl-6+, CD10+, and Bcl-2−, and plasma cells are CD138+ and CD79a+. Immunoglobulin light chain restriction or B-cell monoclonality is observed in malignant marginal zone B cells.

Differential diagnosis: Staging workup including imaging studies must be conducted to exclude cutaneous involvement of other types of marginal zone lymphomas. Secondary involvement of other lymphomas typically effects the head and neck of older adults. Urticaria, arthropod bites, and leukemia cutis should be included in the differential diagnosis.

Management: If there are few lesions, low-dose radiotherapy or excision may be used as treatment along with observation. For multifocal lesions, intralesional corticosteroids or rituximab may be used and result in remission. Rarely, for very extensive or refractory disease, chemotherapy may be used. Cases associated with *B. burgdorferi* require antibiotic therapy.

Course: PCMZL has an excellent prognosis with a 5-year survival rate of 98–100%.

Final comment: PCMZL is a proliferation of B-lymphocytes with an excellent prognosis but must be monitored for extracutaneous disease.

PRIMARY CUTANEOUS FOLLICLE CENTER CELL LYMPHOMA

Synonym: Crosti lymphoma

Definition: Cutaneous follicle center cell lymphoma is a B-cell neoplasm of follicle center cells of the skin, often with a predominance of large centrocytes.

Clinical presentation: Primary cutaneous follicle center cell lymphoma (PCFCL) commonly presents with solitary or grouped papules, plaques, and tumors on the head, trunk, and leg with equal incidence in both genders (Figures 22.12 and 22.13). Grouped lesions may consist of erythematous papules and indurated plaques. Without treatment, existing lesions may increase in size as new nodules appear. The term *Crosti's lymphoma*, or *reticulohistiocytoma of the dorsum*, is used when red plaques and nodules expand around the central tumor.

Laboratory studies: On histology, PCFCL demonstrates follicular or diffuse infiltrates in the dermis without epidermotropism. The nodular infiltrate consists of small, medium, and large centrocytes with multilobed nuclei and centroblasts. The neoplastic follicular structures may lack a well-defined mantle zone and tangible body macrophages. Immunophenotypically, PCFCL B cells express positivity for CD20 and Bcl-6 but not Bcl-2. Additionally, they are CD79a+, MUM1−, and CD5−. CD10 may be seen in follicular growth patterns but not in diffuse growth patterns.

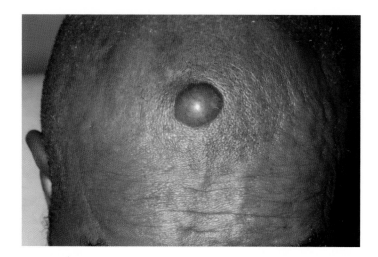

Figure 22.12 Primary cutaneous follicle center cell lymphoma: Solitary tumor on the head of a patient with cutaneous follicle center cell lymphoma.

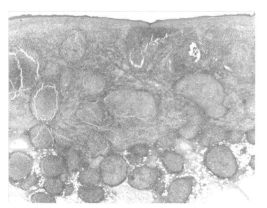

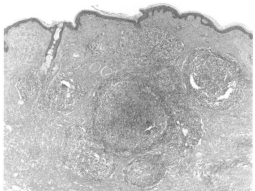

Figure 22.13 Primary cutaneous follicle center cell lymphoma: Dense diffuse infiltrate of atypical lymphocytes indicating follicular center derived B-cell neoplasm.

Differential diagnosis: Staging workup including imaging studies must be conducted to exclude extracutaneous involvement. The differential diagnosis of PCFCL includes arthropod bites, epidermal cysts, acne, lymphoid hyperplasia, and other neoplasms.

Management: Radiotherapy is the mainstay of treatment for solitary or few lesions. Solitary lesions may also be surgically excised with radiation post-excision. Extensive cutaneous disease or systemic involvement may require the use of chemotherapy or monoclonal antibodies, such as rituximab.

Course and/or Prognosis: PCFCLs have a great prognosis with a 5-year survival rate of 94–97%.

Final comment: Although PCFCLs have a favorable prognosis, extracutaneous involvement must be considered.

PRIMARY CUTANEOUS DIFFUSE LARGE B-CELL LYMPHOMA, LEG TYPE

Definition: Primary cutaneous diffuse large B-cell lymphoma, leg type (PCDLBCL-LT) is an aggressive subtype of cutaneous B-cell lymphomas with a diffuse proliferation of large, atypical B-cells usually presenting on the lower legs.

CLINICAL PRESENTATION

PCDLBCL-LT is commonly found on the legs of elderly women and presents as rapidly enlarging solitary or multifocal tumors that are red or bluish-red in color and may ulcerate (Figure 22.14). These lymphomas can occur at other locations and may disseminate to extracutaneous sites.

Laboratory studies: Histologically, PCDLBCL shows diffuse sheets of centroblasts and immunoblasts in the dermis and subcutaneous tissue, without epidermotropism. Markedly atypical

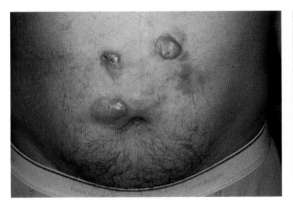

Figure 22.14 Primary cutaneous diffuse large B-cell lymphoma, leg type presenting as an erythematous nodule on left parietal scalp.

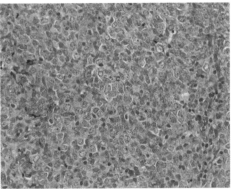

Figure 22.15 Primary cutaneous diffuse large B-cell lymphoma, leg type: The specimen shows a sheet-like diffuse dense proliferate composed of cells with centroblastic morphology and high mitotic activity.

large lymphocytes with many mitoses are seen, but germinal centers are not visible (Figure 22.15). Immunophenotypically, the malignant cells express positivity for MUM1 and Bcl-2. Additionally, they are CD10−, CD20+, and CD79a+. Bcl-6 expression is variable, and Ki-67 proliferation is common.

Differential diagnosis: This includes lymphomatoid granulosis, EBV-positive diffuse large B-cell lymphoma, and diffuse large B-cell lymphoma, not otherwise specified. It is important to differentiate PCDLBCL from other PCBCLs as it is the most aggressive from of PCBCL.

Management: Chemotherapy is used to treat PCDLBCL, particularly R-CHOP (rituximab, cyclophosphamide, hydroxy daunomycin, oncovin/vincristine, and prednisone) regimen. If disease is limited, radiotherapy may be effective. Furthermore, if R-CHOP cannot be done, intralesional rituximab may be therapeutic.

COURSE
PCLBCL has a poor prognosis with a 5-year survival of 55% and adverse risk factors, including multiple skin lesions at diagnosis.

FINAL THOUGHT
PCLBCL is related to systemic diffuse large B-cell lymphoma, the most common form of non-Hodgkin lymphoma, and therefore, systemic involvement must be excluded.

ADDITIONAL READINGS

Cerroni L. Mycosis fungoides-clinical and histopathologic features, differential diagnosis, and treatment. Semin Cutan Med Surg. 2018;37:2–10.

Cook LB, Fuji S, Hermine O, et al. Revised adult T-cell leukemia-lymphoma international consensus meeting report. J Clin Oncol. 2019;37:677–687.

da Silva Almeida AC, Abate F, Khiabanian H, et al. The mutational landscape of cutaneous T cell lymphoma and Sezary syndrome. Nat Genet. 2015;47:1465–1470.

Goyal A, LeBlanc RE, Carter JB. Cutaneous B-cell lymphoma. Hematol Oncol Clin North Am. 2019;33:149–161.

Kim YH, Liu HL, Mraz-Gernhard S, et al. Long-term outcome of 525 patients with mycosis fungoides and Sezary syndrome: clinical prognostic factors and risk for disease progression. Arch Dermatol. 2003;139:857–866.

Larocca C, Kupper T. Mycosis fungoides and Sézary Syndrome: an update. Hematol Oncol Clin North Am. 2019;33:103–120.

Ohtsuka M, Miura T, Yamamoto T. Clinical characteristics, differential diagnosis, and treatment outcome of subcutaneous panniculitis-like T-cell lymphoma: a literature review of published Japanese cases. Eur J Dermatol. 2017;27:34–41.

Pulitzer M. Cutaneous T-cell lymphoma. Clin Lab Med. 2017;37:527–546.

Wilcox RA. Cutaneous B-cell lymphomas: 2019 update on diagnosis, risk stratification, and management. Am J Hematol. 2018;93:1427–1430.

Willemze R, Jaffe ES, Burg G, et al. WHO-EORTC classification for cutaneous lymphomas. Blood. 2005;105:3768–3785.

23 Diseases of the Hair

Rodney Sinclair and Wei-Liang Koh

CONTENTS

Overview: Human hair is important for self-identity and influences our social interaction. Hair disorders include hair loss (nonscarring and scarring alopecias), excessive hair growth (hypertrichosis and hirsutism), and ingrowing hair (pseudofolliculitis). All can result in significant physical and/or psychologic morbidity.

NONSCARRING ALOPECIAS

In this group of hair loss disorders, follicular openings are still patent, and the hair loss is potentially reversible.

Androgenetic Alopecia

Synonym: Common balding

Definition: Androgenetic alopecia (AGA) is a genetically determined condition that is the most common form of hair loss in both men and women.

Overview: AGA is the process whereby genetically predisposed scalp hair follicles miniaturize in response to androgenic influence and presents as male pattern hair loss (MPHL) or female pattern hair loss (FPHL). The incidence of AGA increases with age, affecting 50% of men and 30% of women by age 50.

Clinical presentation: Men develop bitemporal recession, diffuse thinning over the midfrontal scalp and vertex balding (Figure 23.1). In women, especially those with long hair, the first signs are recurrent episodes of increased hair shedding and a reduction in ponytail volume (Figure 23.2). These findings may precede the visible diffuse thinning over the crown by many years (Figure 23.3). Up to 50% of hair can be lost before thinning is noticeable. The severity of MPHL and FPHL is most commonly graded by Hamilton-Norwood scale (Figure 23.4) and Sinclair scale (Figure 23.5), respectively.

Laboratory studies: The diagnosis is established clinically and may be further confirmed by trichoscopy which reveals increased proportion of single hair follicular units, miniaturized vellus-like hairs, and variable hair shaft diameters. A biopsy would reveal reduced terminal: vellus hair ratio (typically <4:1). This is rarely performed, only if the diagnosis is in doubt. Blood tests are not routinely performed, but screening for thyroid dysfunction, iron deficiency anemia, and hyperandrogenism (especially in women with irregular menses, acne, and hirsutism) can be considered if clinical signs and symptoms and signs are present to exclude co-contributory causes.

DOI: 10.1201/9781003105268-23

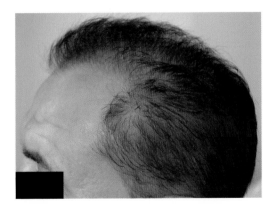

Figure 23.1 Male pattern hair loss with bitemporal recession and reduction in hair density over mid-frontal scalp and vertex.

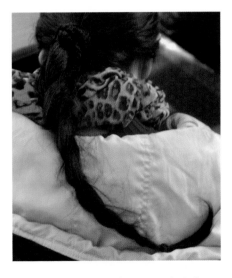

Figure 23.2 Female pattern hair loss with reduction in ponytail volume.

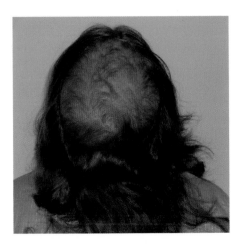

Figure 23.3 Female pattern hair loss with visible diffuse thinning over crown

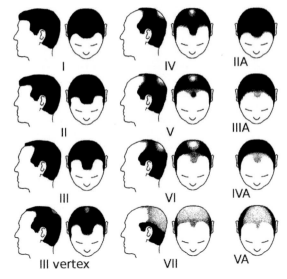

Figure 23.4 The Hamilton-Norwood grading of severity of male pattern hair loss (with stage variants noted in the final column.

Source: From Wikipedia, in the public domain.

Differential diagnosis: These include telogen effluvium, diffuse alopecia areata, sisaipho pattern alopecia areata (with sparing of hair at sides and back of head), and frontal fibrosing alopecia. A detailed history, physical examination, and biopsy for histology will be helpful for distinguishing between these conditions.

Management: For MPHL, topical minoxidil 5% lotion/foam twice daily and/or oral finasteride 1 mg once daily can be considered as first-line treatment. For FPHL, patients can be started on topical minoxidil 2% lotion twice daily or 5% foam once daily. In more severe cases, antiandrogens (e.g., spironolactone, cyproterone acetate, flutamide, bicalutamide) and 5-alpha-reductase inhibitors (e.g., finasteride 2.5–5 mg once daily) can be considered. Low-dose oral minoxidil (0.25–5 mg

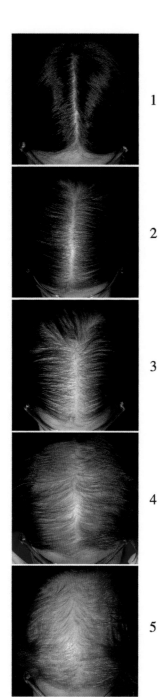

1

2

3

4

5

Figure 23.5 Sinclair hair loss severity scale (a 5-point photographic grading system) for female pattern hair loss based on hair part width.

once daily) can be an option for patients with local side effects or poor adherence to topical minoxidil. Adjunctive treatment with varying degree of success includes platelet-rich plasma injections, low-level light therapy, non-ablative fractionated lasers and microneedling. Camouflage techniques are helpful. Patients with stabilized advanced hair loss can consider hair restoration surgery, usually after the age of 30.

Course: Early onset and rapid progression of AGA predict more severe disease in both sexes, and early treatment improves prognosis. In women, pro-androgen medications (e.g., testosterone), hypothyroidism, obesity-accentuating polycystic ovarian syndrome, and incidental telogen effluvium may accelerate hair loss.

Final comment: The vast majority of patients with AGA can be managed with a combination of medical, surgical, and camouflage techniques. Patients who start treatment early tend to do better and treatment should be continued long-term as hair loss will begin again within few months of stopping therapy

Alopecia Areata

Definition: Alopecia Areata (AA) is a common autoimmune disorder presenting with patchy hair loss.

Overview: AA is a complex polygenic autoimmune hair loss mediated by cytotoxic CD8+ NKG2D+ T cells, in the face of a yet unknown environmental trigger. Although most patients have no systemic signs, there may be underlying thyroid abnormalities or associated vitiligo

Clinical presentation: Patients present with well-demarcated round to oval patches of nonscarring hair loss with no epidermal changes (Figure 23.6). **Exclamation mark** hairs and a positive hair pull test can be present at the periphery of active patches. In a hair pull test, approximately 60 hairs are grasped between the finger and thumb and lifted gently with light traction away from the scalp. The test is positive if 6 or more hairs are released (> 10%). AA can result in total loss of scalp hair (alopecia totalis [AT]) or both scalp and body hair (alopecia universalis [AU]). Other less common variants include ophiasis pattern (with involvement of lateral and occipital scalp margin), sisaipho pattern (inverse of ophiasis pattern), and diffuse pattern (with abrupt, widespread involvement). AA can also affect the eyebrows, eyelashes, and beard. Pitting and trachyonychia of the nails can be present. As the hair regrows, there may be white fine hairs initially before normal hair develops.

Laboratory studies: Diagnosis is usually established clinically, including use of trichoscopy which shows *exclamation mark* hairs, black dots and yellow dots. Scalp biopsy for histology may reveal a lymphocytic peribulbar infiltrate in *a swarm of bees* like appearance preferentially affecting anagen follicles in early stages. A serologic test for syphilis (STS); venereal disease research laboratory (VDRL)/**treponema pallidum hemagglutination (TPHA)** can be considered to exclude secondary syphilis. Screening for autoimmune thyroid disease, diabetes, and pernicious anemia can be performed if the history is suggestive.

Differential diagnosis: These include trichotillomania and secondary syphilis for patchy AA, telogen effluvium for diffuse AA, and MPHL for sisaipho pattern AA.

Management: Spontaneous regrowth is possible but impossible to predict. Choice of treatment depends on the age of the patient, extent of AA and rate of progression. For limited AA, options include topicals (corticosteroids, minoxidil, dithranol [anthralin] and intralesional steroid

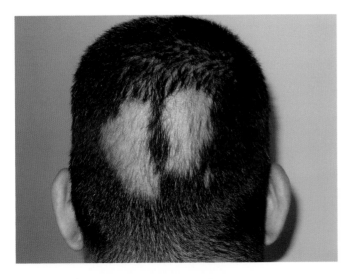

Figure 23.6 Alopecia areata with well-demarcated round to oval patches of nonscarring hair loss.

injections. For more extensive AA (scalp surface area >30%), topical contact immunotherapy (with diphencyprone [DCP] or squaric acid dibutylester [SADBE]), paint psoralen combined with ultraviolet A (paint PUVA), and systemic immunosuppressants (oral corticosteroids, cyclosporin, methotrexate, azathioprine, JAK-inhibitors [e.g. tofacinitib, baricitinib]) can be considered. Rapidly progressive AA may benefit from a course of oral corticosteroids. Cosmetic camouflage is a helpful adjunct.

Course: For unifocal and multifocal AA present for less than 6 months, chances of spontaneous remission are 90% and 65% respectively. Overall, about one-third of cases become chronic (i.e., >1-year duration) and of these cases, approximately 45% progress to AT/AU. Factors associated with poorer prognosis include an ophiasis pattern, nail involvement, young age at onset, personal history of atopy/autoimmune disease, and family history of AA.

Final comment: AA is a common cause of nonscarring alopecia, with a lifetime worldwide incidence of 2%. This autoimmune-mediated form of hair loss has a few distinct clinical presentations and treatment should be individualized.

Telogen Effluvium

Definition: Telogen effluvium (TE) is the diffuse excessive shedding of telogen hairs, which can be secondary to physiologic, physical, or emotional stress.

Overview: Our hair growth cycle consists of an anagen (growth) phase, catagen (transition) phase, and telogen (resting) phase. At any one time, 80–90% of our scalp hair follicles are in anagen phase (which lasts for 2–6 years), while 10–20% of our hair follicles are in telogen phase, where the hairs lie dormant for 2–3 months before eventual release (exogen). In TE, the ratio of anagen to telogen hair is significantly altered, with telogen shedding occurring for several months thereafter.

Clinical presentation: The patient (usually a woman) presents with a history of obvious increased hair shedding above baseline (normal hair shedding approximately 50–150 strands per day). This can be quantified using the Sinclair hair shedding scale (Figure 23.7). On examination, hair part width is usually preserved with mild bitemporal hair thinning. Hair pull test may be positive for telogen club hairs. A history of preceding physiologic stress that may include childbirth, major surgery, significant infection with a high fever, major trauma such as a plane crash, automobile accident, or an occupational catastrophe may have occurred 2–3 months before the onset of TE. Several medications (including lithium, warfarin, valproic acid, phenytoin, and retinoids) may also be implicated. When the process lasts longer than six months, it is considered chronic TE and is usually found in women aged 30–50. Chronic TE can be idiopathic.

Laboratory studies: Blood tests to rule out possible triggers include ferritin, thyroid function panel, complete blood count, liver panel, renal panel, antinuclear antibody, vitamin D, vitamin B12, folate and zinc levels. A scalp biopsy in chronic TE, if performed, shows a normal number of hair follicles, increased number of telogen hairs, and a terminal: vellus hair ratio >8:1.

Differential diagnosis: These include androgenetic alopecia and diffuse alopecia areata.

Management: Identifying and addressing the precipitating factor is key. No treatment is needed, although topical or low-dose oral minoxidil can reduce hair shedding.

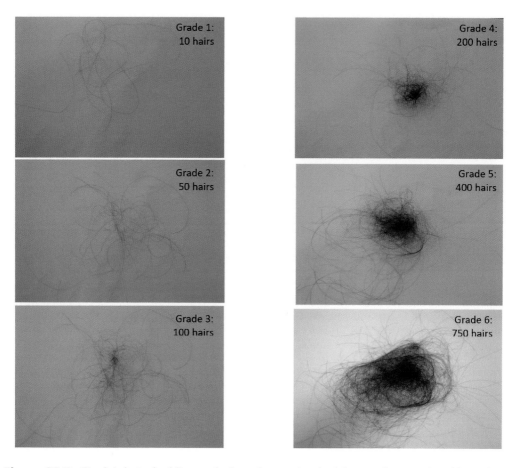

Figure 23.7 Sinclair hair shedding scale (based on patient's estimate of accumulated hair shed over 24 hours).

Course: Once the trigger is removed, hair shedding will usually improve over 3–6 months, before hair density eventually improves. As TE can unmask underlying AGA, not all patients can regain their original hair density. In chronic idiopathic TE, hair shedding can follow a minor fluctuating course for a number of years.

Final comment: TE can be idiopathic or secondary to a wide variety of potential triggers. Management hinges on uncovering the cause if present.

Tichotillomania: see Chapter 26 Psychocutaneous disorders.

Traction Alopecia

Synonyms: Traumatic marginal alopecia, chignon alopecia

Definition: Traction alopecia (TA) is a form of hair loss caused by sustained and repetitive tension on hair follicles.

Overview: TA is nonscarring in early stages but can ultimately eventuate in scarring. It is associated with several hairstyling practices, for example, tight ponytails, plaits, buns, hair extensions, or tight headwear.

Clinical presentation: In its earliest stages, traction folliculitis can be present before progression to hair loss/thinning, most commonly seen at the frontal and lateral scalp areas, (Figure 23.8). Any part of the scalp can be affected depending on the focus of traction. The *fringe sign* may be positive. This is a retained rim of small hairs along the frontotemporal hairline in marginal TA. During the later stages, decreased follicular openings are seen, consistent with scarring alopecia.

Laboratory studies: On scalp biopsy, during the early stage, trichomalacia, increased catagen/telogen hairs, normal number of terminal hair follicles, and preserved sebaceous glands can be seen. During the late stage, scarring alopecia is present. Inflammation is little to absent.

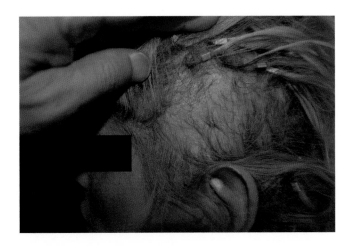

Figure 23.8 Traction alopecia secondary to hair extensions with hair loss over lateral scalp.

Differential diagnosis: These include trichotillomania, alopecia areata, and other scarring alopecias (e.g., frontal fibrosing alopecia).

Management: Cessation of traumatic hair styling practice is key. Topical and/or oral antibiotics, such as doxycycline 100 mg bid or minocycline 100 mg bid for several week can be used to treat any traction folliculitis. Intralesional steroid injections (triamcinolone acetate 10 mg/cc) can be administered to the periphery of alopecic patches. Topical/oral minoxidil can be considered to promote hair regrowth in early stages. Surgical options include hair transplant and scalp reduction surgery.

Course: Early TA is potentially reversible if traction is addressed. Late TA can cause scarring alopecia.

Final comment: In a suspected case of TA, the history of present and past hairstyling practices should be sought. Early cessation of traction is essential to prevent subsequent scarring.

SCARRING ALOPECIAS

In this group of hair loss conditions, the follicular ostia are obliterated and replaced by fibrous scar tissue with irreversible hair loss. These can be primary (where the hair follicle is the primary target of inflammation) or secondary (where the hair follicle undergoes bystander inflammatory damage from a primary process elsewhere, e.g., trauma, burn, infection). Primary scarring alopecias can be further divided histologically into predominantly lymphocytic, predominantly neutrophilic, or mixed inflammatory type. The more common primary scarring alopecias will be discussed in this section.

Discoid Lupus Erythematous

Definition: Discoid lupus erythematous (DLE) is the most frequently encountered form of chronic cutaneous lupus erythematosus, which can present with predominantly lymphocytic scarring alopecia.

Overview: The majority of patients with DLE have just limited cutaneous involvement, with 80% of the scarring localized to the head and neck. Five to 10% of DLE patients can eventually develop systemic lupus erythematous (SLE).

Clinical presentation: Early DLE lesions can present on the scalp as pinkish to erythematous scaly patches or plaques before atrophic scarring develops with loss of hair. This can be associated with follicular plugging and prominent dyspigmentation, usually with central hypopigmentation and a peripheral hyperpigmented rim (Figure 23.9). These lesions may be itchy, painful, or asymptomatic. The face, ears (especially the conchae) and other sun-exposed body areas may show similar lesions.

Laboratory studies: A scalp biopsy will reveal hyperkeratosis, epidermal atrophy, vacuolar interface alteration, thickened basement membrane, increased dermal mucin, perivascular and periadnexal lymphocytic infiltrate, and follicular plugging. In late stages, scarring with loss of appendages is apparent. Direct immunofluorescence (DIF) shows granular deposits of immunoglobulin (Ig) M, IgG and C3 deposition at the basement membrane zone. It is important to screen for underlying SLE at baseline with a full blood count, antinuclear antibody (ANA), and urinalysis.

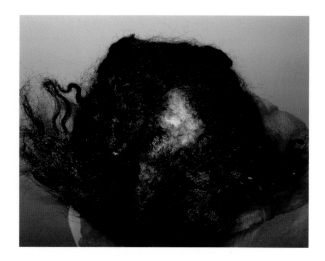

Figure 23.9 Discoid lupus erythematosus with atrophic scarring and prominent surrounding dyspigmentation.

Differential diagnosis: These include scarring alopecias (e.g., lichen planopilaris, central centrifugal cicatricial alopecia, pseudopelade of Brocq) and alopecia areata.

Management: Sun protection is important to reduce flares. Smoking cessation should be encouraged, as smoking can worsen DLE severity and reduce its response to antimalarials. Limited disease can be treated with potent topical/intralesional steroids or topical tacrolimus. Extensive disease can be managed with hydroxychloroquine. Prednisolone can be considered in rapidly progressive cases. Other options include dapsone, retinoids, steroid-sparing immunosuppressants (e.g., methotrexate, azathioprine, mycophenolate mofetil) and belimumab.

Course: Good hair regrowth is possible should patients receive treatment for very early DLE lesions; otherwise, they tend to persist and *burn out* over time into end-stage scarring. Squamous cell carcinoma can potentially arise in very long-standing lesions.

Final comment: DLE is a cause of primary lymphocytic scarring alopecia. DIF findings can be helpful to differentiate from other etiologies of scarring alopecia. Early diagnosis and treatment can be associated with a good prognosis.

Lichen Planopilaris

Definition: LPP, a subtype of lichen planus that predominantly affects the scalp, is the most common cause of primary scarring alopecia

Overview: There are 3 recognized variants of LPP, namely classic LPP, Graham-Little syndrome, and frontal fibrosing alopecia (FFA).

Classic LPP is more commonly found in middle-aged Caucasian women. These patients can present with multifocal scarring alopecic patches that may eventually coalesce over time, typically over the mid-scalp and vertex. Perifollicular erythema and scaling can be seen when the disease is active (Figure 23.10). The hair pull test can be positive for anagen hairs. These patches can be itchy, painful, or asymptomatic. Lichen planus can also involve other sites of the body (flexor of wrists/ankles), oral/genital mucosa and nails in 20–30% of cases. In Graham-Little syndrome, patchy scarring alopecia of the scalp is associated with nonscarring loss of axillary and pubic hair and lichenoid follicular eruption on the body and/or scalp. FFA is mainly found in postmenopausal women, presenting as cicatricial recession of the frontal hair line (Figure 23.11); however, there can also be marginal alopecia over the temporal, lateral, and occipital aspects of the scalp hair line. Loss of sideburns is frequently seen. The band of alopecia seen is often hypopigmented, slightly atrophic, with prominence of underlying veins, and a few *lonely* terminal hairs. Perifollicular erythema and scaling can be seen at the margin of the alopecia. Concomitant AGA is often present. Frequently, there is loss of eyebrows, but hair loss can appear anywhere on the body in FFA. Associated skin-colored or yellowish facial papules can be seen over the forehead and temples.

Laboratory studies: Histopathologic study of a biopsy shows lichenoid dermatitis affecting mainly the upper part of the follicle. In late stages, the scarring is nondescript. Direct immunofluorescence shows deposition of multiple immunoglobulins (usually IgM, occasionally IgG, IgA) and C3 at the colloid bodies in the peri-infundibular/isthmic area and band of fibrin along the basement membrane zone of the affected follicle.

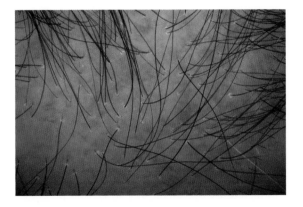

Figure 23.10 Trichoscopic photo of lichen planopilaris showing perifollicular erythema and scaling.

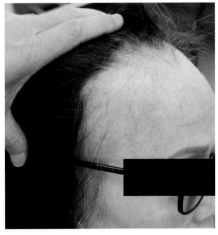

Figure 23.11 Frontal fibrosing alopecia with frontal hair line recession and few lonely terminal hairs remaining in the scarring band of alopecia that is slightly atrophic with prominent underlying veins.

Differential diagnosis: These include other scarring alopecias (e.g. DLE, central centrifugal cicatricial alopecia, pseudopelade of Brocq) and alopecia areata.

Management: This depends on the extent of activity. For limited LPP, potent topical/ intralesional steroids or topical tacrolimus can be used. For extensive LPP, options include hydroxychloroquine, tetracycline antibiotics, short course prednisolone (for rapidly progressive disease/ flares), steroid sparing immunosuppressants (e.g. methotrexate, ciclosporin and mycophenolate mofetil), systemic retinoids and PPAR-g agonists (e.g. pioglitazone). For FFA, 5-alpha-reductase inhibitors (finasteride, dutasteride) can be considered in addition. Adjunctive treatment includes minoxidil to increase background hair density and cosmetic camouflage. Hair transplants can be considered if the disease has been quiescent for at least 2 years.

Course: This is variable, ranging from indolent to rapidly progressive. Many cases progress over the years, with some eventually being *burnt out.*

Final comment: LPP is a primary lymphocytic scarring alopecia with 3 distinct clinical variants. Treatment is largely similar, with the aim of stabilizing progression of hair loss. 5-alpha-reductase inhibitors have been found useful in the setting of FFA.

Central Centrifugal Cicatricial Alopecia

Synonyms: Hot comb alopecia, follicular degeneration syndrome, pseudopelade of the central scalp, pseudopelade in African American patients

Definition: Central centrifugal cicatricial alopecia (CCCA) is a form of predominantly lymphocytic scarring alopecia associated with genetic and exogenous factors.

Overview: CCCA is the most common form of scarring alopecia in women of African ancestry, usually from middle age. Traumatic hair grooming practices can worsen this condition. Certain genetic mutations (e.g. *PADI3*) have been associated with CCCA.

Clinical presentation: CCCA tends to affect the vertex and mid-scalp, with patchy scarring hair loss that slowly and symmetrically expands outwards. During the early stages, hair breakage may be a feature. In the center of the patch, loss of follicular ostia, foci of unaffected hair and polytrichia (≥5 hairs emerging from the same follicular opening) may be seen. Patients can be asymptomatic or complain of mild itch, pain, or burning sensation.

Laboratory studies: Histopathologic examination will show perifollicular infundibular/isthmic lymphocytic inflammation, follicular degeneration, and fibrosis. Premature desquamation of the inner root sheath can be an early feature.

Different diagnosis: These include burnt out stages of LPP and DLE, pseudopelade of Brocq, long-standing TA, trichotillomania, and AGA.

Management: The patient should no longer straighten the hair with hot combs or pull the hair tightly with curlers. For limited disease, potent topical/intralesional steroids or topical tacrolimus can be used. For extensive disease, treatment options with variable success include tetracycline antibiotics, hydroxychloroquine, and immunosuppressants (e.g., cyclosporine and mycophenolate mofetil). Adjunctive treatment may include use of minoxidil and cosmetic camouflage. Hair transplant can be considered if the disease is quiescent for at least 2 years.

Course: Without treatment, the disease runs a chronic progressive course over the years before eventually "burning out," with extensive and permanent hair loss.

Final comment: CCCA is a primary lymphocytic scarring alopecia that is chronic and progressive, most commonly seen in middle-aged women of African descent. Treatment is challenging and aimed at retarding further progression of hair loss.

Folliculitis Decalvans

Definition: Folliculitis decalvans (FD) is an uncommon cause of scarring alopecia that is predominantly neutrophilic.

Overview: FD is chronic progressive inflammatory scalp disease leading to scarring alopecia. It may represent an abnormal immune response to associated *Staphylococcus aureus*.

Clinical presentation: FD affects men more commonly than women. Men may develop this in their teen years and women a decade or so later. This condition tends to affect the vertex. In the early stage, redness, swelling and pustules can be found centered on hair follicles, before scarring alopecia develops as a unifocal expanding patch (Figure 23.12). At the edge of this patch, activity in the form of erythema, pustules, crusting can be present. Scarring in the center tends to be thickened and indurated, rather than atrophic, and there may be tufting of the hair. Patients can present with itch, pain, burning sensation, or bleeding. Multifocal disease is uncommon but possible over time.

Laboratory studies: Histopathologic examination will show polytrichia, upper follicular neutrophilic infiltrate (or mixed acute and chronic inflammation in later stages), granulomatous inflammation secondary to hair-shaft fragments, fibrous tracts, and dermal fibrosis. To exclude bacterial infection, pustules should be swabbed for aerobic culture. To exclude fungal infection, skin scrapings and plucked hairs should be sent for fungal culture.

Differential diagnosis: These include dissecting cellulitis of the scalp, acne keloidalis, erosive pustular dermatosis of scalp, LPP, CCCA, bacterial folliculitis, and tinea capitis.

Management: For mild disease, antiseptic shampoos, topical antibiotics and topical/intralesional steroids can be considered. For extensive disease, options include oral antimicrobials (e.g., tetracyclines, rifampicin, clindamycin, fusidic acid, dapsone), oral retinoids, oral zinc, and short courses of prednisolone (for flares). Cosmetic camouflage can be considered as a useful adjunct. Hair transplant and scalp reduction surgery can be considered if the disease is quiescent for at least 2 years

Course: FD may progress and expand slowly over the years, with on–off flares, before eventually "burning out."

Final comment: FD is a predominantly neutrophilic primary scarring alopecia. Treatment is aimed at stabilizing rate of progression of hair loss, with the mainstay being systemic antibiotics.

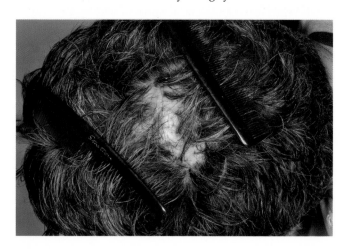

Figure 23.12 Folliculitis decalvans presenting as a unifocal expanding scarring patch over the scalp vertex, with tufting of hair follicles, erythema, and crusting.

Dissecting Cellulitis of the Scalp

Synonyms: Dissecting folliculitis, perifolliculitis capitis abscedens et suffodiens

Definition: Dissecting cellulitis of the scalp (DSC) is a rare severe scarring alopecia that is predominantly neutrophilic.

Overview: DSC affects mainly young men of African ancestry, possibly related to follicular hyperkeratosis, and aggravated by applications of grease. It can be an isolated finding or part of the follicular occlusion tetrad (associated with acne conglobata, hidradenitis suppurativa and pilonidal sinus).

Clinical presentation: DCS tends to affect the vertex and occipital scalp. The patient presents with boggy swellings of the scalp, comprising pustules, nodules, pseudocysts, abscesses, and sinus tracts that can interconnect, and patchy hair loss (Figure 23.13). The scalp swellings can sometimes take on a cerebriform appearance.

Laboratory studies: Histopathologic examination reveals perifollicular inflammatory infiltrate (mixed, predominantly neutrophilic) can be seen at the lower portion of the dermis extending to the subcutis. There can be increased catagen/telogen hairs. In later stages, granulation tissue, sinus tracts, and fibrosis can develop. Negative bacterial cultures and KOH scrapings will assist in confirming the diagnosis.

Different diagnosis: These include FD, acne keloidalis, cutis verticis gyrata, bacterial folliculitis, kerion, and alopecic and aseptic nodules of the scalp.

Management: Isotretinoin is considered the most effective treatment. Other medical options include intralesional steroids, oral antibiotics (e.g., doxycycline, erythromycin, or a combination of clindamycin and rifampicin), and oral zinc. Biologics (e.g., adalimumab, infliximab) can be considered in recalcitrant cases. Physical treatment methods, should medical therapy fail, include laser depilation, CO_2 laser ablation, photodynamic therapy, and external beam radiotherapy. Surgical management may consist of incision and drainage for large cysts and abscesses, and scalp excision with grafting for select cases.

Course: DCS runs a chronic course with on–off relapses, resulting in permanent patchy hair loss.

Final comment: DCS is a rare predominantly neutrophilic primary cicatricial alopecia most commonly seen in young males of African descent. Prompt treatment is necessary to prevent significant scarring.

Pseudopelade of Brocq

Definition: Pseudopelade of Brocq (PPB), a diagnosis of exclusion, is a predominantly lymphocytic scarring alopecia.

Overview: PPB is a controversial entity. Some clinicians see it as a primary lymphocytic scarring alopecia in its own right, while others feel that it is an end-stage/*burnt-out* form of various types of scarring alopecia, for example, LPP, DLE, ad CCCA.

Clinical presentation: PPB tends to affect middle-aged women. Initially, small, round to oval, smooth, soft, slightly atrophic patches of hair loss with loss of follicular ostia ("footprints in snow") can be appreciated primarily over the vertex/parietal scalp (Figure 23.14). These patches

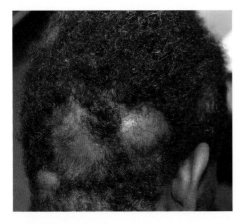

Figure 23.13 Dissecting cellulitis of scalp presenting with boggy swellings and patchy hair loss over the occipital scalp.

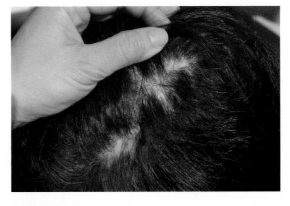

Figure 23.14 Pseudopelade of Brocq presenting with small, smooth skin-colored patches of hair loss ("footprints in the snow"), coalescing to larger patches, over the scalp vertex.

293

can be slightly erythematous initially but usually will be skin-colored to hypopigmented. The patches may coalesce to form larger irregular bald areas. The hair pull test may be positive at the edges of these patches, if active. PPB tends to be asymptomatic.

Laboratory studies: Histopathologic study of a biopsy from the hair bearing edge of the patch will show perifollicular lymphocytic infiltrate in the upper third of the hair follicles. Other histologic features include an atrophic epidermis, sclerotic dermis, fibrotic streams ("follicular ghosts") extending into the subcutis, loss of sebaceous glands. Elastic fiber network is preserved as compared to other scarring alopecias. Direct immunofluorescence is negative.

Differential diagnosis: These include burnt out stages of other scarring alopecia (e.g. LPP, DLE, CCCA, folliculitis decalvans), patchy AA, and secondary syphilis.

Management: Treatment for PPB is met with limited success. For limited disease, use of potent topical/ intralesional steroids and topical tacrolimus may be used. For more extensive disease, systemic oral agents, such as hydroxychloroquine, prednisolone (if rapidly progressive), isotretinoin, and mycophenolate mofetil, have been tried with variable results. Cosmetic camouflage as an adjunct is useful. Hair transplant or scalp reduction surgery can be considered for quiescent disease of at least 2 years.

Course: PPB usually progress in a slow manner over the years before activity ends spontaneously. Some patients may have periods of activity interspersed with periods of dormancy before the disease *burns out.*

Final comment: PPB is a primary lymphocytic scarring alopecia and is still largely a diagnosis of exclusion. Treatment is challenging with limited success.

Pseudofolliculitis

Synonyms: Shaving bumps, razor bumps, ingrown hairs

Definition: Pseudofolliculitis (PF) is an inflammatory dermatosis where ingrown hairs incite an inflammatory foreign-body type reaction.

Overview: PF is more common among men of African ancestry, but any patient with coarse curly hair and a history of inadequate shaving, waxing, or plucking can be affected.

Clinical presentation: Patients present with skin-colored to erythematous folliculocentric papules and pustules, which can be itchy, painful, or easily bled when traumatized (Figure 23.15). This usually affects the anterior neck/under the jawline in men, but any shaved area can be affected. Secondary complications of infection, post-inflammatory hyperpigmentation, scarring and hair loss can ensue.

Laboratory studies: Cultures from pustules can be performed to exclude bacterial and fungal infection.

Differential diagnosis: These include bacterial folliculitis, sycosis barbae, tinea barbae and micropapular sarcoidosis.

Management: Watchful waiting (allowing ingrown hair to grow out by self) with application of warm compresses and avoiding further irritation is an option. Mild topical steroids can be used to reduce inflammation. Topical and/ or oral antibiotics can be prescribed to treat secondary infection and to reduce inflammation. Depilatory creams, laser hair removal (LHR) and intense pulsed

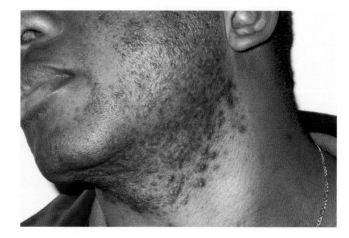

Figure 23.15 Pseudofolliculitis barbae with multiple erythematous to hyperpigmented folliculocentric papules and pustules over the jawline and anterior neck.

light (IPL) can be considered to prevent recurrences. Topical eflornithine may play a role to reduce hair regrowth rate in between hair removal procedures.

Men should be instructed to either shave or not. When shaving, they should use a four or five bladed razor, adequately wet the beard, and shave in all directions. They should not alternate between an electric razor or depilatory and should shave more than once a week.

Course: PF is likely to recur unless proper shaving practices or alternative hair removal methods as above are employed.

Final comment: PF is a common dermatosis usually due to improper shaving. Most patients can improve by adopting proper grooming techniques and using topical treatment. Light-based therapy can help prevent recurrences.

HIRSUTISM AND HYPERTRICHOSIS

Hirsutism

Definition: This is the excessive growth of terminal hairs in androgen-dependent areas in women.

Overview: Hirsutism may occur with or without an increase in circulating androgens. It tends to be more apparent after puberty, but it can occur at any age, should there be ectopic androgen production.

Clinical presentation: Women with hirsutism present with increased terminal hairs in a male pattern, beyond what is considered "normal" for their race/ethnicity (Figure 23.16). Severity can be graded using the modified Ferriman-Gallwey hirsuitism score (Figure 23.17). Other symptoms and signs of hyperandrogenism include history of irregular menses, infertility, acne, FPHL, deepening of voice, increased muscle bulk, and cliteromegaly. Associated causes include polycystic ovarian syndrome (PCOS; with acanthosis nigricans, increased body mass index), nonclassic congenital adrenal hyperplasia (with precocious puberty), androgen-secreting ovarian/adrenal tumors (with acute rapid onset of virilization), Cushing's syndrome (with hypertension, increased fat deposit midsection, face, between the shoulders, skin atrophy, easy bruising, violaceous striae), hyperprolactinemia (with galactorrhea), other endocrine disorders (e.g. acromegaly, thyroid disease), drugs (oral contraceptives, anabolic/androgenic steroids), and pregnancy.

Laboratory investigations: To rule out contributory causes and associations, serum testosterone and sex hormone––binding globulin (SHBG), luteinizing hormone (LH) and follicle-stimulating hormone (FSH), dehydroepiandrosterone sulfate (DHEA-S), 17-hydroxyprogesterone, thyroid function test, prolactin, fasting glucose and lipids, and adrenal/ovarian imaging can be performed.

Management: To reduce existing increased terminal hairs, waxing, shaving, depilatory creams, electrolysis, IPL, and LHR can be considered. Topical eflornithine cream can slow down rate of hair regrowth after depilatory measures. To reduce conversion of vellus to terminal hairs at androgen-dependent sites, medical treatment with oral contraceptives, antiandrogens (e.g., spironolactone, cyproterone acetate, flutamide, bicalutamide) and 5-alpha-reductase inhibitors (finasteride, dutasteride) can be considered. Metformin can be useful to treat associated insulin resistance in PCOS.

Course: This depends on the underlying cause, if any. Hirsutism can be more apparent with age.

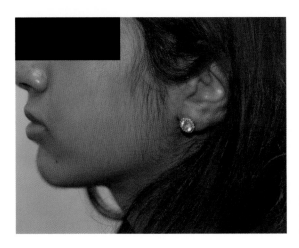

Figure 23.16 Facial hirsutism in a girl with increased terminal hairs over the sides of her face, upper cutaneous lip, and chin.

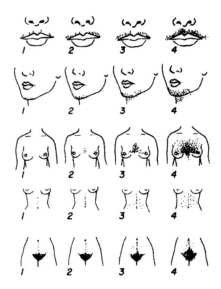

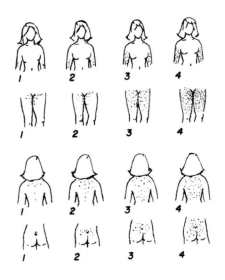

Figure 23.17 Modified Ferriman-Gallwey Score: This score rates hair growth from 0 (no growth of terminal hair) to 4 (extensive growth of terminal hair) over nine body sites (upper lip, chin, periareolar, upper abdomen, lower abdomen, upper arms, upper thighs, upper back, lower back). A score of ≥8 in a Caucasian woman indicates hirsutism.

Source: From Hatch R et al. Hirsutism: Implications, etiology, and management. Am J Obstet Gynecol 1981; 140:815–830, used with permission.

Final comment: Hirsutism can be associated with various causes. Depilatory measures and medical therapy directed to cause are helpful.

Hypertrichosis

Definition: This refers to hair growth in excess of what is expected for an individual age, sex and race/ethnicity, as opposed to hirsuitism.

Overview: Patients with hypertrichosis can present from birth (congenital) or later in life (acquired). Hypertrichosis can be localized or generalized, involving vellus hairs and/ or terminal hairs (Figure 23.18).

Clinical presentation: For congenital localized hypertrichosis, this can be an isolated finding with a discrete circumscribed patch of increased terminal hairs, or associated with a congenital melanocytic nevus, Becker's nevus, or underlying spinal dysraphism (faun tail sign at lumbosacral region). For congenital generalized hypertrichosis, patients rarely can present with increased body hair from birth, either lanugo hair (congenital hypertrichosis lanuginosa) or terminal hair (congenital hypertrichosis terminalis). This can be an isolated finding or associated with other congenital syndromes (e.g., Hurler syndrome, Cornelia de Lange syndrome). For acquired localized hypertrichosis, this can be a feature in porphyria cutanea tarda. This can also occur in pretibial myxedema

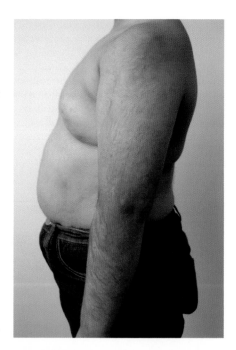

Figure 23.18 Hypertrichosis in a boy with increased terminal hairs seen over the arm and forearm.

plaques, usually associated with Graves's disease. Topical medications, for example, minoxidil, bimatoprost, and potent topical steroids, can induce hair growth. Repetitive rubbing/scratching and application of plaster cast can also result in localized hypertrichosis. For acquired generalized hypertrichosis, this condition can be associated with underlying malignancies ("malignant down," reported rarely in gastrointestinal, lung, breast cancers), hypothyroidism, eating disorders (e.g., anorexia nervosa, bulimia), dermatomyositis, dystrophic epidermolysis bullosa, and certain drugs (e.g., minoxidil, phenytoin, cyclosporine).

Laboratory investigations: Imaging can be considered to rule out spinal dysraphism in a child with lumbosacral hypertrichosis. Targeted investigations can be performed based on systemic review of symptoms and signs.

Management: The underlying cause, if present, should be treated. Depending on the location and extent of hair growth, waxing, shaving, depilatory creams, electrolysis, IPL, and LHR can be considered.

Course: This depends on the underlying cause. Hair tends to grow back after the depilatory measures, but LHR is a more permanent approach.

FINAL THOUGHT

It is useful to classify hypertrichosis based on age of onset and extent when considering possible causes. Depilatory measures are helpful, and treatment should also be directed to cause.

ADDITIONAL READINGS

Bienenfeld A, Azarchi S, Lo Sicco K, et al. Androgens in women: androgen-mediated skin disease and patient evaluation. J Am Acad Dermatol. 2019;80:1497–1506.

Bolduc C, Sperling LC, Shapiro J. Primary cicatricial alopecia: lymphocytic primary cicatricial alopecias, including chronic cutaneous lupus erythematosus, lichen planopilaris, frontal fibrosing alopecia, and Graham-Little syndrome. J Am Acad Dermatol. 2016;75:1081–1099.

Bolduc C, Sperling LC, Shapiro J. Primary cicatricial alopecia: other lymphocytic primary cicatricial alopecias and neutrophilic and mixed primary cicatricial alopecias. J Am Acad Dermatol. 2016;75:1101–1117.

Bridgeman-Shah S. The medical and surgical therapy of pseudofolliculitis barbae. Dermatol Ther. 2004;17:158–163.

Liyanage D, Sinclair RD. Telogen effluvium. Cosmetics. 2016;3:13.

Meah N, Wall D, York K, et al. The alopecia areata consensus of experts (ACE) study: results of an international expert opinion on treatments for alopecia areata. J Am Acad Dermatol. 2020;83:123–130.

Mirmirani P, Khumalo NP. Traction alopecia: how to translate study data for public education closing the KAP gap? Dermatol Clin. 2014;32:153–161.

Starace M, Orlando G, Alessandrini A, et al. Female androgenetic alopecia: an update on diagnosis and management. Am J Clin Dermatol. 2020;21:69–84.

York K, Meah N, Bhoyrul B, et al. A review of the treatment of male pattern hair loss. Expert Opin Pharmacother. 2020;21:603–612.

24 Diseases of the Nails

Robert Baran and Shari Lipner

CONTENTS

Definition: Nails, like hair, represent adaptations of keratins, which in this instance is to protect the distal aspect of the digits.

Overview: Nails grow at the approximate rate of 1 mm each day. Fingernails take six months to progress from the base to the end of the finger, and toenails take nine months to reach the tip of the toe. Figure 24.1 shows components of the nail structure.

Nails often reflect an ongoing dermatologic or systemic disease. For example, pitting of the nails would indicate psoriasis, while clubbing of the finger and rounding of the nail would suggest a pulmonary problem or even a malignancy.

Because there has developed a wealth of information about nails, this chapter focuses on highlights of the nails. For additional information, the reader should refer to one of the additional readings provided.

NAIL TUMORS

Overview: Common nail tumors are numerous. They include benign and malignant lesions. Considering their anatomic localization, a prompt diagnosis followed by appropriate treatment is indispensable.

NAIL BENIGN TUMORS

Definition: Benign tumors (noncancerous tumors) encompass a variety of lesions, including a verruca, distal digital keratoacanthoma, onychomatricoma, pyogenic granuloma, glomus tumor, myxoid cyst, onychopapilloma, exostosis, osteochondroma, enchondroma, and even an epidermoid cyst.

Verrucae

Overview: Different types of HPV are the cause of benign ungual warts. Some others rarely are associated with malignant transformation to squamous cell carcinoma.

DOI: 10.1201/9781003105268-24

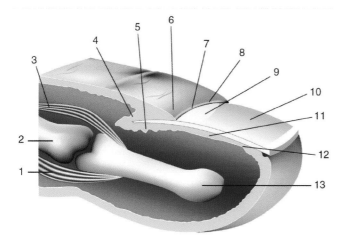

Figure 24.1 Nail structure: (1) anterior ligament; (2) bone, (3) posterior ligament, (4) nail root, (5) nail matrix, (6) proximal nail fold, (7) cuticle, (8) lateral nail fold, (9) lunula, (10) nail plate, (11) nail bed, (12) distal nail fold, (13) phalanx (bone of fingertip)

Source: From Baran R, Rigopoulos D, Nail Therapies, Informa Healthcare, London, 2012, used with permission.

Clinical presentation: Onychophagia (nail biting) often predisposes to periungual warts. A common wart never invades the nail matrix, but may develop underneath the proximal nail fold that appears swollen. Multiple warts distorting the nail apparatus are commonly seen in immunosuppressed patients.

Long-starting periungual warts should alert the physician to the development of Bowen's disease or squamous cell carcinoma. In many cases, HPV16 is then detected.

Management: This may include peeling agents, imiquimod, immunotherapy, viricidal agents, nitric oxide releasing solutions, topical puncture with formic acid 85% solution, bleopuncture, or hydrogen peroxide 45% topical solution in patients younger than 8 years of age. Other therapeutics could include immunomodulators and interferons, cryotherapy, laser surgery, photodynamic therapy, and electrocautery.

Distal Digital Keratoacanthoma

Definition: Distal, digital, subungual, and periungual keratoacanthomas (KA) are rare, benign, rapidly growing lesions usually located beneath the distal portion of the adherent nail plate.

Clinical presentation: If the tumor is located more proximally under the proximal nail fold, it may present as a painful chronic paronychia. Bony involvement is frequent, and a KA may occur as solitary or multiple tumors. There may be an association with incontinentia pigmenti, especially in women who complain of painful tumors. Multiple KAs may be seen in patients receiving cyclosporine and suramin.

Laboratory studies: X-rays may show a well-defined cup-shaped erosion of the underlying bone; however, an MRI is superior to radiographs in detection of an erosion of the distal phalanx.

Differential diagnosis: The three diagnoses to be ruled out are epidermoid implantation cyst, subungual wart, and squamous cell carcinoma. The last is frequently diagnosed histologically as squamous cell carcinoma, KA type, and spontaneous regression is unusual.

Management: Curettage of the cavity is the best treatment, but recurrences may occur. For painful subungual tumors, the first choice of treatment is acitretin.

Onychomatricoma

Clinical presentation: The three main signs are striking enough to make the diagnosis of this benign condition:

1. The nail presents with a yellow-white longitudinal band of variable width

2. There is a tendency toward over curvature

3. The nail is perforated by fibro-epithelial projections of the tumor, making a nail clipping an easy method for making a correct diagnosis (Figure 24.2).

The tumor may involve a finger or toenail; however, it may exceptionally involve several digits.

Laboratory studies: Immunohistochemical analysis may highlight the matrix epithelium.

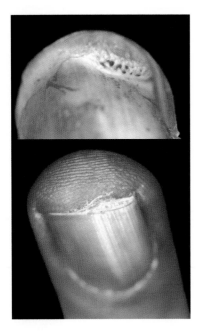

Figure 24.2 Onychomatricoma.

Differential diagnosis: Onychomatricoma associated with longitudinal melanonychia may mimic nail melanoma. Onychomycosis is often associated with onychomatricoma, and one nail sign may mask another. This tumor, when originating from the matrix, can develop in the surrounding epithelial tissue of the nail unit, including the nail bed.

Management: Treatment is surgical.

Pyogenic Granulomas

Clinical presentation: Pyogenic granulomas (PGs) are benign vascular lesions that can result from a large number of etiologic factors.

Management: They can be treated with surgery, cryotherapy, electrodessication, sclerotherapy, or laser surgery. Propranolol 1% cream or timolol 0.5% gel, applied over the paronychia and/or PGs under occlusion for a maximum of 45 days, is often effective. Alternatively, topical ophthalmic betaxolol 0.25% eyedrops once daily is useful for treating relapsing PG-like lesions induced by epidermal growth factor receptor inhibitors.

Glomus Tumor

Definition: These are benign vascular hamartomas containing neuromyoarterial cells of the normal glomus apparatus in the reticular dermis.

Clinical findings: Pain is the main symptom, which is often spontaneous, intense, pulsating in quality, and provoked by the slightness trauma and sometimes worse at night. It may trigger pain radiating up to the shoulder. The vast majority of these tumors are located in the subungual region, which contains a high concentration of glomus bodies. About 75% of glomus tumors occur on the hand.

There are two main clinical presentations:

1. A small reddish or bluish spot <1 mm, seen through the nail, often in the lunula, associated with sharp pain.

2. A longitudinal erythronychia with distal notching glomus tumors, frequently associated with Recklinghausen neurofibromatosis (NF) type I.

Laboratory studies: The patient will experience severe pain when a pin is pressed against the area. The cold test (ice cube) exacerbates the pain. Interestingly, a tourniquet placed at the base of the digit stops the pain. Dermatoscopy may preoperatively localize the tumor, while a flat-plate x-ray should reveal a depression on the dorsal aspect of the distal phalangeal bone or even a cyst in about 50% of cases. If the tumor cannot be localized, an MRI offers the highest sensitivity. Sometimes, the coexistence of several tumors may be diagnosed.

Management: Excision is the recommended treatment.

Myxoid Cyst

Definition: This represents a ganglion of the distal interphalangeal joint, where there is a pocket of synovial fluid that has escaped from the joint and has selected an interstitial location for the accumulation of surrounding structures.

Clinical presentation: There are three types defined by the location of the pocket of synovial fluid. The most common type (A) is on the dorsum of the distal digit. The second-most common type (B) is located beneath the proximal nail fold, above the thin proximal nail plate, which can be indented by the volume of the cyst and production of small ladder-like rungs of the transverse ridge. Type C (myxoid cyst, usually a thumb) is located beneath the matrix, pushing it upwards and increasing the transverse curvature of the nail. In addition, the lunula is red, and over time, pressure under the matrix results in thinning of nail that may disintegrate.

Management: Surgical intervention or injections of a sclerosant, such as polidocanol, are often effective.

Onychopapilloma

Definition: This tumor of the distal matrix and nail bed is usually benign. It shows a monodactylous longitudinal streak beneath the nail plate as an erythronychia or sometimes a leukonychia but rarely as melanonychia.

Clinical presentation: The streak sometimes presents with interrupted hemorrhages. Distally, there may be a hyperkeratotic plug that protrudes from under the nail. Distal splitting of the nail is frequent. Two papillomas on the same nail or onychopapillomas involving several nails are exceptional. Malignancy is rare. In rare instances, lichen planus may be associated leading to an onychopapilloma.

Management: Complete excision is often recommended. This employs a longitudinal nail unit biopsy from matrix to hyponychium that includes the length of the lesion.

For other benign nail tumors, see Table 24.1.

MALIGNANT TUMORS

Overview: These may include basal cell carcinoma, squamous cell carcinoma, Bowen disease, and malignant melanoma, generally requiring histopathologic confirmation.

Basal Cell Carcinoma

Synonym: Basal cell epithelioma

Overview: This tumor is very rare in the nail area, with most presentations occurring on the fingers rather than on the nail.

Clinical presentation: The normal presentation is a chronic paronychia associated with periungual dermatitis. The lesion may show a typical neatly rolled border with erosion of the nail fold and associated transverse ridging of the nail plate. See also Table 24.2.

Management: Surgical excision is the treatment of choice. Sometimes, Mohs micrographic surgery may be required.

Table 24.1 Differential Features for Exostosis, Osteochondroma, Enchondroma, and Epidermoid Cyst

Tumor	Age (years)	Sex Ratio	History of Trauma	Rate of Growth	X-Ray
Exostosis	20–40	F:M 2:1	Occasionally	Moderate	Trabeculated osseous growth with expanded distal portion covered with radiolucent fibrocartilage
Osteochondroma	10–25	M:F 2:1	Often	Slow	
Enchondroma	20–40	M+F	Often	Rapid	Well-defined sessile bone growth with hyaline cartilage cap
Epidermoid cyst	8–83	M:F 2:1	Almost always	Rapid	Lobulated bone cyst showing radiolucent defect, bone expansion, and flecks of calcification
					Radiolucent cyst and no calcification

Source: From Norton LA et al., Nail disorders, JAAD 1980; 2: 451–67, used with permission.

Table 24.2 Association of Localized Longitudinal Erythronychia with Nail Tumors

Basal cell carcinoma	Lichen planus (sometimes polydactylous)
Benign vascular proliferation	Nail melanoma
Bowen disease	Onychopapilloma
Glomus tumor	Verruca
Idiopathic	Warty dyskeratoma

Squamous Cell Carcinoma and Bowen Disease

Overview: The most frequent malignant tumor of the nail unit area is Bowen disease (Figure 24.3), which is squamous cell carcinoma (SCC) *in situ*.

Clinical presentation: Most lesions may appear within the context of human papillomavirus (HPV) infection. One-third of patients with SCC of the nail apparatus have a personal or sexual partner history of HPV-associated genital disease. Other etiologic factors may include exposure to radiation (e.g., physicians, dentists). Consequently, fingers are more frequently affected than toes.

The neoplastic process commonly originates from the nail folds or nail grooves as well from the subungual tissues, as a hyperkeratotic or papillomatous or fibrokeratoma-like growth. The nail bed most commonly involved presents with (in decreasing order): subungual hyperkeratosis, onycholysis, oozing, and nail destruction. Longitudinal melanonychia is present in about 10% of subungual SCC.

Management: Due to the extensive destruction of tissue, Mohs micrographic surgery is often suggested. Radiation therapy is an alternative, as is amputation of the distal phalanx.

Nail Melanoma

Overview: Nail melanoma most commonly occurs on the fingers and toes and in patients with skin of color. It almost always originates from the nail matrix, less frequently from the nail bed and nail folds.

Clinical presentation: In the early period, usually longitudinal melanonychia (melanonychia striata) and mild nail dystrophy are seen, while prominent nail dystrophy, ulceration, and tumoral mass can be observed in the late period. The spread of the pigment in the nail matrix and nail bed to the proximal and/or lateral nail folds over time is called the "Hutchinson sign." This is not pathognomonic for malignant melanoma, as it can be seen in other entities, as demonstrated in Table 24.3.

Laboratory studies: On dermatoscopic examination of nail melanoma presenting with longitudinal melanonychia, there are bands of different thickness and colors, dense dark-colored homogeneous pigmentation, irregular thickness spacing or coloration, and indistinct, disrupted, parallel lines on the lateral borders.

One-quarter of melanomas in the nail unit are amelanotic. In dermatoscopic examination of amelanotic melanoma, atypical vascular structures and irregular pigmentation areas are detected.

Course: The prognosis of malignant melanomas in the nail unit is poor, due to the frequent delay in diagnosis. Histopathologic examination should be performed for diagnosis.

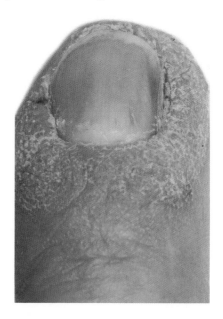

Figure 24.3 Bowen disease with longitudinal melanonychia.

Table 24.3 Nonmelanoma Hutchinson Sign

- *Illusory appearance* (beneath the cuticle)
- *Skin of color pigmentation*
- *Nonmelanoma unit cancer*
  - Bowen disease
  - Basal cell carcinoma
- *Epidermodysplasia verruciformis*
- *Benign tumors of the nail unit*
  - Onychomatricoma
  - Superficial acral fibromyxoma
- *Nail and mucous membrane pigmentation*
  - Laugier disease
  - Peutz-Jeghers syndrome
- *Nail unit nevi*
  - Congenital nevus
  - Acquired nevus
  - Spitz nevus
  - Pigmentation following excision of nevi
  - Regressing nevoid melanosis in childhood
- *Systemic conditions*
  - AIDS
  - Pregnancy
  - Pituitary tumor and Addison's disease
  - Malnutrition
  - Drugs
- *Mycologic and bacterial pigmentation*
  - Black molds, yeasts, dermatophytes
- *Trauma induced pigmentation*
  - Friction
  - Nail biting and picking
  - Boxing
  - Subungual hemorrhage
  - Posttraumatic melanonychia
- *Post-inflammatory pigmentation*
- *Radiation therapy*
- *Silver nitrate staining*

DERMATOSES

Psoriasis

Overview: Up to 50% of psoriatic patients have nail involvement.

Clinical presentation: Nail dystrophy with pitting in patients with psoriasis can be an indicator of ongoing involvement of the distal phalanx. See also Table 24.4.

Management: Triamcinolone acetonide may be used by injecting 0.1 ml of 10 mg/ml into the nail fold or nail bed with regional or digital ring block. Other treatment options for nail psoriasis include topical corticosteroids (with or without occlusion), topical calcipotriol (with or without occlusion), topical tazarotene, acitretin, methotrexate, cyclosporine, phototherapy (e.g., PUVA), and the biologic agents.

Lichen Planus

Overview: Nail changes may be the sole manifestation of this disease in 75% of adults, with an even higher proportion in children. See also Table 24.5.

Management: Intralesional triamcinolone acetonide into the nailbed may be useful.

Table 24.4 Anatomic Origin of Psoriatic Clinical Nail Signs (Figure 24.4)

Nail Bed and Hyponychium Disease	Nail Matrix Disease	Proximal Nail Involvement
- Onycholysis - Splinter hemorrhages - Subungual hyperkeratosis - Oil drops (Salmon patch dyschromia) - Yellow-green discoloration (due to serum glycoproteins) or secondary infection (yeasts or Pseudomonas)	- Pitting - Leukonychia - Red spots in the lunula - Crumbling	- Chronic paronychia with loss of the cuticle

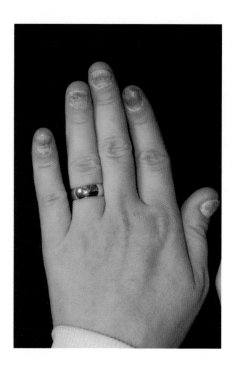

Figure 24.4 Nail findings due to psoriasis.

Source: Courtesy of Istanbul Medeniyet University Dermatology Clinic.

Table 24.5 Anatomic Origin of Lichen Planus Nail Signs (see Figure 24.5)

Proximal Nail Fold	*Nail Matrix*
Bluish red discoloration	Fragmentation, increased longitudinal ridging
Dorsal pterygium	Idiopathic nail atrophy
	Leukonychia
Nail bed	Longitudinal melanonychia
Bullous lichen planus	Nail shedding
Onycholysis	Onychorrhexis, crumbling
Permanent anonychia	Pitting
Subungual hyperkeratosis	Split nail
	Twenty nail dystrophy
Nail unit	Thinning or thickening of the nail
Nail deglovement	Transient or permanent longitudinal melanonychia
	Yellowish nail

Dermatitis

Overview: A variety of dermatitides may afflict the nails. These include allergic or irritant contact dermatitis associated with housework, hair and nail care, or manual labor. Atopic dermatitis is a common cause for nail problems in children.

Clinical presentation: When there is pruritus, superinfection due to *Staphylococcus aureus* is common. The nails are shiny and buffed from constant rubbing. Additional complications include bacterial paronychia and even underlying osteomyelitis.

Identification of the offending allergen is desirable every time it is possible.

Management: This involves complete protection by wearing two pairs of gloves; cotton beneath vinyl gloves or nitrile gloves offer complete protection. Judicious use of topical corticosteroids or calcineurin agents, such as tacrolimus or picerolimus may be prescribed, but the agents should be applied to the surrounding skin. Because nail is dead tissue, applying the medication to the nail itself would be for naught.

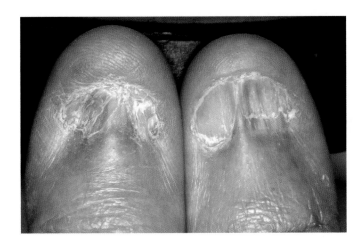

Figure 24.5 Pterygium and nail dystrophia due to lichen planus.

Brittle Nail Syndrome

Overview: Nail fragility results from an alteration in the consistency of the nail.

Clinical presentation: There are several presentations ranging from shallow parallel furrows running in the superficial layer of the nail, sometimes resulting in a split of the free edge, to a single longitudinal split involving the entire nail or multiple crenelated splitting. There can be lamellar splitting of the free edge into fine layers or transverse splitting of the lateral edge. Another finding may be friable nails often confined to the surface. See also Table 24.6.

Table 24.7 shows some common benign nail pathologies.

Table 24.6 Differential Diagnosis of Polydactylous Longitudinal Erythronychia

Acantholytic dyskeratotic epidermal nevus (as a mosaic form of Darier's disease)

Acantholytic epidermolysis bullosa

Acrokeratosis verruciformis of Hopf

Darier's disease (figure 24.6)

Graft-versus-host disease

Hemiplegia

Idiopathic

Primary amyloidosis (sometimes monodactylous)

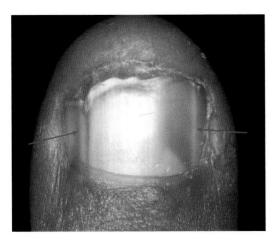

Figure 24.6 Darier Disease

Table 24.7 Common Benign Nail Pathologies

Splinter hemorrhage (Figure 24.7)	It is a linear red-brown splinter-like lesion located longitudinally under the nail plate.
	It occurs as a result of capillary damage and bleeding in the nail bed.
	It often occurs in healthy people due to minor trauma. Numerous diseases can cause splinter hemorrhage, such as lupus erythematosus, rheumatological diseases, subacute bacterial endocarditis, and chronic renal failure.
Clubbing (Hippocratic finger; Figure 24.8)	It is the convex dome-shaped appearance of the nails due to soft tissue hypertrophy at the fingertips. It can be familial as well as cause lung, heart, and gastrointestinal diseases. It may also develop depending on the pachydermoperiostosis syndrome.
Koilonychia (spoon nail; Figure 24.9)	It is the concave shape of the middle of the nail plate, which is more depressed than its edges. It can be found physiologically in childhood and old age. It is most often associated with iron deficiency anemia. It may be due to trauma (nail biting), many systemic diseases (hematologic, cardiovascular, gastrointestinal), and endocrinological diseases.
Ingrown toenail (Figure 24.10)	It occurs when the nail plate is embedded in the surrounding soft tissue (unguis incarnatus) or this soft tissue covers the nail plate (onychocryptosis). It is often seen in the big toenail. Especially wearing tight shoes and deep cutting of the nail are facilitating factors.
Beau's lines (Figure 24.11)	These are transverse grooves on the nail plate. It occurs due to nail matrix damage. With the extension of the nail, the grooves move distally. It occurs due to trauma such as cuticle, onychophagia or inflammation of the proximal nail fold such as eczema, psoriasis, chronic paronychia. Presence of Beau's lines at the same level on all nails indicates systemic disease.
Onycholysis (Figure 24.12)	Distal and/or lateral nail plate detachment from the nail bed as a result of nail bed damage. Hyperthyroidism, thyrotoxicosis, and porphyria are the most common systemic diseases.

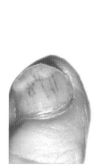
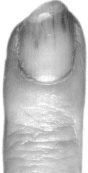
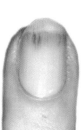

Figure 24.7 Splinter hemorrhage.

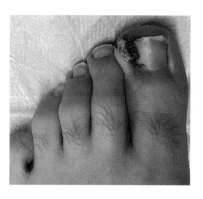

Figure 24.8 Clubbing.

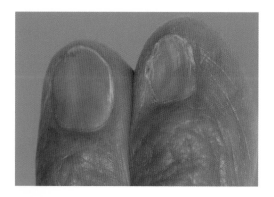

Figure 24.10 Ingrown toenail.

Source: Courtesy of Ayşe Serap Karadağ.

Figure 24.9 Koilonychia.

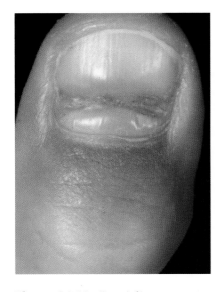

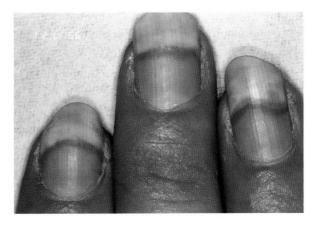

Figure 24.12 Onycholysis.

Figure 24.11 Beau's line.

CONGENITAL NAIL DISEASES

Overview: These often appear in several groups.

Clinical presentation: Genetic disorders restricted to the nail apparatus (nonsyndromic congenital nail disorders), such as leukonychia, koilonychia, anonychia, micronychia, or fourth convex toenails (Figure 24.13).

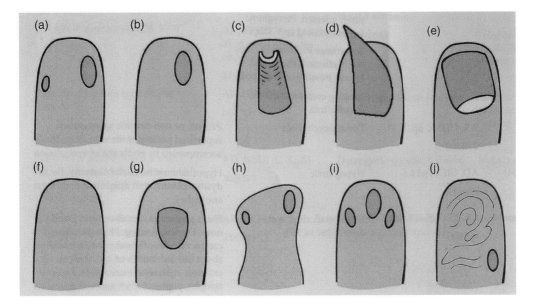

Figure 24.13 Types of micronychia and other dystrophies are seen particularly in congenital onychodystrophy of the index finger (COIF): (a) Polyonychia in COIF; (b) micronychia in COIF; (c) "rolled" micronychia in COIF, (d) hemionychogryphosis in COIF; (e) malalignment in COIF; (f) anonychia in COIF; (g) usual micronychia; (h) polyonychia in syndactyly; (i) polyonychia in congenital skin disease; (j) onychoheterotopia (Ohya's type).

Source: From Baran R, de Berker D, Holzberg M, et al., eds, Baran & Dawber's Diseases of the Nails and their Management, 5th edn, Wiley, Chichester, 2018, used with permission.

Iso-Kikuchi Syndrome

Synonym: Congenital onychodysplasia of the index fingers (COIF)

Overview: There are different dystrophies involving mainly the index fingers (see Figure 24.13a–24.13h).

Laboratory studies: An x-ray may show a Y-shaped bifurcation of the distal phalanx, while arteriography may reveal stenosis in the radial aspect of the palmar digital artery.

Genetic diseases with nail involvement and limited to skin manifestations only (various forms of *Epidermolysis bullosa*).

Genetic diseases involving the nail and other organs. Fingernails are affected in 98% of the patients.

Nail Patella Syndrome

Definition: This is a rare autosomal dominant disease characterized by nails with triangular lunula, alone or in combination with missing dorsal creases of the distal finger joint, a micronychia with hemionychia (thumb > index finger > other fingers), fissures, and/or anonychia. The patella is aplastic or luxated as well as the radial head. Bilateral posterior iliac horns are a pathognomonic sign. Nephropathy is frequent.

Genetic Disorders in Which the Nail Might Be Involved

Clinical presentation: The nail in **Darier-White disease** usually presents with longitudinal white and red streaks, associated with wedge-shaped distal subungual keratosis and splinter hemorrhages. Flat keratotic papules can be observed on the proximal nail fold.

Hailey-Hailey disease (familial benign pemphigus) may show longitudinal white streaks of the nail, prevalent in the thumbnails and observed in more than half of the patients.

Tuberous sclerosis: It is characterized by multiple hamartomas evident in the first years of life with elongated nails (leaf rowen). Koenen's tumors appear as firm masses that are ovoid, white, or pinkish, which never appear before the age of 5. They usually produce a longitudinal groove, splinter hemorrhages, longitudinal leukonychia (rarely), and sometimes "red comets" in the fingernails. Angiofibromas often involve the face.

Koenen periungual fibromas develop in about 50% of patients with tuberous sclerosis. They appear between the age of 12–14 years and increase in size and number as the child grows older. They can be found more frequently on the toes than on the fingers.

Surgical excision from its base is the best treatment. Occasionally, sirolimus, when used for facial angiofibromas, may be useful.

Dactylitis (sausage finger) is swelling of an entire finger or toe, as found in psoriasis; there is occasional nail involvement (see Table 24.8).

FINAL THOUGHT

Afflictions of the nails may reflect underlying disease or occur without any systemic findings.

Table 24.8 Possible Etiologies of Dactylitis

One Digit	Multiple Digits
With blisters	Primary skin disease
Group A, beta hemolytic strep	Psoriasis
Without blisters	Methacrylic acid burns from nail primers
Pseudomonas (usually toes)	Allergic contact dermatitis from nail polish
Haemophilus influenza (sickle cell disease)	*Veillonella* infection of the newborn
Mycobacteria tuberculosis	Systemic diseases
Parakeratosis pustulosa	Acrodermatitis enteropathica
	Systemic candidiasis
	Reactive arthritis
	Dermatomyositis

ADDITIONAL READINGS

Baran R, de Berker DAR, Holzberg M, et al. Baran and Dawber's Diseases of the Nails and their Management. 5th ed. Oxford: Wiley-Blackwell; 2018.

Baswan S, Kasting GB, Li SK, et al. Understanding the formidable nail barrier: a review of the nail microstructure, composition and diseases. Mycoses. 2017;60:284–295.

Bloom A, Blanken B, Schlakman B, et al. A review of nail dystrophies for the practitioner. Adv Skin Wound Care. 2020;33:20–26.

Chessa MA, Iorizzo M, Richert B, et al. Pathogenesis, clinical signs and treatment recommendations in brittle nails: a review. Dermatol Ther (Heidelb). 2020;10:15–27.

Cohen PR. The color of skin: blue diseases of the skin, nails, and mucosa. Clin Dermatol. 2019;37:468–486.

Golińska J, Sar-Pomian M, Rudnicka L. Dermoscopic features of psoriasis of the skin, scalp and nails—a systematic review. J Eur Acad Dermatol Venereol. 2019;33:648–660.

Logan IT, Logan RA. The color of skin: yellow diseases of the skin, nails, and mucosa. Clin Dermatol. 2019;37:580–590.

Martin-Playa P, Foo A. Approach to fingertip injuries. Clin Plast Surg. 2019;46:275–283.

Muneer H, Masood S. Psoriasis of the nails. 2020 Aug 8. In: StatPearls [Internet]. Treasure Island, FL: StatPearls Publishing; 2021 Jan. PMID: 32644686.

Wollina U, Abdel-Naser MB. Drug reactions affecting hair and nails. Clin Dermatol. 2020;38:693–701.

25 Disorders of Pigmentation

Michael Joseph Lavery, Charles Cathcart, and Hasan Aksoy

CONTENTS

Overview: Melanocytes are dendritic cells derived from the neural crest. They are located in the basal layer of the epidermis but may also be observed in the eye, inner ear and leptomeninges of the brain. Melanocytes serve three important functions: production of melanin, protection from ultraviolet-associated mutations, and absorption of ultraviolet radiation (UVR).

Melanin is derived from phenylalanine and passes through several steps before forming pheomelanin, eumelanin, or neuromelanin (Figure 25.1). Pheomelanin produces yellow-red pigment, and eumelanin produces brown-black pigment. The process of determining which pigment is produced is controlled by the melanocortin-1 receptor (MC1R). A loss of function in this receptor leads to increased production of pheomelanin and can increase the risk of melanoma from ultraviolet radiation. Genetic variations in the *MC1R* gene have been identified in malignant melanoma and oculocutaneous albinism.

Melanin synthesis is controlled by the melanocyte-stimulating hormone (MSH), which is derived from propiomelanocortin (POMC). POMC is also the precursor for adrenocorticotropic hormone (ACTH), which is raised in Addison's disease. This accounts for the cutaneous hyperpigmentation seen in this condition. Once synthesized, melanin is then packaged into melanosomes and transported to neighboring keratinocytes.

Higher Fitzpatrick phototypes have increased melanocyte size and distribution rather than increased melanocyte density. An increase in the number of melanosomes may be present in darker skin types.

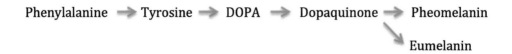

Figure 25.1 Phenylalanine forms tyrosine through phenylalanine hydroxylase. Tyrosine forms DOPA and dopaquinone through the action of copper-dependent enzyme tyrosine. The melanocortin-1 receptor determines the type of melanin produced.

DOI: 10.1201/9781003105268-25

GENERALIZED HYPOPIGMENTATION

Albinism

Definition: Albinism is a genetic condition that results in either minimal or loss of pigmentation in the hair, skin, or eyes.

Overview: Oculocutaneous albinism is the most common form of albinism, which is inherited in an autosomal recessive pattern. The lack of pigment is the result of deficiency in tyrosinase, which renders the individual unable to synthesize melanin despite maintaining the same number of basal melanocytes.

Clinical presentation: Affected individuals present with a pale-pink skin complexion, white or yellow colored hair, and light blue or occasionally pink eyes. The skin of affected individuals is unable to absorb UVR, resulting in extreme photosensitivity, sunburn, and an increased risk of developing skin cancers. Patients with albinism often suffer from visual impairment (due to refractive errors), photophobia, nystagmus, and strabismus. The psychological impact of the condition must also be taken into account, because affected individuals are at higher risk of social isolation due to the associated stigma.

Differential diagnosis: Other forms of albinism are described in Table 25.1.

Management: Patients with albinism require education on the importance of sun avoidance and protection to guard against the harmful effects of UVR. Patients should wear sun protective clothing and eyewear and apply high-protective factor sunscreens. Regular self-examination for abnormal skin growths and clinical examinations with a dermatologist are paramount. Patients may also require specialist input from other health care professionals (e.g., ophthalmology, hematology, neurology, and psychiatry).

LOCALIZED HYPOPIGMENTATION/DEPIGMENTATION

Vitiligo

Definition: Vitiligo is an acquired skin disorder secondary to the autoimmune destruction of melanocytes.

Overview: Vitiligo often presents in childhood and can be triggered by periods of emotional stress. Vitiligo occurs in 1–2% of the population with equal incidence in men and women. A positive family history of vitiligo or other autoimmune diseases, including thyroid disease, alopecia areata, and diabetes, is often present.

Clinical presentation: Individuals present with well-defined patches of depigmentation. Any anatomic site may be affected, but periocular, perioral, and acral site involvement confers a poor response to treatment. The affected patches of skin are symmetric and located on sun-exposed sites or in skin creases (Figure 25.2). Different patterns have been described, including segmental, nonsegmental, mixed, and unclassified.

Depigmented patches of skin can also occur over sites of previous injury, such as areas of trauma, operative scars, or burns, which is known as the Koebner phenomenon. The depigmentation is more prominent during the summer months, when the surrounding skin takes on more pigment giving a stark comparison. Hair and nails may also be affected (leukotrichia and

Table 25.1 Rare Types of Albinism

Disorder	Comment
Hermanski-Pudlak syndrome	Oculocutaenous albinism with a bleeding abnormality secondary to platelet dysfunction.
Griscelli Syndrome	Lack of pigment in the hair and skin associated with neurological abnormalities. High infant mortality.
Chediak-Higashi syndrome	Oculocutaneous albinism with neurological symptoms and immunodeficiency, resulting in frequent infections.
Cross Syndrome	Lack of pigment in the hair and skin associated with small eyes and corneal opacities.

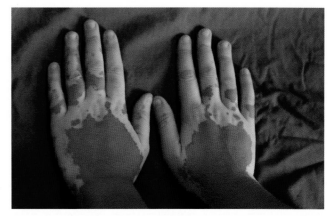

Figure 25.2 Vitiligo. Well-demarcated depigmented patches on the dorsum of the hands.

Source: Courtesy of Istanbul Medeniyet University Dermatology Clinic.

leukonychia, respectively). Vitiligo can be classified as stable (no progression in the preceding 6 months) or unstable (progression of depigmented patches within the preceding 6 months) which is important when determining management options.

Differential diagnosis: Piebaldism is a rare autosomal dominant disorder due to mutation in the KIT-proto-oncogene. It is characterized by a white forelock and depigmented patches, which are commonly located on the forehead. The presence of a white forelock, a depigmented patch, sensorineural deafness, and iris heterochromia are consistent with Waardenburg's syndrome. The differential diagnosis of localized hypopigmentation is summarized in Table 25.2.

Management: Spontaneous repigmentation may occur but is uncommon. Treatment options include topical therapy (e.g., topical corticosteroids and calcineurin inhibitors), phototherapy,

Table 25.2 Causes of Localized Hypopigmentation

Differential Diagnosis of Localized Hypopigmentation	
Tinea versicolor	A superficial yeast infection, caused by *Malassezia furfur*; hypopigmented scaly patches commonly on the trunk and neck. Wood's lamp examination shows yellow-green fluorescence.
Pityriasis alba	Hypopigmented patches with overlying fine scale, more noticeable in spring/summer. It is more common in darker skin phototypes.
Leprosy	Caused by mycobacterium leprae. Five categories: tuberculoid leprosy (TT), borderline tuberculoid (BT), borderline borderline (BB), borderline lepromatous (BL) and lepromatous leprosy (LL); hypopigmented macules and patches, which may be hypoanesthetic and hypohidrotic. Thickened peripheral nerves may also be present
Tuberous sclerosis	Inherited in an autosomal recessive fashion; oval-round hypopigmented macules/patches "ash-leaf macules" (Figure 25.3), connective tissue nevus (shagreen patch), facial angiofibromas, and periungual/subungual fibromas. Ocular, neurologic, cardiac, gastrointestinal, pulmonary, and renal involvement
Nevus anemicus	A vascular malformation caused by catecholamine-induced vasoconstriction; hypopigmented macules and patches that are less visible with diascopy. Rubbing surrounding skin and the nevus anemicus simultaneously will result in reactive erythema in the surrounding skin only.
Nevus depigmentosus	Decreased melanin synthesis; irregular depigmented macule or patch. Rubbing the nevus depigmentosus area results in reactive erythema. Wood's lamp examination reveals an "off-white" fluorescence.
Other	
Halo nevus (Sutton nevus)	Medication (e.g., immunotherapy)
Idiopathic guttate hypomelanosis	Post-inflammatory hypopigmentation
Hypopigmented mycosis fungoides	Chemical toxicity (e.g., rubber, arsenic)
Hypomelanosis of Ito	

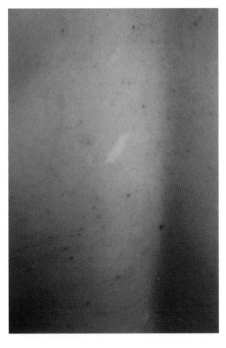

Figure 25.3 Hypopigmented macules (ash-leaf macules) in tuberous sclerosis.

Source: Courtesy of Istanbul Medeniyet University Dermatology Clinic.

immunosuppression (especially in unstable vitiligo), and grafts. The use of cosmetic camouflage is often useful, and it can provide psychologic support.

Course: Vitiligo is a difficult condition to manage. Periocular, perioral, and acral site involvement confer a poor response to treatment.

Final comment: Vitiligo is a common condition encountered in dermatology practice. Patients should be educated on the condition and physicians should discuss treatment expectations with each patient. Integrated psychologic care should be considered in management plans.

HYPERPIGMENTATION

Overview: Skin color is predominantly determined by the quantity or distribution of melanin. Hyperpigmentation is typically secondary to melanin overproduction but sometimes develops due to an increase in active melanocytes. Skin color changes may also occur via different mechanisms due to medications or heavy metals. Hyperpigmentation can be localized (e.g., melasma, nevus of Ota; Figure 25.4) or generalized (e.g. Addison disease) in distribution, and circumscribed, linear, or reticulate in configuration.

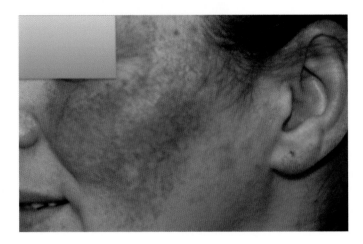

Figure 25.4 Nevus of Ota in a Fitzpatrick Type IV Skin Phototype.

313

Pigmentary Demarcation Lines

Synonyms: Voigt lines, Futcher lines

Definition: Pigmentary demarcation lines (PDLs) are a physiologic pattern of pigmentation that is mostly seen in individuals with skin of color. The contrast between the darker dorsal surfaces and lighter ventral surfaces seems more prominent.

Clinical presentation: PDLs can be found on the anterolateral aspects of the arms (Type A), posterior medial aspects of the thighs (Type B), parasternal area (Type C), paraspinal area (Type D), lateral aspects of the chest (Type E), and face, in a symmetric distribution.

Course: PDLs are usually noticed in childhood and remain throughout life.

POST-INFLAMMATORY HYPERPIGMENTATION

Definition: Post-inflammatory hyperpigmentation (PIH) is an acquired pigmentation that develops as a consequence of inflammatory skin conditions, cutaneous injuries, or therapeutic interventions. It can be observed in all skin phototypes, but it is more common in individuals with darker skin (Fitzpatrick skin types III–VI) due to their greater melanocyte reactivity.

Overview: PIH is caused by increased melanocyte activity and melanin overproduction, which are triggered by inflammatory mediators. Excessive melanin can be transferred to the epidermal keratinocytes to form epidermal hypermelanosis or released to the dermis and phagocytized by melanophages to develop a more resistant clinical form of dermal hyperpigmentation.

Clinical presentation: PIH presents with hyperpigmented macules or patches corresponding to the distribution of the preceding inflammatory skin disease or injury (Figure 25.5). If the hyperpigmentation is epidermal, then the color of the lesions is tan to dark brown, whereas dermal hyperpigmentation appears as a blue/gray to darker brown coloration. The diagnosis is usually based on visual assessment. Epidermal PIH accentuates and appears darker during Wood's lamp examination.

Laboratory studies: Histopathology shows increased melanin in the epidermis and melanophages in the superficial dermis.

Differential diagnosis: The differential diagnosis includes other hyperpigmentation disorders (Table 25.3).

Management: The management of PIH involves the treatment of the predisposing inflammatory dermatosis, protection against prolonged sun exposure, and treatment of the pigmentation. Topically, hydroquinone 4% alone or in combination with tretinoin (0.025%, 0.05%) and corticosteroid (fluocinoloneacetonide 0.01% [modified Kligman formula]) can be used as first-line therapy.

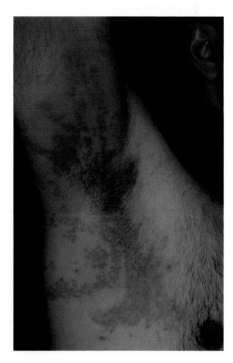

Figure 25.5 Post-inflammatory hyperpigmentation on the axilla and lateral aspect of the trunk developed due to laser treatment.

Source: Courtesy of Istanbul Medeniyet University Dermatology Clinic.

Table 25.3 Differential Diagnosis of Localized or Circumscribed Hyperpigmentation

Post-inflammatory hyperpigmentation

Melasma

Erythema dyschromicum perstans

Idiopathic eruptive macular pigmentation

Cutaneous amyloidosis

Drug-induced hyperpigmentation

Pityriasis versicolor

Fixed drug eruption

Pigmented contact dermatitis (Riehl melanosis)

Exogenous ochronosis

Lichen planus pigmentosus

Nevus of Ota

Nevus of Becker

Cutaneous mastocytosis

Pigmentary demarcation lines

Topical therapy includes topical retinoids (e.g., tretinoin, adapalene, tazarotene) and azelaic acid. Chemical peels such as salicylic, glycolic, or trichloroacetic acid, along with laser/light-based treatments, can be used by experienced physicians. Caution must be taken against skin irritation and subsequent worsening of the PIH.

Final comment: Epidermal PIH usually resolves or improves within a few months to one year, and dermal PIH can be more resistant.

Melasma

Definition: Melasma is a common hyperpigmentation disorder characterized by irregular hyperpigmented patches that involve sun-exposed sites. It particularly affects women (9:1 ratio) and those with darker skin phototypes (Fitzpatrick skin types III–VI).

Overview: Pregnancy is a well-known triggering factor. It is also associated with prolonged UVR, the use of hormonal therapies, cosmetics, photosensitizing drugs or anticonvulsants, thyroid dysfunction, and genetic predisposition.

Clinical presentation: Clinically, asymptomatic, light to dark brown patches with irregular borders are observed (Figure 25.6). The lesions are symmetrically located on the face and sometimes on the neck. Three clinical patterns of distribution include: centrofacial (the most common clinical pattern), malar, and mandibular.

Laboratory studies: The diagnosis is usually made clinically. Epidermal lesions of melasma intensify under a Wood lamp examination. Histopathology reveals increased epidermal melanin deposits and number of melanocytes, disruption of basal membrane and protrusion of melanocytes into the dermis, superficial and mid-dermal melanophages, increased mast cell count, and vascularization in the dermis.

Differential diagnosis: Differential diagnosis includes the disorders in Table 25.3.

Management: Avoidance of sunlight exposure and the use of high-SPF (≥50) sunscreens are pivotal in the management. Topical therapy includes hydroquinone (2%, 4%), retinoids,

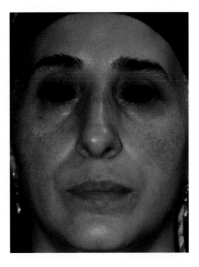

Figure 25.6 Melasma. Light brown macules and patches on the zygomatic region and dorsum of the nose.

Source: Courtesy of Istanbul Medeniyet University Dermatology Clinic.

315

azelaic acid, tranexaminic acid, and triple combination creams consisting of hydroquinone, treti-noin, and topical corticosteroids (i.e., modified Kligman formula). Cosmeceuticals containing kojic acid, ascorbic acid (vitamin C), *Polypodium leucotomos*, or niacinamide can also be beneficial.

Chemical peels such as glycolic acid or salicylic acid, may not be superior to hydroquinone, but can be preferred as second-line therapy. Laser and light-based therapies have had mixed outcomes but can deliver significant improvement by trained physicians, especially in concert with topical or oral therapies. In moderate to severe and recalcitrant cases, oral tranexamic acid (500–1500 mg daily) can be a safe and efficacious therapeutic option.

Course: Despite the use of appropriate treatment, melasma often recurs during the summer months.

Drug-Induced Hyperpigmentation

Definition: Drug-induced hyperpigmentation is an acquired and usually diffuse cutaneous hyperpigmentation caused by medications. Antineoplastic drugs, antimalarials, minocycline, zidovudine, amiodarone, analgesics, anticoagulants, hormones, metals, anticonvulsants, pheno-thiazines (chlorpromazine), and tricyclic antidepressants (imipramine, desipramine) are the most commonly reported agents to cause hyperpigmentation.

Overview: Various mechanisms, such as drug-induced stimulation of melanogenesis (either directly or via inflammation), deposition of a stable drug-melanin complex within the dermis, direct accumulation of the responsible drug itself, drug-induced production of nonmelanin pig-ments, or drug-induced damage of dermal vessels, may play a role in pathogenesis.

Clinical presentation: Drug-induced hyperpigmentation often begins insidiously and exhib-its a gradual progression over months or years after drug initiation. The lesions can be brown or blue-gray in color and primarily involve sun-exposed areas. Mucosa or nails may also be affected. Clinical manifestation can vary, depending on the drug, as summarized in Table 25.4.

Table 25.4 Common Causes of Drug-Induced Pigmentation and Localization or Pattern of Pigmentation

Medication	Localization/pattern
Bleomycin	Flagellate pigmentation, localized pigmentation overlying small joints, transvers melanonychia
Cyclophosphamide	Palmoplantar pigmentation, nail pigmentation, mucosal pigmentation
Dactinomycin	Generalized, mostly facial pigmentation
Daunorubicin	Hyperpigmentation in sun exposed sites, transvers melanonychia
Doxorubicin	Palmoplantar pigmentation, localized pigmentation overlying small joints, mucosal pigmentation, nail pigmentation
Antimalarials	Brown to blue-gray pigmentation affecting the face, neck, lower limbs and forearms, mucosal pigmentation (hard palate), nail pigmentation
Minocycline	Cutaneous, ungual, mucosal, and dental pigmentation (≥100 mg/day).
	Type 1: Blue-gray pigmentation on the sites of previous inflammation (face) and in normal skin
	Type 2: Pigmentation affecting the shins, calves, and forearms
	Type 3: Diffuse smudgy brown pigmentation exacerbated with sunlight
Zidovudine	Flagellate pigmentation, nail pigmentation (longitudinal > transverse or diffuse melanonychia), mucosal pigmentation
Amiodarone	Blue-gray pigmentation in sun exposed sites
Estrogen	Melasma-like pigmentation
Silver (argyria)	Generalized gray to blue pigmentation. Nails and mucosa are also affected.
Iron	Permanent brown pigmentation at the sites of intramuscular injection. Diffuse slaty pigmentation with intravenous infusion.
Gold	Permanent blue-gray pigmentation in sun exposed sites (periorbital), nail pigmentation
Anticonvulsants	Melasma-like pigmentation
Psychotropic drugs	Slaty to brown discoloration in sun-exposed sites
Hydroquinone	Exogenous ochronosis
Psoralens	Diffuse pigmentation after oral psoralen + UVA exposure, nail pigmentation

Management: Establishing a causal relationship between the medication and hyperpigmented lesions can be difficult. Current and previous medications should be reviewed. Although not specific, histology may provide clues regarding the mechanism by which the suspected drug caused the hyperpigmentation. When the diagnosis is made, the associated drug should be discontinued.

Erythema Dyschromicum Perstans

Synonym: Ashy dermatosis

Definition: Erythema dyschromicum perstans (EDP) is a progressive disorder characterized by brown to gray, "ashy" patches on the trunk and extremities. It is a rare disease worldwide but may be more common in Hispanics and individuals with darker skin phototypes (Fitzpatrick skin types III–V).

Overview: The etiology of EDP is uncertain, but it may be associated with the use of some medications (e.g., penicillin, omeprazole, fluoxetine, benzodiazepines, ethambutol), ingestion of chemicals (e.g., barium sulfate, ammonium nitrate, chlorthalonil), infections (e.g., hepatitis C), infestations (e.g., nematodes), endocrinopathies (e.g., hypothyroidism, diabetes), and cobalt allergy.

Clinical presentation: EDP presents with asymptomatic shapeless ash-brown to blue-gray macules or patches affecting the trunk, proximal extremities, and, occasionally, the neck and face. An erythematous border may exist in early lesions. Dermatoscopy shows brown or gray-blue dots (corresponds to dermal melanophages) over a pigmented background in crista cutis, which forms a marble-like appearance.

Laboratory studies: EDP is diagnosed by its clinical and histologic features. Histologically, epidermal papillomatosis, vacuolization of the basal cell layer (in early lesions), pigment incontinence and melanophages, and mononuclear infiltrate in the papillary and subpapillary dermis can be detected.

Differential diagnosis: Lichen planus pigmentosus, PIH, contact dermatitis, argyria, morphea, hemochromatosis, mastocytosis, arsenicism, and fixed drug eruption should be considered in the differential diagnosis.

Management: There is no effective treatment for EDP. Current therapeutic options that are based on small series include topical corticosteroids, topical tacrolimus, dapsone, clofazimine, and narrow-band UVB phototherapy.

Final comment: EDP usually persists in adults whereas spontaneous resolution may be seen in children.

Cutaneous Amyloidosis

Definition: Cutaneous amyloidosis is a group of disorders characterized by dermal deposition of amyloid without any systemic involvement.

Overview: Macular amyloidosis and lichen amyloidosis are the most common subtypes of primary cutaneous amyloidosis that cause localized hyperpigmentation.

Clinical presentation: Macular amyloidosis presents with dark brown and moderately pruritic patches mostly located on the upper part of the back (Figure 25.7a). Lichen amyloidosis manifests as severely pruritic, discrete, and hyperpigmented papules usually affecting the lower extremities. Itching is typically the presenting symptom of cutaneous amyloidosis, and this leads to rubbing, which plays a role in the development of lesions. Hyperpigmentation represents a rippled pattern in both subtypes (Figure 25.7b).

Laboratory studies: Histopathology reveals melanophages, and amorphous, eosinophilic amyloid deposits that stain orange-red with Congo red stain in the superficial dermis.

Management: Oral colchicine, ablative laser treatments and topical application of dimethyl sulfoxide are a few of the therapeutic options that have shown to achieve improvement in the hyperpigmentation of cutaneous amyloidosis.

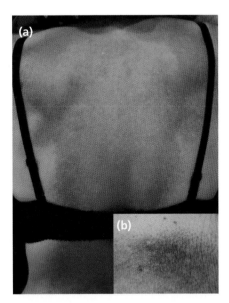

Figure 25.7 Macular amyloidosis: (a) Light to dark brown patches on the back; (b) note the rippled pattern of pigmentation.

Source: Courtesy of Istanbul Medeniyet University Dermatology Clinic.

317

Peutz-Jeghers Syndrome

Definition: Peutz-Jeghers Syndrome (PJS) is an uncommon autosomal dominant genodermatosis characterized by mucocutaneous pigmented macules, gastrointestinal hamartomatous polyposis, and a predisposition for occurrence of malignancies. Mutation of a tumor suppressor gene, the *STK11/LKB1* on chromosome 19, is implicated in the majority of cases.

Overview: The most frequent neoplasms associated with this syndrome are gastrointestinal (colorectal, pancreatic, gastric), genitourinary (uterine, cervical, testicular, ovarian), breast, and bronchial cancers.

Clinical presentation: Mucocutaneous hyperpigmented lesions manifest as 2–5-mm sized brown to black macules distributed on the lips, buccal mucosa, perioral region, eyelids, nostrils, fingertips, hands, feet, and perianal region in early childhood. Pigmentary lesions, except those on the buccal mucosa and fingers, may fade later in life. Longitudinal melanonychia may also occur.

Differential diagnosis: Carney complex (spotty hyperpigmentation, cardiac myxoma, endocrine hyperactivity, and schwannomas) and Laugier-Hunziker syndrome (hyperpigmented macules on the lips, in the mouth, and genitalia, plus dark nail streaks) should be considered in the differential diagnosis of the pigmented macules.

Management: Management of PJS should involve the evaluation and screening for neoplasms. Laser and light-based therapies can be used to treat the hyperpigmented lesions.

Addison Disease

Definition: Addison disease is an acquired primary adrenocortical insufficiency mostly caused by autoimmunity. It is characterized by diffuse hyperpigmentation and symptoms of electrolyte imbalance, such as malaise, nausea, vomiting, and diarrhea.

Overview: Insufficient secretion of glucocorticoids and mineralocorticoids results in overproduction of ACTH, which stimulates melanogenesis via MC1R.

Clinical presentation: Hyperpigmentation is usually generalized but more prominent in the sites of sun-exposure, chronic pressure (e.g. elbows, knees), trauma, and scars. Palm lines, areolas, nipples, armpits, and genitalia are other typical locations.

Laboratory studies: Histopathology reveals increased melanin within the melanocytes and dermal melanophages. Hyponatremia, hyperkalemia, and elevated blood urea nitrogen are expected in laboratory findings. Specific endocrinologic tests are employed to make the diagnosis.

Genetic Reticulate Pigmentary Disorders

Dowling-Degos Disease

Definition: Dowling-Degos disease (DDD) is a rare autosomal-dominant disorder characterized by reticulate hyperpigmentation affecting the flexural sites.

Overview: Loss-of-function mutation in the keratin 5 gene is implicated in the etiology.

Clinical presentation: The onset of DDD is typically during young adulthood. Symmetrical brown reticular macules or papules initially appear in the axillae and groins, which then spread to the inframammary and intergluteal folds, neck, and trunk. Additional findings, such as pitted perioral scars, comedo-like lesions on the neck and back, and epidermoid cysts may also be found.

Laboratory studies: Histopathology reveals hypermelanosis in the basal layer, branch-like elongation of the rete ridges and follicular infundibulum with hypermelanotic tips, and dermal melanophages.

Differential diagnosis: These include other reticulate pigmentary disorders (Table 25.5). *Galli-Galli Disease* has similar features to DDD; however, there are some distinctive features, such as erythematous–brown keratotic papules with suprabasal acantholysis in histopathologic evaluation. It is considered a variant of DDD. *Haber's syndrome* is also manifested by a reticulate pigmentation, comedo-like lesions, and pitted scars, but it can be distinguished by a photosensitive, facial rosacea-like rash that occurs in childhood.

Management: There is no curative treatment, and hyperpigmentation progresses over the years. Therapeutic options include topical hydroquinone, adapalene, tretinoin, corticosteroids, and laser treatment.

Reticulate Acropigmentation of Kitamura

Definition: Reticulate acropigmentation of Kitamura (RAK) is an uncommon autosomal-dominant disorder caused by the loss-of-function mutation in *α disintegrin and metalloproteinase domain-containing protein 10*, also known as ADAM10.

Table 25.5 Differential Diagnosis of Reticulate Pigmentary Disorders

Dowling-Degos disease
Galli-Galli disease
Kitamura reticulate acropigmentation
Haber syndrome
Confluent and reticulated papillomatosis
Erythema ab igne
Prurigo pigmentosa
Naegeli-Franceschetti-Jadassohn syndrome
Dermatopathia pigmentosa reticularis

Clinical presentation: RAK is clinically characterized by reticulated, slightly depressed, hyperpigmented macules on the dorsa of the hands and feet, palmar pits, loss of fingerprint lines, and inclusion cysts. Hyperpigmented lesions manifest in childhood and spread over within years.

Laboratory studies: Histologically, epidermal atrophy, elongated rete ridges with increased melanin at the tips, and an increase in melanocyte number can be demonstrated.

Management: Therapeutic choices are similar to those for DDD.

FINAL THOUGHT

- Oculocutaneous albinism is an autosomal recessive disorder characterized by a normal number of melanocytes but a deficiency in tyrosinase enzyme. Individuals present with fair skin, blue eyes, and white hair. Sun protection is paramount.

- Vitiligo presents as well-defined depigmented patches. Woods lamp will assist in distinguishing depigmentation from hypopigmentation. It affects 1–2% of the population and may be associated with other autoimmune conditions. Treatment involves topical therapies, phototherapy, immunosuppression, and surgical treatments.

- Generalized hyperpigmentation is usually caused by melanin overproduction but sometimes develops due to an increase in active melanocytes. Hyperpigmentation can be localized or generalized in distribution and circumscribed, linear, or reticulate in configuration.

- Hyperpigmentation may be caused by melasma, medications, genetic disorders, systemic disease or may occur as post-inflammatory pigmentation.

ADDITIONAL READINGS

Chang MW. Disorders of hyperpigmentation. In: Bolognia J, Schaffer JV, editors. Dermatology. 4th ed. Philadelphia: Elsevier Saunders; 2018. p. 1115–1143.
Errichetti E, Angione V, Stinco G. Dermoscopy in assisting the recognition of ashy dermatosis. JAAD Case Rep. 2017;3:482–484.
Handel AC, Miot LD, Miot HA. Melasma: a clinical and epidemiological review. An Bras Dermatol. 2014;89:771–782.
Marks R, Motley R. Common Skin Diseases. 18th ed. London: CRC Press; 2011.
Nahhas AF, Braunberger TL, Hamzavi IH. An update on drug-induced pigmentation. Am J Clin Dermatol. 2019;20:75–96.
Nicolaidou E, Katsambas AD. Pigmentation disorders: hyperpigmentation and hypopigmentation. Clin Dermatol. 2014;32:66–72.
Rodrigues M, Pandya AG. Hypermelanoses. In: Kang S, Amagai M, Bruckner AL, et al., editors. Fitzpatrick's Dermatology. 9th ed. New York: McGraw-Hill; 2019. p. 1361–1389.
Silpa-Archa N, Kohli I, Chaowattanapanit S, et al. Postinflammatory hyperpigmentation: a comprehensive overview: epidemiology, pathogenesis, clinical presentation, and non-invasive assessment technique. J Am Acad Dermatol. 2017;77:591–605.
Weidner T, Illing T, Elsner P. Primary localized cutaneous amyloidosis: a systematic treatment review. Am J Clin Dermatol. 2017;18:629–642.
Zhang J, Li M, Yao Z. Updated review of genetic reticulate pigmentary disorders. Br J Dermatol. 2017;177:945–959.

26 Psychocutaneous Disorders

Kristen Russomanno and Vesna M. Petronic-Rosic

CONTENTS

Overview: Psychocutaneous diseases are commonly seen in dermatologic practice, and thus both recognizing these entities and understanding treatment options are important for physicians who may receive skin complaints. Oftentimes, patients affected by psychocutaneous diseases initially present to dermatology rather than psychiatry because they may not be aware of the psychiatric component of their condition. Treatment is often difficult, and many patients are lost to follow-up; however, disease management is possible with the correct approach.

DELUSIONS OF PARASITOSIS

Synonyms: Psychogenic parasitosis, delusional infestation, Ekbom syndrome, Morgellons disease (a variant)

Definition: This is a rare type of delusional disorder that is defined by the fixed, false belief of a skin infestation that is maintained despite evidence to the contrary. It is classified in the *Diagnostic and Statistical Manual of Mental Disorders*, 5th Edition (*DSM-5*) as a somatic type of delusional disorder. Individuals affected by this disorder firmly believe that they have a skin infection of parasites, mites, bacteria, worms, bugs, or other types of organisms. They are resistant to alternative explanations for their symptoms and lack insight into the possibility that they are not infested. Primary delusions of parasitosis occur in the absence of underlying systemic or psychiatric diseases that may mimic the condition. Secondary delusions of parasitosis occur when the delusions and/or abnormal skin sensations are attributable to an underlying condition and/or the use of medications or illicit drugs.

Clinical presentation: Delusions of parasitosis classically presents with various symptoms including pruritus and abnormal skin sensations which are typically described as "crawling, stinging, or biting." Although the condition has been reported in all age groups and both genders, middle-aged women are most commonly affected. The average age of onset is 57 years old.

At presentation, symptoms have often persisted for several months or longer and have been refractory to various treatments. Patients frequently seek the help of multiple medical professionals and may have been treated with both topical and systemic antibiotics and steroids without significant improvement. They may have attempted treatment by using disinfectants and/or pesticides, moving locations, and hiring exterminators without improvement. Patients often provide detailed accounts of the organisms that they are infested with, including in-depth descriptions of their appearance, timing of their infestation, and behavior. They frequently present with collections including fragments of skin, lint, and other debris, which they believe to be organisms or proof of infestation. This behavior is referred to as the "matchbox," "Ziploc bag," or "specimen" sign (Figure 26.1). In up to 25% of cases, family members or friends may also be drawn into the delusions in a *folie a deux* phenomenon.

Morgellons disease is a condition characterized by a similar constellation of symptoms; however, it is controversial and poorly understood. Patients experience similar abnormal skin sensations, but they specifically report the emergence of small fibers protruding through the skin. Many similarities have been observed between patients affected by delusions of infestation and Morgellons disease, which is the reason that some physicians believe it may be a subset of the former rather than its distinct entity. Unlike delusions of parasitosis, the disease is not recognized by the *DSM-5*.

Laboratory studies: Primary delusion of parasitosis is a diagnosis of exclusion, and other etiologies of abnormal skin sensation must be ruled out. A thorough physical examination should be

DOI: 10.1201/9781003105268-26

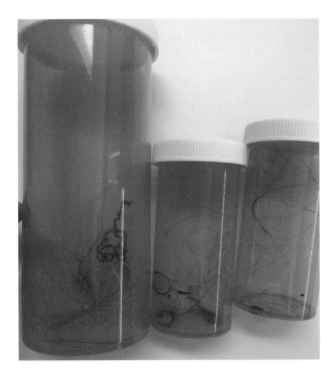

Figure 26.1 Samples of materials believed to be evidence of an infestation, provided by a patient with delusions of parasitosis.

performed to evaluate for a true infestation (e.g., scabies, pediculosis). Skin scrapings prepared with mineral oil may aid in the detection of organisms. Microscopic examination of patient-provided skin samples may be performed to confirm the lack of organisms. Although rarely required, a skin biopsy may be necessary if there is a concern for an alternative dermatologic diagnosis.

If pruritus is a prominent symptom and infestation has been excluded, a workup should rule out a systemic cause for pruritus. The investigation should exclude renal and/or liver disease, endocrine disorders, nutritional deficiencies, anemia, malignancies, neurologic diseases, lupus erythematosus, infections (e.g., syphilis, HIV), and heart failure. An exhaustive medication and social history should be obtained to determine if the abnormal sensations are attributable to drug side effects. Illicit drugs, especially amphetamines and cocaine, can cause both abnormal skin sensations and psychiatric disturbances, including hallucinations. Medications, particularly anticholinergics, angiotensin-converting enzyme inhibitors, antiepileptics, stimulants, antimicrobials, and dopamine agonists may cause itching and/or abnormal skin sensation.

Finally, an in-depth psychiatric history should be obtained, and other disorders including schizophrenia, psychoses, dementia, depression, and obsessive-compulsive disorder should be excluded.

Differential diagnosis: This includes true infestation or infection, as well as secondary causes of abnormal skin sensation mimicking parasitosis including psychiatric disease, substance abuse, or systemic medical conditions. The use of amphetamines, cocaine, and alcohol, in addition to withdrawal from alcohol, can precipitate hallucinations and abnormal skin sensations.

Psychiatric diseases, including bipolar disorder, schizophrenia, obsessive-compulsive disorder, generalized anxiety disorder, and major depressive disorder may cause secondary delusions of parasitosis. Medical conditions, including neurologic disorders, nutritional deficiencies (e.g., B12 and folate deficiency), infections (e.g., HIV, syphilis, tuberculosis), thyroid dysfunction, anemia, malignancies, systemic lupus erythematosus, liver, kidney or pancreatic disease, and diabetes mellitus, may cause abnormal skin sensation.

Certain medications have been known to cause side effects that may mimic delusions of parasitosis. These include but are not limited to anticholinergics, stimulants, antiepileptics, angiotensin-converting enzyme inhibitors, antimicrobials, and dopamine agonists.

Management: The most important facet in approaching a patient with delusions of parasitosis is to first develop a strong therapeutic relationship before developing a treatment plan. Patients often refuse to consider that their condition is psychiatric, and the suggestion of such may cause further frustration, isolation, and depressive symptoms. Neutrality should be maintained, and directly challenging the patient's beliefs should be avoided. In addition, the provider should not make any statements that support the delusion and perpetuate the false belief of an infestation. Once a trusting relationship has been established with the patient, a treatment regimen may be recommended.

Second-generation antipsychotics (e.g., risperidone, olanzapine) have become the first-line treatment for delusions of parasitosis, and atypical antipsychotics have also been used successfully. In small case reports and case series, risperidone and olanzapine have shown to be effective and well tolerated. Risperidone is typically initiated at a dose of 0.25 or 0.5 mg/day and can be titrated up to 6 mg/day. Patients may require between 2–4 mg/day for symptom benefit, and at least partial response may be achieved within a few weeks to months of treatment. Initiation of olanzapine at a dose of 5 mg/day, titrated up to as high as 20 mg/day may be effective within 1–3 months. Severe side effects of second-generation antipsychotics include extrapyramidal symptoms, hyperprolactinemia, neuroleptic malignant syndrome, tardive dyskinesia, agranulocytosis, and metabolic syndrome. Baseline bloodwork and close monitoring are recommended.

As an adjunct to antipsychotic treatment, abnormal skin sensations can be managed with topical anti-itch lotions/creams, including those containing menthol or pramoxine. Systemic medications, such as gabapentin and antihistamines, may also reduce itch and other sensations; however, limited data are supporting their use in this condition.

If the patient is willing, a multidisciplinary approach to treatment with the input of psychiatry is ideal; however, patients are often reluctant and refuse evaluation by psychiatry, and thus, this is rarely practical.

Course: The treatment of delusions of parasitosis is challenging given patients often refuse psychiatric care and/or the initiation of antipsychotic medications. Patients are often lost to follow-up, and therefore, the course and prognosis of the disease are poorly understood. In those agreeable to pharmacologic therapy, the response to treatment with antipsychotic medications is typically adequate. If compliant, patients may experience a partial or complete response within weeks to months; however, achieving a sustained response is difficult because many patients are ultimately lost to follow-up.

Final comment: Delusions of parasitosis is a disorder defined by a firm belief of infestation/ infection with a parasite or other organism in the absence of any underlying drug side effects, psychiatric conditions, or medical illnesses to explain the symptoms. The condition is distressing to patients and can be challenging to treat. After exclusion of a true infestation, underlying systemic or psychiatric disease, and side effects from drugs, the diagnosis of primary delusions of parasitosis can be made. By building a strong therapeutic alliance with affected patients and selecting an appropriate antipsychotic medication, the disease can be managed.

EXCORIATION DISORDER

Synonyms: Dermatillomania, psychogenic excoriation, skin-picking disorder, neurotic excoriation disorder

Definition: Excoriation disorder (ED) is categorized in the *DSM-5* under "obsessive-compulsive and related disorders," and is defined by (1) recurrent skin picking resulting in skin lesions, (2) repeated attempts to decrease or stop the behavior, (3) significant distress or impaired functioning related to the behavior, and 4) no underlying medical condition or other psychiatric disorder that explains the behavior.

Clinical presentation: ED is characterized by the conscious, repetitive, and poorly controlled desire to pick the skin which leads to compulsive picking, digging, squeezing, or scratching. This behavior causes significant distress for affected patients in contrast to those who have a controllable behavioral tendency toward skin picking. Patients may present with skin lesions that are *de novo* or that have evolved from the handling of primary skin lesions, such as those in acne or insect bites. Acne excorieé is a specific subset of ED that describes the compulsive picking of acne lesions specifically. The prevalence of ED is about 1–5% and is reported to occur at any age; however, it most frequently occurs during childhood or adolescence. Studies have shown a female predominance.

Visualized lesions vary in distribution but are most commonly seen on the face, arms, and legs (Figure 26.2). Lesions may vary in size and morphology, ranging from a few millimeters to several centimeters in diameter and often are in different stages of healing. They may be geometric erosions or deep ulcerations, which often scar. Sparing of the upper portion of the back, referred to as the *butterfly sign*, is indicative of self-inflicted lesions because this area is typically unreachable.

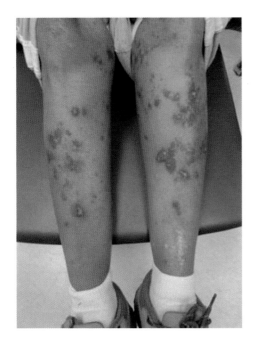

Figure 26.2 Hyperpigmented nodules with central erosion on the legs due to persistent excoriation and manual manipulation.

Patients may describe a variety of negative emotions as triggers for the behavior, including depression, anxiety, or boredom. They often experience shame, anxiety, or depressive symptoms secondary to their inability to stop. Many psychiatric conditions occur in association with ED and may be evident on evaluation. Affected patients have higher rates of depression, obsessive-compulsive disorder, substance dependence, body dysmorphic disorder, and bipolar disorder, among other conditions.

To diagnose ED, a thorough physical examination should be performed to rule out other dermatologic or systemic conditions. Investigation into associated distress and any detriment to the quality of life should be conducted with an understanding that many affected patients experience a great amount of shame and embarrassment.

If pruritus is a significant symptom, then a full workup for underlying systemic etiologies as alternative diagnoses should be pursued and an exhaustive medication and social history review should be completed. (See the laboratory studies/evaluation section under delusions of parasitosis.)

Differential diagnosis: Repetitive behaviors, such as skin picking and hair pulling, should be differentiated from stereotypic movement disorders that may occur in the setting of certain neurodevelopment disorders and an autism spectrum disorder. Other psychocutaneous disorders should be excluded, including delusions of infestation and factitial dermatitis. If pruritus is present, primary causes such as systemic diseases or adverse effects from medications or illicit drugs should be ruled out. Dermatoses that may cause abnormal skin sensation and/or pruritus should be evaluated for including, but not limited to, eczema, psoriasis, and prurigo nodularis. If the face is affected, the trigeminal trophic syndrome should be considered in the correct clinical context.

Management: This is most challenging, and studies suggest that a multidisciplinary approach is often necessary to optimize symptomatic relief and disease control. Cognitive-behavioral therapy, specifically habit reversal training, is efficacious. Habit reversal training consists of training in self-awareness, stimulus control, competing response, and relaxation. Other nonpharmacologic approaches, including acceptance and commitment therapy, psychodynamic psychotherapy, mindfulness-based therapy, and progressive muscle relaxation are helpful.

At present, there is no Food and Drug Administration–approved treatment specifically for ED. There are mixed results for selective serotonin reuptake inhibitors (SSRIs), selective serotonin-norepinephrine inhibitors (SNRIs), tricyclic antidepressants (e.g., doxepin), and antipsychotics. N-acetylcysteine may improve symptoms after 12 weeks of treatment with doses ranging from 1200–3000 mg/day. Some reports also show the efficacy of N-acetylcysteine in combination with other medications, including SSRIs and antipsychotics. Fluoxetine, an SSRI at doses ranging from 20 mg/day to 80 mg/day may be beneficial in addition to escitalopram at doses up to 20–40 mg/

day, fluvoxamine 25–50 mg/day, and various doses of sertraline. Much of this literature reports improvement of symptoms in 12 weeks with the use of SSRIs.

As an adjunct to treatment for the psychologic component of the condition, cutaneous symptoms can be managed with topical anti-itch lotions/creams, including those containing menthol or pramoxine. Antihistamines may reduce the sensation of itching and provide a sedating effect at night.

Course: The course of ED is chronic, and symptoms often persist with fluctuating severity for many years.

Final comment: Excoriation disorder is classified as an obsessive-compulsive and related disorder that is characterized by the conscious, repetitive, and poorly controlled desire to pick the skin, which ultimately results in significant distress for affected patients. Diagnosis requires the exclusion of other dermatoses. The condition is chronic, and a combination of pharmacologic and non-pharmacologic approaches may be used to address both psychologic and cutaneous components.

FACTITIAL DERMATITIS

Synonyms: Dermatitis artefacta, factitious skin disorder

Definition: This is a psychocutaneous condition classified as a factitious disorder under "somatic symptom and related disorders" in the *DSM-5*. The condition is defined by the self-infliction of cutaneous lesions to satisfy a psychologic need or unconscious motive and subsequent denial of the self-inflicted nature of the condition.

Clinical presentation: Factitial dermatitis has been reported to affect women more commonly than men and the typical onset occurs in late adolescence and early adulthood. The prevalence is difficult to estimate due to a lack of studies.

Affected patients present with a wide variety of cutaneous lesions that often fail to heal. Classic lesions have geometric and/or unusual shapes with angulated edges which suggest an external etiology. Lesions may be inflicted in various ways, including burning or injecting the skin with foreign materials and/or chemicals and manipulating the skin with sharp objects. For this reason, the morphology and distribution of lesions are often highly variable. Lesions may consist of abrasions, ulcerations, excoriations, urticarial type plaques, scars, nail/hair abnormalities, or vesicles/bullae. The most commonly affected site is the face followed by the legs (Figures 26.3–26.5).

Patients may have comorbid psychiatric diseases including depression, personality disorders, or neuroses. Alternatively, patients may describe recent stressors, and a variety of contributing etiologies have been identified including unconscious motivations, impaired interpersonal relationships, and psychosocial conflicts. Patients will not take responsibility for the lesions they present with, and they may not be consciously aware of the triggers and goals that drive the process.

Laboratory studies: This is one of exclusion, and thus, alternative organic etiologies must be ruled out. Primary dermatoses that may mimic the condition must be excluded including

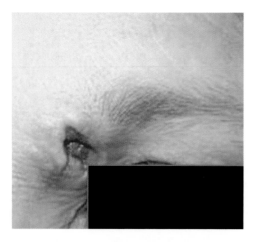

Figure 26.3 Factitial dermatitis presenting as an angulated erythematous ulceration of the lateral nasal root.

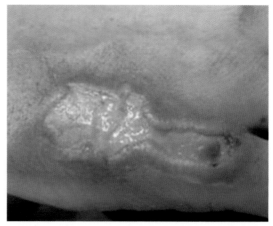

Figure 26.4 Factitial dermatitis presenting as a geometric and angulated ulceration of the dorsal aspect of the hand.

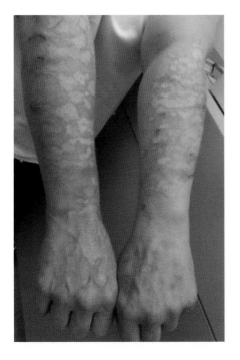

Figure 26.5 Unusually shaped, geometric, and atrophic plaques on the forearms consistent with scarring from factitial dermatitis.

various types of vasculitis, ulcerating disorders, collagen vascular diseases, and arthropod infestations. Although a skin biopsy is often not necessary, it may be performed when the diagnosis is unclear.

Differential diagnosis: This includes primary dermatoses, such as blistering disorders, vasculitides, ulcerating disorders, panniculitis, arthropod bites, alopecias, and drug eruptions. Other alternative psychocutaneous conditions should be considered, including delusions of parasitosis and excoriation disorder. Nonsuicidal self-injury and malingering must also be on the differential. Unlike malingerers, patients with factitial dermatitis are not consciously seeking secondary gain.

History should be obtained to evaluate for the presence of any comorbid psychiatric conditions. Healing a lesion that was refractory to other treatments by covering it with occlusive dressing is of diagnostic value given that this suggests an external process.

Management: This consists of addressing both the cutaneous manifestations of the disease and the underlying psychologic disorder. First and foremost, it is important to establish a trusting relationship with the patient to improve the likelihood that they will accept treatment options. Although a multidisciplinary approach in coordination with both dermatology and psychiatry is ideal, it is often not possible to convince patients to seek psychiatric care.

Patients may be amenable to topical treatment with antibiotics, emollients, dressings, and other wound care products which may facilitate the healing of lesions. Occlusive dressings can prevent further manipulation of the skin and may be of diagnostic value as above.

Antidepressants, including SSRIs, anxiolytics, and low-dose antipsychotics (e.g., aripiprazole, pimozide, risperidone, olanzapine) can be useful in the management of underlying depression, anxiety, and/or obsessive-compulsive behaviors respectively. Dosing of 0.5–1 mg/day of pimozide, risperidone 0.5–2 mg/day, or aripiprazole 2–5 mg/day may be beneficial; however, it is often difficult to approach the subject of these treatments given that patients often lack awareness and/or acceptance of an underlying psychologic etiology.

Course: Factitial dermatitis is a chronic disorder and relapses are common. Although there is no specific cure, improving outcomes with treatment and close follow-up is possible. Oftentimes, patients are lost to follow up, are not compliant with treatment regimens, and experience frequent relapses. The prognosis is poor for many patients, and the disease severity tends to wax and wane.

Final comment: This is a factitious disorder in which affected patients self-inflict skin lesions to fulfill internal psychologic motives and subsequently deny any responsibility. The condition is a diagnosis of exclusion. Patient denial of responsibility and a lack of acceptance of psychiatric care renders treatment difficult.

TRICHOTILLOMANIA

Synonyms: Trichotillosis, hair-pulling disorder

Definition: Trichotillomania is classified in the *DSM-5* under obsessive-compulsive and related disorders. It is defined by "recurrent pulling out of one's hair, resulting in hair loss" despite "repeated attempts to decrease or stop hair pulling." The pulling cannot be explained by the symptoms of another psychiatric or medical disorder, and the urges cause significant distress and/or impairment in social, occupational, and/or other important areas of functioning.

Clinical presentation: Patients affected by trichotillomania are commonly older children and adolescents who are an average of 13 years of age at the onset of disease. The prevalence is thought to be between 1–4%, and girls and women are more commonly affected. Despite the strong psychiatric component of the diagnosis, patients often initially present to a dermatologist for evaluation of hair loss.

Patients may present with hair thinning and patches of alopecia anywhere on the body; however, the scalp is most commonly affected (Figure 26.6). The distribution of hair loss is often irregular and geometric, and hairs are characteristically broken at various lengths. Oftentimes, patients will not admit to pulling their hair out, either because they are unaware of the behavior or they are embarrassed. Patients may describe a lack of ability to grow hair longer than a few centimeters in length.

There is typically a trigger that leads to the pulling behavior, which may be emotional, cognitive, or sensory. Upon questioning, patients may reveal awareness of circumstances that heighten their urges to pull. Patients often have low self-esteem and poor quality of life, which may be related to the hair pulling itself or secondary to comorbid psychiatric conditions. They often have concomitant depression, obsessive-compulsive disorder, eating disorders, anxiety, substance use disorders, and/or other behavioral issues. Affected individuals are more likely to engage in other similar compulsive behaviors, such as skin picking or nail biting which may be clinically apparent.

Hairs are sometimes ingested causing a mass within the intestines which is referred to as a trichobezoar. In severe cases, trichobezoars may obstruct the intestines and cause associated gastrointestinal symptoms that may be apparent on evaluation.

Laboratory studies: Physical examination and obtaining a thorough history are key in the evaluation and diagnosis of trichotillomania. Trichoscopy (i.e., dermatoscopic examination of the hair and scalp) may be helpful for supporting the diagnosis. Under magnification, hairs of various lengths can be appreciated in addition to other diagnostic clues, including flame hairs (i.e., remnants of anagen hairs), coiled hairs, and the v-sign (i.e., two small hairs emerging from one follicle). If there is diagnostic uncertainty, then a scalp biopsy may be performed to support the diagnosis.

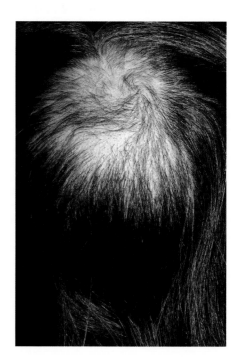

Figure 26.6   Trichotillomania presenting as an alopecic patch with hairs of multiple different lengths and perifollicular erythema and hemorrhage.

Further investigation may be pursued by shaving a small area of the scalp and subsequently observing if hairs grow back in normal fashion before growing long enough to pull out. This diagnostic tool is referred to as a "hair growth window."

Differential diagnosis: The differential diagnosis includes other types of hair loss, and trichotillomania is often confused for alopecia areata given the geometric patches of hair loss. Other entities that may occur in both adolescence and adulthood that may mimic the diagnosis include traction alopecia, telogen effluvium, and tinea capitis. Pressure alopecia, temporal triangular alopecia, and some structural hair abnormalities, including pili torti and monilethrix, should also be considered.

Trichotillomania may be also be mistaken for other psychiatric conditions, most commonly obsessive-compulsive disorder; however, anxiety disorders and other psychiatric conditions may present similarly.

A thorough psychiatric and medical history should be obtained to evaluate for comorbid conditions that may contribute to the overall distress of the patient. Consideration should be given for any other psychiatric conditions that may be present, either in association with trichotillomania or as a mimicker.

Management: Patients often do not seek treatment for their condition, which is partly due to embarrassment and/or fear that their condition is not treatable or is poorly understood by medical professionals; however, there are options available that have shown to be efficacious in improving symptoms. Provider must first focus on building strong and trusting relationships with patients and their families and delivering treatment options in a neutral and supportive way.

Given the lack of data to widely support pharmacologic therapies, behavioral treatment is considered the first line. Cognitive behavioral therapy, specifically habit reversal training, is effective, especially in children. Habit reversal training consists of training in self-awareness, stimulus control, competitive response, and relaxation. Its effectiveness relies on social support; therefore, the provider needs to promote both family and social support in the care of the patient.

There are no medications approved for use in treating trichotillomania, and despite the efficacy of SSRIs in many other psychiatric conditions, there is no substantial evidence to support their use in the treatment of trichotillomania.

N-acetylcysteine dosed at 1200 mg twice daily is effective after 9 weeks of treatment. Other options include olanzapine dosed at a mean of 10.8 mg daily for 12 weeks, as well as dronabinol dosed at a mean of 11.6 mg daily for 12 weeks.

Course: With increasing age, prognosis typically worsens, and full recovery is less common. Many patients experience a chronic waxing and waning disease course over many years. Complications of severe disease include gastrointestinal symptoms associated with trichobezoars; otherwise, specifics regarding the morbidity and mortality of the condition are largely unknown.

Final comment: Trichotillomania is a chronic disorder in which patients pull out their hair, often in association with external stressors. The disorder is recognized by the DSM-5, and the diagnosis can be made clinically. The condition is chronic and typically waxes and wanes over many years. Treatment is challenging given the strong psychiatric component of disease and lack of widely accepted pharmacologic therapies. Cognitive-behavioral therapy is efficacious; however, patients must be willing to accept the psychiatric component of the disease to benefit.

FINAL THOUGHT

Psychocutaneous diseases are commonly encountered in dermatologic practice and management is complex. Diagnosis is often one of exclusion after other mimicking conditions have been ruled out. Treatment consists of addressing both the underlying condition as well as associated symptoms. In general, patients affected by psychocutaneous diseases should be approached with neutrality, and a trusting relationship should be established before suggesting treatment options. Although improvement may be possible, many patients are resistant to addressing the underlying psychologic component of their condition and are ultimately lost to follow-up.

ADDITIONAL READINGS

American Psychiatric Association. Diagnostic and Statistical Manual of Mental Disorders (DSM 5). Arlington: American Psychiatric Association; 2013.

Campbell EH, Elston DM, Hawthorne JD, et al. Diagnosis and management of delusional parasitosis. J Am Acad Dermatol. 2019;80:1428–1434.

Grant JE, Chamberlain SR. Trichotillomania. Am J Psychiatry. 2016;173:868–874.

Gupta MA, Vujcic B, Pur DR, et al. Use of antipsychotic drugs in dermatology. Clin Dermatol. 2018;36:765–773.

Henkel ED, Jaquez SD, Diaz LZ. Pediatric trichotillomania: review of management. Pediatr Dermatol. 2019;36:803–807.

Jafferany M, Patel A. Skin-picking disorder: a guide to diagnosis and management. CNS Drugs. 2019;33:337–346.

Jones G, Keuthen N, Greenberg E. Assessment and treatment of trichotillomania (hair pulling disorder) and excoriation (skin picking) disorder. Clin Dermatol. 2018;36:728–736.

Koblenzer CS, Gupta R. Neurotic excoriations and dermatitis artefacta. Semin Cutan Med Surg. 2013;32:95–100.

Kuhn H, Mennella C, Magid M, et al. Psychocutaneous disease: clinical perspectives. J Am Acad Dermatol. 2017;76:779–791.

Lavery MJ, Stull C, McCaw I, et al. Dermatitis artefacta. Clin Dermatol. 2018;36:719–722.

27 Sexually Transmitted Diseases

Aarthy K. Uthayakumar and Christopher B. Bunker

CONTENTS

Overview: The global health burden of sexually transmitted infections (STIs) remains large and increasing. In developed countries, education and sexual health are more widely available, but the burden is greatest in resource-poor countries where health care is limited. STIs are caused by a wide range of microorganisms, and many have asymptomatic early infection which favors onward transmission. They are a potential cause of serious morbidity and mortality, with late complications including in pregnancy. Furthermore, coinfection with HIV affects transmission rates. Ease of diagnostic testing, combined with early and effective treatment and increased public education, are vital for gaining control.

SYPHILIS

Definition: This is an infectious disease caused by the spirochete *Treponema pallidum*. It is usually acquired through sexual transmission, though can also be transmitted transplacentally causing congenital syphilis. It can evolve through various stages, separated by variable periods of latency.

Clinical presentation: The incubation period is 9–90 days. Primary syphilis is characterized by the appearance of a chancre, representing the site of inoculation. This is a painless, firm, ulcer of variable size, between 0.5–3 cm in diameter, with a sloughy and indurated base. It is usually on the glans penis, prepuce, or shaft in men and the vulva in women; it can also appear in and around the mouth and around the anus in men who have sex with men (MSM). Chancres heal without scarring after 3–8 weeks if left untreated.

The latent period between primary and secondary syphilis can range between 2 months to 3 years. Approximately 25% of individuals with untreated primary syphilis will develop an illness representing secondary syphilis.

Secondary syphilis involves a wide range of symptoms and signs so is called a great imitator, including systemic upset with fever, headache, mild arthralgia, and generalized lymphadenopathy. Cutaneous manifestations include an early widespread macular eruption early on, typically involving the palms and soles, with asymptomatic copper-colored or red-brown lesions (Figure 27.1). Pustular, lichenoid, or papular eruptions can occur later on, as well as psoriasiform lesions on the palms. There may patchy hair loss with a "moth-eaten" appearance (Figure 27.2). Mucosal involvement includes condylomata lata (thickened warty lesions) that appear in warm, moist sites including the mouth and perianal areas (Figure 27.3), and white *snail-trail ulcers* on the oral mucosa (Figure 27.4). In immunocompromised patients, more severe ulcerative skin lesions can occur, termed *lues maligna* (Figure 27.5). Secondary syphilis lesions resolve spontaneously without scarring, and patients subsequently enter the latency period.

Latent syphilis is subdivided into early latent syphilis (infection within the previous 12 months) and late latent (infection after 12 months), which is not considered infectious. There are no clinical features; however, serologic tests will remain reactive. Vertical transmission can still occur in early latency, although in the absence of mucocutaneous lesions, sexual transmission is less likely.

Tertiary syphilis can occur after an asymptomatic latent period ranging between 5–50 years. It includes such cardiovascular manifestations as aortic aneurysm formation, central nervous system involvement, including paresis and tabes dorsalis, and gummatous disease of the skin, subcutaneous tissues, or bones. Cutaneous signs involve asymptomatic nodular lesions, which typically

DOI: 10.1201/9781003105268-27

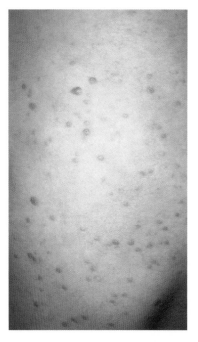
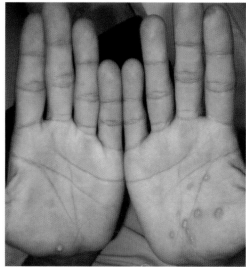

Figure 27.1 Erythematous copper-colored macules and papules on (a) the torso and (b) palms in secondary syphilis.

Source: Courtesy of Jorge Navarette, MD, Santiago, Chile.

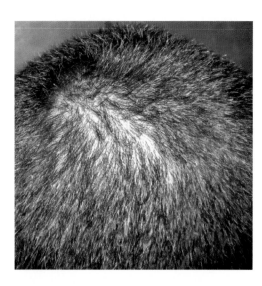
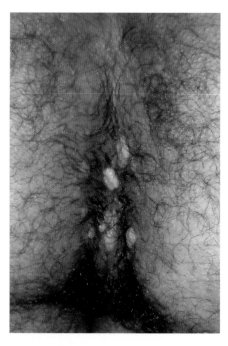

Figure 27.2 Alopecia in secondary syphilis.

Source: Courtesy of Jorge Navarette, MD, Santiago, Chile.

Figure 27.3 Perineal condyloma lata in secondary syphilis.

Source: Courtesy of Jorge Navarette, MD, Santiago, Chile.

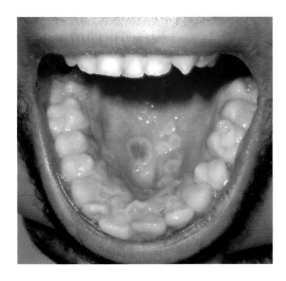

Figure 27.4 Oral ulcers in secondary syphilis.

Source: Courtesy of Jorge Navarette, MD, Santiago, Chile.

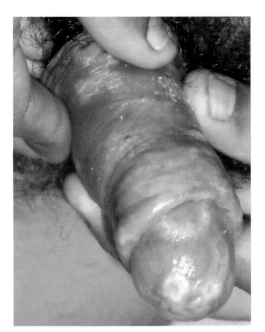
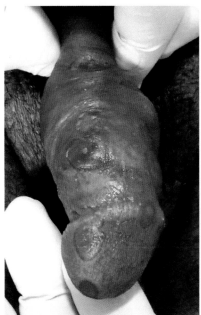

Figure 27.5 Lues maligna: Ulcerative lesions on the glans and penile shaft in secondary syphilis in HIV.

Source: Courtesy of Jorge Navarette, MD, Santiago, Chile.

involve the extensor surface of the arms, back, and face, which may be grouped, often in a circinate arrangement. In contrast, a gumma is often a single lesion, composed of granulomatous plaques or nodules irregularly shaped. There is often central ulceration that is usually painless, plus peripheral healing

Congenital syphilis occurs due to transplacental transmission or at delivery. During pregnancy, it can lead to fetal loss or stillbirth, prematurity, neurologic impairment including deafness, and bone and dental deformities (Hutchinson's teeth, Mulberry molars). Mucous membrane involvement with syphilis rhinitis, described as "snuffles," is common and manifests as profuse nasal discharge containing a high concentration of *T. pallidum*. Cutaneous manifestations are similar to those seen in secondary syphilis.

Laboratory studies: The diagnosis is most commonly made serologically, using a technique first described by August von Wasserman (1866–1925) in 1906. The 2 types of serologic tests include nontreponemal and treponemal specific tests. Non-treponemal tests are cheaper and therefore more commonly used—usually the rapid plasma reagin (RPR) or venereal disease research laboratory tests, which detect the titer of antibody present. Treponemal tests are serologic tests which once positive, remain positive for life, and therefore cannot be used to confirm possible reinfection of syphilis in prior treated disease. Darkfield microscopy can be used in primary, secondary, or tertiary syphilis to identify the *T. pallidum* organism and its characteristic corkscrew movements.

Histologic features in secondary syphilis include a perivascular infiltrate of lymphocytes and plasma cells and psoriasiform hyperplasia of the epidermis. Spirochaetes can be demonstrated with immunohistochemistry, predominantly within the epidermis.

Differential diagnosis: Syphilis is known as the "Great Imitator" due to the variety of clinical presentations. Differential diagnoses are vast and include other sexually transmitted genital infections such as chancroid, *Herpes simplex* infection, genital warts, and other viral infections such as measles, rubella, and EBV (Epstein-Barr virus), as well as all causes of ulceration, papulosquamous eruptions, and granulomatous disease.

Management: A single dose of intramuscular benzathine penicillin G 2.4 million units is the treatment of choice for all stages of syphilis, with more prolonged treatment indicated in late latent, tertiary syphilis, and HIV patients (3 doses of 2.4 million units benzathine penicillin G, weekly for 3 weeks). Alternatives include oral doxycycline 100 mg twice daily for 14 days, erythromycin 500 mg four times daily for 14 days or ceftriaxone 500 mg intramuscularly or intravenously.[4]

Course: Patients should be monitored clinically and serologically to ensure a curative treatment response. The cure rates with initial treatment of early syphilis are greater than 95%. The Jarisch-Herxheimer reaction is an acute, self-limiting, febrile reaction, occurring usually within 24 hours of treatment in 10–35% of cases. An adequate serologic response is demonstrated by a greater than a fourfold decline in antibody titers.

GONORRHEA

Synonym: Clap

Overview: It is caused by the gram-negative bacterium *Neisseria gonorrhea* and remains a global public health concern. It usually causes mucosal infections of the urogenital tract, most frequently resulting in urethritis and cervicitis, the latter can be asymptomatic. Gonorrhea also facilitates the transmission of other sexually transmitted diseases (STDs), including HIV.

Clinical presentation: The incubation period for urogenital gonorrhea ranges from 2–8 days. In men, the majority of infections are symptomatic, presenting with urethral discharge and dysuria. More women are asymptomatic, and although vaginal discharge may be reported, this is unreliable for diagnosis. Infection of the oropharynx and rectal mucosa can also occur.

Hematogenous spread can occur in approximately 0.5–3% of cases, leading to disseminated gonococcal infection. This typically presents with a dermatitis-arthritis syndrome with systemic upset, including fever.

Cutaneous lesions occur in crops, commonly near affected joints. They are initially maculopapular and then develop a central vesicle or pustule with necrosis. A migratory polyarthritis affecting peripheral joints can occur in addition to tenosynovitis.

Laboratory studies: Gram staining the discharge is central to diagnosis; gram-negative diplococci can also be detected on culture; nucleic acid amplification tests (NAATs) from urine (men) or swabs detect *N. gonorrhoeae* DNA or RNA.

Differential diagnosis: This includes other STDs such as *Chlamydia, Trichomonas vaginalis*, and genital herpes, urinary tract infection, non-specific urethritis, and pelvic inflammatory disease.

Management: In the UK, single-dose intramuscular ceftriaxone 1g is the first-line recommended treatment for uncomplicated infection. In the United States, the Centers for Disease Control recommends treatment with single-dose IM ceftriaxone 250 mg in combination with 1 g oral azithromycin. The rationale for dual antimicrobial therapy is to address *Chlamydia trachomatis* coinfection, which occurs in 10–40% of patients. Complicated infections should be treated with oral doxycycline 100 mg twice daily for 14 days. In pelvic inflammatory disease, metronidazole 400 mg twice daily for 14 days is also recommended. Ciprofloxacin may also be used provided that the organism is susceptible, as resistance to ciprofloxacin is high.[10]

Course: Uncomplicated urethritis and pharyngeal infection can spontaneously clear within a few months; however, the complication rate may be greater than 20%. Ascending infection in men causes acute prostatitis or epididymis-orchitis, and in women, it can lead to pelvic inflammatory disease, with resultant fertility issues. Local abscess formation, including periurethral, can lead to fistula formation, deformities such as the *saxophone penis* and urethral strictures on resolution. Another complication is the development of antimicrobial resistance, an increasing problem with cephalosporins in many parts of the world.

CHANCROID

Synonym: Soft chancre

Overview: This acute ulcerative condition is caused by the gram-negative bacillus *Haemophilus ducreyi*. It is rare in most developed countries, but it remains an important co-factor in the transmission of HIV.

Clinical presentation: Following a short incubation period between 3–10 days, a painful, soft ulcer forms at the site of inoculation (Figure 27.6). This may start as an inflammatory papule that progresses to form central necrosis and ulceration. Autoinoculation can lead to kissing ulcers. Lesions are more common in uncircumcised men, and perianal lesions can occur in MSM. Inguinal lymphadenitis occurs in more than 30% of patients, is usually unilateral, and can progress to suppurating bubo formation.

Laboratory studies: As *H. ducreyi* is difficult to culture, the mainstay of diagnosis is by polymerase chain reaction (PCR). Direct microscopy that shows a classic *shoal of fish* pattern is no longer recommended due to low sensitivity and specificity.

Differential diagnosis: Other STIs to be ruled out include primary syphilis, herpes progenitalis, granuloma inguinale, and traumatic-induced ulceration.

Management: Single-dose ceftriaxone 250 mg IM or azithromycin 1 g orally is first line, although the latter should be avoided in HIV co-infected patients. Second-line treatment is either oral ciprofloxacin 500 mg BID for 3 days or erythromycin 250 mg TID for 7 days.

Course: HIV transmission is increased with chancroid infection. Other complications include phimosis and chronic ulceration, with genital deformity as a result of secondary infection.

LYMPHOGRANULOMA VENEREUM

Overview: Lymphogranuloma venereum (LGV) is caused by 3 serovars (L1–L3) of the intracellular bacterium *Chlamydia trachomatis*. It is most common in tropical and subtropical countries, but it is an increasing problem in developed countries with MSM, often found with HIV coinfection.

Clinical presentation: There are 3 stages to infection. The primary stage is characterized by small ulcers at the site of inoculation, occurring after an incubation period of 3–12 days. These may painful or asymptomatic and heal spontaneously. They are commonly found in the penile coronal sulcus and posterior vaginal wall or vulva.

The secondary stage occurs 2–6 weeks later and is due to direct lymphatic involvement of regional draining nodes, with tender lymphadenopathy. Abscesses or buboes may form from

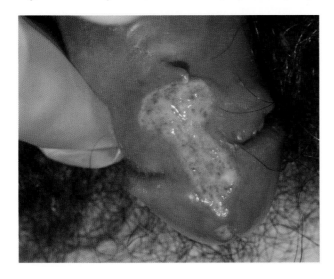

Figure 27.6   Chancroid ulcer.

Source: Courtesy of Andres Fuentes, MD, Santiago, Chile.

coalesced lymph nodes, with systemic features including fever. Proctocolitis can present with rectal discharge, anal pain, constipation, or tenesmus. Rarely, oropharyngeal involvement can occur.

Tertiary stage infection (genito-anorectal syndrome) occurs years after chronic untreated infection, due to a granulomatous process with lymphatic obstruction. It involves subsequent complications including strictures, fistula formation, and genital elephantiasis.

Laboratory studies: Diagnosis is achieved by NAAT from swabs or tissue from active genital, rectal, lymph node, or pharyngeal lesions. Serologic testing is available, but it cannot reliably distinguish current from the previous infection; it can help diagnose late-presenting disease.

Differential diagnosis: During the primary stage with ulceration, the differential is fairly wide, including other STDs, namely, *Herpes simplex* progenitalis, syphilis, and chancroid. Proctocolitis may be misdiagnosed as inflammatory bowel disease.

Management: First-line treatment of all stages of LGV infection is doxycycline 100 mg twice daily for 21 days. Second-line treatment is with a macrolide antibiotic such as azithromycin 1 g orally weekly for 3 weeks or erythromycin 500 mg QDS for 21 days.

Course: Antibiotic treatment is curative and minimizes chronic damage. Complications due to tertiary infection and fibrosis include fistulas, strictures, and genital elephantiasis. Other rare complications to be considered include reactive arthritis and cardiac involvement.[7]

GRANULOMA INGUINALE

Synonym: Donovanosis

Overview: This is a genital ulcerative condition caused by the bacterium *Klebsiella granulomatis*, formerly known as *Calymmatobacterium granulomatis*. It is rare in Western countries, but it can be seen in small endemic foci in some tropical countries.

Clinical presentation: The incubation period can vary between 1 day to 1 year. Four clinical presentations of ulcers at the site of inoculation, are described. The commonest type includes

- Ulcerogranulomatous, presenting with beefy red ulcers;

- Hypertrophic lesions present with a raised irregular edge;

- Necrotic lesions often due to secondary infection; and

- Sclerotic lesions that are cicatricial and fibrotic.

All manifestations are classically painless. Intra-abdominal dissemination has been described.

Laboratory studies: Biopsy allows microscopic identification of intracellular Donovan bodies, with a typical *safety-pin* appearance, and is diagnostic. The organism is difficult to culture. Serologic tests and PCR are not yet available.

Differential diagnosis: Additional diagnoses to consider include such other causes of genital ulceration including primary syphilis, chancroid, LGV, and *Herpes simplex* progenitalis. Other granulomatous diseases or malignancy may also be considered.

Management: This involves prolonged antimicrobial therapy for at least 3 weeks until all lesions have healed. The first-line treatment is with azithromycin 1 g once weekly. Alternative regimens with doxycycline 100 mg twice daily, ciprofloxacin 750 mg twice daily, erythromycin 500 mg four times a day, or co-trimoxazole 160 mg/800 mg can be used.

Course: Persistent granulomas leading to lymphatic constriction can lead to genital scarring.

CONDYLOMATA ACUMINATA

Synonym: Genital warts

Overview: These have become increasingly common over the past 50 years, with the highest incidence in young adults. The causative organism is the human papillomavirus (HPV), usually low-risk subtypes (HPV 6 and 11 most frequently). Other HPV subtypes cause different types of warts (Table 27.1). Genital warts are highly infectious and transmitted by direct skin contact. They are frequently transmitted through sexual contact. Anogenital warts in children can raise concerns over possible sexual abuse; however, transmission can occur through infection from the mother's genital tract at delivery.

Clinical presentation: These are often asymptomatic, with varied clinical appearances, affecting the genitals or groin. They can be flesh-colored, erythematous, or hyperpigmented and can be soft, flat, filiform, or pedunculated lesions, ranging from a few millimeters to several centimeters in size. They are usually multiple and can be symptomatic with discomfort, discharge, or

Table 27.1 Human Papillomavirus (HPV) Types and the Common Clinical Varieties of Warts with which They Are Associated

Clinical Type	The Most Common HPV Subtype Associated
Verruca vulgaris (common warts of hands and fingers)	2, 4
Deep plantar warts (myrmecia warts)	1
Plane warts	3, 10
Mosaic warts	2
Epidermodysplasia verruciformis	5, 8 (although many others have been isolated)
Condyloma acuminatum	6, 11, 16, and 18 on occasion—associated with cervical cancer
Laryngeal papilloma	6, 11

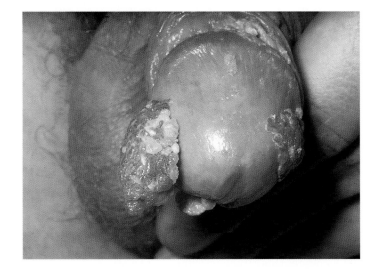

Figure 27.7 Condylomata acuminata on the glans.

bleeding (Figure 27.7). Small black dots representing thrombosed capillaries may be visible. The most common sites in men are the frenulum, corona, and glans, and in women, the posterior fourchette—this is likely due to these areas being sites of most friction. HPV can also enter an asymptomatic latent phase. The usual incubation period in condylomata acuminata is 3 weeks to 8 months.

High-risk HPV subtypes (HPV 16 and 18 in 70–80%) are associated with anogenital and oropharyngeal intraepithelial and invasive neoplasia. Other epidemiologic associations, particularly in cervical premalignant and malignant disease, include the age of first intercourse, number of sexual partners, and history of STDs. In addition to sexual practices, HIV coinfection, particularly with low CD4 counts, can increase the risk of infection with multiple HPV subtypes. The main factors associated with the development of HPV-related anogenital precancers are the presence of high-risk HPV subtypes, the site of infection (mainly cervix and anus), and clinical and molecular persistence of HPV. The transformation zones within anal and cervical epithelia are highly susceptible to HPV-mediated dysplasia. The introduction of HPV vaccination will hopefully lead to a reduction in the incidence of these conditions. High-risk HPV can also be associated with some squamous cell carcinomas or Bowen disease of the fingertip for example.

Laboratory studies: Diagnosis is typically made clinically; however, histologic features with HPV immunostaining can be confirmatory and differentiate from premalignant disease. Histologic features are seen are extreme acanthosis and papillomatosis and koilocytosis. Dermal capillaries are often tortuous and increased in number.

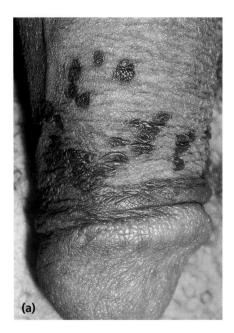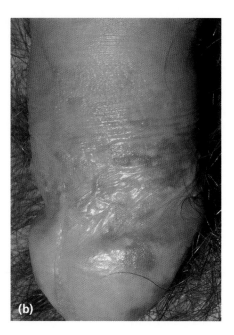

(a)   (b)

Figure 27.8   Bowenoid papulosis: (a) Pigmented lesions; (b) Erythematous lesions.

Differential diagnosis: Other diagnoses to consider are seborrheic keratoses, particularly with pigmented lesions, and intraepithelial neoplasia (Bowenoid papulosis; Figure 27.8). Malignant change should be considered particularly with large protuberant masses induration, pain, or serosanguinous discharge. Other differentials include verrucous carcinoma (Buschke-Lowenstein tumor) that can be misdiagnosed as genital warts. Florid genital warts should raise suspicions of underlying immunodeficiency.

Management: Anogenital warts can spontaneously resolve; however, treatment is recommended, as they can spread or enlarge. The first-line topical treatment of condylomata acuminata is podophyllotoxin or imiquimod, with antiproliferative and immunomodulatory effects, respectively. Podophyllotoxin is applied twice daily for 3 consecutive days, and the course is repeated weekly for 4 weeks. It is contraindicated in pregnancy. Imiquimod is applied 3 times per week until there is clearance, for a maximum of 16 weeks. Second-line treatment includes cryotherapy, surgical removal, laser surgery, or photodynamic therapy.

Course: Latent HPV infection adjacent to warts leads to recurrence of lesions, expected in approximately 25% of cases. The duration can vary from a few weeks to several years. The introduction of HPV vaccination (now built into immunization schedules) will likely lead to a reduction of the incidence of anogenital warts and other HPV-related infections. There are three vaccines currently available; the quadrivalent HPV vaccine (Gardasil), which targets subtypes 6,11,16, and 18; Gardasil 9, which additionally targets HPV 31, 33, 45, 52, 58; and the bivalent vaccine (Cervarix), which targets HPV 16 and 18. Routine vaccination is recommended at age 11–12 years, although is approved up to the age of 45.

HUMAN IMMUNODEFICIENCY

Overview: Human immunodeficiency virus (HIV) is a retrovirus that primarily infects CD4 T cells and was first identified in the 1980s. There are 2 subtypes, HIV-1 and HIV-2, that can be transmitted sexually, from blood or blood products, or vertically from an infected mother. HIV causes variable presentation of disease; dermatologic involvement is recognized in a wide range of dermatoses.

Clinical presentation: Dermatologic manifestations of HIV vary depending on the stage of infection and degree of immunosuppression and are listed in Table 27.2. HIV and its associated immune dysfunction can lead to opportunistic infections, skin cancers, and other more severe variants of common dermatoses that can be treatment-resistant.

Table 27.2 Dermatologic Indicators of HIV Infection

Classic	Pathognomonic (Figure 27.10)	Extended
Seborrheic dermatitis	Eosinophilic folliculitis	Pruritus/xerosis/ichthyosis
Herpes zoster	Oral hairy leukoplakia	Urticaria
Herpes simplex infection	Kaposi's sarcoma	Vasculitis
Psoriasis		Nodular prurigo
		Pruritic papular eruption
		Granuloma annulare
		Drug eruptions
		Viral warts
		Mollusca
		Oral and vaginal candidosis
		Tinea
		Scabies
		Basal cell carcinoma
		Squamous cell carcinoma
		Photosensitivity

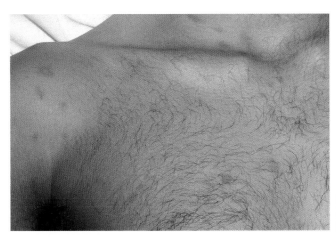

Figure 27.9 HIV Seroconversion Erythematous Maculopapular Eruption.

Primary infection: Acute primary HIV infection can be asymptomatic in 10–60%, with an incubation period of approximately 2–4 weeks; however, a variety of signs and symptoms can be associated with acute infection. The most common systemic features are fever, lymphadenopathy, weight loss, myalgia, or arthralgia; sore throat and headache can also occur. Dermatologically, the most common (occurring in up to 75% of people during seroconversion) manifestation is asymmetrical maculopapular erythematous exanthem (Figure 27.9), with particular involvement of the face, palms, and soles. Occasionally, there may be perifollicular erythematous papular, urticarial, or vesicular lesions, and alopecia. Other dermatologic manifestations of seroconversion are urticaria, toxic erythema, erythema multiforme, oropharyngeal candidosis, acute genito-crural intertrigo, plus oral and genital ulceration.

AIDS-defining conditions: Acquired immunodeficiency syndrome (AIDS) occurs when the CD4 T cell count drops below 200×10^6/L. Certain conditions are indicator conditions or "AIDS-defining." These include invasive deep fungal infections, such as cryptococcosis, bacterial infections, such as *Pneumocystis jiroveci* pneumonia; malignancy, including non-Hodgkin lymphoma and Kaposi sarcoma; and cognitive impairment. There are some cutaneous presentations of AIDS-defining conditions that are important to mention. Kaposi sarcoma (Figure 27.10) can present as single or multiple purple papules, plaques, or nodules. Invasive *Herpes simplex* infection may

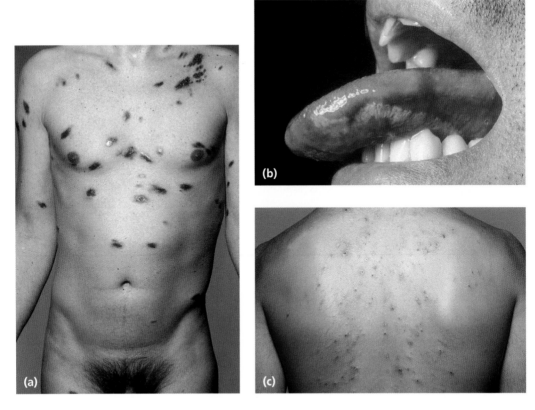

Figure 27.10 Pathognomic signs of HIV: (a) Kaposi sarcoma; (b) oral hairy leukoplakia; (c) eosinophilic folliculitis.

present with mucocutaneous ulceration for more than 1 month (Figure 27.11) and may also lead to pulmonary or esophageal involvement.

HIV and other infections: HIV infection leads to an increased incidence of common bacterial infections—staphylococcal folliculitis, including methicillin-resistant staphylococcal aureus infections being high in prevalence. Coinfection with HIV can impact treatment options in other venereal diseases. The atypical mycobacterial disease is usually secondary to *Mycobacterium avium-intracellulare*, and it can occur at very low CD4 T-cell counts (<50 × 10⁶/L), presenting with disseminated infection.

Viral infections, such as *Herpes simplex*, warts, and molluscum contagiosum, are of increased incidence and severity. Herpes zoster reactivation can be severe in HIV infection, affecting multiple dermatomes. Other viral reactivation diseases, such as cytomegalovirus (CMV), with CD4 counts less than 50 × 10⁶/L, can lead to systemic involvement, with ocular, gastrointestinal, and neurologic complications.

Superficial fungal infections, including candidosis (Figure 27.11) and dermatophyte infection, are common in HIV infection. Disseminated infection tends to occur with low CD4 counts and are indicator conditions in AIDS, for example, candidosis and cryptococcal infection.

Differential diagnosis: One of the most common manifestations in patients with HIV is pruritus; it may be idiopathic or, secondary to xerosis, an underlying dermatosis, such as neurodermatitis or seborrheic dermatitis or as a side effect of antiretroviral (ARV) medications. Systemic causes of pruritus that include hepatic or renal impairment and lymphomas should be excluded.

Seborrheic dermatitis is very common in patients with HIV, occurring in 20–85% of patients, compared with 1–3% of the general population.[3] Psoriasis in patients with HIV can be more severe and atypical; patients benefit from conventional therapy, including phototherapy and biologics.

ARV therapy has reduced the incidence of eosinophilic folliculitis (Figure 27.10), which occurs at CD4 counts of 250–300 × 10⁶/L. It presents as perifollicular pruritic, erythematous papules

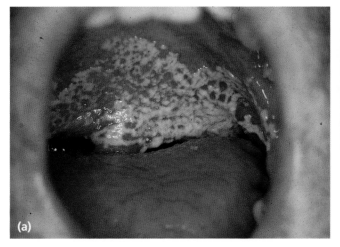
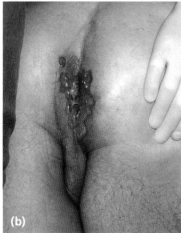

Figure 27.11 (a) Oral candidosis in HIV; (b) chronic herpes simplex virus in HIV.

occurring centripetally. It can mimic bacterial folliculitis, seborrheic folliculitis, or acne vulgaris. Phototherapy is a useful treatment, in addition to potent topical steroids, topical tacrolimus, and oral antibiotics, including macrolides and tetracyclines.

The pruritic papular eruption is another common cutaneous manifestation of HIV, and presents as erythematous, urticarial papules with associated eosinophilia, and tends to occur at CD4 counts below $100-200 \times 10^6/L$.

HIV and neoplasms: HIV patients are found to have a 2-fold increased risk for skin cancer.[3] Kaposi sarcoma, caused by *Human herpesvirus 8* (HHV-8), can be disseminated in the context of HIV or AIDS, with gastrointestinal and pulmonary involvement. Cutaneous lesions can involve the oral mucosa and genitals (Figure 27.10). Localized treatments include cryotherapy, radio-therapy, topical retinoids, or surgical removal, for example, with curettage and electrodesiccation. Systemic chemotherapy is required for advanced stage Kaposi sarcoma. With the introduction of ARV, the incidence of Kaposi sarcoma has declined; however, non-AIDS-defining cancers, of which skin cancer is the most common, are increasing. Actinic keratoses are extremely common, and both basal cell cancer (BCC) and squamous cell cancer (SCC) may present at younger ages and with an atypical appearance. Melanoma may be more common and more dangerous in HIV.

Laboratory studies: HIV diagnosis is now widely achieved through detection of HIV-1/2 anti-bodies, HIV-1 p24 antigen, or viral RNA, in serum, saliva, or urine (Table 27.3). Point of care tests is also available, allowing rapid diagnosis. The CD4 T cell count is also measured on serum and routinely performed at diagnosis. Seroconversion is diagnosed by positive HIV PCR with nega-tive serology tests. Histologic features of acute HIV seroconversion are often nonspecific, showing spongiosis, apoptosis, interface dermatitis, and mild perivascular inflammatory infiltrate.

Table 27.3 Diagnosis of HIV Infection

Essential Assays
- Fourth generation HIV-1/2 immunoassay (includes HIV-1 p24 antigen testing)
- HIV RNA PCR

Supplementary Tests after Inconclusive ELISA Results
- Quantitative RNA PCR
- T-cell subset enumeration
- Exclusion of other viral illnesses, e.g., CMV, EBV

Point-of-Care Tests
- Finger prick or saliva (antibody tests that require subsequent confirmation by ELISA/ western blot)

Abbreviations: HIV, human immunodeficiency virus; PCR, polymerase chain reaction; ELISA, enzyme-linked immunosorbent assay; CMV, cytomegalovirus; EBV, Epstein-Barr virus.

Table 27.4 Differential Diagnoses of Primary HIV Infection

- Toxic erythema (and associated differential diagnosis, drugs, infections, connective tissue disease
- Urticaria (and associated differential diagnosis, drugs, infections, connective tissue disease, neoplasia)
- Erythema multiforme (and associated differential diagnosis)
- Orgenital ulceration (and associated differential diagnosis, drugs, infections, connective tissue disease, immunobullous disease, Bechet syndrome, Stevens-Johnson syndrome)
- Pityriasis rosea
- Guttate psoriasis
- Reactive arthritis
- Still disease
- Infections: EBV CMV, parvovirus B19, HSV, HTLV1/2, Hepatitis A, B, C, gonococcaemia, syphilis, rheumatic fever, toxoplasmosis, causes of meingoencephalitis and pneumonitis
- Drug reactions

Abbreviations: HIV, human immunodeficiency virus; CMV, cytomegalovirus; EBV, Epstein-Barr virus.

Differential diagnosis: Many dermatologic manifestations of primary HIV infection are nonspecific, and so the differential diagnosis can be wide (Table 27.4).

Management: ARV has revolutionized HIV treatment and prognosis, by preserving and restoring immune function, achieving an undetectable viral load, reducing morbidity associated with chronic HIV infection including opportunistic infections, and reducing onward transmission. The drug classes used are protease inhibitors (PI), nucleoside reverse transcriptase inhibitors (NRTIs) and non-nucleoside reverse transcriptase inhibitors (NNRTI), and integrase inhibitors (INI). Combination treatment is initiated, usually with two NRTIs (typically tenofovir and emtricitabine) in addition to a third drug (either NNRTI, INI, or PI).

Many ARV medications have significant dermatologic side effects, including severe drug reactions: Stevens Johnsons syndrome/ Toxic epidermal necrolysis (especially nevirapine), and drug reaction with eosinophilia and systemic symptoms (DRESS).

Subsequent immune restoration following ARV therapy can lead to immune reconstitution-associated diseases (IRADs), also known as immune reconstitution inflammatory syndrome (IRIS). This refers to a worsening of preexisting often opportunistic infection in the setting of improving immunologic function. There is a temporal association between initiation of ARVs and clinical manifestations of an inflammatory condition, in the absence of drug allergy, drug-resistant infection, and bacterial superinfection. Common causes are *Mycobacterium tuberculosis, Mycobacterium avium complex*, cytomegalovirus, *Cryptococcus neoformans, Pneumocystic jirovecii*, and *Herpes simplex* (Figure 27.12). IRADs can be a diagnostic challenge, and over 50% are estimated to have dermatologic presentations.

HIV prevention with increased education on sexual practices, access to health services, and behavioral interventions, have led to reduced transmission in low- and middle-income countries by 30%.[3] ARV treatment can decrease HIV transmission by 96%. The use of preexposure prophylaxis (PrEP) in patients at higher risk of HIV acquisition, in both heterosexual and MSM populations, is now recommended. Combination therapy with oral tenofovir-emtricitabine taken daily or on-demand prior to potential risk, is highly efficacious in preventing HIV infection in MSM; 86% in 2 phase 3 randomized controlled trials.[2]

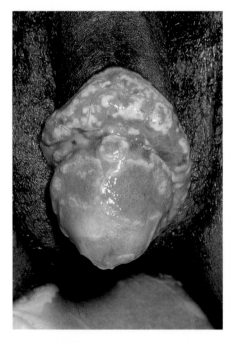

Figure 27.12 IRAD secondary to *Herpes simplex* virus.

Course: HIV is a chronic condition, that no longer carries the same mortality and morbidity once feared with the use of ARV. HIV-infected adults with CD4 > 500×10^6/L continuing on long-term combination treatment have the same mortality rates as the general population. Treatment failure can be attributed to several reasons, including poor compliance and drug adherence. There are second-and third-line treatments in addition to salvage therapy.

There are some factors that influence and can help predict the rate of disease progression to AIDS. These include CD4 T cell count, viral load, later age of onset at infection, and clinical indicators such as symptomatic primary infection, development of oral thrush, oral hairy leukoplakia, herpes zoster, and constitutional symptoms.

FINAL THOUGHT

The management of sexual health in the United Kingdom is primarily carried out by specialists within genitourinary medicine in public health clinics. In the United States, a variety of medical professionals in public health clinics and specialties including dermatology, infectious diseases, urology, obstetrics, and gynecology are involved in the management of STDs.

ADDITIONAL READINGS

BHIVA guidelines—ARV. Available from: www.bhiva.org/file/RVYKzFwyxpgiI/treatment-guidelines-2016-interim-update.pdf

BHIVA guidelines—PreP. Available from: www.bhiva.org/file/5b729cd592060/2018-PrEP-Guidelines.pdf

Bunker CB, Piquet V. HIV, and AIDS. In: Griffiths C, Barker J, Bleiker T, et al., editors. Rook's Textbook of Dermatology. 9th ed. Oxford: Wiley-Blackwell; 2016, Ch. 31, p. 1–37.

CDC guidelines—g inguinale. Available from: www.cdc.gov/std/tg2015/donovanosis.htm

CDC Guidelines—syphilis. Available from: www.cdc.gov/std/tg2015/syphilis.htm#latent

Kinghorn GR, Briggs A, Gupta NK. Other Sexually transmitted bacterial diseases. In: Griffiths C, Barker J, Bleiker T, et al., editors. Rook's Textbook of Dermatology. 9th ed. Oxford: Wiley Blackwell; 2016, Ch. 30, p. 1–27.

Kinghorn GR, Omer R. Syphilis and congenital syphilis. In: Rook's Textbook of Dermatology. 9th ed. Oxford: Wiley-Blackwell; 2016, Ch. 29, p. 1–35.

Meites E, Szilagyi PG, Chesson HW, et al. Human papillomavirus vaccination for adults: updated recommendations of the Advisory Committee on Immunization Practices. Am J Transplantation. 2019;19:3202–3206.

Meys R, Gotch FM, Bunker CB. Human papillomavirus in the era of highly active antiretroviral therapy for human immunodeficiency virus: an immune reconstitution-associated disease? Br J Dermatol. 2010;162:6–11.

Unemo M, Seifert HS, Hook EW, et al. Gonorrhoea. Nat Rev Dis Primers. 2019;5:1–23.

28 Pregnancy and Skin Disease

Tugba Kevser Uzuncakmak, Ozge Askin, and Yalçın Tüzün

CONTENTS

THE PREGNANT STATE

Overview: Pregnancy is a unique time in a woman's life when many hormonal, immunologic, and metabolic physiologic changes occur. Inherent changes in hormones, increased intravascular volume, the pressure exerted by the growing fetus and uterus, and immunologic processes required for fetal development may present with different clinical adjustments. Recognition of these clinical scenarios and awareness of the physiologic modifications can prevent unnecessary treatment and anxiety. They can also facilitate early diagnosis and treatment when necessary.

PHYSIOLOGIC CHANGES DUE TO PREGNANCY

Overview: The most common physiologic skin changes occurring during pregnancy can be grouped under the categories of pigmentary variations, vascular proliferation or congestive anomalies, alterations in nevi, mucosa, hair, and nails, and connective tissue alterations. Although some of these changes may regress completely after pregnancy, others become permanent. Therapeutic interventions are mostly for cosmetic purposes, and unfortunately, many have not been proven to be safe during pregnancy or lactation.

PIGMENTARY CHANGES DURING PREGNANCY

Overview: Pigmentary abnormalities observed in the skin and mucous membranes during pregnancy represent the most common physiologic changes. They are reported to occur in 85–90% of patients, especially in the second half of pregnancy. Although the reasons behind the pigmentary alterations are not clear, hormonal factors, genetic predisposition, and ultraviolet exposure may play a role. Increased α and β melanocyte-stimulating hormones, estrogen, progesterone, and β-endorphin levels can stimulate melanocytes and increase melanin production. Placental lipids, which are rich in bioactive lipids, can also augment melanin synthesis with their tyrosinase-stimulating effects.

Although the increase in pigmentation may be generalized throughout the body, it is frequently seen in physiologically darker areas, such as the nipples, periumbilical region, groin, and intertriginous areas. Acanthosis nigricans may also accompany these pigmentary changes.

Clinical presentation: Linea nigra is the darkening of the line-shaped linea alba that runs through the midline between the lower part of the abdomen and the suprapubic area (Figure 28.1). The hyperpigmented line often extends from the umbilicus to the symphysis pubis. It regresses spontaneously from the sixth month after pregnancy without treatment.

DOI: 10.1201/9781003105268-28

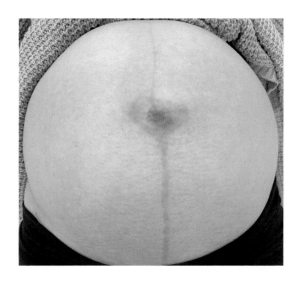

Figure 28.1 Linea nigra: Darkening of the linea alba in the midline between the lower part of the abdomen and the suprapubic area.

Pigmentary demarcation lines, also known as Futcher's (Voight) lines, are infrequent manifestations. These are characterized by lighter and darker pigmented areas with linear extensions, which follow the innervation lines of peripheral nerves. They are often seen on the arms and posterior aspects of the legs.

Chloasma, also known as the mask of pregnancy, is the counterpart of melasma in pregnant women. It is said to be seen in up to 70% of pregnancies, especially in women with darker skin. It often appears as symmetrical, sharply circumscribed brown patches on much of the face, mandibular areas, or centrofacial region, including the chin, nose, upper lip, cheeks, and forehead. This condition, which becomes prominent in the second half of pregnancy, can be found more frequently in patients using oral contraceptives before pregnancy. For the treatment of melasma, which may partially regress spontaneously in the first postpartum year, recommendations include using sunscreens containing mineral filters, avoiding irritant cosmetics, and preventing prolonged exposure to ultraviolet radiation. Treatment regimens can include lasers and applications of topical 4% hydroquinone, often combined with tretinoin and corticosteroids applied in the postpartum period after cessation of breast-feeding.

CHANGES IN NEVI DURING PREGNANCY

Overview: During pregnancy, there can be changes in the color and size of nevi, which are believed to be hormonal fluctuations. In histologic studies, the rate of dermal mitosis in nevi increases during pregnancy, and areas with eosinophilic cytoplasm and large epithelioid melanocytes have been named superficial micronodules of pregnancy. In lesions suspicious for melanoma following clinical, dermatoscopic, and histologic examination, a biopsy should be performed, especially when there is growth, alterations, and ulcerations, regardless of location or the week of gestation. Recent studies, fortunately, suggest that the prognosis for melanoma during pregnancy is no worse than for nonpregnant women.

VASCULAR CHANGES DURING PREGNANCY

Overview: There is an increase in vascular volume during pregnancy which can cause edema and the development of varicose veins, especially in the legs. The effects of hormones can create vascular changes, such as spider angiomas, telangiectasias, pyogenic granulomas, and palmar erythema. Irregularities in the vasomotor system can contribute to flushing, the cold–hot sensation disorder, and cutis marmorata.

Clinical presentation: With the increased vascular pressure during pregnancy, nonpitting edema can be found on the legs, face, and hands. Partial relief can often be achieved with bed rest and lying laterally, leg elevation, and compression stockings. When there is persistent edema in the face and hands, preeclampsia should be considered, and the internist should be immediately consulted.

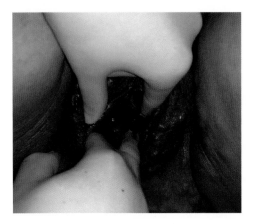

Figure 28.2 Jacquemier's sign: Varicose veins in the vagina and vulva.

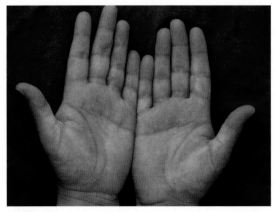

Figure 28.3 Palmar erythema: An erythematous area separated by sharp borders from normal skin in the hypothenar or thenar region.

Increased venous pressure due to compression of the growing uterus on the femoral and pelvic vessels can often contribute to the development of varicose veins in the legs. Varicosities, which occur in approximately 40% of pregnant women, may lead to vascular thrombosis. Symptomatic treatment is indicated, including the use of compression stockings and leg elevation.

Another problem that can develop due to venous congestion is hemorrhoids (Figure 28.2). These venous pouches, which are common during pregnancy, may be associated with constipation, high birth weight, and prolonged delivery, and they can create pain and bleeding. Treatment involves taking sitz baths, applying topical anesthetics, and following a stool softening protocol often with laxatives.

Spider angioma and telangiectasias can develop and increase in number due to the high estrogen levels. These lesions are more common in fair-skinned individuals. Preexisting hemangiomas, subcutaneous hemangioendothelioma, glomangiomas, petechiae, and purpura may worsen with pregnancy. Although routine treatment is not required for such lesions, elective cryotherapy, electrocauterization, and vascular laser treatment are alternatives if only for aesthetic purposes.

Pyogenic granulomas are some of the most common vascular lesions occurring during pregnancy and are known as granuloma gravidarum. These fast-growing lesions are characterized by benign papillary hyperplasia that is red to purple, lobulated, and often pedunculated in appearance. They often develop in the third month of pregnancy and are found in approximately 0.5–5% of pregnant women. They may develop and then regress spontaneously after birth due to the effect of increasing vascular endothelial growth factor and estrogen during pregnancy. When there are pain or bleeding and a large diameter, intralesional steroid application, cryotherapy, electrocauterization, laser treatment, or surgical excision may be recommended.

Palmar erythema is characterized by an erythematous area that is sharply demarcated from normal skin in the hypothenar or thenar region of the palms. Rarely, there can be diffuse involvement. Palmar erythema often begins in the first trimester, only to rapidly regress in the first postpartum week (Figure 28.3). This commonly found redness is attributed to increased estrogen levels.

CHANGES IN THE MUCOSAL SURFACES DURING PREGNANCY

Overview: Bluish discoloration can be observed. The vaginal mucosa may become bluish due to the increased blood flow and vascularity, along with edema occurring within the first 4–8 weeks of pregnancy, known as Chadwick's sign. The cervical softening is called Hegar's sign, while the bluish discoloration is known as the Goodell sign. Another observation, called Jacquemier's sign, is the varicose veins in the vagina and vulva (Figure 28.2). These varicosities occur in about 8–23% of pregnant women, are frequently present before pregnancy, and become more lobulated and deeper in color during pregnancy. Compression of the growing uterus on the pelvic and femoral

Table 28.1 Changes in Mucosal Surfaces during Pregnancy

Mucosal Changes	Clinical Findings
Chadwick's sign	Bluish discoloration observed in vagina mucosa due to increased blood flow, increased vascularity, and edema usually seen within the first 4–8 weeks of pregnancy
Hegar's sign	
Goodell's sign	Softening in the cervix
Jacquemier's sign	Bluish discoloration in the cervix
Hemangiomas	Varicose veins in the vagina and vulva usually seen late terms of pregnancy
Vulvar melanosis	
Hyperemia and edema of the gingiva	Usually develops on the lips and gums in approximately 2% of pregnant women and may cause pain and bleeding
Pyogenic granuloma	

veins can ultimately lead to tension and pain. Other findings include vaginal and vulvar hemangiomas and melanosis (Table 28.1).

Hyperemia and edema of the gingiva, which starts around the second month of pregnancy, leads to gingivitis. Pyogenic granulomas may develop on the lips and gums in approximately 2% of pregnant women. When there is pain, bleeding, and larger lesions, intralesional steroids, cryotherapy, electrocauterization, laser treatment, or even surgical intervention may be recommended.

CHANGES IN SEVERAL GLANDS

Overview: During pregnancy, increased activity is observed in the eccrine sweat glands, which may cause dyshidrosis, hyperhidrosis, and miliaria. A decrease in activity is also seen in the apocrine sweat glands. This can provide relative relief in those women who have hidradenitis suppurativa and Fox-Fordyce lesions. Sebaceous glands can also become more active, as seen with Montgomery tubercles, which are the small papules on the areola that provide lubrication during breastfeeding and are now enlarged. Increased activity in the sebaceous glands may also cause acne flares.

CHANGES IN CONNECTIVE TISSUE DURING PREGNANCY

Overview: During pregnancy, stretch marks, also called striae gravidarum, may occur due to hormonal factors, genetic predisposition, and mechanical stress. Striae occur in 60–90% of pregnant women and represent one of the most common skin findings of pregnancy. Contributing factors include the weakening of the connections between collagen fibers in areas of tension, such as breasts, abdomen, and hips. With the effect of increased corticosteroids, estrogen, and relaxin, the elastic fibers in the reticular dermis may rupture or fracture. Striae rubrae, which are clinically pink to purple, linear bands, develop and can later become ivory-colored, atrophic lesions, known as overtime, but they do not disappear completely. Striae development is known to occur more frequently in young primiparous women with a high body-mass index, plus excessive weight gain during pregnancy, carrying macrosomic babies, and a personal or family history of striae.

Physical tension in the skin and mucous membranes can also cause itching of the scalp, abdomen, anal area, and vulva. Patients with neurofibromas, keloids, leiomyomas, dermatofibromas, and cellulite, may observe growth during pregnancy.

Another finding may be molluscum fibrosum gravida that becomes noticeable during the second trimester. These pedunculated, skin-colored soft lesions with a diameter of 1–5 mm, often seen on the neck, axillae, and inframammary region, my regress postpartum. They are easily eliminated with cryosurgery, electrodesiccation, or snipping.

CHANGES IN HAIR DURING PREGNANCY

Overview: During pregnancy, varying degrees of hirsutism and/or hypertrichosis can be seen. These are characterized by the terminal or vellus-type hair growth on the face, the lower part of the abdomen, chest, legs, arms, back, and buttocks, being more prominent in darker-skinned women. Midline hypertrichosis may appear in the suprapubic region due to the increase in ovarian androgen. These usually regress within 6 months postpartum. Excessive hirsutism may be suggestive of lutein cysts, luteoma, and androgen-secreting tumors.

The effects of hormones can cause hair shaft thickening and prolongation of the anagen phase. With postpartum hormonal changes, hair rapidly transitions from anagen to the telogen phase. This telogen effluvium can be seen in 1–5% of women postpartum.

CHANGES IN NAILS DURING PREGNANCY

Overview: Nail changes occur anywhere from a 2–40% of women. There is increased nail growth, both nail problems can occur. These include leukonychia, onycholysis, ingrown toenails, distal onycholysis, longitudinal melanonychia, transverse furrowing, and subungual hyperkeratosis. Occasionally, there may be a benign, uniform, symmetrical hyperpigmentation observed in the postpartum period. In patients with clinically and dermatoscopically irregular pigmentation, melanoma can be considered, requiring immediate evaluation

GESTATIONAL DERMATOSES

Overview: Gestational dermatoses include a heterogeneous group of pruritic inflammatory diseases that occur during pregnancy and the early postpartum period. There are four dermatoses of pregnancy: Polymorphic eruption of pregnancy (PEP), an atopic eruption of pregnancy (AEP), pemphigoid gestationis (PG), and intrahepatic cholestasis of pregnancy (Table 28.2, Figure 28.4).

POLYMORPHIC ERUPTION OF PREGNANCY

Definition: Pruritic urticarial papules and plaques of pregnancy (PUPPP) and PEP are two synonymous names for this gestational dermatosis that is characterized by a multitude of presentations, which largely consist of nondescript pruritic papules and plaques.

Overview: The incidence of PEP has been estimated at 0.5%, and it is more common in primiparous women. Various studies have also reported that it may occur frequently in multiple pregnancies, male fetus pregnancy, and after cesarean delivery. Although the mechanism of PEP is not clear, maternal immune hyperreactivity, placental or fetal factors, sex hormones, and beta-human chorionic gonadotropin levels have been thought to be contributing factors.

Clinical presentation: Typical lesions are pruritic, urticarial papules, and plaques that begin in the third trimester of pregnancy or the postpartum period. These lesions can occur on the lower part of the abdomen, especially over any striae, and typically, the periumbilical region, face, palmoplantar region, and mucous membranes are not involved (Figure 28.5). Lesions may spread to the rest of the trunk, arms, and legs. Fifty percent of those afflicted will have eczematous, vesicular, or targetoid lesions.

Laboratory studies: The diagnosis is typically made by patient history and clinical findings. Laboratory tests are not needed, and findings from a skin biopsy are generally nonspecific. The histologic examination will reveal edema of the epidermal and upper portion of the dermis, focal spongiosis, and parakeratosis, along with perivascular infiltrates of neutrophils, lymphocytes, mast cells, and eosinophils.

Differential diagnosis: Atopic eruption of pregnancy, intrahepatic cholestasis of pregnancy, and early lesions of herpes gestations should be excluded. Urticaria, atopic or contact dermatitis, and viral exanthema may also be considered in the diagnosis.

Management: Because the diagnosis has no negative effect on the pregnancy or fetus, treatment is largely symptomatic. In mild disease, topical steroids, moisturizers, and antihistamines may be

Table 28.2 Classification and Clinical Findings of Pregnancy Dermatoses

Dermatoses	Onset	Clinical Findings
Polymorphic eruption of pregnancy	Third trimester, postpartum	Urticarial papules and plaques, often starting from striae gravidarum
Atopic eruption of pregnancy	First and second trimester	Eczematous plaques on the face, neck, and extremity
Pemphigoid gestationis	Second and third trimester	Urticaria papules and plaques, vesicles, and blisters
Impetigo herpetiformis	Third trimester	Papules, pustules in flexural areas
Intrahepatic cholestasis of pregnancy	Second and third trimester	Pruritus, excoriations, prurigo nodularis–like papulonodular lesions

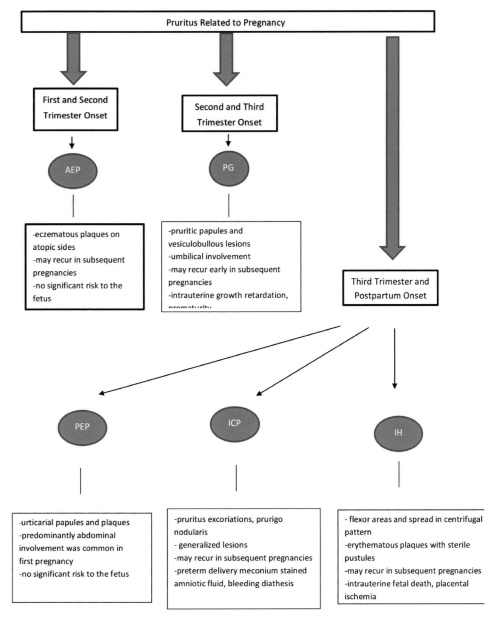

Figure 28.4 Differential diagnosis of pruritus-related to pregnancy (AEP: Atopic eruption of pregnancy, PG: Pemphigoid gestationis, PEP: Polymorphic eruption of pregnancy, ICP: Intrahepatic cholestasis of pregnancy, IH: Impetigo herpetiformis) (see further refs 3,5,9)

helpful. Systemic corticosteroid therapy (20–30 mg/day prednisolone) and phototherapy (narrowband ultraviolet B [UVB]) can be initiated in refractory cases with severe pruritus; however, phototherapy may be more appropriate for generalized lesions.

Prognosis: PEP does not tend to recur in subsequent pregnancies or with hormonal exposures. It also has no negative effects on the pregnancy or fetus.

Final comment: Polymorphic eruption of pregnancy has a typical clinical appearance with erythematous urticarial plaques starting over the striae in the umbilicus usually appearing in the last trimester. It can be controlled with local or systemic steroids, depending on the severity of the disease. There is no prominent maternal or fetal risk during pregnancy and recurrence is not common in subsequent pregnancies or with hormonal exposures.

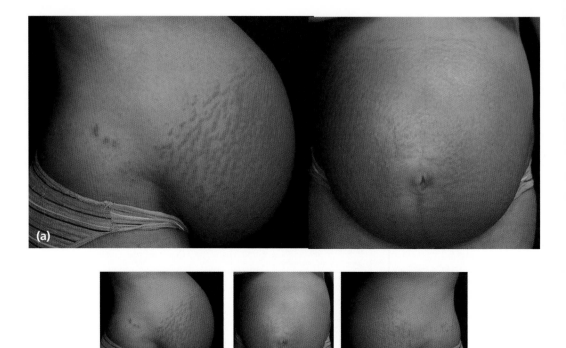

Figure 28.5 (a, b) Polymorphic eruption of pregnancy: Pruritic urticarial papules and plaques on striae, typically affecting the periumbilical region.

Source: Courtesy of the Istanbul Medeniyet University Dermatology Clinic.

ATOPIC ERUPTION OF PREGNANCY

Definition: AEP is also known as prurigo of pregnancy, pruritic folliculitis of pregnancy, and eczema in pregnancy. AEP is characterized by eczematous or papular lesions.

Overview: AEP typically occurs in patients with a history of atopic dermatitis or new-onset atopic dermatitis during pregnancy. AEP is the most common cause of pruritus during pregnancy with an incidence of 5–20%. Although its etiology is not fully elucidated, it is believed that in individuals with a personal or familial history of atopy, suppressed cellular immunity during pregnancy, as well as the dominant Th2 cytokine pathway and humoral immunity, may play a role.

Clinical presentation: AEP is frequently seen in the first or second trimester of pregnancy. Erythematous, pruritic, and scaly lesions can present on the face, eyelids, neck, and flexural surfaces of the arms and legs (Figure 28.6). About one-third of patients may have small papular or prurigo nodularis–like lesions. The lesions typically disappear after pregnancy.

Laboratory studies: The diagnosis is mostly based on clinical characteristics. The histopathology of AEP is nonspecific, and there are no specific laboratory abnormalities, except for an occasional elevation in serum IgE.

Differential diagnosis: Polymorphic eruption of pregnancy, intrahepatic cholestasis of pregnancy, early lesions of herpes gestations, and contact dermatitis should be excluded.

Management: Treatment of AEP is based on the control of pruritus and xerosis. Emollients and topical corticosteroids are first-line therapies. When topical treatment is not sufficient, narrowband UVB therapy can be effective and safe during pregnancy. Systemic corticosteroids can be considered for severe disease.

Prognosis: AEP does not cause any risks to the pregnancy or fetus. It may recur in subsequent pregnancies.

Final comment: Atopic eruption of pregnancy is usually seen in the first or second trimester of pregnancy. Clinically eczematous lesions are commonly located on the flexural surfaces as typically seen in the adult type of atopic dermatitis. Topical corticosteroids are the first-line therapy,

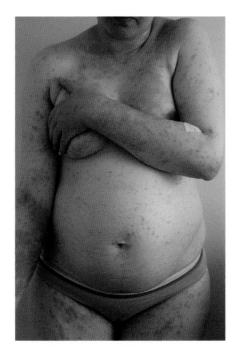

Figure 28.6 Atopic eruption of pregnancy: Erythematous pruritic eczematous lesions suggesting atopic dermatitis.

Source: Courtesy of the Istanbul Medeniyet University Dermatology Clinic.

but in severe or generalized involvement, narrowband UVB therapy, systemic corticosteroids, and even systemic cyclosporine can be considered.

PEMPHIGOID GESTATIONIS

Definition: PG is a rare autoimmune disease associated with pregnancy that can be intensely pruritic. It has also been called herpes gestationis; however, it is not related to any herpes virus infection.

Overview: PG can rarely be seen together with choriocarcinoma, trophoblastic tumors, and mole hydatidiform. Although the pathogenesis of PG is not fully established, it is believed to be a similar entity to bullous pemphigoid. Autoantibodies against (BP)180 (BPAG2), type XVII collagen, and, less frequently, BP230 can be observed.

Clinical presentation: PG typically develops in the second trimester of pregnancy, but it can also occur in the third trimester or even in the postpartum period. The disorder generally recurs with an even earlier onset with each subsequent pregnancy. It is characterized by pruritic papular and vesiculobullous lesions that begin in the periumbilical area and rapidly spread to the trunk, abdomen, arms, and legs (Figure 28.7). Mucosal lesions and facial involvement are rarely seen.

Laboratory studies: Although the patient's history and clinical findings are helpful for diagnosis, direct immunofluorescent (DIF) examination is diagnostic. Linear deposition of IgG (Ig G1 and G3), IgA, and C3 have may be demonstrated by DIF. Histologic findings vary according to the stage of the disease. Results of routine laboratory tests are typically normal but, peripheral eosinophilia can be seen.

Differential diagnosis: Bullous pemphigoid (BP), cicatricial pemphigoid, linear IgA dermatosis, PEP, acute urticaria, erythema multiforme, allergic contact dermatitis, dermatitis herpetiformis, and scabies should be considered in the differential diagnosis.

Management: Spontaneous remission without scarring within weeks to months following delivery is common. The primary goal of treatment is to reduce pruritus. Although topical corticosteroids, emollients, and antihistamines are sufficient for limited disease, systemic steroids may be required in severe cases. PG can typically be controlled with prednisone (20–40 mg daily, but 1–2 mg/kg/d may be required for refractory cases). New blister formation should be stabilized for 2 weeks before trying to taper the dose of prednisone. In conjunction with prednisone, intravenous IgG can be used during pregnancy and the postpartum period for refractory cases. Immunosuppressive agents, such as azathioprine and rituximab, can be used in cases of severe postpartum exacerbation and inadequate suppression with steroids. Lesions may recur during the menstrual cycle and with the use of oral contraceptives.

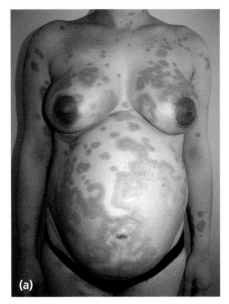

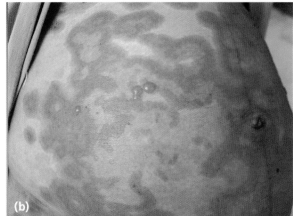

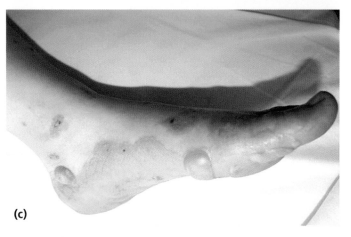

Figure 28.7 Pemphigoid gestationis: Pruritic papular and vesiculobullous lesions on (a, b) the periumbilical area, trunk, abdomen, and (c) extremities.

Source: Courtesy of the Istanbul Medeniyet University Dermatology Clinic.

Prognosis: The prognosis of PG is variable, and it may recur in subsequent pregnancies. If so, it may start earlier and progress more significantly. During the follow-up of pregnant women diagnosed with PG, care should be taken in terms of intrauterine growth retardation, prematurity, and low-birth-weight babies. PG may also be associated with other autoimmune diseases, such as pernicious anemia and Graves' disease, in the following period.

Final comment: Pemphigoid gestationis is a rare autoimmune disease of pregnancy that can be intensely pruritic. It has similar clinical and histopathological findings with bullous pemphigoid. Topical and systemic corticosteroids are the first-line therapeutics according to disease severity. In refractory cases, intravenous Ig in conjunction with prednisone can be used during pregnancy and the postpartum period. Immunosuppressive agents, such as azathioprine and rituximab, can be also used in cases of severe postpartum exacerbation and inadequate suppression with steroids. Lesions may recur during the menstrual cycle and with the use of oral contraceptives.

IMPETIGO HERPETIFORMIS

Definition: Impetigo herpetiformis (IH) is a rare dermatosis of pregnancy that is generally considered to be a form of generalized pustular psoriasis.

Overview: IH typically presents in the third trimester of pregnancy and typically resolves after delivery; however, there is the possibility of recurrence in any subsequent pregnancies.

Although the etiopathogenesis is not clear, it is accepted as pustular psoriasis that develops secondary to hypoparathyroidism, hypocalcemia, and hypoalbuminemia observed during pregnancy in individuals with a genetic predisposition. Patients with PPP often lack a previous or family history of psoriasis. The previous history of psoriasis has been reported in almost one-third of the patients. In addition to this finding, in a study conducted in patients with generalized pustular psoriasis, it was reported that unlike patients with classic psoriasis vulgaris, there was a homozygous or compound heterozygous mutation in the IL-36 receptor antagonist in the IL36RN gene. As part of the IL36 signaling pathway, *IL36RN* is involved in the epithelial barrier and local inflammatory response. Similarly, homozygous or heterozygous mutations in the IL36RN gene were reported in two patients with impetigo herpetiformis, and it was emphasized that impetigo herpetiformis might be associated with generalized pustular psoriasis rather than classical psoriasis. Most of the patients do not have a personal or family history of psoriasis, and the subsequent development of chronic plaque-type psoriasis is not observed.

Clinical presentation: IH is characterized by symmetric erythematous plaques studded with sterile pustules along the border in a circinate pattern. Lesions tend to begin in flexural areas and then spread centrifugally with new pustules at the margins, while older central pustules dry with collarettes of scale or crust. Systemic symptoms, such as nausea, vomiting, fever, chills, diarrhea, hypovolemic shock, and malaise, can be seen.

Laboratory studies: Clinical examination is typically all that is required for diagnosis. Possible laboratory findings in IH include leukocytosis, elevated ESR, hypocalcemia, hypoalbuminemia, and iron deficiency anemia.

Differential diagnosis: Clinical history, morphology, histopathology, and negative immunofluorescence can help to differentiate IH from impetigo, subcorneal pustular dermatosis, dermatitis herpetiformis, and acute generalized exanthematous pustulosis.

Management: If present, fluid and electrolyte imbalances should be corrected, especially hypovolemia and hypocalcemia. Low levels of vitamin D can also be treated. Topical or systemic corticosteroid therapy can be given for improvement, and cyclosporine may be used in severe cases, especially when systemic corticosteroids fail.

Prognosis: Maternal risk factors are typically related to deficiencies in treatment and complications of hypocalcemia. Intrauterine fetal loss may occur as a result of placental ischemia. IH may recur in subsequent pregnancies and can start earlier on.

Final comment: IH is a rare dermatosis of pregnancy that is considered as a form of generalized pustular psoriasis. It is characterized by symmetric erythematous plaques studded with sterile pustules along the border in a circinate pattern. Patients should be examined for hypoparathyroidism, hypocalcemia, hypoalbuminemia, and iron deficiency anemia. Patients should be carefully followed up for fetal and maternal complications and should be warned for recurrence in subsequent pregnancies that may start earlier on.

INTRAHEPATIC CHOLESTASIS OF PREGNANCY

Definition: Intrahepatic cholestasis of pregnancy (ICP), also known as pruritus gravidarum and obstetric cholestasis, is a liver disorder that typically develops in genetically predisposed individuals in the third trimester.

Overview: The prevalence of ICP is estimated to be about 1%. Hormonal changes, genetic predisposition, and exogenous factors play roles in the pathogenesis of ICP. Genetic predisposition has been blamed for the increased incidence in patients with a family history of ICP and monozygous twins. The most studied biliary proteins are ABCB4, ATP8BI, and ABCBII. As a result of the mutations observed in the genes encoding these proteins, the transfer of biliary acids in the canalicular membranes of hepatocytes is impaired, and there is an increase in the levels of bile acids (e.g., cholic acid, chenodeoxycholic acid). While toxic bile acids can cross the placenta to cause severe pruritus in the mother, they can also cause acute placental anoxia and cardiac depression in the fetus.

Clinical presentation: ICP typically presents with sudden-onset severe pruritus without primary skin lesions. In most cases, pruritus starts on the palms and soles but later spreads to the shins, forearms, buttocks, and abdomen. Secondary skin lesions. such as excoriations and prurigo nodules, which can develop due to scratching. Jaundice, due to concomitant extrahepatic cholestasis, occurs in only 10% of patients. The clinical manifestations typically disappear after delivery, but they may persist for weeks in some cases. ICP may occur in subsequent pregnancies or with the use of oral contraceptives.

Laboratory studies: The clinical diagnosis of ICP is based on the presence of severe pruritus and elevated bile acids in the absence of any other signs or symptoms of liver disease. Total bile acids >11.0 µmol/L can confirm the diagnosis. Alkaline phosphatase, aspartate aminotransferase, alanine aminotransferase, gamma-glutamyl transferase, and bilirubin levels may be elevated. Histopathology is nonspecific and immunofluorescence studies are negative in ICP.

Differential diagnosis: With the clinical and laboratory findings, ICP can be differentiated from scabies, an atopic eruption of pregnancy, polymorphic eruption of pregnancy, and early lesions of herpes gestations.

Management: Ursodeoxycholic acid is used to relieve pruritus and to improve fetal prognosis. The dosing varies, but it has been given as 10–20 mg/kg/day or 1–2 g/day, divided into 1–3 doses. UVB phototherapy can be used in refractory cases. Cholestyramine, antihistamines, and oral corticosteroids have been used, but they do not seem to be significantly effective and do not improve the fetal prognosis.

Prognosis: Early diagnosis and treatment are especially important in ICP. Maternal and fetal prognosis varies according to serum bile acid levels. Pregnant women with ICP have an increased risk for preterm delivery, meconium-stained amniotic fluid, and fetal loss during delivery. It has been observed that the frequency of fetal loss increased around or after 38 weeks gestation; therefore, labor induction is recommended before this time point. In severe or prolonged ICP, cholestasis might also cause vitamin K deficiency and coagulopathy in both the patients and their babies.

FINAL THOUGHT

In pregnant women who have severe itching without any lesions on the skin, intrahepatic cholestasis should be considered. Serum bilirubin levels mildly increase, and bile acids have increased significantly in the laboratory. Ursodeoxycholic acid is the main treatment agent for decreasing maternal and fetal risks in pregnant women with intrahepatic cholestasis.

ADDITIONAL READINGS

Ambros-Rudolph CM, Müllegger RR, Vaughan-Jones SA, et al. The specific dermatoses of pregnancy revisited and reclassified: results of a retrospective two-center study on 505 pregnant patients. J Am Acad Dermatol. 2006;54:395–404.

Bechtel MA, Plotner A. Dermatoses of pregnancy. Clin Obstet Gynecol. 2015;58:104–111.

Bieber AK, Martires KJ, Driscoll MS, et al. Nevi and pregnancy. J Am Acad Dermatol. 2016;75:661–666.

Geraghty LN, Pomeranz MK. Physiologic changes and dermatoses of pregnancy. Int J Dermatol. 2011;50:771–782.

Kroumpouzos G. Advances in obstetric dermatology. Clin Dermatol. 2016;34:311–436.

Lehrhoff S, Pomeranz MK. Specific dermatoses of pregnancy and their treatment. Dermatol Ther. 2013;26:274–284.

Motosko CC, Bieber AK, Pomeranz MK, et al. Physiologic changes of pregnancy: a review of the literature. Int J Womens Dermatol. 2017;3:219–224.

Oumeish OY, Parish JL. Pregnancy and the skin. Clin Dermatol. 2005;24:78–141.

Sävervall C, Sand FL, Thomsen SF. Dermatological diseases associated with pregnancy: pemphigoid gestationis, polymorphic eruption of pregnancy, intrahepatic cholestasis of pregnancy, and atopic eruption of pregnancy. Dermatol Res Pract. 2015;2015:979635.

Tyler KH. Physiological skin changes during pregnancy. Clin Obstet Gynecol. 2015;58:119–124.

29 Systemic Diseases and the Skin

Jana Kazandjieva, Razvigor Darlenski, and Nikolai Tsankov

CONTENTS

Overview: Skin changes often mirror a systemic disease. Dermatologists can observe variations in skin color, modification of skin structure, hair alterations, and changes in facial feature. Specific syndromes may be associated with a variety of typical signs.

SKIN MARKERS OF MALIGNANT DISEASES

Overview: Skin markers of malignant diseases may have characteristic skin manifestation, pointing to specific malignant tumors in the internal organs. The recognition of these paraneoplastic syndromes may help in making an earlier diagnosis and even complete elimination of the malignant disease

Acanthosis Nigricans

Definition: Acanthosis nigricans (AN) is the symmetrical asymptomatic areas of hyperpigmented, hyperkeratotic plaques with velvety appearance occurring on the nape, axillae, or groin.

    Overview: The pathophysiology of AN consists of multifactorial stimulation and proliferation of epidermal keratinocytes and dermal fibroblasts.

Table 29.1 Skin Markers of Malignant Diseases

Skin Markers	Short Description	Localization	Associated Malignant Tumors
Acanthosis nigricans	Hyperpigmented, hyperkeratotic plaques with velvety appearance	Skin folds	Bile duct cancer, Breast cancer Endometrial cancer, Gastric malignancy, Hodgkin disease, Liver cancer, Lung cancer, Mycosis fungoides, Ovarian cancer, Pancreatic cancer, Prostate cancer Thyroid cancer
Leser-Trelat sign	Numerous seborrheic keratosis with waxy or velvety texture	Symmetric pattern on the back	Breast cancer Gastric adenocarinoma Lymphoproliferative disorders
Bazex syndrome	Acral psoriasiform changes	Earlobes, helix, nasal tip, fingertips, and the nails Palms and soles Trunk	Squamous cell carcinoma of the upper gastro-intentinal tract
Tripe palms	Rugose thickening of the palms with an accentuation of the dermatoglyphic ridges and sulci	Palms	Gastric malignancy Lung cancer
Necrolytic migratory erythema	Ring-shaped erythema with centrifugal growth and irregular edges	In areas of increased friction and pressure—genital and anal regions, buttocks, groin, and legs	Glucagonoma
Erythema gyratum repens	Wood-grain pattern composed of erythematous concentric bands	Trunk, extremities	Breast cancer Esophagus cancer Lung cancer

Clinical presentation: AN usually occurs in the skin folds. The dark, rough, and thickened skin areas have poorly defined border. Acrochordons are often found in and around the affected areas. AN might also be observed on the nipple areola, oral, nasal, and laryngeal mucosae as well as in the esophagus. Mucosal involvement is suggestive for the malignant form.

It is well established that AN has a significant ethnic predisposition, being rare among Caucasians but more common among Native Americans and African Americans and is especially prevalent among Asians and individuals of mixed ancestry.

The disease is associated with various benign and malignant conditions and accordingly is divided into seven types: **Obesity-associated** AN (considered a marker of insulin resistance), **syndromic** AN (Cushing syndrome, polycystic ovary syndrome, hyperinsulinemia acromegaly, alstrom telangiectasia, Barter syndrome, Beare-Stevenson syndrome, benign encephalopathy, Bloom syndrome, Capozucca syndrome, chondrodystrophy with dwarfism, Costello syndrome, Crouzon syndrome, dermatomyositis, familial pineal body hypertrophy, gigantism, Hashimoto thyroiditis, Hirschowitz syndrome, Lawrence-Moon-Bardet syndrome, Lawrence-Seip syndrome, lipoatrophic diabetes mellitus, lupoid hepatitis, lupus erythematosus, phenylketonuria, pituitary hypogonadism, pseudoacromegaly, Prader-Willi syndrome, pyramidal tract degeneration, Rud syndrome, scleroderma, Stein-Leventhal syndrome, Type A syndrome [HAIR-AN syndrome], Werner syndrome, Wilson syndrome), **benign** AN, **drug-induced** AN (nicotinic acid, insulin, pituitary extract, systemic corticosteroids, diethylstilbestrol), **familial** AN, **malignant** AN, and **mixed-type** AN.

In nearly one-third of the patients with malignant acanthosis nigricans, the skin changes usually occur before any clinical signs of the malignancy. Skin changes develop rapidly and are often escorted by mucous membrane involvement, seborrheic keratoses, acrochordons, and tripe palms. The malignant type is usually due to a gastric malignancy but may result from other malignancies. carcinoma uteri, hepatic carcinoma, carcinoma of the gut, ovaria, and lungs. Tumors creating AN are often very aggressive.

Laboratory studies: Screening for diabetes, insulin resistance, and internal malignancy is required. The histopathology shows hyperkeratosis, hyperpigmentation of the basal cell layer, and papillomatosis, without a dermal inflammatory infiltrate.

Dermatoscopy will demonstrate linear crista cutis and sulcus cutis with scattered black or dark brown dots and globules. Dots or globules vary in size and take the diverse shapes according to their orientation of pigment in the papillary structures.

Differential diagnosis: Diseases to be considered include atopic dermatitis, confluent and reticulated papillomatosis, Addison's disease, hemochromatosis, pellagra, erythrasma, ichthyosis, and pellagra.

Management: Managing the accompanying disease may eliminate AN. Nonparaneoplastic AN may be addressed by appropriate weight reduction and diabetes control.

Bazex Syndrome

Synonym: Acrokeratosis paraneoplastica

Definition: Bazex syndrome (BS) represents an acral psoriasiform eruption associated with internal malignancies, most frequently squamous cell carcinoma of the upper gastrointestinal tract.

Clinical presentation: BS predominantly affects are Caucasian men in their 40s and appears in 3 stages: (1) psoriasiform changes affecting the earlobes and helix, nasal tip, fingertips, and the nails; (2) palms and soles showing psoriasis-like and hyperkeratotic changes; and (3) involvement of the trunk as the tumor progresses. Unlike in psoriasis, the ear helix and nasal tip are affected. Alopecia and onychodystrophy are common and can be early findings.

Laboratory studies: Histopathologic examination will show epidermal spongiosis, vacuolar degeneration and dyskeratotic keratinocytes, while the dermis may contain a lichenoid infiltrate and papillary dermal fibrosis.

Differential diagnosis: Other conditions to be considered are lupus erythematosus, psoriasis, contact dermatitis, or a drug eruption.

Management: Treating the underlying malignancy will reduce or eliminate the cutaneous changes. A reoccurrence of the syndrome may indicate tumor recurrence.

Tripe Palms

Synonym: Acanthosis palmaris; acanthosis nigricans of the palms

Definition: Tripe palms (TP) is a cutaneous paraneoplastic syndrome characterized by a curious rugose thickening of the palms with an accentuation of the normal dermatoglyphic ridges and sulci.

Clinical presentation: In most patients with TP, there is an association with carcinomas of the gastrointestinal tract and lung, the most common malignancy being pulmonary carcinoma (53% of cases). TP often occurs simultaneously with other paraneoplastic syndromes, including AN and the sign of Leser-Trélat. The onset of TP precedes malignancy in more than 40% and follows the presence of malignancy in 19% or concurrent within 1 month of the diagnosis of malignancy in 37% of all patients.

Laboratory studies: Histopathologic findings consists of hyperkeratosis, acanthosis, and papillomatosis. There may be deposition of mucin in the dermis in 20% of the patients.

Differential diagnosis: Other conditions to be considered include pachydermoperiostosis, acromegaly, thyroid acropachy, and keratosis palmaris et plantaris.

Management: With the surgical removal of the underlying tumor, TP should disappear.

Necrolytic Migratory Erythema

Synonym: Erythema necrolytic migrans

Definition: Necrolytic migratory erythema (NME) is usually part of the glucagonoma syndrome, a paraneoplastic syndrome which includes the triad of diabetes mellitus, NME, and weight loss.

Clinical presentation: Initially, there is ring-shaped erythema with centrifugal growth and irregular edges. The skin lesions gradually blister, erode, and crust over. As the central portion of the wound heals, the surrounding erythema may expand outward. The eruption is prominent in areas of increased friction and pressure—the genital and anal regions, the buttocks, groin, and legs. The skin lesions become quite itchy and painful. Trauma can exacerbate the condition or even promote the formation of new lesions, each of which can be complicated by infections with *Staphylococcus aureus* or *Candida albicans*.

Laboratory studies: Histopathologic changes are limited entirely to the epidermis with necrosis of the spinous layer. There may be confluent parakeratosis and irregular acanthosis with loss of the granular layer.

Additional studies should include a complete blood count, glucose tolerance test, liver function tests, serum glucagon levels, amino acids levels, serum insulin, gastrin, and vasoactive intestinal peptide levels. An MRI is required to detect the glucagonoma, an alpha-cell tumor of the pancreatic islets usually located in the tail of the pancreas.

Differential diagnosis: Other diagnoses to consider include acrodermatitis enteropathy, annular lupus erythematosus, a drug reaction, contact dermatitis, erythrokeratoderma, erythema gyratum repens, and erythema elevatum diutinum.

Management: NME usually resolves once the glucagonoma tumor has been surgically removed.

Erythema Gyratum Repens

Definition: Erythema gyratum repens (EGR) demonstrates a specific wood-grain pattern composed of erythematous concentric bands that are mildly scaling.

Clinical presentation: There is rapid migration (up to 1 cm/d) of the bands on the trunk and extremities. EGR tends to spare the face, hands, and feet. The eruption is intensely pruritic. In 80% of patients, there is an association with a variety of malignancies, most notably lung, esophagus, and breast cancers. EGR has a propensity for Caucasians, with a male to female ratio of 2:1.

Laboratory studies: The histologic features of EGR. Investigations should include a malignancy screening (chest x-ray, mammogram, cervical smear, tumor markers, CAT scan of the chest/abdomen/pelvis and, if indicated, endoscopy or colonoscopy)

Differential diagnosis: Disease to be considered are erythema annulare centrifugum, erythema necrolyticum migrans, erythema multiforme, granuloma annulare, and subacute cutaneous lupus erythematosus

Management: EGR usually resolves within 6 weeks once the malignant tumor has been removed.

ENDOCRINE DISEASES AND THE SKIN

Definition: There are several cutaneous findings that are due to or associated with endocrine abnormalities (see Table 29.2).

DERMATOLOGIC MANIFESTATIONS OF THYROID DISEASE

Overview: Skin manifestations of thyroid dysfunction may be classified into 2 main groups: direct action of the thyroid hormone on skin and autoimmune skin disease associated with thyroid dysfunction. *Direct action of thyroid hormone on skin tissues:* Both hypothyroidism and hyperthyroidism are known to have cutaneous manifestations.

Clinical presentation: In hyperthyroidism (Graves's disease), the skin is most commonly warm, sweaty, soft, and velvety. Palmoplantar hyperhidrosis, facial flushing, skin pigmentation and exophthalmos; fine, soft, and thinned scalp hair; thyroid acropachy (distorted and overgrown nails); and onycholysis are also associated with hyperthyroidism. The explanation of hyperpigmentation in hyperthyroid patients is the increased release of pituitary adrenocorticotropic hormone compensating for accelerated cortical degradation. In addition, pruritus is a common presenting complaint. Thyroid dermopathy is almost always associated with ophthalmopathy (Figure 29.1).

In hypothyroidism, the skin is cold, dry, and pale with widespread xerosis, especially on the extensor surfaces. In addition, there may be carotenemia, dry, coarse, brittle hair, diffuse loss of the scalp hair, loss of the outer third of the eyebrows, and thin, striated, brittle, slow growing nails.

Pretibial myxedema or the newer term *thyroid dermopathy* is a classic cutaneous sign of hypothyroidism. It refers to increased glycosaminoglycan deposition in the skin, often with a peau d'orange appearance on the surface due to the prominent hair follicles. The lesions are most commonly found on the pretibial areas, having a waxy appearance and being light to yellowish brown.

Thyroid acropachy is most often occurring in patients with a long history of active hyperthyroidism disease. Thyroid acropachy is a triad consisting of digital clubbing, soft tissue swelling of the hands and feet, and periosteal new bone formation with possible pain in the digits. Thyroid acropachy is an indicator of severity of dermopathy and ophthalmopathy.

Table 29.2 Endocrine Diseases and the Skin

Endocrine Disease		Skin Peculiarity	Skin Appendages
Disorders of the thyroid gland	Hyperthyroidism	Warm, sweaty, soft skin; skin hyperpigmentation;	Fine, soft, and thinned scalp hair; thyroid acropachy, onycholysis palmoplantar hyperhidrosis;
	Hypothyroidism	Cold, dry, pale skin; pretibial myxedema; thyroid acropachy; carotenemia	dry, coarse, brittle hair; loss of the outer third of the eyebrows; thin, striated, slow-growing nails
Disorders of the pancreas. Diabetes mellitus	Diabetic dermopathy	Multiple discretely erythematous, coin-shaped macules located on the pretibial areas	Thinned, fragile and sparse hair on the scalp; corporal vellus hairs are also affected; onychodystrophies and onychomycoses are frequent; sweating is reduced on the lower extremities
	Diabetic acanthosis nigricans	Brown to gray-black, velvety, papillomatous thickening of the skin in the folds; associated skin tags	
	Rubeosis faciei diabeticorum	Erythrosis reaction commonly present on the face	
	Necrobiosis lipoidica	Infiltrated yellow-brown plaques, located on the shins	
Disorders of the adrenal gland	Cushing's syndrome	Violaceous striae, steroid acne, acanthosis nigricans, hyperpigmentation, purpura and easy bruisability	Hypertrichosis, hirsutism, alopecia
	Addison's disease	Skin hyperpigmentation with muddy appearance, most visible on scars; intraoral pigmentation; vitiligo, occurs in 10–20%	Hair hyperpigmentation, longitudinal bands on nails
Disorders of androgen excess	Hirsutism		Excessive male pattern hair in women after puberty;

Laboratory studies: These include thyroid-stimulating hormone (TSH), T_4, T_3, and thyroid antibody tests. The histopathologic findings for pretibial myxedema typically show deposition of mucin (glycosaminoglycans) throughout the dermis and subcutis. In thyroid acropachy plain radiographs show a solid periosteal reaction that tends to be bilateral and generally symmetrical involving the tubular bones of the hands and feet.

Differential diagnosis: The most commonly autoimmune diseases associated with thyroid dysfunction include vitiligo, urticaria, and alopecia areata. There is a strong association of vitiligo with autoimmune thyroid disorders, in particular with Hashimoto thyroiditis and hyperthyroidism with a possible sharing of a subset of susceptibility genes.

Pretibial myxedema may be confused with erythema nodosum, lichen myxedematous, lichen planus hypertrophicus, neurodermatitis, necrobiosis lipoidica diabeticorum, or stasis dermatitis.

Thyroid acropachy may resemble hypertrophic pulmonary osteoarthropathy, pachydermoperiostosis, or voriconazole induced periostitis.

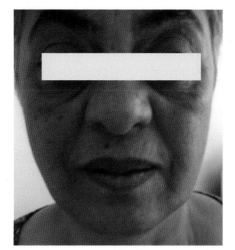

Figure 29.1 54-year-old woman with hyperthyroidism, ophthalmopathy, and periorbital hyperpigmentation.

Management: Initial treatment should be directed to the underlying cause. Pretibial myxedema may be reduced with corticosteroids locally, systemically, or intralesionally, pentoxifylline 400 mg tid may be beneficial.

There is no specific therapy for thyroid acropachy.

DERMATOLOGIC MANIFESTATIONS OF DIABETES

Several dermatoses are routinely associated or influenced by diabetes mellitus (Table 29.3). Skin manifestations, characteristic for diabetes, are often seen in patients with chronic diabetes and occasionally in prediabetics. The prompt recognition of these frequently underestimated entities is extremely important.

Diabetic Dermopathy

Definition: Diabetic dermopathy (pretibial pigmented patches) is the most common dermatologic manifestation found in 9–55% of diabetics.

Overview: The skin lesions are usually associated with the dysregulated vascular regeneration (diabetic microangiopathy) and observed in patients with long-standing disease and poor glycemic control.

Clinical presentation: Diabetic dermopathy presents with multiple discretely erythematous, coin-shaped lesions, which regress after a few years, leaving well-circumscribed atrophic, hyperpigmented macules located most commonly on the pretibial areas. The lesions may be asymptomatic. Generally, the lesions last approximately 18–24 months, but new lesions may develop as the old ones resolve.

Diabetic dermopathy has an unfavorable association with the 3 most common microangiopathic complications of diabetes mellitus: neuropathy, nephropathy, and retinopathy.

Laboratory studies: Skin biopsies from the lesions demonstrate diabetic microangiopathy, epidermal atrophy with flattening of the rete ridges and dermal fibroblastic proliferation.

Differential diagnosis: This includes pretibial myxedema, lichen planus, necrobiosis lipoidica, stasis dermatitis, post inflammatory hyperpigmentation, purpura pigmentosa chronica, and lichen amyloidosus

Management: There is no effective therapy. The condition heals by itself, leaving depressed, atrophic, hyperpigmented scars.

Rubeosis Faciei Diabeticorum

Definition: Rubeosis faciei is a relatively common but often unnoticed complication of diabetes mellitus.

Overview: The prevalence of rubeosis faciei is 7% in patients with type 1 diabetes and 21–59% in patients with type 2 diabetes. There is a chronic flushed appearance on the face, neck, and upper extremities. Telangiectasias may also be visible (Figure 29.2).

Clinical presentation: The vascular changes are caused by diabetic microangiopathy, as well as by dilatation of the superficial veins of the face. The condition can be exacerbated by hypertension. Rubeosis diabeticorum may be associated with other microangiopathic complications, such as retinopathy.

Rubeosis faciei tends to be more easily observed in Fitzpatrick skin types 1 and 2, because the increased melanin in the other Fitzpatrick skin types can obscure the coloration.

Laboratory studies: None.

Differential diagnosis: Other conditions that could be similar include rosacea, systemic lupus erythematosus, and seborrheic dermatitis.

Table 29.3 Dermatologic Manifestations of Diabetes

Noninfectious Manifestations	Infectious Manifestations
• Acanthosis nigricans	• Bacterial infections
• Diabetic dermopathy	• Erysipelas
• Rubeosis faciei	• Cellulitis
• Diabetic foot ulcer	• Folliculitis
• Diabetic bullae	• Diabetic foot infections
• Scleredema diabeticorum	• Necrotizing fasciitis
• Eruptive xanthomas	• Erythrasma
• Granuloma annulare	• Fungal infections
• Necrobiosis lipoidica	• Candidosis
• Perforating dermatosis	• Dermatophyte infections

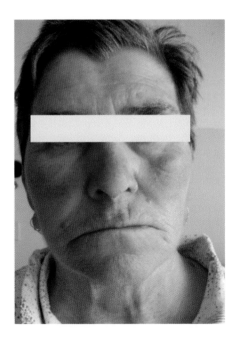

Figure 29.2 Rubeosis faciei diabeticorum in a 72-year-old woman.

Management: With better diabetic control, much of the redness may disappear. If there are residual telangiectasias, light electrodessication, or laser surgery with intense pulsed light sources, Nd: YAG, or pulsed dye lasers may be considered.

Necrobiosis Lipoidica

Definition: Necrobiosis lipoidica (NL) is a granulomatous skin disease characterized by circumferential red-brown bilateral plaques with a firm yellow-brown waxen atrophic center containing telangiectasias.

Clinical presentation: The well-circumscribed infiltrated yellow-brown lesions usually are found on the shins. They tend to expand to several centimeters in diameter. Ulcerations can occur in about one-third of lesions. Additional complications include secondary infections and the development of squamous cell carcinoma. Less than 1% of all diabetic patients have NL. NL can occur in both type 1 and type 2 diabetes, although this association is currently debated. There is no proven relationship between the level of glycemic control and the likelihood of developing this collagen degeneration.

It is three times more common in women than in men.

Laboratory studies: Histologic examination of a cutaneous biopsy will reveal palisading granulomatous inflammation, necrobiotic collagen, and mixed inflammatory infiltrate.

On dermatoscopy, there will be shows arborizing telangiectasias, hairpin vessels, and a yellowish background.

Differential diagnosis: Conditions that may mimic this condition include granuloma annulare, sarcoidosis, and xanthomas.

Management: Topical and intralesional steroids are sometimes helpful, as are calcineurin inhibitors. Pentoxifylline at 400 mg tid or 600 mg bid may be considered.

ADRENAL GLAND DISEASES

Definition: The adrenal gland is made up of the cortex and medulla. The cortex produces steroid hormones including glucocorticoids, mineralocorticoids, and adrenal androgens, and the medulla produces the catecholamines, epinephrine, and norepinephrine.

Overview: The adrenal gland, although small in size, provides a major power to human metabolism. Aldosterone regulates the body sodium content affecting the blood pressure. Cortisol contributes to the regulation of glucose and protein metabolism. Adrenal diseases are generally rare, but diseases like Addison's disease and Cushing's syndrome that affect the normal levels of these hormones can lead to potentially life-threatening consequences.

Cushing's Syndrome

Definition: Cushing's syndrome is a rare condition characterized by increased glucocorticoid levels. Both exogenous and endogenous types of Cushing's syndrome cause a variety of skin conditions.

Overview: Skin manifestations include violaceous striae (Figure 29.3), acne, facial plethora, hypertrichosis, hirsutism, acanthosis nigricans, fungal infections, hyperpigmentation, alopecia, purpura and easy bruisability.

Clinical presentation: Skin striae due to hypercortisolism are often wide and purple, although light-colored striae can persist for years depending on the age of the patients. Acne and hirsutism are attributed to increased adrenal androgen and/or cortisol secretion. Superficial fungal infections are caused by cortisol-induced immune suppression and glucose intolerance. Facial plethora is another characteristic sign probably due to increase perfusion of the face under the influence of excess glucocorticoids.

Management: The best therapy for iatrogenic Cushing's syndrome is slowly tapering the exogenous steroids. Hypercortisolism due to an adrenal tumor or ectopic tumor is best treated with surgical resection.

Addison's Disease

Definition: This is a traditional term for primary adrenal insufficiency. It results from bilateral adrenal cortex destruction leading to decreased production of adrenocortical hormones.

Overview: The presentation of adrenal insufficiency depends on the rate and extent of adrenal function involvement.

Clinical presentation: Hyperpigmentation is considered a hallmark for Addison's disease, which is related to ACTH melanogenesis. The pigmentary changes create a very characteristic "muddy" appearance and are present in about 95% of the patients (Figure 29.4).

Intraoral pigmentation is considered the initial sign and develops earlier than the dermatologic pigmentation. Skin hyperpigmentation is most visible on scars (Figure 29.5), skin folds, pressure points, and lips. It is generally more prominent on sun-exposed skin. Vitiligo may also be seen in association with hyperpigmentation in idiopathic Addison's disease, due to autoimmune destruction of the melanocytes.

Laboratory studies: Blood levels of sodium, potassium, cortisol, and adrenocorticotropic hormone should be measured. ACTH stimulation test and CT scan are necessary for diagnosis establishment.

Differential diagnosis: Hyperpigmentation may be due to a variety of conditions including: melasma, hemochromatosis, post inflammatory hyperpigmentation, metallic deposition of, porphyria cutanea tarda, or drug induced hyperpigmentation.

Management: Patients with Addison's disease should be treated with mineralocorticoid and glucocorticoid replacement therapy for life. The treatment goal is to reduce the drive for excess production of adrenocorticotropic hormone and melanocyte-stimulating hormone.

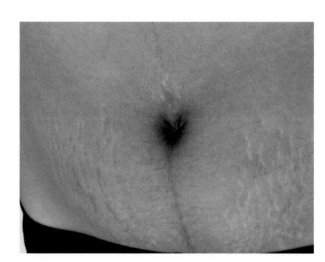

Figure 29.3 Striae cutis distensae as a dermatologic manifestations of Addison's disease.

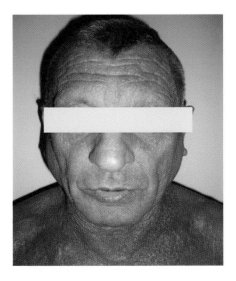

Figure 29.4 63-year-old patient diagnosed with Addison's disease 3 years prior. He developed gradual skin hyperpigmentation, severe pruritus, chronic fatigue, and weakness.

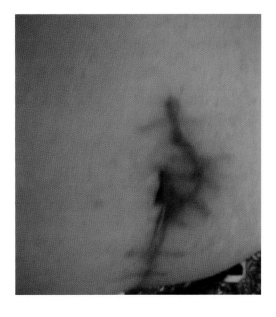

Figure 29.5 Skin hyperpigmentation is most visible on scars.

Androgenization

Synonym: Virilization

Definition: Hirsutism and hypertrichosis are two distinct conditions. Hirsutism is defined as the presence of excessive male pattern hair in women after puberty (Figures 29.6 and 29.7). Hypertrichosis is defined as an excessive growth in body hair beyond the normal variation compared with individuals of the same age, race, and sex.

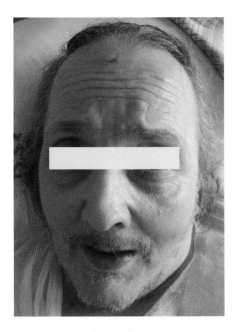

Figure 29.6 Hirsutism—excessive male pattern hair in a woman.

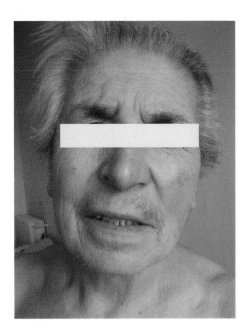

Figure 29.7 Hirsutism—excessive male pattern hair distribution in a woman.

361

Table 29.4 Causes of Hirsutism

Causes	Specific Features
Androgen-producing tumors	Androgen secreting tumors of the ovaries or adrenal glands (most common virilizing ovarian tumors are Sertoli Leydig cell tumors)
Congenital adrenal hyperplasia	Most frequent caused by 21-hydroxylase deficiency
Hyperandrogenic-insulin resistant-acanthosis nigricans syndrome	Characterized by hyperandrogenism, insulin resistance, and acanthosis nigricans
Hyperprolactinemia	Increased levels of adrenal dihydroepiandrosterone sulfate
Polycystic ovarian syndrome	Irregular or prolonged menstrual cycles; elevated levels of male hormones; polycystic ovaries
Idiopathic hirsutism	Normal androgen levels and ovarian function

Overview: Increased androgen levels in women may be due to Cushing's disease, androgen-producing tumors, congenital adrenal hyperplasia, most commonly caused by 21-hydroxylase deficiency, hyperandrogenic-insulin resistant-acanthosis nigricans syndrome (HAIRAN), hyperprolactinemia due to increasing adrenal dihydroepiandrosterone sulfate production, polycystic ovarian syndrome (Stein-Leventhal syndrome; PCOS), or an ovarian tumor. Idiopathic hirsutism with normal androgen levels and ovarian function may be probably to disorders in peripheral androgen activity, while androgenic drugs such as anabolic steroids may be the cause.

Clinical presentation: While the condition would not be recognizable in men, women so afflicted may develop male pattern baldness, excessive facial hair particularly above the upper lip, and increased body hair.

Laboratory studies: Laboratory testing should be based on the patient's history and physical findings, but screening for levels of serum testosterone and 17α-hydroxyprogesterone are indicated.

Differential diagnosis: These include androgen-secreting adrenal tumors, exogenous androgens, including illicit or herbal forms of androgens, 21-hydroxylase deficiency, 11-β hydroxylase deficiency, 3 beta-hydroxysteroid dehydrogenase deficiency, and drug-induced hypertrichosis due to cyclosporine, benoxaprofen, acetazolamide, oral contraceptives, corticosteroids, danazol, streptomycin, phenytoin, methoxypsoralen, penicillamine, interferon-alpha, and epidermal growth factor receptor inhibitors.

Management: It takes up to 6 months before a significant difference in hair growth is noticed. Drugs such as oral contraceptives, androgen receptor blockers, 5-alpha reductase inhibitors, and systemic glucocorticoids are indicated for treatment when hyperandrogenism is confirmed by various laboratory tests. Antiandrogens are indicated for moderate to severe hirsutism, with spironolactone being the first-line antiandrogen and finasteride and cyproterone acetate being second-line antiandrogens. Due to its risk for hepatotoxicity, flutamide is not considered a first-line therapy. Gonadotropin-releasing hormone analogs and glucocorticoids are only recommended in specific circumstances.

Local intervention may include laser epilation, electrolysis, shaving, bleaching, and waxing. Eflornithine cream may reduce the facial hair up to 50%, but it is not popular due to its price. The patient should be advised that contrary to hearsay, there is no way of making the hair grow more or less.

GASTROINTESTINAL DISEASES AND THE SKIN

Definition: The skin and the gastrointestinal tract possess many common features—specific microbiota, rich vasculature, and important barrier functions. Practically, the skin and the gastrointestinal tract are the two main barrier between outside agents and the human organism.

Overview: Skin diseases linked to the gastrointestinal tract may be divided into four groups:

1. Genodermatoses and gastrointestinal diseases

2. Skin diseases closely related to specific changes in the gastrointestinal tract

3. Skin changes characteristic for some gastrointestinal diseases

4. Skin diseases due to the changes in gastrointestinal microbiota

GENODERMATOSES AND GASTROINTESTINAL DISEASES

Table 29.5 Genodermatoses Closely Related to Gastrointestinal Diseases

Diagnosis	Common Features
Focal palmoplantar keratoderma	Focal hyperkeratotic changes on the palms and soles and esophageal cancer
Blue rubber bleb nevus syndrome	Multifocal venous malformation of the skin, gastrointestinal tract, and soft tissues
Gardner syndrome	Intestinal polyposis, desmoids, osteomas, epidermoid cysts
Peutz-Jeghers syndrome	Polyps throughout the gastrointestinal tract and mucocutaneous pigmentation
Acrodermatitis enteropathica	Periorificial dermatitis, alopecia, and diarrhea
Osler-Weber-Rendu disease	Multiple mucocutaneous telangiectasias, epistaxis, visceral telangiectasias

Focal Palmoplantar Keratoderma

Synonyms: Howel-Evans syndrome, tylosis

Definition: This represents the combination of focal hyperkeratotic palmar and plantar changes and an esophageal malignancy.

Overview: This syndrome, resulting from an autosomal dominant inheritance (genes TOC; *RHBDF2*) represents thickening of the palms and soles.

Clinical presentation: The keratoderma may begin in childhood (5–10 years) and involve only small areas of pressure points of the palms and soles (focal keratoderma). As the patient matures, esophageal malignancy develops with patients older than 65 having esophageal carcinoma, often with buccal leukokeratosis.

The diagnosis is made on the basis of a positive family history, characteristic clinical features, including focal palmar and plantar hyperkeratosis plus esophageal lesions, and mutations in *RHBDF2* located on 17q25.

Laboratory studies: The histologic findings from a skin biopsy include acanthosis, hyperkeratosis, and hypergranulosis without parakeratosis or spongiosis. The diagnosis of the associated esophageal malignancy is made by performing an esophagogastroscopy and biopsy.

Differential diagnosis: Other syndromic palmoplantar keratodermas (PPK)—PPK with deafness, PPK with cardiac involvement and woolly hair, PPK with erythroderma and hyper-IgE (SAM syndrome), PPK with periodontitis (Papillon-Lefèvre syndrome and Haim-Munk syndrome), Richner-Hanhart syndrome, punctate PPK with calcinosis cutis (Cole disease), striate PPK with woolly hair, and PPK with pigment anomalies and cutaneous carcinoma.

Management: Early detection and treatment of the esophageal malignancy is necessary. Application of emollients, particularly ones with urea, are helpful. Podiatric care and specialized shoes are often required. More specific treatment for the thick skin is available in the form of oral retinoids such as etretinate and acitretin. These treatments can be effective in causing the thick skin to regress but unfortunately side effects are common.

Blue Rubber-Bleb Nevus Syndrome

Definition: The multifocal venous malformation of the skin, gastrointestinal tract, and soft tissues was originally described by William Bennett Bean (1909–1989).

Overview: The syndrome, with autosomal dominant inheritance, consists of numerous blue to purple nodules of varying size (Figure 29.8).

Clinical presentation: The "blue rubber-bleb nevi" may be located in the oral and anal mucosa. Gastrointestinal lesions develop later in live, but they are more clinically relevant, due to gastrointestinal bleeding. Patients require lifelong treatment with iron and blood transfusions.

Laboratory studies: Histopathologic examination reveals a large blood filled, ectatic vessels, lined by a single layer of endothelium and surrounding thin connective tissue.

Differential diagnosis: Other diseases to be considered include Kaposi sarcoma, hemangiomas, familial glomangiomatosis, and mucosal venous malformation syndrome.

Management: Treatment of blue rubber-bleb nevus syndrome is largely symptomatic. The most important step is monitoring the evolution of gastrointestinal lesions and preventing severe bleeding. Various treatment options are sclerotherapy, laser surgery, and surgical excision. Sirolimus

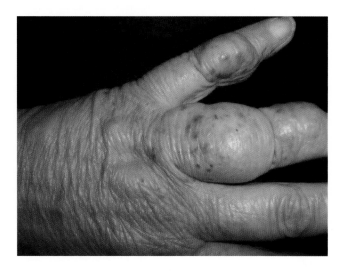

Figure 29.8 Blue rubber-bleb nevus syndrome.

and the second generation of c-kit-specific inhibitors may prove to be helpful; however, the doses and treatment duration remain uncertain.

Gardner Syndrome

Definition: This syndrome, described by John Elton Gardner (1909–1987), includes multiple polyps in the colon accompanied by desmoids, osteomas, and epidermoid cysts.

Overview: A genetic connection to the development of Gardner syndrome has been shown within band 5q21, which is associated with the adenomatous polyposis coli gene.

Clinical findings: The development of intestinal polyposis and colorectal adenocarcinoma are key features of Gardner syndrome. Osteomas, cutaneous cysts, atypical skin pigmentation, and abnormal dental findings or radiographic lesions can precede by many years the development of intestinal polyposis.

Laboratory studies: Genetic testing is the most efficient mode of identifying gene carriers. Biopsies of abnormal plaques of tissue or random biopsies of duodenal mucosa are indicated to rule out any malignancy.

Differential diagnosis: These include other variants of familial adenomatous polyposis, such as Turcot syndrome (colorectal cancer with primary brain tumors), and attenuated forms of familial polyposis.

Management: Treatment should focus on the internal problems and include proctocolectomy or a permanent terminal ileostomy, if there are more than 20 polyps are present. The cutaneous cysts are treated as any other cyst with various types of surgical intervention. Osteomas may require resection if they interfere with function.

Peutz-Jeghers Syndrome

Definition: This autosomal dominant condition includes gastrointestinal polyposis, mucocutaneous pigmentation, and a predisposition to malignancies. It was described by John Law Peutz (1886–1957) and Harold Jeghers (1904–1990)

Overview: Peutz-Jeghers syndrome is due to germ-line mutations in the *STK11* (*LKB1*) on chromosome 19p13.3.

Clinical presentation: Mucocutaneous pigmented lesions are seen in about 95% of patients who develop in childhood dark blue to dark brown macules around the mouth, eyes, and nose, as well as in the perianal area and on the buccal mucosa. Some of these macules may fade in puberty and adulthood.

Women with Peutz-Jeghers syndrome are also at risk for developing ovarian sex cord tumors with annular tubules and mucinous tumors of the ovaries and fallopian tubes. Men with Peutz-Jeghers syndrome are at risk for developing Sertoli cell tumors of the testes.

Laboratory studies: The histopathology of the pigmented macules will reveal increased melanin in the basal cells. On dermatoscopy, melanin deposits will appear in a parallel ridge pattern.

Differential diagnosis: Other syndromes to be considered are Bannayan-Riley Ruvalcaba syndrome (childhood onset, cutaneous lipomas, macrocephaly, intestinal polyps, developmental delay), Laugier-Hunziker syndrome (hereditary pigmentary disorder characterized by a unique expression of pigmentation over the mucosal, nail, and acral sites), and Cowden Syndrome (multiple hamartoma syndrome with mucocutaneous lesions and macrocephaly, associated with an increased risk of breast, thyroid, and endometrial cancers).

Management: Genetic counseling is recommended, followed by prevention of the manifestations, and treatment of complications. It is imperative to evaluate the small intestine with upper endoscopy in addition to colonoscopy beginning at early adolescence, magnetic resonance cholangiopancreatography, and/or endoscopic ultrasound beginning at 25–30 years old, 6-month clinical breast examination beginning at age 25, annual testicular examination, and yearly ultrasound beginning at age 10. Endoscopic treatment of the polyps is the main therapy, but endoscopy combined with laparoscopy or surgical treatment should be performed when complications occurred or the polyps are too large.

Acrodermatitis Enteropathica

Definition: Acrodermatitis enteropathica represents dermatitis due to an inherited form of zinc deficiency, resulting from a defect in zinc absorption and due to mutations in the zinc transporter gene *SLC39A4*.

Overview: The classic clinical triad of periorificial dermatitis, alopecia, and diarrhea is complete in only 20% of patients with acrodermatitis enteropathica.

Clinical presentation: The clinical picture includes sharply demarcated, dry, scaly erythematous plaques that are found around the mouth or in the anogenital are. There may be diffuse alopecia, loss of eyelashes and eyebrows, glossitis, gingivitis, angular stomatitis, and onychodystrophy. The severity of the skin lesions is variable. Diarrhea is the predominant extracutaneous symptom followed by irritability and growth retardation.

Laboratory studies: Serum, urine, and hair examination will reveal markedly lowered zinc levels. The levels of alkaline phosphatase can also be depleted. Genetic tests are precise, but not routinely available. An important diagnostic test is the rapid clinical response to zinc supplementation. Histopathologic study is nonspecific and is generally indistinguishable from those of other forms of vitamin deficiency dermatitis.

Differential diagnosis: Other conditions that might be considered include psoriasis, atopic dermatitis, seborrheic dermatitis, contact dermatitis, mucocutaneous candidosis, Langerhans cell histiocytosis, maple syrup disease, and cystic fibrosis.

Management: Oral lifelong zinc supplementation given daily, which leads to dramatic disappearance of the symptoms within a few days. The recommendation is of one dose between 1–3 mg/kg/day of elemental zinc. Zinc sulfate is preferred and most tolerated oral formulation—4 mg of zinc sulfate contains about 1 mg of elemental zinc. Zinc chloride is preferred for parenteral supplementation.

Osler-Weber-Rendu Disease

Synonym: Hereditary hemorrhagic telangiectasia (HHT)

Definition: This is an autosomal dominant disorder characterized by multiple mucocutaneous telangiectasias.

Overview: Patients typically present with nose bleeds, gastrointestinal bleeds, and iron deficiency anemia.

Clinical presentation: There are two main types of HHT: HHT1, characterized by a mutation in endoglin, and HHT2, with a mutation in activin A receptor-like type 1. Women with HHT1 are at a higher risk of developing pulmonary and cerebral arterial venous malformations (AVMs). Patients with HHT2 have a higher risk of developing liver AVMs. The diagnosis is made by the presence of epistaxis, mucocutaneous telangiectasias, visceral lesions, and an autosomal dominant inheritance.

Laboratory studies: The histopathology of the telangiectasias is characterized by dilated capillaries lined with flat endothelial cells. AVMs are seen with an admixture of thick and thin-walled vessels in the dermis.

Differential diagnosis: Diseases to be considered include: CREST syndrome (calcinosis, Raynaud's phenomenon, esophageal dysmotility, sclerodactyly, and telangiectasia), spider angiomas (also known as spider nevus or spider telangiectasia), ataxia-telangiectasia (cerebellar atrophy with progressive ataxia, cutaneous telangiectasias, higher incidence of lymphoid malignancy, radiosensitivity, immune deficiency, recurrent sinopulmonary infections, and high levels of alpha-fetoprotein in serum), Bloom syndrome (growth deficiency, unusual facies, sun-sensitive telangiectatic erythema, immunodeficiency, predisposition to cancer), and Rothmund syndrome (poikiloderma associated with short stature; sparse hair, eyelashes, and/or eyebrows; juvenile cataracts; skeletal and dental abnormalities; radial ray defects; premature aging; increased risk for cancer, especially osteosarcoma).

Management: Transcatheter embolotherapy is recommended for all adults and symptomatic children with pulmonary AVMs. Gastrointestinal AVMs can be managed by endoscopic cauterization.

SKIN DISEASES CLOSELY RELATED TO SPECIFIC CHANGES IN THE GASTROINTESTINAL TRACT

Papulosis Atrophicans Maligna

Synonym: Degos's disease, Lethal cutaneous and gastrointestinal arteriolar thrombosis, Fatal cutaneointestinal syndrome

Definition: This represents a rare, chronic, thrombo-obliterative vasculopathy of unknown cause.

Overview: It affects the skin, gastrointestinal tract, and central nervous system. The disease usually affects young men, with an age of onset between 20–40 years. There are two types: benign variant (involving only the skin for many years) and malignant variant (with multivisceral involvement being life-threatening).

Clinical presentation: The skin changes are disseminated on the trunk and arms and are characterized by rose colored papules with a diameter of 2–5 mm. These asymptomatic papules have a central porcelain-white atrophy with a surrounding telangiectatic rim. There is involvement of the gastrointestinal tract and other organs in at least 50–60% of the patients. Most often the small bowel is affected with characteristic micro perforation due to vascular changes. Occlusion of cerebral blood vessels can lead to strokes, headaches, epilepsy, or nonspecific neurologic findings.

Laboratory studies: The histologic findings of a skin biopsy include wedge-shaped connective tissue necrosis, due to thrombotic occlusion of the small vessels deep in the dermis. Additional examinations may include an MRI of the brain, chest x-ray, gastroscopy, colonoscopy, or abdominal ultrasound to assess the long-term prognosis.

Differential diagnosis: Other diseases to be considered include systemic lupus erythematosus, lichen sclerosus, antiphospholipid antibody syndrome, and atrophie blanche.

Management: An early diagnosis is very important to stem the dissemination of the disease. Drugs like aspirin and dipyridamole may reduce the number of new lesions in some patients. Anticoagulants such as heparin or fibrinolytic agents achieved a partial regression of the skin lesions in single cases; therefore, these agents can be used only as a first therapeutic approach on a newly diagnosed patients. Subcutaneous treprostinil (vasodilator, synthetic analog of prostacyclin) has been tested successfully in one case with intestinal and central nervous system manifestations.

Pyoderma Gangrenosum

Definition: This is an inflammatory cutaneous disease in the spectrum of the neutrophilic dermatoses.

Overview: There are ulcerations that commonly occur on the legs. Contrary to the name, it is not a bacterial infection. Inflammatory bowel disease is present in up to 30% of all patients.

Clinical presentation: Pyoderma gangrenosum occurs most commonly on the pretibial region. Several clinical subtypes have been described: classic, bullous, superficial granulomatous, pustular, peristomal, and malignant. The classic. presentation begins as a small follicular pustule with rapid growth. After several days, a deep painful ulcer with raised and violaceous borders appears (Figure 29.9).

The surrounding skin is erythematous and indurated. The ulcers heal with characteristic cribriform or "cigarette paper–like" scars. The transition from elevated to more flat borders with string-like growths of epithelium between them is denoted as "Gulliver's sign" (Figure 29.10).

Many of the lesions are precipitated by minor trauma or previous surgical manipulation. This phenomenon is known as *pathergy* to indicate pathologic hyper-reactivity to *normal* stimuli.

Laboratory studies: The histopathology is not specific. Early lesions may reveal deep folliculitis with neutrophilic infiltration and purulent material.

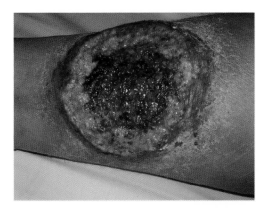

Figure 29.9 Pyoderma gangrenosum.

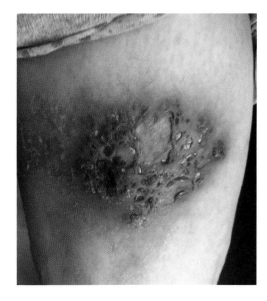

Figure 29.10 "Gulliver's sign" in pyoderma gangrenosum.

Table 29.6 Skin Changes Characteristic for Some Gastrointestinal Diseases

Diagnosis	Etiology	Clinical Presentation
Histamine intolerance	Impaired ability to metabolize ingested histamine	Urticaria, diarrhea, headache, rhino conjunctival symptoms, asthma, hypotension, arrhythmia, pruritus, flushing
Erythema necrolyticum migrans	In most cases associated with glucagonoma	Ring-shaped erythema with centrifugal growth and irregular edges
Carcinoid syndrome	Release of serotonin and other substances from well-differentiated neuroendocrine tumors	Flushing, tachycardia, and diarrhea
Skin changes in liver cirrhosis	Hepatic cirrhosis	Telangiectasia, palmar erythema, pink distal nail plate, leukonychia
Hemochromatosis	Inherited autosomal recessive disease	Cirrhosis, diabetes mellitus, skin hyperpigmentation, cardiac failure

Differential diagnosis: A wide variety of diseases may give similar presentations. These include antiphospholipid antibody syndrome, anthrax, arterial insufficiency, Sweet syndrome, traumatic ulceration tubercular or syphilitic gumma atypical mycobacterial infections, or verrucous carcinoma.

Management: Appropriate wound care is required. Surgical debridement can aggravate the condition. An occlusive dressing with antimicrobial coverage when required can be helpful. Pentoxifylline at 400 mg TID may be useful.

Hereditary Hemochromatosis

Definition: This is an inherited disease, caused by mutations in the hemochromatosis gene (HFE) protein.

Overview: Excess iron is usually metabolized and excreted from the body, but in hemochromatosis, excess iron is deposited in the liver, pancreas, heart, endocrine glands, and joints. The classic tetrad consists of cirrhosis, diabetes mellitus, skin hyperpigmentation, and cardiac failure.

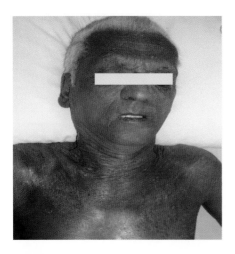

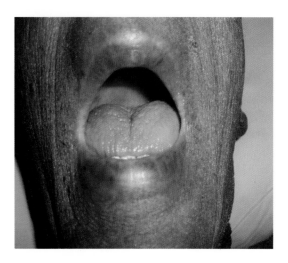

Figure 29.11a 68-year-old Caucasian man—since age of 25 years he has gradually developed skin darkening, diabetes mellitus, and hepatomegaly.

Figure 29.11b Skin darkening on the lips of the same patients.

Clinical presentation: The hyperpigmentation usually develops in patients at least 40 years or older. The skin hyperpigmentation is one of the earliest signs and is seen in more than 90% of patients (Figure 29.11a).

The color varies from brownish bronze to slate gray and is caused by hemosiderin deposition (Figure 29.11b).

The different types of hereditary hemochromatosis include Type 1, classic autosomal recessive form HFE-related; Type 2a (mutations of hemojuvelin gene) and Type 2b (mutations of the hepcidin gene), autosomal recessive disease with age of onset—15–20 years; Type 3 (mutations of transferrin receptor-2 gene), autosomal recessive disease with age of onset—30–40 years; and Type 4 (mutations of the ferroprotein gene), autosomal dominant disorder with age of onset—10–80 years.

Laboratory studies: The disease can be found in its preclinical stage by routine measurement of serum transferrin saturation or serum ferritin concentration. Genetic testing for the characteristic mutations will confirm the diagnosis in more than 90% of patients. Liver enzymes and fasting blood glucose will be elevated. Additional tests include MRI of the liver for iron content, echocardiogram for cardiomyopathy, chest radiograph for cardiomegaly, hormone levels to evaluate hypogonadism, and bone densitometry to check for osteoporosis.

Differential diagnosis: Other disease to be considered are porphyria cutanea tarda, iron overload from chronic transfusions, nonalcoholic fatty liver disease, excessive iron supplementation, and Laennec's cirrhosis.

Management: Phlebotomy is usually performed once or twice weekly to obtain a ferritin level of less than 50 mcg/L. Although chelation is not the most effective treatment method, deferoxamine, deferiprone, and deferasirox are used for some patients.

SKIN DISEASES DUE TO THE CHANGES IN GASTROINTESTINAL MICROBIOTA

Bowel-Associated Dermatosis-Arthritis Syndrome

Synonyms: BADAS, bowel bypass syndrome

Definition: Bowel-associated dermatosis-arthritis syndrome (BADAS) is a noninfectious neutrophilic dermatosis that occurs in multiple conditions, including intestinal surgery and inflammatory bowel diseases. The syndrome was first described in patients with jejunoileal bypass surgery for obesity.

Clinical presentation: The most common explanation for BADAS is a bacterial overgrowth in the bowel loop. This overgrowth leads to immune response to bacterial antigens and release of immune complexes consisting of antibodies to *Escherichia coli* and *Bacteroides fragilis*. These complexes enter the circulation and cause such systemic manifestations as fever and arthralgia.

The skin changes are disseminated on the arms, legs, and the upper part of the trunk. The initial skin lesions are small asymptomatic, pruriginous, or painful erythematous macules. They may become vesicular and pustular lesions, as well as purpuric papules or erythema nodosum–like nodules. The lesions generally heal without scarring within 2 weeks. Joint manifestations are episodic, migratory, and polyarticular, with involvement of the fingers and accompanying tenosynovitis.

Laboratory studies: No key test is available. Histopathologic findings include marked neutrophilic infiltrates, resembling those associated with Sweet syndrome.

Differential diagnosis: This includes Sweet syndrome, pyoderma gangrenosum, leukocytoclastic vasculitis, and dermatitis herpetiformis.

Management: The most common treatment employs antimicrobials, such as tetracycline or metronidazole, and both systemic corticosteroids and nonsteroidal anti-inflammatory drugs. In some patients, cyclosporine or mycophenolate are used to reduce the steroid dose.

HEMATOLOGIC DISEASES AND THE SKIN

Overview: Cutaneous manifestations of hematologic diseases fall into four main groups:

Clinical presentation: The skin disorders due to vascular changes include dilatation, occlusion, and inflammation:

- Spontaneous hemorrhages in the skin in the form of petechiae (usually appear in disorders of hemostasis)

- Neutrophilic dermatoses (mostly associated with myelodysplastic syndromes):

  - Vasculitis

  - Skin ulcerations (sickle cell anemia, thalassemia, antiphospholipid antibody syndrome, heparin necrosis, protein C deficiencies)

Anemia can cause changes in the appearance of the skin, nails, tongue, and hair. The common skin manifestations in patients with anemia are (Table 29.7):

- Pallor of the skin (especially palmar creases), mucocutaneous membranes, and conjunctiva

- Glossitis

- Poikilodermatous hypopigmentation

- Brittle nails

Table 29.7 Common Skin Manifestations in Anemia

Anemia	Skin Manifestations	Mucosal Changes	Hair and Nail Changes
Hemolytic anemia	Jaundice; petechiae and hemosiderosis	Pallor of lips and oral mucosa; oral petechiae	Fragile nails
Iron deficiency anemia	Pallor (not usually visible unless hemoglobin falls to 7 g/dL)	Pallor of lips and oral mucosa; angular stomatitis; atrophy of filiform tongue papillae	Diffuse hair thinning; fragile nails with longitudinal ridges; koilonychia
Pernicious anemia	Skin tends to have a yellowish hue; late-onset vitiligo is reported in 10% of the patients	Red, cobblestone-appearing tongue	Some Latin American patients may display reddish hair discoloration
Sickle cell anemia	Occurrence of leg ulcerations in the ankle area—the size of the ulcers varies from a few millimeters to large circumferential lesions	Dentofacial deformities—increased thickening of the skull, mandibular infarction, orofacial pain, enamel hypo-mineralization and diastema	
Fanconi anemia	Pigmentation abnormalities—cafe au lait spots, diffuse hyperpigmentation, hypopigmented macules		
Aplastic anemia	Facial petechiae	Oral petechiae, gingival hyperplasia, spontaneous gingival bleeding	
Megaloblastic anemia		Atrophy of the entire oral mucosa and atrophic glossitis, recurrent aphthous lesions	Brittle nails

Table 29.8 Cutaneous Manifestations of Hematologic Malignancies

Cutaneous Manifestations	Hematologic Disease
Malignancy-associated Sweet syndrome	Myelodysplastic syndrome, acute myeloid leukemia, polycythemia vera, myelofibrosis, myelo-proliferative neoplasms
Pyoderma gangrenosum	Acute myeloid leukemia; chronic myeloid leukemia; multiple myeloma; monoklonal gammopathie, lymphomas, myelodysplastic syndrome, polycythemia vera, essential thrombocythemia, myelofibrosis
Neutrophilic eccrine hidradenitis	Acute myeloid leukemia, chronic myeloid leukemia
Paraneoplastic pemphigus	Non-Hodgkin's lymphoma, chronic lymphocytic leukemia, Castleman's disease
Leukemia cutis (myeloid or granulocytic sarcoma)	Acute myeloid leukemia, chronic myelogenous leukemia, myelodysplastic syndromes
Amyloid deposition in blood vessels	Multiple myeloma
Necrobiotic Xanthogranuloma	Monoclonal gammopathy, multiple myeloma
Paraneoplastic pruritus	Lymphoma
Dermatomyositis	Non-Hodgkin lymphoma
Leser-Trelat syndrome	Lymphoma
Sclerodema of Buschke	Paraproteinemia, multiple myeloma, Waldenström's macroglobulinemia
Paraneoplastic vasculitides Cutaneous small-vessel vasculitis	Acute myeloid leukemia, chronic myeloid leukemia, myelofibrosis, polycythemia vera, essential thrombocytopenia
Paraneoplastic vasculitides Polyarteritis nodosa	Hairy cell leukemia, myelodysplastic syndrome, chronic myelomonocytic leukemia
Schnitzler syndrome	Monoklonal gammopathie IgM; Waldenström's macroglobulinemia
Reactive granulomatous dermatitis	Myelodysplastic syndrome

Polycythemia vera is an example of a chronic myeloproliferative disorder of myeloid cells that results in an increased red cell mass. The vascular complications in patients with polycythemia vera include a plethora and flushing of the face and palms, aquagenic pruritus associated with a hot shower in 40% of patients), erythromelalgia, livedo reticularis, acrocyanosis, and pyoderma gangrenosum.

There may be nonspecific signs, such as paleness or those due to opportunistic infections, including recurrent cutaneous infections.

The paraneoplastic skin disorders are listed in Table 29.8.

The skin manifestations of acute and chronic graft versus host disease may occur in recipients of allogeneic hematopoietic stem cell transplants induced by immune-competent donor cells attacking host tissues. GVHD signs and symptoms appearing within the first 100 days after transplantation are considered acute, whereas those occurring beyond 100 days are categorized as chronic. Acute GVHD presents with erythematous maculopapular eruptions starting on the face, ears, palms, and soles. Follicular erythema is a frequent acute GVHD early manifestation

Lichen planus–like and lupus erythematous–like eruptions, as well as poikiloderma, are the most typical skin changes in the nonsclerotic chronic GVHD. Lichen sclerosus and morphea or deep and disseminated mimicking systemic scleroderma changes are the main characteristic of the sclerotic chronic GVHD.

Laboratory studies: A skin biopsy will likely provide a more accurate histologic, immunocyto-chemical and microbiologic analysis. Polymerase chain reaction–based molecular techniques will improve the accuracy of the diagnosis, when bacterial, fungal, and viral infections are suspected.

Management: Cutaneous manifestations of hematologic diseases require the treatment of the underlying hematologic malignancy.

FINAL THOUGHT

The skin, as the largest organ of the body, covers the surface; this results in skin diseases being called superficial and even dermatologists being so labeled. For example, since the last decade of the 20th century, the concept that psoriasis is a systemic disease has been discussed and increasingly accepted. The advent of the biologics has provided support for the systemic nature of skin diseases. Nowadays this concept is accepted from the scholars all over the world. The skin markers of systemic diseases help us better understand this process.

ADDITIONAL READINGS

Abreu Velez AM, Howard MS. Diagnosis and treatment of cutaneous paraneoplastic disorders. Dermatol Ther. 2010;23:662–675.

Afifi L, Saeed L, Pasch LA, et al. Association of ethnicity, Fitzpatrick skin type, anhirsutism: a retrospective cross-sectional study of women with polycystic ovarian syndrome. Int J Womens Dermatol. 2017;3:37–43.

Begbie ME, Wallace GM, Shovlin CL. Hereditary haemorrhagic telangiectasia (Osler-Weber-Rendu syndrome): a view from the 21st century. Postgrad Med J. 2003;79:18–24.

Beggs AD, Latchford AR, Vasen HF, et al. Peutz-Jeghers syndrome: a systematic review and recommendations for management. Gut. 2010;59:975–986.

Binus AM, Qureshi AA, Li VW, et al. Pyoderma gangrenosum: a retrospective review of patient characteristics, comorbidities and therapy in 103 patients. Br J Dermatol. 2011;165:1244–1250.

Erfurt-Berge C, Dissemond J, Schwede K, et al. Updated results of 100 patients on clinical features and therapeutic options in necrobiosis lipoidica in a retrospective multicentre study. Eur J Dermatol. 2015;25:595–601.

Gu GL, Wang SL, Wei XM, et al. Diagnosis and treatment of Gardner syndrome with gastric polyposis: a case report and review of the literature. World J Gastroenterol. 2008;14:2121–2123.

Karadağ AS, You Y, Danarti R, et al. Acanthosis nigricans and the metabolic syndrome. Clin Dermatol. 2018;36:48–53.

Murphy-Chutorian B, Han G, Cohen SR. Dermatologic manifestations of diabetes mellitus. Endocrinol Metabol Clin N Amer. 2013;42:869–898.

Powell LW, Seckington RC, Deugnier Y. Haemochromatosis. Lancet. 2016;388:706–716.

30 Diseases of Infancy and Childhood

Serap Utaş

CONTENTS

Definition: In newborns, the transition from an intrauterine to extrauterine environment brings immediate physiologic and anatomic changes to multiple organ systems, including the skin. Newborn skin differs from adult skin by being thinner, having less hair, producing less sweat and sebaceous gland secretions, and possessing fewer intercellular attachments and melanosomes. An infant's body surface area–to–weight ratio is up to five times that of an adult. As a result, infants have increased risks for skin damage, infections, and percutaneous toxicity from topically applied agents. Newborn skin must adapt and mature to protect against many infections, toxins, ultraviolet radiation, temperature changes, and transepidermal water loss.

 Overview: Skin diseases in neonates are usually benign and self-limited, but they may also signal the existence of underlying systemic diseases, syndromes, or severe infections. Those may be life-threatening in nature. A careful examination is crucial, and an accurate and prompt diagnosis is necessary. Awareness of the normal phenomena, as well as their differentiation from more significant cutaneous disorders of the newborn, is important.

 Several skin diseases are more common or specific in infants and children and may present with different characteristics than in adults. Treatment and management may also differ. Children should not be considered little adults for medical management, as had occurred in the 19th century.

TRANSIENT ERUPTIONS OF THE NEWBORN

During the neonatal period, newborn skin shows many physiologic changes (Table 30.1). These temporary conditions are important to recognize and should be differentiated from more significant skin disorders, such as bacterial, viral, and fungal infections or inflammatory skin conditions.

DOI: 10.1201/9781003105268-30

Table 30.1 Transient Benign Cutaneous Lesions of Newborns

Physiologic desquamation

Sebaceous hyperplasia

Erythema toxicum neonatorum

Transient neonatal pustular melanosis

Suction blisters

Milia

Oral mucosal cysts (Epstein's pearls, Bohn's nodules)

Miliaria crystalina/rubra

Rubor

Cutis marmorata

Acrocyanosis

Harlequin color change

Hypertrichosis

Physiologic jaundice

Vernix Caseosa

Vernix caseosa is a physiologic biofilm that covers the neonatal skin. The appearance of the vernix is creamy, viscous, and thick, with a chalky-white color (Figure 30.1). Vernix is produced by desquamated fetal epithelial cells and sebaceous glands that cover the fetus during the third trimester in utero. It may protect the epidermis from the amniotic fluid while promoting epidermal cornification and stratum corneum formation.

The composition of vernix is 80% water, 10% protein (e.g., cathelicidins, defensins, cystatin A), and 10% lipids (e.g., ceramides, cholesterol, free fatty acids, phospholipids). Apart from its natural moisturizing abilities, vernix has various functions during the fetal transition (from an intrauterine to an extrauterine environment). It lubricates the birth canal during delivery, provides temperature regulation and innate immunity, stimulates intestinal development, and creates a barrier to prevent water loss.

Neonatal Desquamation

The skin of the full-term infant is normally soft and smooth. Increased desquamation can be present at birth due to post maturity or dysmaturity. Desquamation of neonatal skin generally takes place within 24–48 hours following delivery and may not be complete until the third week of life.

For physiologic desquamation, differential diagnosis includes congenital ichthyosis and X-linked recessive hypohidrotic dysplasia.

Erythema Toxicum Neonatorum

Synonyms: Erythema neonatorum allergicum, toxic erythema

Erythema toxicum neonatorum (ETN) is an inflammatory reaction that is benign and self-limited. It can affect up to 31–72% of full-term infants and usually affects both sexes equally. ETN is characterized by 1–3 mm erythematous papules and sterile pustules on a blotchy erythematous base. Lesions can affect the trunk, face, and extremities (Figure 30.2) but typically spare the palmoplantar areas. They can appear at 48–72 hours of life and regress in 3–14 days without scarring. Some studies have shown activation of immune response in the lesions, which suggests that this may represent an inflammatory reaction of the skin to microbial colonization occurring at birth.

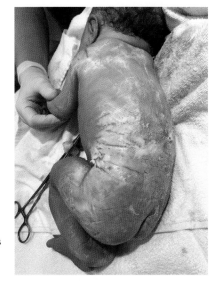

Figure 30.1 Vernix caseosa. Newborn's skin in the first minutes of life. White, cheesy, greasy layer covering the skin, which has protected the fetus in utero.

373

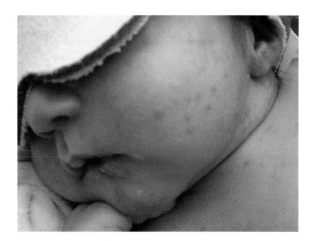

Figure 30.2 Erythema toxicum neonatorum. Erythematous papules and sterile pustules on the cheeks, chin, neck, and trunk.

ETN can usually be diagnosed by the clinical appearance alone. A Tzanck smear may reveal numerous eosinophils and occasional neutrophils. ETN may be differentiated from other neonatal pustular dermatoses, including miliaria, transient neonatal pustular melanosis, infantile acropustulosis, bacterial, *Candida spp.*, or *Malassezia furfur* pustulosis, and neonatal *Herpes simplex* infection. Treatment is not required. Recovery generally takes place spontaneously.

Transient Neonatal Pustular Melanosis

Transient neonatal pustular melanosis (TNPM) is a rare disease of unknown cause that occurs in less than 5% of neonates. It is more prevalent in African American newborns of both sexes. TNPM is characterized by superficial and fragile pustules on a non-erythematous base. These can be easily ruptured which leads to a collarette of scale. Subsequently, hyperpigmented brown macules may appear. Lesions are always present at birth and may appear anywhere on the body, including palmoplantar areas and genitalia.

The diagnosis is made clinically, and on most occasions, only hyperpigmented macules with collarettes of scale may be seen. A Tzanck smear of the pustules can show polymorphonuclear neutrophils. The differential of TNPM includes ETN, miliaria, acropustulosis of infancy, infectious eruptions, such as staphylococcal impetigo, neonatal candidosis, *Herpes simplex* infection, and varicella-zoster. No specific therapy is indicated for TNPM, as it resolves spontaneously. The pigmented macules may take weeks to months to fade.

Milia

Milia are common transient skin disorders in neonates, being present in up to 30–50% of babies. These are white or yellowish smooth-surfaced 1–2 mm papules that are visible on the face, scalp, upper aspect of the trunk, and arms. There is no significant racial or sex difference (Figure 30.3).

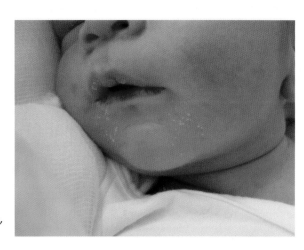

Figure 30.3 Milia: Multiple, tiny, white, smooth-surfaced papules on the chin.

Milia may be present at birth or occur within a few months. Milia are seen as few or numerous, discrete papules that disappear spontaneously.

The main differential diagnosis is sebaceous hyperplasia, which appears as follicular, grouped, pinpoint whitish-yellow papules around the nose and upper lip. Milia may be a feature of many genodermatoses, such as epidermolysis bullosa. Although rarely required, incision and excretion of the typical keratinous debris can confirm the diagnosis. Similar inclusion cysts may be seen on the palate (Epstein's pearls) or alveolar ridges (Bohn's nodules), and these also resolve within weeks to months.

Miliaria

Synonyms: Heat rash, prickly heat

Miliaria, a common term used for obstruction of the eccrine ducts, is frequently characterized by superficial vesicles. It generally originates from sweat retention due to obstruction of the sweat glands or ducts within the stratum corneum or deeper in the epidermis. Ductal blockage can be caused by cutaneous debris or bacterial biofilms. Miliaria is common in newborns due to humidity, warmth, excessive clothing, febrile periods, and immaturity of the sweat pores.

Miliaria crystallina (sudamina) is the most common form, which presents with pinpoint vesicles that can be easily ruptured. They are generally found on the face, neck, trunk, and axillae (Figure 30.4). Miliaria rubra is characterized by numerous erythematous 1–3-mm papules, papulopustules, or grouped pruritic papulovesicles. These may be pustular in occluded skin areas and are not follicular.

Differential diagnosis: This includes varicella, *Herpes simplex*, TNPM, ETN, and neonatal acne. Miliaria is usually self-limited and heals without treatment. Keeping the room cooler and avoiding overdressing the infant can be helpful.

Sebaceous Hyperplasia

Sebaceous hyperplasia is a common and benign condition of the sebaceous glands. In neonates, it results from exposure to maternal hormones. These are multiple white-yellowish tiny papules that commonly occur around the nose and upper lips of full-term infants. Lesions gradually involute, which usually happens within the first few weeks of life.

Cutis Marmorata

Cutis marmorata is a reticulated, blanchable, violaceous mottling of the neonatal skin seen on the trunk and extremities. This phenomenon is a physiologic response of the neonate to cooling, which causes dilation of capillaries and venules. It rapidly disappears as the infant is rewarmed. Treatment is unnecessary. Its distinction from cutis marmorata telangiectasia congenita should be made, because the latter is a vascular malformation that persists for several years in the form of well-defined large patches.

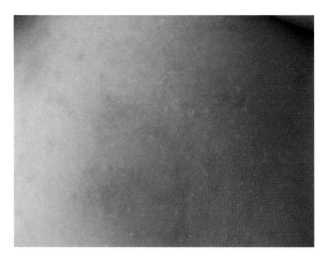

Figure 30.4 Miliaria crystalline (sudamina). Translucent, thin roofed, delicate 1–2-mm diameter vesicles on the face.

Harlequin Color Change

Harlequin color change (HCC) is a rare condition in newborns, which is characterized by episodes of suddenly forming, transient, well-demarcated erythema. It generally occurs on the dependent half of the body with visible pallor on the upper half. HCC may be observed transiently in up to 10% of healthy newborns, but it is more common in premature infants. HCC generally occurs on the third or fourth day of life, with the color change seen for between 30 seconds and 20 minutes. An affected newborn may experience 1–12 HCC episodes within a day.

HCC is a benign idiopathic condition, which does not require treatment and resolves on its own. Reasons for HCC remain unclear; however, functional immaturity in the hypothalamus leading to dysfunction in peripheral capillary bed tonus control is suspected.

DISEASES OF INFANCY AND CHILDHOOD VESICULOPUSTULAR ERUPTIONS INFANTILE ACROPUSTULOSIS

Synonym: Acropustulosis of infancy

Infantile acropustulosis (IA) is characterized by extremely pruritic, sterile vesiculopustules that occur on the palms and soles. Lesions generally appear in crops every 2–4 weeks, with individual lesions lasting for 5–10 days. Its characteristics and course are generally typical. It may occur from birth up to one year of age and generally resolves spontaneously by 2–3 years of age.

The reason for IA remains unclear; however, a probable link with preceding scabies infestation in some has been suggested. A Tzanck smear reveals large numbers of neutrophils and occasionally eosinophils. ETN, TNPM, scabies, pustular psoriasis, and impetigo should be taken into account in the differential diagnosis. Treatment is often unnecessary due to the self-limiting nature of IA. Low-potency topical corticosteroids, such as hydrocortisone 2.5% cream applied twice per day, can be helpful.

COLLAGEN VASCULAR DISEASE NEONATAL LUPUS ERYTHEMATOSUS

Neonatal lupus erythematosus (NLE) is an uncommon autoimmune disease that occurs due to transplacental transmission of maternal antibodies. The mother sometimes has systemic lupus erythematosus (SLE) or Sjögren syndrome.

Frequent clinical manifestations include congenital heart block and cutaneous lupus erythematosus. Other manifestations, such as hematologic disease, hepatobiliary disease, and central nervous system involvement, may also occur.

The lesions are generally not present at birth but develop soon after the first month of life. NLE appears as an inflammatory and superficial macular erythema of the upper eyelids and scalp (Figure 30.5), which often causes a raccoon-like appearance in the periorbital area. The extremities or trunk may also be affected, which is possibly due to photosensitivity.

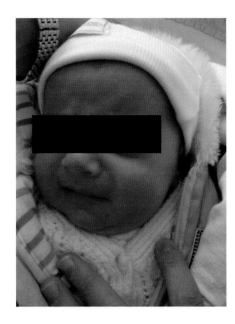

Figure 30.5 Neonatal lupus erythematosus in girl born by Cesarean section to a 27-year-old mother. There were erythematous scaly lesions more prominent on the cheeks and eyelids. She required a pacemaker for a complete AV block. She also had ANA (+), Anti SSA (+), Anti PCNA (+) and Anti dsDNA (+).

NLE is related to the anti-Ro/SSA (Sjogren syndrome autoantigen type A-SSA) antibody in more than 90% of patients. Occasionally, patients only have anti-La/SSB (Sjogren syndrome autoantigen type B-SSB) or anti-U1RNP (small nuclear ribonucleoprotein-associated with U1 spliceosomal RNA) antibodies. The presence of these antibodies should be screened in infants with NLE. Laboratory investigations may reveal pancytopenia, thrombocytopenia, leukopenia, or elevated transaminase level.

With the exception of cardiac involvement, NLE usually resolves spontaneously. Protection from sunlight is advised and hydrocortisone 2.5% or fluticasone cream can be used.

THE INBORN DISORDERS OF METABOLISM

Acrodermatitis Enteropathica

Zinc is an important trace element that has a vital role in the development, growth, and differentiation of various tissues. Zinc deficiency can occur due to inadequate intake, malabsorption, or a combination of these factors caused by genetic or acquired conditions. Acrodermatitis enteropathica is an autosomal recessive disorder that is caused by defects in *SLC39A4* located on chromosome 8q24.3, which codes for the zinc transporter protein, *ZIP4*. Patients have reduced zinc absorption in the small intestine. Acquired zinc deficiency is usually caused by low birth weight, prematurity, maternal zinc deficiency, malabsorption syndromes, poor feeding, and Kwashiorkor.

Cutaneous manifestations of zinc deficiency are characterized as sharply circumscribed, psoriasiform, or eczematous plaques, which frequently have peripheral scaling and crusts (Figure 30.6, 30.7). Pustules and vesicles may subsequently appear. The lesions occur in acral, periorificial, and anogenital areas. Alopecia, diarrhea, irritability, growth retardation, photophobia, conjunctivitis, and blepharitis may also be seen.

The diagnosis is clinical but may be confirmed by findings of low serum zinc level or alkaline phosphatase. Inherited zinc deficiency should be considered if there is relevant family history or recurrence following cessation of zinc supplementation. Confirmation of a genetic deficiency requires genetic testing.

Rare metabolic diseases, psoriasis, seborrheic dermatitis, and candida infections should be considered in the differential diagnosis. Management includes administration of oral zinc sulfate or gluconate 1–3 mg/kg/per day. Cutaneous resolution occurs within 1–2 weeks with irritability being the first symptom to respond. Lifelong therapy may be required depending on the cause.

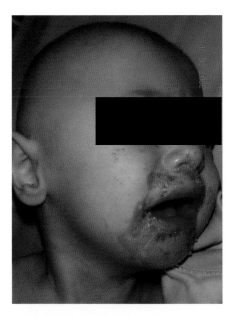

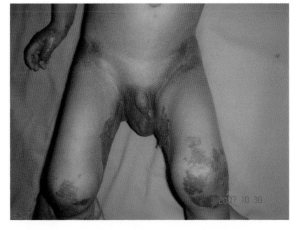

Figure 30.6 Acrodermatitis enteropathica. Erythematous, scaly, erosive plaques and superficial erosions involving the perioral and periorbital areas with diffuse alopecia of the scalp.

Figure 30.7 Acrodermatitis enteropathica. Circumscribed brownish-red eczematous lesions, with peripheral scaling on the hands, thighs, buttocks, and knees, plus superficial erosions on the scrotal area.

Langerhans Cell Histiocytosis

Langerhans cell histiocytosis (LCH) is an inflammatory neoplasia that primarily affects children. It has a peak incidence in patients aged 1–3 years and is most common in Caucasian boys. LCH may appear as a single cutaneous lesion or can affect many body systems, such as the skin, bone, lymph nodes, liver, lung, spleen, brain, pituitary gland, and bone marrow. LCH classically presents with a cutaneous eruption or painful osteolytic lesion. Systemic symptoms may also be present.

Cutaneous involvement is present in approximately 40% of patients. Common skin manifestations include seborrheic dermatitis–like dermatitis; erythematous, scaly red-brown papules; crusted papules on the palms and/or soles; vesiculopustular lesions; and red nodules or plaques (Figures 30.8 and 30.9). The affected areas usually involve the scalp, chest, back, abdomen, and intertriginous areas, which may be more severe due to the risk of ulceration. Gingival erythema, erosions, and petechiae may also be visible. Skin lesions are usually pruritic.

Diagnosis is dependent on clinical and histologic findings. Histology can show infiltration of typical Langerhans cells (confirmable by positive CD1a, S100, or langerin immunostaining). The differential diagnosis includes seborrheic dermatitis, candidal diaper dermatitis, atopic dermatitis, scabies, psoriasis, and mastocytosis.

Treatment is dependent on the localization and extent of the disease. If only limited to the skin, watchful waiting may suffice, since the lesions can spontaneously resolve. In cases of severe skin disease, systemic therapies used for the treatment of multiorgan LCH could be employed. Topical corticosteroids, topical tacrolimus, topical nitrogen mustard, psoralen plus ultraviolet A treatment, and systemic corticosteroids may be used in patients with symptomatic or recalcitrant skin lesions. Single bone lesions may also resolve spontaneously. Painful bone lesions may be treated with curettage and/or intralesional steroid injection. Localized radiotherapy could be another treatment option. First-line treatment for patients with multisystemic LCH is prednisone and vinblastine combination. Mercaptopurine is added for patients with risk organ involvement. The second-line treatment choice is cytarabine. Targeted treatments such as vemurafenib, trametinib, and cobimetinib may be used for refractory multisystemic LCH involving risk organs. Prognosis is dependent on the involvement of organs and response to initial systemic therapy.

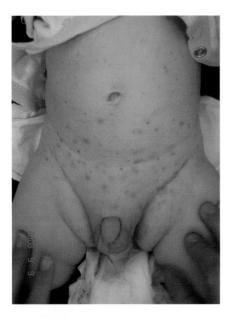

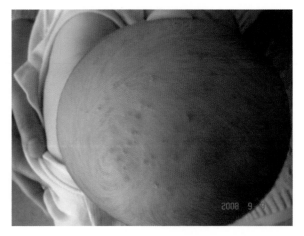

Figure 30.8 Langerhans cell histiocytosis. Erythematous papules on the abdomen and inguinal folds.

Figure 30.9 Langerhans cell histiocytosis. The child also has erythematous, scaly papules on the scalp mimicking seborrheic dermatitis.

DISORDERS OF THE SEBACEOUS GLANDS: PEDIATRIC ACNE

Although acne is usually a disorder of adolescents and young adults, neonates, and infants can also be occasionally affected.

Neonatal Acne

Neonatal acne may be observed at birth or after 2 weeks. Clinically, there are tiny comedones and papulopustules on the cheeks and nasal bridge and is more common in boys. It generally disappears within three months, but infrequently, it may progress to erythematous papules, pustules, and scarring cysts over the neck and upper parts of the trunk.

Neonatal acne develops due to excessive sebum production from hormonal stimulation of the sebaceous glands and possible colonization by the Malassezia species. The differential includes neonatal cephalic pustulosis, TNPM, ETN, nevus comedonicus, milia, miliaria, and sebaceous hyperplasia. Medical therapy is generally not required, and the use of daily cleansers with water may be all that is needed. Neonatal acne typically resolves within 3–6 months. In persistent or more inflammatory cases, a low-strength (2.5–5%) benzoyl peroxide gel or topical antibiotic (e.g., erythromycin gel) could be employed.

Infantile Acne

Infantile acne typically presents later than neonatal acne. It may occur anytime between 6 weeks and 1 year of age. It is more frequent in males. It shows typical acneiform lesions, including open or closed comedones, inflammatory papules, pustules, nodules, and cysts (Figure 30.10). It generally affects the face and to a lesser extent, the chest or back. In contrast to neonatal acne, infantile acne may be persistent, lasting from 6 months to several years.

Treatment of infantile acne is not different from common acne. Topical tretinoin, benzoyl peroxide, or erythromycin can be used. Oral therapy can be used for larger papulonodules or pustules that may scar. Erythromycin may be used for severe involvement. Infantile acne usually does not have an underlying endocrinologic cause.

Childhood Acne

Mid-childhood acne occurs between 1–7 years of age. Its frequency is quite rare. It presents with comedonal and inflammatory lesions on the face. In this age group, acne may be a sign of underlying androgen excesses, such as congenital adrenal hyperplasia and true precocious puberty. Patients should have an endocrinologic assessment, as secretion of androgens is rare for children in this age group.

Angiofibromas, verruca plana, molluscum contagiosum, corticosteroid-induced acne, and demodicosis can be considered in the differential. Treatment for this age group should rather focus on determining the underlying cause. Options for acne treatment are parallel to those for infantile acne.

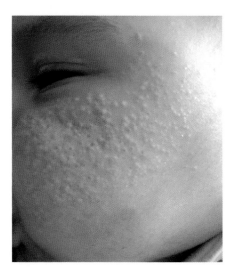

Figure 30.10 Infantile acne. Multiple open and closed comedones on the cheeks and chin.

Neonatal Cephalic Pustulosis

Neonatal cephalic pustulosis (NCP) is an inflammatory condition arising from the reaction of the skin to the *Malassezia* species. It generally occurs within the first 3 weeks of life. Lesions are typically localized to the cheeks, eyelids, chin, and sometimes the neck and upper portions of the chest. NCP is characterized by erythematous papulopustules with an erythematous halo (Figure 30.11). The absence of comedones and the presence of pustules surrounded by the erythematous halo help distinguish NCP from neonatal acne. NCP typically resolves on its own within 3 months; however, application of topical ketoconazole 2% twice per day for 1 week can offer improvement of the symptoms. Low-potency topical corticosteroids can be used in unresponsive patients.

DERMATITIS IN CHILDHOOD

Diaper Dermatitis

Synonym: Napkin dermatitis

Diaper dermatitis (DD), as the name suggests, occurs in the diaper area. With the advent of disposable diapers, it has not been as intense as when cloth diapers were covered by rubber protectives. The primary contributing factors are occlusion, friction, and maceration, which are augmented by the presence of urine and feces and potential bacterial and/or fungal infections (Figure 30.12, 30.13). Irritant contact dermatitis is most frequently observed directly where the diaper touches the skin and does not extend much beyond this area. The inguinal creases and gluteal cleft are usually spared.

The differential diagnosis includes infantile seborrheic dermatitis, intertrigo, psoriasis, allergic contact dermatitis, atopic dermatitis, candidiasis, perianal streptococcal dermatitis, Langerhans cell histiocytosis, and acrodermatitis enteropathica. Prevention is the best management strategy. The ABCDE rule (mnemonic for air, barrier, cleansing, diapering, education) can be considered for prevention. Leaving the diaper area open to the environment can speed up recovery; however, if this is not feasible, then diaper changes should occur more frequently. It is important to wash the area with warm water or to wipe it with a cotton swab. Cleansing wipes containing harsh chemicals and scents should be avoided. Applying a thick layer of an emollient or a zinc oxide paste is recommended for barrier protection. If there is no improvement despite

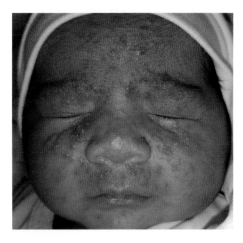

Figure 30.11 Neonatal cephalic pustulosis. Erythematous papulopustules, surrounded by an erythematous halo, on the forehead, cheeks, chin, and eyelids. No comedones are seen.

Source: Courtesy of Filiz Cebeci, MD-Istanbul Medeniyet University, Department of Dermatology, Istanbul, Turkey.

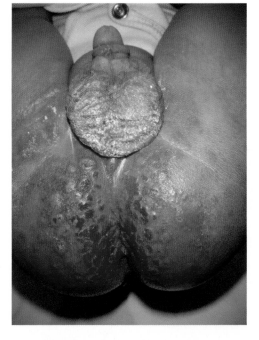

Figure 30.12 Severe diaper dermatitis, with erosions, raised papules, and nodules.

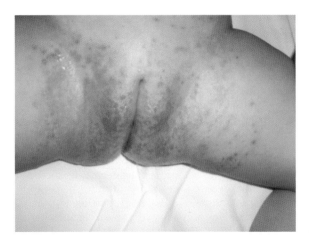

Figure 30.13 Diaper dermatitis. Erythematous papules and small erosions on the diaper area. Satellite papules also appear outside of the lesions.

the previously mentioned applications, or in case of resistance, low-potency topical corticosteroids can be used twice per day.

Infantile Seborrheic Dermatitis

Synonym: Cradle cap

Infantile seborrheic dermatitis (ISD) is a self-limited, inflammatory, and scaling skin condition that causes erythema and greasy yellowish scaling in infants and young children. There is typically no pruritus. The exact etiology of ISD remains unknown, with hormonal fluctuations and colonization by *Malassezia* species being suggested.

ISD occurs within the first 3 months of life and generally self-resolves by the first year. ISD tends to occur on skin where sebaceous glands are more common, especially the scalp, eyebrows, and nasolabial folds. ISD frequently begins on the scalp, which is commonly known as cradle cap. This is characterized by greasy, adherent, thick, yellowish scales on the vertex and frontal area of the scalp (Figure 30.14). Atopic dermatitis, psoriasis, contact dermatitis, and Langerhans cell histiocytosis can be considered in the differential diagnosis. Conservative management involves gentle emollients and frequent shampooing, occasionally involving removal of scales with soft brushes. More extensive or resistant cases may require low-potency topical corticosteroid (e.g., hydrocortisone 1%) or azole (e.g., ketoconazole 2%).

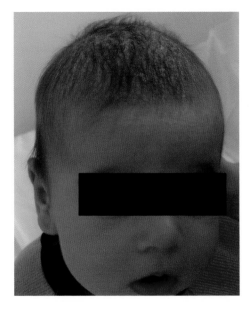

Figure 30.14 Infantile seborrheic dermatitis (cradle cap) with adherent, yellowish, greasy scales

Juvenile Plantar Dermatosis

Synonyms: Atopic winter feet, sweaty-sock dermatitis

Juvenile plantar dermatosis (JPD) is a common dermatitis of the feet that manifests with cracks and fissures. It generally affects children who are 3–14 years old and is more prevalent in boys than girls. The cause is often blamed on the occlusive effects of synthetic socks and plastic shoes, repetitive frictional movements, and excessive sweating followed by quick drying. JPD tends to follow a better course in the winter and then deteriorates in the summer.

Both feet are symmetrically affected. Lesions appear as shiny and glazed erythematous plaques on the weightbearing areas of the plantar surface and toes (especially the first toes). There is usually sparing of the toe webs and instep. Painful fissures can be present. The diagnosis of JPD is clinical. Skin scrapings to exclude tinea pedis and patch testing to exclude a contact allergy can be useful. Tinea pedis, plantar psoriasis, atopic dermatitis, and allergic contact dermatitis should be considered in the differential diagnosis. Wearing thicker and more absorbent cotton socks and more breathable shoes may improve the condition. Emollients and mid- to high-potency topical corticosteroids (e.g., mometasone furoate, methylprednisolone aceponate) or topical calcineurin inhibitors (e.g., tacrolimus ointment) can reduce inflammation. The disease may take several weeks to resolve.

EXANTHEMATOUS DISEASES OF CHILDHOOD: GIANOTTI-CROSTI SYNDROME

Synonyms: Papular acrodermatitis of childhood, infantile papular acrodermatitis

Gianotti-Crosti syndrome is a benign and self-limited condition that is commonly seen in children who are 1–6 years old. It mostly occurs sporadically in the spring and summer. There is no gender or racial predilection. The exact pathophysiology of the syndrome is unknown; however, various viral infections, including hepatitis B, Epstein-Barr virus, cytomegalovirus, Coxsackie A, parvovirus B19, and parainfluenza, and vaccinations have been implicated. The condition may develop due to an immunologic response to the infection rather than the infection itself.

Gianotti-Crosti syndrome presents with an acute onset of a symmetrically distributed papular or papulovesicular eruption (Figure 30.15). Lesions are acrally distributed, monomorphic papules or papulovesicles with an absence of extensive truncal lesions. The eruption usually presents on extensor surfaces of the extremities, buttocks, and face. Its association with systemic findings is rare; however, fever, lymphadenopathy, and upper respiratory symptoms precede the eruption. No laboratory examinations are required. The differential includes hand-foot-mouth disease, erythema infectiosum, erythema multiforme, papular purpuric gloves and sock syndrome, papular urticaria, frictional lichenoid dermatitis, molluscum contagiosum, lichen planus, and nonspecific viral exanthems. Treatment is generally not required, because it is a benign, self-limited condition.

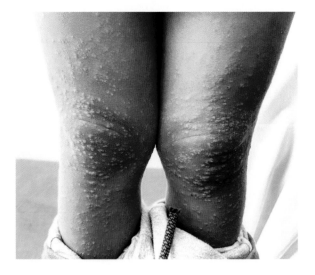

Figure 30.15 Gianotti-Crosti syndrome. Symmetric, flat-topped, discrete, skin-colored to erythematous, 2–10-mm papules and papulovesicles on the legs

Source: Courtesy of Demet Kartal, MD- Erciyes University, Department of Dermatology, Kayseri, Turkey.

PAPULOSQUAMOUS DISORDERS

Pediatric Psoriasis

Psoriasis is a common and chronic inflammatory disorder that affects the skin, nails, and joints. Almost one-third of cases begin in childhood; however, onset may occur at any age, including infancy. The commonly reported median age for pediatric psoriasis is 7–10 years.

Plaque psoriasis is the most common form of pediatric psoriasis which may not have the same appearance as in adults. Compared to adults, the erythematous plaques are usually thinner, smaller, and have less scaling (Figure 30.16). Lesions are often localized on the face, scalp, and flexural areas. In pediatric psoriasis, pruritus is more common, and provocative factors can be more frequently identified. Guttate psoriasis is the second-most common form, with napkin psoriasis being the most common form in infants younger than 2 years of age (Figure 30.17). There can be the presence of characteristic psoriatic plaques with umbilical involvement. Pustular (Figure 30.18) and erythrodermic psoriasis are rarely seen in childhood.

Differential diagnosis should be based on the clinical type of psoriasis. Common differential diagnoses include atopic dermatitis, nummular dermatitis, tinea corporis, DD, seborrheic dermatitis, pityriasis rosea, viral infections, and drug eruptions.

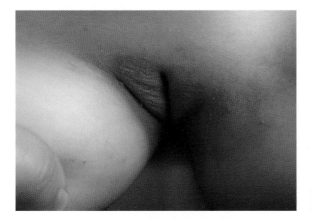

Figure 30.16 Anogenital psoriasis: Red scaly lesions with sharp borders.

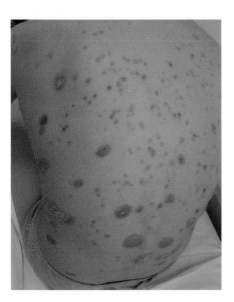

Figure 30.17 Childhood psoriasis: Guttate, nummular, and plaques.

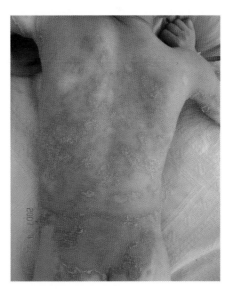

Figure 30.18 Pustular psoriasis: Erythematous and desquamated plaques with superficial yellowish-white pustules on the back, neck, arms, and buttocks.

Parent and patient education regarding the chronic nature of the disorder are crucial. Topical treatments are considered first-line treatment in children, which include topical corticosteroids, topical calcineurin inhibitors, vitamin D analogs, and keratolytic. Emollient and low-potency topical corticosteroids are safe for children under 2 years of age, whereas mid-potency topical corticosteroids may be used for children between 2–12 years of age. Topical corticosteroid use should be limited on the face and groin and should only last for the minimum required duration. Alternating with topical steroid-sparing agents can help reduce side effects and optimize disease maintenance. Phototherapy and systemic medications are generally only used for refractory or extensive psoriasis. For these children, methotrexate (0.2–0.7 mg/kg/weekly or 10–15 mg/m^2/weekly), acitretin (0.25–1 mg/kg/day), and cyclosporine (1.5–5 mg/kg/day) may be used. For children with severe psoriasis who have not responded to, or cannot receive, other systemic therapies or phototherapy, biologic medications may be considered. Etanercept, adalimumab, and ustekinumab are licensed biologics for childhood psoriasis. Etanercept is licensed from 6 years of age (0.8 mg/kg/weekly—*max 50 mg*—or 0.4 mg/kg/ twice a week sc injection), adalimumab from four years of age (24 mg/m^2—*max 40 mg*—every 2 weeks sc injection) and ustekinumab from 12 years of age (0.75 mg/kg baseline, 4 weeks, every 12 weeks; usually 45- or 90-mg sc injection).

FINAL THOUGHT

A wide variety of skin diseases can be seen in infants/children of all age groups from birth. Some of these diseases may be specific to infancy/childhood. Whereas some of these disorders are localized to the skin, some of them could be the signs of life-threatening conditions. Physicians should be aware of the diagnosis, differentiation, and treatment of pediatric skin diseases. Through such awareness, correct diagnosis and treatment may be achieved and the family members could be correctly informed and relieved.

ADDITIONAL READINGS

Bronckers IM, Paller AS, van Geel MJ, et al. Psoriasis in children and adolescents: diagnosis, management and comorbidities. Paediatr Drugs. 2015;17:373–384.

Coughlin CC, Eichenfield LF, Frieden IJ. Diaper dermatitis: clinical characteristics and differential diagnosis. Pediatr Dermatol. 2014;31:19–24.

Glutsch V, Hamm H, Goebeler M. Zinc and skin: an update. J Dtsch Dermatol Ges. 2019;17:589–596.

Klunk C, Domingues E, Wiss K. An update on diaper dermatitis. Clin Dermatol. 2014;32:477–487.

Krooks J, Minkov M, Weatherall AG. Langerhans cell histiocytosis in children: history, classification, pathobiology, clinical manifestations, and prognosis. J Am Acad Dermatol. 2018;78:1035–1044.

Leung AKC, Sergi CM, Lam JM, et al. Gianotti-Crosti syndrome (papular acrodermatitis of childhood) in the era of a viral recrudescence and vaccine opposition. World J Pediatr. 2019;15:521–527.

Maroñas-Jiménez L, Krakowski AC. Pediatric acne: clinical patterns and pearls. Dermatol Clin. 2016;34:195–202.

Paller AS, Mancini AJ. Cutaneous disorders of newborn. In: A Textbook of Skin Disorders of Childhood and Adolescence. 5th ed. Philadelphia: Elsevier Saunders; 2016. p. 11–37.

Que SK, Whitaker-Worth DL, Chang MW. Acne: kids are not just little people. Clin Dermatol. 2016;34:710–716.

Relvas M, Torres T. Pediatric psoriasis. Am J Clin Dermatol. 2017;18:797–811.

31 Nutritional Diseases

Chelsea Kesty, Madeline Hooper, Erin McClure, Emily Chea, and Cynthia Bartus

CONTENTS

Synonym: Nutritional deficiency, malnutrition

Overview: Nutrition-related skin disease occurs in the setting of either deficiency or excess of essential nutrients needed to maintain biologic function. These essential nutrients include macronutrients (e.g., protein, carbohydrates, fats) and/or micronutrients (e.g., vitamins and minerals). Dietary intake, comorbid conditions, metabolic aberrancy, and underlying illnesses are factors associated with nutrition-related skin disease.

MACRONUTRIENTS

Kwashiorkor

Definition: Kwashiorkor, also known as edematous malnutrition, is a form of severe protein malnutrition that results from numerous weeks of severe lack of protein in the diet.

Clinical presentation: Kwashiorkor is mainly found in populations with limited resources and access to protein (e.g., developing countries and food deserts within developed countries) and is especially prevalent in children who have sufficient daily caloric intake but insufficient daily protein intake (e.g., the so-called rice diet). Patients will present with fatigue, a swollen abdomen (Figure 31.1), growth retardation, and impaired immunity that may manifest as recurrent infections. Cutaneous findings include flaking or peeling skin (Figure 31.2), dyschromia, and changes in hair color (bands of light and dark).

Laboratory studies: Patients will demonstrate hypoglycemia and hypoalbuminemia.

Management: Slow increase of caloric intake of carbohydrates and fats with gradual increase of protein intake over several weeks. Goal intake rates are 175 kcal/kg/d and 4 g/kg/d of protein for children and 60 kcal/kg/d and 2 g/kg/d of protein for adults.

Course: Treatment in early stages of disease will produce prompt recovery, although growth potential may never be recovered. Treatment in later stages is more challenging, and some effects may be irreversible. Without protein supplementation, the disease may be fatal.

Final comment: Kwashiorkor is a disease of severe protein malnutrition found mainly in children of developing countries, which can be fatal if not treated with adequate protein supplementation.

DOI: 10.1201/9781003105268-31

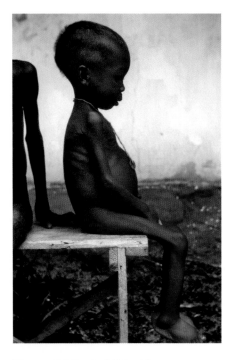

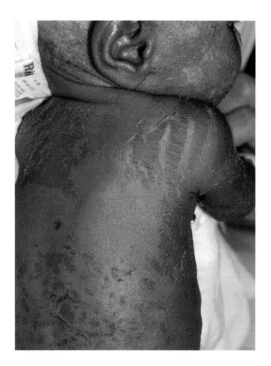

Figure 31.1 A child with a protuberant, swollen abdomen was found to have Kwashiorker.

Source: Courtesy of Dr Lyle Conrad and Public Health Image Library, Centers for Disease Control and Prevention.

Figure 31.2 An infant with flaking and peeling dermatitis was found to have Kwashiorker

Source: From VisualDx, used with permission.

Marasmus

Definition: Marasmus is a state of severe caloric deficit diet, which results in body weight less than 60% of age-appropriate normal range.

Clinical presentation: Marasmus is frequently seen in impoverished populations with limited access to food to provide sufficient caloric intake. Children are more commonly affected than adults. It presents with overt fat and muscle loss, irritability, diarrhea, failure to thrive, and eventual cardiovascular dysfunction. Cutaneous findings include thin, dry, pale wrinkled skin with emaciated facies due to loss of buccal fat pads. Impaired hair growth or lanugo-like hair may also be observed.

Laboratory studies: Anemia, hypokalemia, and elevated cortisol may be present.

Management: After initial stabilization, total caloric intake should be gradually increased. Rapid increase poses risk for refeeding syndrome.

Course: Adequate nutritional rehabilitation will lead to complete recovery of growth in most cases. If not treated, the condition is fatal.

Final comment: Marasmus arises from months of severe caloric deficit commonly seen in impoverished children, which is reversible with nutritional rehabilitation.

Eating Disorders

Definition: These are characterized as psychiatric disorders with nutritional-based imbalances. Dermatologic manifestations can occur in various conditions, such as anorexia and bulimia.

Clinical presentation: Patients with anorexia may present with lanugo-like hairs, especially on the face and arms. Patients with bulimia may exhibit Russel's sign, which are calluses or scars on the dorsal hands from repeated self-induced vomiting (Figure 31.3). Such patients also may have hypertrophic salivary glands and erosion of the tooth enamel.

Final comment: Recognition of the dermatologic signs can aid in diagnosis. Management is guided by mental health professionals.

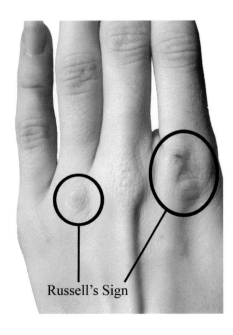

Figure 31.3 Patient with bulimia and Russell's Sign defined by hypertrophic calluses on the dorsal surface of the hand from repetitive self-induced vomiting.

Source: From Wikimedia Commons.

Russell's Sign

MICRONUTRIENTS

Vitamin A

Definition: Vitamin A encompasses a group of fat-soluble vitamins, such as retinol. It functions in the body as an essential factor for vision and immune function.

Overview: Vitamin A is an essential factor in growth and development, reproduction, vision, and immune function. It is found in dairy, produce, and liver. Vitamin A is also obtainable in the form of beta-carotene from carrots, tomatoes, and other vegetables.

Clinical presentation: Vitamin A deficiency is rare; however, it may be pronounced in periods of high nutritional demand, such as pregnancy, childhood, infancy, and lactation, or in conditions associated with pancreatic insufficiency, such as cystic fibrosis. Clinical findings include diarrhea, xerophthalmia (with characteristic night blindness and corneal deposits, known as Bitot spots; Figure 31.4), and ultimately blindness. Cutaneous manifestations include follicular hyperkeratosis and roughening of the skin (phrynoderma), xerosis cutis, and acneiform lesions.

Vitamin A excess can lead to pseudotumor cerebri, dizziness, headaches, liver damage, and even death. Cutaneous signs of hypervitaminosis A include pruritus, widespread erythema, peeling of the palms and soles, alopecia, and epistaxis. Similar findings are seen with retinoid toxicity.

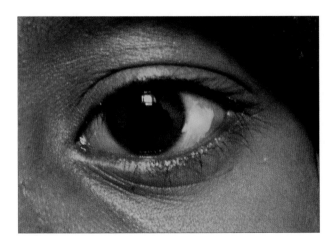

Figure 31.4 Close-up of patient with Bitot spot secondary to vitamin A deficiency.

Source: From Sharma A, Aggarwal S, Sharma V. Bitot's Spots: Look at the Gut. Int J Prev Med. 2014 Aug;5(8):1058–9, used under Creative Commons license.

387

Laboratory studies: Vitamin A deficiency is defined as laboratory values of <0.7 micromoles/L.

Management: Vitamin A supplementation at 700–900 mcg daily (2000–3000 IU) is recommended with a maximum of 3000 mcg/d. Toxicity concerns arise with daily doses of approximately 7000 mcg (25,000 IU) or greater.

Course: Vitamin A deficiency arising in young infants may result in chronic eye, gastrointestinal, and pulmonary disease. In most cases, adequate supplementation corrects vitamin A deficiency and its manifestations without long term sequelae.

Hypervitaminosis A can be deadly. It is important to correct toxic over-supplementation and monitor systemic retinoid patients. The incurred liver damage may be irreversible, and women of childbearing potential may risk fetal defects.

Final comment: Vitamin A is essential in periods of growth (e.g., pregnancy, lactation, infancy/childhood). Long-term sequelae of deficiency and excess are profound, and appropriate intake is essential.

Beta-Carotene

Definition: This is a red-orange pigment found in colorful vegetables and fruits. Beta-carotene-rich foods include carrots, sweet potatoes, and dark leafy greens.

Overview: It is a provitamin A that is converted to retinol after ingestion. It serves as an antioxidant and is often taken as a supplement to aid in lung, skin, eye, and cognitive health.

Clinical presentation: Hyper-beta-carotenemia does not have the toxic consequences of hypervitaminosis A; however, carotenoderma may result from over-supplementation. This manifests as yellow-orange discoloration, most notably on the palms, soles, and central portion of the face (Figure 31.5).

Management: Ceasing or greatly decreasing beta-carotene supplementation is generally all that is required.

Course: Once supplementation is discontinued, the skin discoloration will gradually resolve.

Final comment: Beta-carotene is a provitamin A supplement that, when taken in excess, may harmlessly cause yellow-orange discoloration of the skin. It is not associated with the toxic effects of excess vitamin A.

Vitamin B7

Synonym: Biotin

Definition: Biotin acts as a cofactor in carboxylation reactions integral for gene regulation and cell signaling.

Overview: It is found in high concentrations in foods, such as liver and eggs. Biotin deficiency is very rare in individuals who consume a well-balanced diet.

Clinical presentation: Patients with biotin deficiency may present with periorificial dermatitis, perianal dermatitis, alopecia, brittle nails, and, in severe cases, neurologic dysfunction. Populations at risk for biotin deficiency include infants born with biotinidase deficiency, pregnant and lactating women, and those with chronic alcohol consumption, which can decrease the

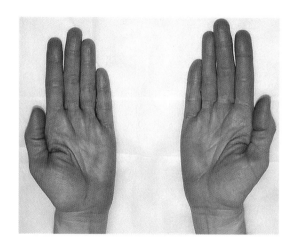

Figure 31.5 Patient with cutaneous findings of carotenemia that include yellow-orange discoloration of the palms as pictured.

Source: Courtesy of Samuel Freire da Silva, MD, from www.atlasdermatologico.com.br.

absorption of dietary biotin. It is frequently used as a supplement for hair and nail growth, but there are limited data to support this.

Laboratory studies: Newborns are screened for biotinidase deficiency, which is an autosomal recessive inherited defect in the *BTD* gene.

Management: Supplementation with biotin, usually at a dose of 10 mg/day, is recommended. Dosing up to 50 mg/day is nontoxic.

Final comment: Biotin supplementation, even as low as one dose of 10 mg, may interfere with several laboratory tests, including troponin, pro-BNP, and thyroid function studies. It is recommended that patients wait a minimum of 8 hours after consuming >5 mg of biotin prior to blood collection for laboratory tests.

Selenium

Definition: This is a trace element involved in antioxidant defense, thyroid hormone metabolism, and DNA synthesis.

Overview: Selenium proteins are cofactors for glutathione peroxidase and iodothyronine deiodinases. Deficiency is implicated in thyroiditis, cancer, immune dysfunction, and poor glucose metabolism. If a deficiency occurs in combination with secondary physiologic stress, then Keshan cardiomyopathy may develop. Both deficiency and toxicity (selenosis) are rare.

Clinical presentation: Selenium deficiency is associated with myriad symptoms, including myalgias, depression and anxiety, macrocytosis, immune dysfunction, and whitened nail beds. Deficiency is typically seen in severely malnourished patients and those receiving total parenteral nutrition. Selenosis secondary to overconsumption of selenium manifests with gastrointestinal upset, fatigue, peripheral neuropathy, and hair and nail changes.

Laboratory studies: Serum, scalp hair, and nail bed selenium levels may be tested; however, these values are not frequently obtained in a clinical setting.

Management: Diet should include foods that contain selenium, such as Brazil nuts, sardines, tuna, kidney, and liver meats. Supplementation ranges from 20 mcg daily in young children to 50–75 mcg daily in adults.

Prognosis: Selenium deficiency responds well to dietary management. This poses less risk for toxicity compared to inorganic supplementation.

Final comment: Issues with selenium levels are rare in individuals with normal diets.

Vitamin B1

Synonym: Thiamine

Definition: It is a water-soluble vitamin critically involved in the tricarboxylic acid (TCA) cycle and nerve impulse propagation.

Overview: Thiamine levels are sensitive to heavy alcohol consumption, malnutrition, and malabsorptive states. Deficiency is identified in two phenotypes: beriberi and Wernicke-Korsakoff encephalopathy.

Clinical presentation: Dry beriberi presents with symmetric mixed peripheral neuropathy, loss of deep tendon reflexes, paralysis, confusion, and vomiting. Wet beriberi involves edema and dilated cardiomyopathy. Wernicke-Korsakoff encephalopathy is a neurologic syndrome that presents acutely with reversible confusion, oculomotor dysfunction, and ataxia (Wernicke), and chronically with confabulations, hallucination, amnesia, disorientation, and personality changes (Korsakoff). Korsakoff changes are usually irreversible.

Laboratory studies: Thiamine supplementation should trigger an increase in RBC transketolase activity.

Management: Oral thiamine supplementation is used to manage beriberi with 5–30 mg per dose daily to 3 times daily (TID) depending on severity of illness. Wernicke encephalopathy is immediately managed with 500 mg IV thiamine TID in combination with other B vitamins. Glucose administration must follow thiamine supplementation in severely malnourished patients. Korsakoff encephalopathy is treated with oral vitamin B1 supplementation to help prevent further deterioration of mental status. Lifetime abstinence from alcohol is crucial in Wernicke-Korsakoff syndrome.

Course: Early recognition and treatment of beriberi results in a favorable prognosis; nerve and cardiac function is responsive to thiamine supplementation. Wernicke encephalopathy is usually reversible with prompt therapy; however, Korsakoff-related changes are irreversible.

Final comment: Thiamine deficiency is significant in malnourished and severely alcoholic patients, and it is implicated in beriberi and Wernicke-Korsakoff encephalopathy.

Vitamin B2

Synonym: riboflavin

Definition: This is a water-soluble vitamin with important roles in reduction-oxidation reactions in its active forms of flavin adenine dinucleotide (FAD) and flavin mononucleotide (FMN).

Overview: Riboflavin deficiency is relatively rare, but it can occur in malnourished patients (anorexia nervosa, malignancy, and malabsorptive state, such as celiac disease and short bowel syndrome), long-term users of phenobarbital, and patients with very restricted diets. It may also be found in breastfed infants whose mothers are riboflavin deficient. Symptoms are nonspecific, and riboflavin deficiency is usually accompanied by other coexisting vitamin deficiencies.

Clinical presentation: Riboflavin deficiency may manifest clinically as the oral-ocular-genital syndrome, which includes cheilitis, glossitis, angular stomatitis, pharyngitis, corneal vascularization, seborrheic dermatitis, and genital dermatitis. Normocytic-normochromic anemia may be present.

Laboratory studies: Erythrocyte glutathione reductase activity coefficient can be measured in presence and absence of FAD (FAD is a necessary coenzyme of glutathione reductase); coefficient will increase with addition of FAD in riboflavin deficiency.

Management: Riboflavin 5–10 mg/day can be administered orally until recovery. Intramuscular forms are available. There should also be supplementation of other B vitamins.

Course: Deficiency responds well to supplementation. The constellation of signs and symptoms likely benefits from supplementation of all B vitamins.

Final comment: Riboflavin deficiency manifests as nonspecific mucocutaneous findings that are responsive to supplementation.

Vitamin B3

Synonym: Niacin

Definition: This is a generic term for nicotinic acid and nicotinamide. Niacin is naturally found in meats, fish, fortified cereals, and legumes. Niacin can also be synthesized from tryptophan in the liver. Niacin biologically acts as an essential cofactor in several reduction-oxidation reactions and as a component of nicotinamide adenine dinucleotide (NAD) and nicotinamide adenine dinucleotide phosphate (NADP).

Overview: Niacin is absorbed in the small intestine, and deficiency may be encountered in patients with decreased intake and absorption of niacin, chronic and excessive alcohol intake, malabsorption syndromes, and anorexia. Deficiency may be induced by medications that decrease absorption, such as 5-fluorouracil, azathioprine, and isoniazid. Hartnup disease, a congenital defect in neutral amino acid absorption, presents similarly to niacin deficiency due to the reduced absorption of tryptophan. Niacin has been shown to increase high-density lipoproteins (HDL) and decrease triglycerides; it can be prescribed for those patients with hyperlipidemia.

Clinical presentation: Cutaneous manifestations may include erythema, hyperpigmentation of sun exposed skin, and the broad collar sign or dermatitis in a C3/C4 dermatome, also known as Casal's necklace (Figure 31.6). Pellagra, a consequence of long-term B3 deficiency, is a constellation of symptoms, including dermatitis, diarrhea, dementia, and mucosal ulcers that can ultimately cause death. Niacin taken in excess may cause cutaneous flushing, pruritus, and acanthosis nigricans. Sustained high levels of niacin may lead to jaundice and hepatotoxicity.

Laboratory studies: Levels of tryptophan, NAD, NADP, and niacin can be examined to determine the extent of deficiency.

Management: Supplementation can be performed with 250–500 mg/day orally in the form of nicotinamide to avoid flushing reaction. Recommended daily

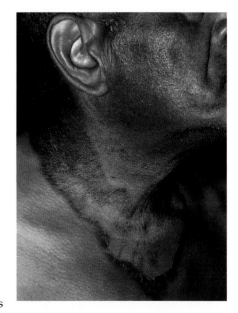

Figure 31.6 Patient displaying signs of pellagra (B3 deficiency) with the characteristic Casal's necklace in the C3/C4 dermatome as well as photosensitive dermatitis on the face

Source: From VisualDx, used with permission.

dosing range depends on age and other conditions. Children require between 2–16 mg/day. Adults may range from 14–18 mg/day depending on sex and child-bearing status.

Course: Deficiency is preventable with adequate diet. Patients may opt to supplement or engage fortified foods if at risk for deficiency. Reversal of manifestations may be seen as early as weeks to months after adequate supplementation. If left untreated for approximately four years, niacin deficiency may result in death.

Final comment: Niacin deficiency is a rare entity in industrialized nations, although it may be seen in specific populations, such as alcoholics and patients with malabsorption syndromes. It is imperative to identify these patients by their unique clinical presentation and treat in a timely manner as death may result.

Vitamin B6

Definition: This includes a group of closely related compounds, notably pyridoxine.

Overview: Pyridoxine deficiency and toxicity can occur. Primary deficiency is rare, but secondary causes include heavy alcohol consumption, isoniazid use, oral contraceptive use, chronic hepatitis, chronic renal failure, and malnutrition. Toxicity occurs secondary to over-supplementation (>500 mg/day).

Clinical presentation: Signs of deficiency include a pellagra-like syndrome (cheilosis, stomatitis, glossitis) and peripheral neuropathy. Severe deficiency involves seizures, sideroblastic anemia, and seborrheic dermatitis. Toxicity causes photosensitivity, dermatosis, and potentially irreversible peripheral neuropathy.

Management: This may be treated with supplements of pyridoxine 50–100 mg/day. Patients taking isoniazid should supplement with pyridoxine 30–50 mg/day for the duration of their treatment to prevent deficiency.

Prognosis: Vitamin B6 deficiency is responsive to oral supplementation; however, irreversible neuropathy can occur due to toxicity.

Final comment: While pyridoxine should be supplemented in deficient patients and those undergoing isoniazid therapy, daily limits should not be exceeded so as to precipitate toxicity.

Vitamin B9

Synonym: Folic acid

Definition: Vitamin B9, also known as folate, is critical for DNA synthesis and amino acid metabolism. It is found in several foods, including leafy green vegetables, beans, and whole grains.

Overview: Folate deficiency presents with megaloblastic anemia and can cause neural tube defects in developing fetuses. Folate deficiency often coincides with vitamin B12 deficiency; as such, the two vitamins should be assessed together. Folic acid deficiency occurs secondary to malabsorptive states, malnutrition, increased requirements (pregnancy), and certain drugs (e.g., phenytoin, methotrexate, trimethoprim). Deficiency is more prominent in patients with goat milk in their diets.

Clinical presentation: Worsening signs of anemia, including pallor and fatigue, combined with glossitis or angular cheilitis suggest folate deficiency. Other common cutaneous signs include hyperpigmentation of the hands, nails, face, palmar creases, and intertriginous sites, as well as hair depigmentation (cannities). Fetal spina bifida and anencephaly noted on ultrasound are indicative of maternal folate deficiency.

Laboratory studies: Patients with folate deficiency will demonstrate elevated homocysteine, normal methylmalonic acid, low hemoglobin with increased mean corpuscular volume, and a peripheral blood smear with hyper-segmented polymorphonuclear leukocytes.

Management: Supplementation with 1–5 mg/day of folate orally should be prescribed. Standard obstetric prophylaxis is 0.4 mg/day orally.

Course: Folate serum levels typically return to normal range after 1 month of supplementation.

Final comment: Folate deficiency results in megaloblastic anemia, and obstetric prophylaxis is suggested to reduce the likelihood of neural tube defects.

Vitamin B12

Synonym: Cobalamin

Definition: This is an essential cofactor for methionine synthase and plays an important role in DNA synthesis. Vitamin B12 deficiency is characterized by neurologic, hematologic, and psychiatric findings.

Overview: While the true prevalence remains unknown, the incidence appears to rise with age. Low vitamin B12 levels are generally due to either nutritional deficiency or malabsorption.

A noteworthy cause of malabsorption is pernicious anemia, which results from impaired uptake of vitamin B12 due to lack of intrinsic factor. Pernicious anemia can be inherited or acquired later in life.

Clinical presentation: Vitamin B12 deficiency is a common cause of megaloblastic anemia and initially presents with fatigue, glossitis, anorexia, and diarrhea. Long-term deficiencies can manifest with peripheral neuropathy, impaired memory, depression, dementia, irritability, and hair and nail changes. Cutaneous symptoms include skin hyperpigmentation, vitiligo, angular stomatitis, atopic dermatitis, and acne. Severe deficiencies can cause pancytopenia and subacute combined degeneration. This deficiency can also produce hyperhomocysteinemia, which is a risk factor for atherosclerosis.

Laboratory studies: In addition to low vitamin B12 levels, patients with this vitamin deficiency will demonstrate elevated homocysteine and methylmalonic acid levels. This is a distinguishing feature from folate deficiency, which demonstrates elevated homocysteine levels with normal methylmalonic acid levels.

Management: Oral supplementation of 1000–2000 mcg/QID for 1–2 weeks followed by a maintenance dose of 1000 mcg/day or intramuscular (IM) injection of 100–1000 mcg/daily to every other day for 1–2 weeks followed by 100–1000 mcg/every 1–3 months for maintenance. After initiation of treatment, laboratory studies should be rechecked in 1–2 weeks in severe anemia and 2–3 months in milder forms.

Course: Megaloblastic anemia responds well to treatment; however, nerve damage may be permanent. Earlier detection and treatment results in better outcomes.

Final comment: Vitamin B12 deficiency is typically seen in the elderly and may present with anemia and neuropathies, which are treated with either oral or intramuscular vitamin B12 supplementation.

Vitamin C

Synonym: Ascorbic acid

Definition: It is a water-soluble compound that is an essential cofactor for the hydroxylation of proline and lysine in collagen synthesis and for dopamine beta-hydroxylase, which catalyzes the conversion of dopamine to norepinephrine.

Overview: Vitamin C deficiency is more common in developing countries or areas with limited access to vitamin C-rich foods. Risk factors for deficiency include inadequate dietary intake of fresh fruits and vegetables, alcoholism, smoking, type 1 diabetes, gastrointestinal malabsorption diseases, and iron overload.

Clinical presentation: Vitamin C deficiency is also known as scurvy, and classic symptoms include corkscrew hairs (Figure 31.7), gingival bleeding (Figure 31.8), and perifollicular

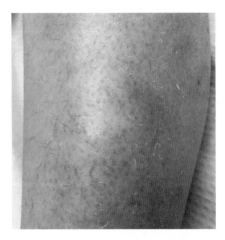

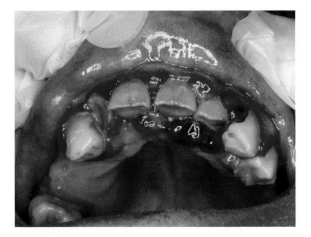

Figure 31.7 Corkscrew hairs and perifollicular erythema of the right leg with evidence of vitamin C deficiency.

Source: Courtesy of Lehigh Valley Health Network, Department of Dermatology.

Figure 31.8 Patient with scurvy secondary to Vitamin C deficiency with classic gum findings of hypertrophy and bleeding.

Source: From VisualDx, used with permission.

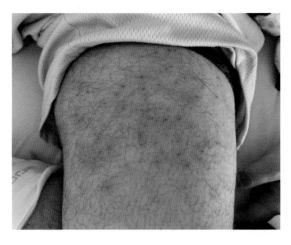

Figure 31.9 Prominent perifollicular erythema and hyperkeratotic papules of the anterior part of the left thigh in a patient with vitamin C deficiency.

Source: Courtesy of Lehigh Valley Health Network, Department of Dermatology.

hemorrhage. Initial symptoms of irritability and anorexia develop after 2–3 months of inadequate vitamin C intake. These symptoms are followed by the classic scurvy findings as well as impaired wound healing, tooth loss, ecchymosis, petechiae, hyperkeratosis (first cutaneous sign; Figure 31.9), koilonychia, splinter hemorrhages, hemarthrosis, brittle bones, and subperiosteal hemorrhages.

Laboratory studies: Measurement of plasma ascorbic acid levels can confirm deficiency.

Management: For adults, oral vitamin C 500–1000 mg/day can be administered for 30 days or until symptoms resolve. For children, dosing can be 300 mg/day for 30 days. Labs can be rechecked at one month and then every 3–6 months thereafter.

Course: Prognosis is excellent with improvement in constitutional symptoms within 24 hours and improvement in bleeding diathesis in several days to weeks. Corkscrew hair completely resolves after 3 months.

Final comment: Vitamin C deficiency is found in individuals with insufficient vitamin C intake or suffering from malabsorption. Symptoms range from irritability to bone fractures, and most symptoms resolve over the span of a couple of months with appropriate treatment.

Vitamin D

Definition: This is a fat-soluble molecule that is integral in bone metabolism and calcium homeostasis. The two most important forms of vitamin D are vitamin D_3 (cholecalciferol) and vitamin D_2 (ergocalciferol). Individuals with vitamin D deficiency may develop hypocalcemia but are generally asymptomatic.

Overview: Approximately 1 billion people are vitamin D deficient, and about half of the global population is vitamin D insufficient. Prevalence is higher in the elderly, breastfed infants, nursing home and hospitalized patients, and obese individuals. Vitamin D deficiency can be caused by decreased dietary intake/absorption, limited endogenous synthesis, and limited sun exposure. It can also be a result of end organ resistance and increased hepatic catabolism by CYP450-inducing medications (e.g., phenobarbital, dexamethasone, and rifampin). Vitamin D deficiencies that are severe enough to trigger secondary hyperparathyroidism as a result of hypocalcemia will experience accelerated bone resorption and phosphaturia. This leads to osteomalacia and osteoporosis in adults and rickets in children.

Clinical presentation: Long-term deficiency manifests as osteoporosis and secondary hyperparathyroidism, which presents as arthralgia, myalgia, bone pain, muscle weakness, and fasciculations. Children may experience developmental delay, irritability, fractures, and fatigue. Vitamin D is also responsible for regulating the proliferation, differentiation, and apoptosis of keratinocytes. Vitamin D deficiency disrupts these processes, which increases the risk of developing psoriasis and atopic dermatitis. Alopecia is an important cutaneous finding in vitamin D deficiency.

Laboratory studies: Measurements can include serum 25-hydroxyvitamin D, serum PTH, and serum calcium levels.

Management: Adults can be treated with oral vitamin D_3 6000 IU/day or 50,000 IU/week for 8 weeks followed by a daily maintenance dose of 1000–2000 IU/day. Children require 2000 IU/day or 50,000 IU/week for 6 weeks followed by 1000 IU/day for maintenance. Calcitriol or calcidiol can be considered in patients with persistent deficiencies, fat malabsorption, or liver disease.

Course: Vitamin D_3 supplementation has been shown to reduce mortality, falls, and fractures. Bodily stores of vitamin D are generally restored over 8–12 weeks of appropriate treatment; however, pathologic bone lesions due to vitamin D deficiency can take many months to resolve.

Final comment: Vitamin D deficiency is most common in individuals with limited sun exposure and dietary intake, which can disrupt calcium and keratinocyte homeostasis, leading to increased risk of osteomalacia, rickets, psoriasis, and dermatitis. Oral supplementation for 8–12 weeks can correct serum vitamin D levels and restore bone mass over the course of several months.

Vitamin E

Definition: This is a group of 8 fat-soluble compounds, with the most biologically active being alpha-tocopherol. It has antioxidant, antiplatelet, and immunomodulation effects. Deficiencies can present with ataxia and vision changes.

Overview: Vitamin E deficiency is rare and is present in only 0.1% of the adult population in the United States. It is more commonly observed in children.

Clinical presentation: Deficiency is usually caused by fat malabsorption, genetic defects in the alpha-tocopherol transfer protein (ataxia with vitamin E deficiency), or severe malnutrition. This deficiency can cause red blood cell hemolysis, night blindness, decreased upward gaze, peripheral neuropathy, spinocerebellar ataxia, and myopathy. The most severe symptom is cardiomyopathy, which can be lethal. In excess vitamin E consumption, cutaneous signs may include petechiae and ecchymosis.

Laboratory studies: Serum alpha-tocopherol levels can be measured.

Management: Supplementation includes oral alpha-tocopherol 15–25 mg/kg/day or mixed tocopherols 200 IU.

Course: If left untreated, vitamin E deficiency results in progressive neurologic disease. Mild symptoms quickly resolve after treatment. Progressive disease has limited potential for recovery.

Final comment: Vitamin E deficiency is rare but may result in lethal cardiac complications. If treated early, patients can expect a rapid and full recovery.

Vitamin K

Definition: This is a fat-soluble compound that is primarily involved in coagulation. Vitamin K deficiency can lead to bleeding, increased risk for cardiovascular disease, osteoporosis, and poor bone development. Vitamin K is responsible for maturation of the following coagulation factors: II, VII, IX, X, protein C, and protein S.

Overview: All neonates are born with low levels of vitamin K. Approximately 8–31% of healthy adults are vitamin K deficient. Severe deficiencies with clinically significant bleeding are limited to individuals taking vitamin K antagonists, such as warfarin, and those with malabsorption syndromes. Adults can acquire vitamin K deficiency through diseases of fat malabsorption (e.g., celiac disease and cystic fibrosis), inadequate dietary intake (typically seen in vegans), antibiotic regimens (that decrease gut bacteria responsible for vitamin K production), or vitamin K–inhibiting anticoagulation therapy.

Clinical presentation: Low vitamin K levels cause an increased risk of bleeding, which can manifest as easy bruising, mucosal bleeding, and splinter hemorrhages in the nails. Severe vitamin K deficiencies can cause life-threatening hemorrhaging.

Laboratory studies: Prothrombin time and PIVKA-II levels can be checked.

Management: Newborn vitamin K prophylaxis consists of an intramuscular injection of 1 mg vitamin K1 within the first hour of birth. Vitamin K deficiency in adults is treated with oral replacement of 120 ug/day for men and 90 ug/day for women.

Course: Prophylaxis in newborns significantly reduces the incidence of vitamin K deficiency–related bleeding. Adults treated with nutritional supplementation have an excellent prognosis.

Final comment: Vitamin K deficiency is typically observed in neonates, malabsorptive diseases, and individuals taking vitamin K antagonists. It presents with an increased risk of bleeding, which is effectively treated with oral or intramuscular injection of vitamin K.

Zinc

Definition: Zinc is an essential mineral, and its deficiency is characterized primarily by loss of appetite, immunosuppression, and delayed growth. Cutaneous manifestations include hair loss, dermatitis, and nail dystrophy.

Overview: Zinc deficiency is most prevalent in sub-Saharan Africa and South Asia while relatively rare in North America. Groups most at risk for zinc deficiency include pregnant and lactating women due to increased zinc demand, as well as vegetarians, alcoholics, and people with digestive disorders (e.g., Crohn's disease and ulcerative colitis) due to decreased absorption or parenteral feeding. Acrodermatitis enteropathica is an inherited or acquired disorder associated with zinc deficiency and is characterized by periacral and periorificial dermatitis, alopecia, and diarrhea. Primary acrodermatitis enteropathica is an autosomal recessive disorder caused by a loss-of-function mutation of the *SLC39A4* gene located on chromosome 8q24.3, which codes for the zinc transporter protein ZIP4. This mutation results in a decrease in zinc absorption across the mucosa of the small intestine.

Clinical presentation: Depending on the severity, individuals with zinc deficiency can present with stunted growth, diarrhea, depressed immune function, impaired wound healing, weight loss, and eye and skin lesions. Cutaneous findings include alopecia, nail dystrophy, stomatitis, angular cheilitis, and periorificial, acral, and anogenital dermatitis. The classic triad of dermatitis, diarrhea, and depression is seen in about 20% of patients. Symptoms of zinc deficiency can manifest within days to weeks after birth in formula-fed infants or shortly after weaning of breast-fed infants (Figure 31.10–31.11).

Laboratory studies: Measurements include plasma zinc and serum alkaline phosphatase levels. Pathology is characteristic of nutritional deficiencies in general (Figure 31.12).

Management: The recommended dietary allowance (RDA) of zinc is 11 mg/day for men and 8 mg/day for women. Oral replacement of 2–3 times the RDA for 6 months is recommended to treat mild zinc deficiency and 4–5 times the RDA for 6 months is recommended for moderate to severe deficiency.

Course: With adequate treatment, individuals with zinc deficiency have a quick and complete recovery. Cutaneous lesions typically resolve within 1–2 weeks, and diarrhea ceases within 24 hours.

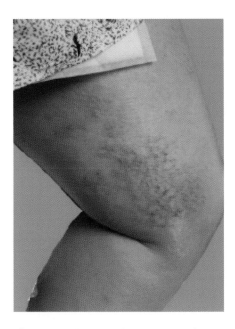

Figure 31.10 Erythematous, scaly plaques on the left thigh with edema and serous drainage. Patient was found to have multiple vitamin deficiencies including zinc, vitamin A, and vitamins B1 and B6.

Source: Courtesy of Lehigh Valley Health Network, Department of Dermatology.

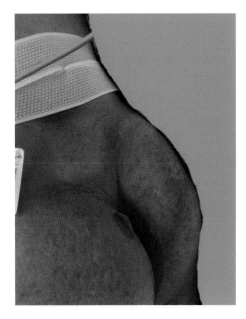

Figure 31.11 Gluteal cleft with desquamation over an erythematous patch. Patient was found to have deficiencies including zinc, vitamin B1, vitamin B6, and vitamin A.

Source: Courtesy of Lehigh Valley Health Network, Department of Dermatology.

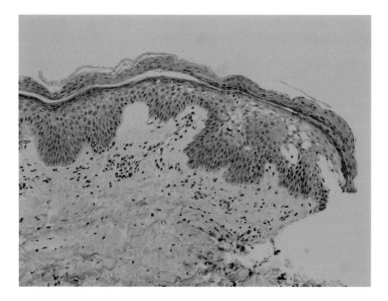

Figure 31.12 Biopsy from the anterior proximal area of the right thigh shows patchy vacuolation and pallor of the upper epidermis, overlying parakeratosis, papillary dermal and dermal edema with superficial and deep, predominantly perivascular, lymphohistiocytic inflammation (hematoxylin and eosin 20×).

Source: Courtesy of Lehigh Valley Health Network, Department of Dermatology.

Table 31.1 Overview of Vitamin and Mineral Biologic Function, Cutaneous Manifestations of Deficiencies, and Associated Significant Complications of Deficiencies

Vitamin/ Mineral	Biologic Function	Cutaneous Manifestations of Deficiency	Significant Complications of Deficiency
Iron	Essential component of hemoglobin	Pallor Dry or rough skin Atrophic glossitis with loss of tongue papillae Angular cheilitis Koilonychia Alopecia Chlorosis	Iron deficiency anemia
Selenium	Antioxidant defense Thyroid hormone production	Hypopigmentation of nail beds	Skeletal muscle dysfunction Cardiomyopathy Mood disorders Impaired immune function
Vitamin A (Retinol)	Protein synthesis in the eye Enhances immune system and keratinocyte function	Xerosis cutis Acneiform lesions Follicular keratosis	Nyctalopia Keratomalacia Immunosuppression
Vitamin B1 (Thiamine)	Essential cofactor involved in NADPH synthesis, macromolecule aggregation, and neural function.	Wet beriberi: edematous skin with subsequent breakdown and glossitis	Wernicke-Korsakoff syndrome Dry beriberi Wet beriberi

Table 31.1 (Continued)

Vitamin/ Mineral	Biologic Function	Cutaneous Manifestations of Deficiency	Significant Complications of Deficiency
Vitamin B2 (Riboflavin)	Essential cofactor in redox reactions, FAD and FMN are derivatives	Cheilosis Angular stomatitis Keratitis Seborrheic dermatitis Scrotal dermatitis	Normocytic-normochromic anemia Oral-ocular-genital syndrome
Vitamin B3 (Niacin)	Essential cofactor in redox reactions, NAD is a derivative	Erythema Hyperpigmentation of sun-exposed skin Dermatitis with a C3/C4 dermatome circumferential broad collar rash Seborrheic dermatitis Scrotal dermatitis Glossitis	Pellagra
Vitamin B6 (Pyridoxine)	Cofactor for more than 140 enzymes	Eczematous or seborrheic dermatitis Scrotal dermatitis Angular cheilitis Stomatitis Glossitis Intertrigo	Convulsions Peripheral neuropathy Sideroblastic anemia
Vitamin B7 (Biotin)	Cofactor for carboxylation enzymes	Dermatitis around the eyes, nose, and mouth Alopecia	Hallucinations
Vitamin B9 (Folate)	Essential for methylation reactions and DNA/RNA synthesis	Glossitis	Megaloblastic anemia
Vitamin B12 (Cobalamin)	Cofactor for methionine synthase Important for DNA synthesis	Skin hyperpigmentation Vitiligo Angular stomatitis Atopic dermatitis Acne Hair and nail changes	Megaloblastic anemia Subacute combined degeneration
Vitamin C (Ascorbic acid)	Essential cofactor for hydroxylation of proline and lysine in collagen synthesis Necessary for dopamine B-hydroxylase Facilitates iron absorption	Swollen gums Ecchymosis Petechiae Poor wound healing Perifollicular and subperiosteal hemorrhages Corkscrew hair	Scurvy Weakened immune response
Vitamin D	Aids in intestinal absorption of calcium and phosphate Bone mineralization and bone resorption	Increased risk of psoriasis and atopic dermatitis	Rickets Osteomalacia
Vitamin K	Necessary for the maturation of clotting factors II, VII, IX, X, protein C, protein S	Easy bruisability Mucosal bleeding Splinter hemorrhages	Hemorrhage

(Continued)

Table 31.1 (Continued)

Vitamin/ Mineral	Biologic Function	Cutaneous Manifestations of Deficiency	Significant Complications of Deficiency
Zinc	Essential trace element required for metalloproteinases and transcription factors to function in wound repair, immune responses, and reproduction Antioxidant properties against UV radiation damage	Periorificial, acral, and anogenital dermatitis Alopecia Nail dystrophy Stomatitis Angular cheilitis	Acrodermatitis enteropathica

Abbreviations: NADPH; FAD, flavin adenine dinucleotide; FMN, flavin mononucleotide; NAD, nicotinamide adenine dinucleotide; UV, ultraviolet.

FINAL THOUGHT

Zinc deficiency is due to either intake insufficiency or malabsorption. It is more commonly found in developing countries and is rapidly and effectively treated with oral zinc supplementation.

ADDITIONAL READINGS

Benjamin O. Kwashiorkor. In: StatPearls [Internet]. Treasure Island, FL: StatPearls Publishing; 2020 July 19. Accessed 2021 Mar 28. Available from: www.ncbi.nlm.nih.gov/books/NBK507876/

Eden RE. Vitamin K deficiency. In: StatPearls [Internet]. Treasure Island, FL: StatPearls Publishing; 2020 Nov 21. Accessed 2021 Mar 28. Available from: www.ncbi.nlm.nih.gov/books/NBK536983/#:~:text=Introduction-,Vitamin%20K%20refers%20to%20a%20group%20of%20fat%2Dsoluble%20compounds,osteoporosis%2C%20and%20increased%20cardiovascular%20disease

Kemnic TR. Vitamin E deficiency. In: StatPearls [Internet]. Treasure Island, FL: StatPearls Publishing; 2020 July 10. Accessed 2021 Mar 28. Available from: www.ncbi.nlm.nih.gov/books/NBK519051/

Mock DM. Biotin. In: Ross AC, Caballero B, Cousins RJ, et al., editors. Modern Nutrition in Health and Disease. 11th ed. Baltimore, MD: Lippincott Williams & Wilkins; 2014. p. 390–398.

Office of Dietary Supplements. Vitamin D. NIH Office of Dietary Supplements. 2018 Mar 2 [updated 2021 Mar 26]. Accessed 2021 Mar 28. Available from: https://ods.od.nih.gov/factsheets/VitaminD-HealthProfessional/

Office of Dietary Supplements. Zinc. NIH Office of Dietary Supplements. 2018 Mar 2 [updated 2021 Mar 26]. Accessed 2021 Mar 28. Available from: https://ods.od.nih.gov/factsheets/Zinc-HealthProfessional/#:~:text=Zinc%20deficiency%20is%20characterized%20by,8%2C27%2C28%5D

Pazirandeh P, Burns D. Overview of water soluble-vitamins. In: Post TW, editor. UpToDate. Waltham, MA: UpToDate; 2021.

Publishing HH. Vitamin B12 deficiency. Harvard Health. Accessed 2021 Mar 28. Available from: www.health.harvard.edu/a_to_z/vitamin-b12-deficiency-a-to-z

Ross CA. Vitamin A. In: Coates PM, Betz JM, Blackman MR, et al., editors. Encyclopedia of Dietary Supplements. 2nd ed. London and New York: Informa Healthcare; 2010. p. 778–791.

Titi-Lartey OA. Marasmus. In: StatPearls [Internet]. Treasure Island, FL: StatPearls Publishing; 2021 Feb 6. Accessed 2021 Mar 28. Available from: www.ncbi.nlm.nih.gov/books/NBK559224

Index

Note: Page locators in **bold** indicate a table. Page locators in *italics* indicate a figure.

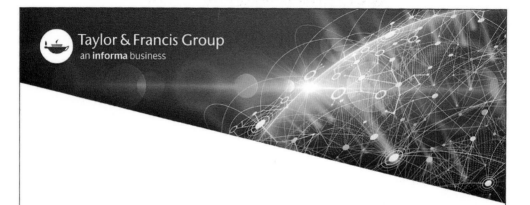
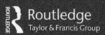
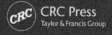